CREEK'S

Occupational Therapy and Mental Health

CREEK'S

Occupational Therapy and Mental Health

SIXTH EDITION

Wendy Bryant, DipCOT, MSc, PGCert (TLHE), PhD
Honorary Professor in Occupational Therapy
School of Health and Human Sciences
University of Essex
Essex, UK

Jon Fieldhouse, BA (Hons), DipCOT, MScOT, PGCert (TLHE), DPhil
Senior Lecturer, School of Health & Social Wellbeing – Faculty of Health & Applied Science
University of the West of England
Bristol, UK

Nicola Ann Plastow, BSc (OccTher), PGCert (TLHE), MSc (PHS), PhD (Clinical Sciences)
Associate Professor and Head of Division: Occupational Therapy
Department of Health and Rehabilitation Sciences
Faculty of Medicine and Health Sciences, Stellenbosch University
Cape Town, South Africa

ELSEVIER

For new editions, list copyright history of previous editions below.
First edition 1990
Second edition 1996
Third edition 2002
Fourth edition 2008
Fifth edition 2014

Notices

Practitioners and researchers must always rely on their own experience and knowledge in evaluating and using any information, methods, compounds or experiments described herein. Because of rapid advances in the medical sciences, in particular, independent verification of diagnoses and drug dosages should be made. To the fullest extent of the law, no responsibility is assumed by Elsevier, authors, editors or contributors for any injury and/or damage to persons or property as a matter of products liability, negligence or otherwise, or from any use or operation of any methods, products, instructions, or ideas contained in the material herein.

ISBN: 978-0-7020-7745-6

Content Strategist: Trinity Hutton
Content Project Manager: Kritika Kaushik
Design: Margaret Reid
Marketing Manager: Belinda Tudin

Printed in India

Last digit is the print number: 9 8 7 6 5 4 3 2

Working together
to grow libraries in
developing countries

www.elsevier.com • www.bookaid.org

CONTENTS

FOREWORD BY JENNIFER CREEK

The first edition of *Occupational Therapy and Mental Health* was commissioned in 1986 and published in 1990 by the Edinburgh-based publisher, Churchill Livingstone. As the first editor, I had a vision from the beginning of a comprehensive textbook covering the theory and practice of occupational therapy in the field of mental health that would be a source of essential information for students and practitioners. In the preface to that first edition, I wrote that

> 'my primary intention in compiling this textbook has been to communicate to students and professionals the enormous potential of occupational therapy and to give them a clear picture of the scope of the profession (and) a firm grounding that will allow them to enter the profession with confidence and build on this knowledge as they gain experience'.

It has been more than three decades since that aspiration was articulated, and the scope of occupational therapy has expanded more than anyone could have imagined. In editions two and three of the book, the authors and I sought to keep up with this expansion, adding chapters on new areas of practice and including key developments in theory. We wanted to look forward, thinking at least as much about where the profession might be in five years' time as about current practice. This means that for every edition, the content and scope of the book were examined, modified and updated.

One of the principles the book is based upon is that practice chapters should be authored or co-authored by practitioners. Occupations are performed within, and shaped by, social, physical and temporal contexts, and occupational therapy practice is always situated in particular contexts. Only current practitioners can capture the essentially contextual nature of practice and the everyday challenges and affordances that the occupational therapist has to work with. Another principle underpinning the book is that occupational therapists should not limit themselves to learning a finite number of supposedly universal, profession-specific models for practice but feel free to draw on a wide range of theories: from psychoanalytical theory to social cognitive theory, from biomedical theory to occupational science and from complexity theory to social practice theory.

In 2005, while the fourth edition of the book was in progress, my daughter died and I was unable to continue working. Lesley Lougher, an experienced occupational therapy author and textbook editor, kindly stepped in to complete the editing process. One of the innovations we introduced in that edition was to invite service users to comment on chapters. We felt that the people who use occupational therapy services should have the last word on how useful and appropriate those services are. The idea was good but, for that edition, we only managed to elicit commentaries on three chapters.

For some years I had been trying to find someone willing to take over the book so that I could retire from editing. Lesley had the idea of bringing together an editorial team, and we invited Wendy Bryant, Jon Fieldhouse and Katrina Bannigan to edit the fifth edition. They all agreed to take it on, with some support from Lesley and me, and that edition was published in 2014. The editors remained true to the guiding principles of the book, bringing in new authors and introducing several new areas of practice. They also managed to include service user commentaries on 13 of the chapters—a great achievement. In my foreword to the fifth edition, I wrote that 'the book does not present instructions for doing occupational therapy but aims to provide practitioners with a range of tools and techniques, including tools to support their thinking, from which they can select those most appropriate to particular contexts'.

For this edition of the book, the sixth, Wendy and Jon invited South African occupational therapist, Nicola Plastow, to be their co-editor. Prior editions included chapters by authors from different countries but having a non-UK, non-European editor on the team represents an important step forward. Some of the most exciting developments of recent years in occupational therapy theory and practice have been emerging from Southern Africa and South America, where practitioners are responding in innovative ways to the major social, health and occupational needs of those regions. These fresh, creative approaches to occupational therapy are revitalizing the profession, supporting both our growth within mainstream services and our expansion into other, more marginal settings.

Producing a major textbook requires the editors to have a sound understanding of the field, up-to-date knowledge of current practice and a good grasp of the professional knowledge base. They also have to be skilled in organizing huge amounts of material and presenting complex ideas in ways that are accessible and comprehensible for readers. Furthermore, the editors have to stay abreast of the rapidly changing ways in which academic materials are published, stored, advertised, accessed and consumed. The quality of a textbook is judged by the people who read it, not by those who produce it.

For the sixth edition of *Creek's Occupational Therapy and Mental Health*, Wendy, Jon and Nicola have had to make some big decisions about the content, style and presentation of the book. For example, they have restructured how the knowledge base of occupational therapy is presented, capturing both the essence of the profession as an entity, its form, and the complexity of occupational therapy as an intervention, its performance. The essence of the profession is found in our focus on the ordinary things that people do in their everyday lives and in our commitment to equity of access to occupation for all people. The complexity of intervention is expressed in the flexibility of the occupational therapist's reasoning and capacity to respond swiftly to changes in clients' circumstances, whether those clients are individuals, groups or populations.

In this edition, there are commentaries by service users on 22 of the 29 chapters. For me, this is one of the most exciting features of the book: the authors and editors are confident enough in their knowledge and purpose to submit their work for critique by the people who use occupational therapy services.

It has been 37 years since Churchill Livingstone wrote to ask me if I would be interested in editing a new textbook on occupational therapy in the field of mental health. While the profession is still recognizably the same one in terms of its purpose and many of its methods, much has changed. It is satisfying to see that Wendy, Jon and Nicola have kept the focus on the book on current and future theorizing and practice, updating the text to provide a solid grounding for students and a reference for practitioners.

The profession of occupational therapy is still expanding into new fields and new countries. The theories, approaches and methods presented in this book are intended to be adaptable for different contexts. They will support practitioners in providing services that meet health-related occupational needs in ways that are effective, culturally relevant and acceptable to the people who use them.

JENNIFER CREEK

FOREWORD BY ALISON FAULKNER

Many years ago, when attending a therapeutic community-style day service, I met my first occupational therapist. I can still see her in the art room, standing over or emptying the kiln or sharing out the art materials. She was clearly a junior member of the team; she remained very quiet in team meetings, only speaking when spoken to. But when one of us was painting or working with clay, she was there in the background, someone to talk to, a nonjudgemental presence in an atmosphere that seemed to me to be all about judgement and fitting in.

Looking back on my experience of mental health services since (and that first experience was some 40 years ago), I have rarely encountered an occupational therapist. Days on inpatient wards were relentlessly boring. In Chapter 21: The Acute Setting, Katherine L Sims presents the role for occupational therapy as part of the multidisciplinary team for people in inpatient care, often focusing on 'specific skills in individual and/ or group sessions, aiming to prepare for discharge, prevent relapse and promote recovery and social inclusion'. In my experience of inpatient care, some patients talked about attending groups, but I didn't know what or where they were. There was either a selection process going on behind the scenes or just limited resources.

I came to think of occupational therapy, if I thought about it at all, as a poor relation of the mental health service. But then, in those days of relentless boredom on an inpatient ward, I had work to go back to – and perhaps that says it all, as is very well documented in Chapter 10: Perspectives on Using Services. The authors, Anne Laure-Donskoy and Rosemarie Stevens, discuss the responsibilization agenda, the co-option of recovery and welfare to work policies, which shift the focus from occupation as a vehicle for recovery to occupation as a route into paid work. This is not a direction that many of us, as service users or survivors, would advocate. The underlying agenda, to move people back into paid work, speaks to a neo-liberal policy of productivity, as against seeking to understand and support someone in their mental health, community and life context. Of course, the essence of occupational therapy is to understand 'occupation' in its broader sense: as '*all activities that are necessary for survival and human flourishing*' (Chapter 2). In this same Chapter, Wendy Bryant and Nicola Plastow explore ways of understanding the person holistically using the 'doing-being-becoming-belonging' framework that incorporates basic needs as well as, for example, spiritual and creative needs. It is not all about engaging in paid work.

The depth and breadth of the experiences, subjects, settings and interests covered in these chapters suggest a mature and learning profession. In the Occupations section, chapters cover physical activity, life-long learning, client-centred groups, creative activities, play, self-care, nature-based practice and work. The breadth of these activities is encouraging in the sense that you can feel the potential for everyone to find something to engage with. It is important to be aware of this potential, even if the reality of resources and austerity in recent years will have had a significant impact on what is available to an individual.

On a good day, then, occupational therapy clearly constitutes far more than the arts and crafts that I first encountered 40 years ago: it is about understanding people within their life context, engaging people in the community and rediscovering hope and meaning. I think it is significant that occupational therapists are encouraged to engage in reflective practice (see Chapter 3: Being a Therapist) and in understanding the meaning of 'occupation' in people's lives. Indeed, reading this chapter made me think that many other mental health practitioners could learn something from the training of occupational therapists. I was particularly interested to read this definition of occupational justice from the World Federation of Occupational Therapists, 2019:

> 'the fulfilment of the right for all people to engage in the occupations they need to survive, define as meaningful, and that contribute positively to their own well-being and the well-being of their communities.'
>
> *[Chapter 2]*

A recent development in community mental health services is the community mental health transformation programme, as is touched on by Hazel Parker and Simon Hughes in Chapter 22: Community Practice. The transformation programme aims to create a more integrated service for people experiencing mental health difficulties in the community, merging primary and secondary care mental health teams with social care and local community voluntary sector organisations. There is an intention to create a local and less diagnosis-based service with greater connection to local communities (see www.england.nhs.uk/wp-content/uploads/2019/09/community-mental-health-framework-for-adults-and-older-adults.pdf). In the words of Parker and Hughes, the programme:

> 'presents opportunities and challenges for occupational therapists to develop practice beyond addressing existing health problems and disability, for example, by working in a more proactive way within primary care services and particularly non-statutory services'.

I have recently been involved in an evaluation of the community mental health transformation programme in one locality. I found occupational therapists to be enthusiastic supporters of a process that gave them the opportunity to link proactively with local community groups and services in the interests of promoting a wider understanding of the social determinants of mental health. One of the key contributions that they can make is that they are ahead of the game in thinking outside of the diagnostic box and focusing on people's skills, interests and strengths. Perhaps with the status of diagnosis in mental health services potentially waning, the role and value of practitioners such as occupational therapists can be seen more clearly. If the transformation programme is implemented and resourced well, it could mean a significant opportunity for the occupational therapists of the future.

If you are one of those occupational therapists of the future, then I commend you to read this book, as and when a chapter becomes relevant to you, your mental health or your work.

ALISON FAULKNER, SURVIVOR RESEARCHER

PREFACE

T hank you for choosing to read this edition of *Creek's Occupational Therapy and Mental Health*. In this preface, the editors will orientate you to the enduring focus of these textbooks, what is new for this edition and the context for it.

Like the previous five editions, this textbook offers diverse and critical perspectives on occupational therapy and mental health, rather than being a manual for practice. The chapters are organized with increasingly specific content, starting with how occupational therapy and mental health are understood across practice settings, the context for professional practice and groups of occupations often used in therapy. Then, details of people and settings are explored in the final nine chapters. Brief definitions in the glossary orientate the reader to terms used in occupational therapy and mental health. Rather than starting from a diagnosis, readers are guided to reflect on the people they are working with and their context and relevant occupations. For any practice scenario, insights into how to think and act can be gained from several chapters. Therefore the structure of the textbook reflects how occupational therapists consider a situation from many perspectives, centred on those of people engaging with occupational therapy to promote or address their mental health. Regardless of the practice setting or diagnosis (if there is one) of the people they are working with, mental health is a concern for every occupational therapist.

In updating this book, other enduring aspects have been protected. People with direct experience of occupational therapy as service users, patients and carers have been involved as authors and commentators. Their experiences are also included with extracts and references to blogs and other published sources. Many of these sources show how practice and theory are not separate but intertwine with very real implications for people's lives. As with previous editions, many of our authors are practitioners who have written their chapters while also doing their job. To create and revise chapters which explore contemporary theory and practice in a clear and accessible way, the editorial process has involved many dialogues between us.

There are four new chapters in this edition. Three chapters replace the two theory chapters in previous editions. The theoretical grounds for occupational therapy and mental health are discussed in Chapter 2, followed by what is involved in being a therapist in Chapter 3. Structures for practice, such as the occupational therapy process, models and frames of reference, are explored in Chapter 4. The other new chapter is in the people and settings section, focused on eating disorders (Chapter 28). In many chapters, current themes in mental health and occupational therapy have been discussed, such as trauma-informed care approaches, social prescribing and recovery-oriented practice. To encourage critical engagement with these and other established approaches and ideas, there are now questions for the readers at the end of every chapter.

Recognizing the international audience for this textbook, we encouraged authors to engage with more international sources and think beyond their own immediate practice context. We are delighted to be working with Nicola Plastow from Stellenbosch University, South Africa, as co-editor for this edition, who energized our efforts to question our sources and assumptions. With her involvement, new authors were recruited, so in this edition a third of them are based in countries other than the United Kingdom. We also aimed to recruit as many service user commentators as we could. Twenty-two of the chapters have commentaries, a big step forward in Jennifer Creek's vision that people who have engaged with occupational therapy could share their thoughts and feelings on every aspect of it. The response to our regular appeals for volunteer commentators was so encouraging, and we particularly want to thank everyone who expressed interest as well as those people who became involved in drafting and finalizing a commentary.

Three other people joined the editorial team in their spare time with our invitation, bringing fresh eyes to the book and occupational therapy: Chris Sexton, an economist; Carey Brown, a charity administrator; and Rebecca Wynne, a recent graduate currently working for another publisher. First on board in early 2019 was Chris, who read through many drafts of chapters and suggested helpful clarifications and revisions. We discussed the importance of writing about what occupational therapists do, rather than what they should or could do, to strengthen and clarify understandings of the profession. From later that year, Carey supported people who volunteered to write commentaries, guiding them through the sometimes long process of choosing a chapter and drafting a commentary. Once the commentary was completed, she put these new contributors in touch with Elsevier. From 2020 Rebecca read every chapter in the book with great focus so she could revise the glossary and draft the questions for authors. She helped us clarify the differences between lay and profession-specific understandings of particular terms and issues. Chris, Carey, and Becca were very

supportive and helpful not only drawing our attention as co-editors to where clarity was needed for people who are new to the profession, but also in recognizing the scale and importance of the book for occupational therapists.

One particular challenge for this book has been the pandemic, which started early in 2020. Some chapters were completed by this stage. Others became severely delayed as dramatic changes occurred in people's lives and jobs. This textbook is a large project and so, since signing the contracts with Elsevier from early 2018, many life events have disrupted and influenced writing and editing. We want to thank those who became involved as authors, for their hard work and willingness of many to engage in new writing partnerships. We also want to thank Jennifer Creek, who generously put aside her many other writing projects to help with editing, especially in 2021. Her warm encouragement and clear guidance enabled us to realize the idea of the new Chapters 2, 3 and 4, which we feel set the scene for occupational therapy and mental health in a new and refreshing way.

WENDY BRYANT
JON FIELDHOUSE
NICOLA ANN PLASTOW

CONTRIBUTORS

JUANITA BESTER, BOccTHER, BSc (HONS), MPHIL, PGDME
Senior Lecturer, Department of Health and
    Rehabilitation Sciences – Faculty of Medicine and
    Health Sciences, Stellenbosch University,
Stellenbosch, South Africa

MARY BIRKEN, BSc (OT), MSc (OT), PHD
Research Fellow, Division of Psychiatry, University
    College London
London, UK

SALLY BRAMLEY, BA (HONS), DIPCOT, MA
Consultant Occupational Therapist
Vocational Rehabilitation & Mental Health (Retired)
Sheffield, UK

ROB BROOKS, PHD
Associate Professor, Faculty of Health Studies,
    University of Bradford
Bradford, UK

**WENDY BRYANT, DIPCOT, MSc, PGCERT
(TLHE), PHD**
Honorary Professor in Occupational Therapy
School of Health and Human Sciences
University of Essex
Essex, UK

**THEODORA MILDRED CHIKWANHA, BSc (HONS),
MPH, PGCERT (HEALZ), PHD (OT)**
Senior Lecturer, Rehabilitation Sciences Unit
Department of Primary Health Care Sciences,
    Faculty of Medicine Health Sciences, University of
    Zimbabwe
Harare, Zimbabwe

**ELSPETH CLARK, BSc (HONS), MSc (CLINICAL
RESEARCH)**
Specialist Occupational Therapist, Devon Partnership
    Trust
Devon, UK

**FIONA COLE, BSc (HONS), DIPCOT, MSc,
PGCERT (TLHE)**
Senior Lecturer in Occupational Therapy, Institute of
    Health, University of Cumbria
Carlisle, UK

MARILYN B. COLE, MS, OTR/L, FAOTA
Professor Emerita of Occupational Therapy
Quinnipiac University
Hamden, Connecticut, USA

BOB COLLINS, BSc (HONS)
Occupational Therapist/Recovery Coordinator
Bradford and Airedale Early Intervention Team
Bradford District Care Trust
Bradford, UK

**KEVIN CORDINGLEY, DIPCOT, MScOT, PGCERT
(TLHE), PGCERT (ARM), PHD**
Senior Lecturer, Department of Sport, Health
    Sciences and Social Work, Faculty of Health & Life
    Sciences
Oxford Brookes University
Oxford
Oxford, UK

JENNIFER CREEK, DIPCOT, FRCOT, PHD
Honorary Senior Lecturer, School of Health and
    Social Care
University of Essex
Colchester, UK

ANNE-LAURE DONSKOY, MA, MPHIL (PSYCH)
Doctoral Researcher (Gender and Politics), University
    of Bristol
Research Partner, Health and Life Sciences
University of the West of England
Bristol, UK

MADELEINE DUNCAN, MSc, BA (HONS), DIpOT,
BAOT, DPHIL
Associate Professor, Division of Occupational
    Therapy, Department of Health and Rehabilitation
    Sciences, Faculty of Health Sciences, University of
    Cape Town
Cape Town, South Africa

CAROLYN DUNSFORD, DIpCOT, MSc, PHD
Division Lead for Occupational Therapy, Department
    of Health Sciences, College of Health
Medicine and Life Sciences, Brunel University
London, UK

BRID DUNNE, BA, MA, MScOT (PQ), PHD
Occupational Therapist, Health Service Executive and
    School of Allied Health
University of Limerick
Limerick, Ireland

JON FIELDHOUSE, BA (HONS), DIpCOT, MScOT,
PGCERT (TLHE), DPHIL
Senior Lecturer, School of Health & Social Wellbeing,
    Faculty of Health & Applied Science
University of the West of England
Bristol, UK

ELLIE FOSSEY, DIpCOT (UK), MSc
(HEALTH PSYCHOL), PHD (MELBOURNE)
Professor and Head, Department of Occupational
    Therapy
School of Primary and Allied Health Care
Monash University – Peninsula campus
Frankston, Australia

ROSHAN GALVAAN, BSc (HONS), MScOT, PHD
(OT) UCT
Professor, Division of Occupational Therapy,
    Department of Health & Rehabilitation Sciences,
    Faculty of Health Sciences
University of Cape Town
Cape Town, South Africa

SUSAN HARDIE, BEd, HBSc, MSW, PHD
Executive Director, Canadian Centre on Disability
    Studies Inc. operating as Eviance
Adjunct Professor, School of Health Policy and
    Management, Faculty of Health, York University
Toronto, Canada

DEBORAH HARRISON, BSc (HONS), DIpCOT, MSc
Associate Tutor, School of Health Sciences
University of East Anglia
Norwich, UK

JACKIE PARSONAGE HARRISON, BSc (HONS OT),
MRESCP, PHD
Oxford Brookes University
Oxford, UK

SIMON HUGHES, MA (ADVANCING PRACTICE),
DIpCOT
Specialist Occupational Therapist
Tees Rehabilitation and Recovery Services
Tees, Esk and Wear Valleys

CLAIRE KEMBLE, BSc (HONS) OT, MSc OT
Aylesbury, UK

JENNY LANCASTER, DIpCOT, PGDIPLOMA IN
OCCUPATIONAL THERAPY
Occupational Therapist
Joint Community Rehabilitation Team
East Sussex Health Care NHS Trust
East Sussex, UK

DINAH LAPRAIRIE, BA
Formerly Executive Director NISA/Northern
    Initiative for Social Action
Sudbury, Ontario, Canada

CLARE LAWRENCE, BSc (HONS), PGDIP (OT)
Manager of Mental Health Services, Bath Spa
   University
Bath, UK

REBECCA LICORISH, BSc (HONS), MScOT
CAMHS Crisis Practitioner
South London and Maudsley NHS Trust
London, UK

JESSICA LING, BA (HONS), MScOT
Senior Occupational Therapist, Essex County Council
Colchester, UK

ESTE LOUW, BACHELOR OF OCCUPATIONAL THERAPY
Occupational Therapist, Bophelong Psychiatric
   Hospital
Mahikeng, North West Po, South Africa

HELEN MASON, BSc (HONS), PGCERT, HCPC REG
CEO/Founder, Animation Therapy Ltd
Consultant Occupational Therapist
South West England, UK

SARAH MCAULEY, BSc (HONS) OT, BPSYCH,
PGDIP (SENSORY INTEGRATION)
Operational Manager, Avon and Wiltshire Mental
   Health Partnership NHS Trust
Swindon, UK

TOM MILLS, BSc (HONS) OT
Occupational Therapist
Wickham Low Secure Unit, Avon and Wiltshire
   Mental Health Partnership
Bristol, UK

MARINA MORROW, PHD
Professor & Chair
School of Health Policy & Management, Faculty of
   Health, York University
Toronto, Canada

EVA NAKOPOULOU, BSc (HONS)
Specialist Children's Occupational Therapist and
   Team Lead
Sirona Care & Health
Bristol, UK

CLEMENT NHUNZVI, BSc HOT, MScOT, PHD (OT)
Lecturer & OT Programme Coordinator
Rehabilitation Sciences Unit, Department of Primary
   Health Care Sciences, Faculty of Medicine &
   Health Sciences
University of Zimbabwe
Harare, Zimbabwe

LANA VAN NIEKERK, B (OCCTHER), M (OCCTHER)
(UOFS), PHD (UCT)
Associate Professor, School of Health &
   Rehabilitation Sciences, Faculty of Medicine and
   Health Sciences
Stellenbosch University
Parow, South Africa

HAZEL PARKER, BSc (HONS) OT, MA (ADVANCING
PRACTICE)
Advanced Practitioner/Occupational Therapist
Tees, Esk and Wear Valleys NHS Foundation Trust
Redcar and Cleveland, UK

JUDITH PETTIGREW, DIPCOT, BSCOT, MA, PHD
Associate Professor, Occupational Therapy
School of Allied Health, University of Limerick
Limerick, Ireland

NICOLA ANN PLASTOW, BSc (OCCTHER), PGCERT
(TLHE), MSc (PHS), PHD (CLINICAL SCIENCES)
Associate Professor and Head of Division:
   Occupational Therapy
Department of Health and Rehabilitation Sciences
Faculty of Medicine and Health Sciences,
   Stellenbosch University
Cape Town, South Africa

MATUMO RAMAFIKENG, BSCOT, MScOT, PHD
Lecturer in Occupational Therapy
School of Health and Social Care
University of Essex
Colchester, UK

NATHAN REEVE, BSc (HONS) OT, SROT
Quality Improvement Lead, Secure Services, Bristol,
   Avon and Wiltshire Mental Health Partnership
   NHS Trust
Swindon, UK

GABRIELLE RICHARDS, BSc (OT), MSc, FCOT
Head of Inclusion, Recovery, Professional Head of
    Occupational Therapy and AHPs
South London and Maudsley NHS Foundation Trust
London, UK

KATIE ROBINSON, BSc (Cur. Occ.), MSc, PhD
Senior Lecturer, Occupational Therapy,
School of Allied Health, University of Limerick
Limerick, Ireland

JOE SEMPIK, BSc, MSc, PhD
Former Senior Research Fellow
University of Nottingham
Nottingham, UK

KATHERINE L. SIMS, MScOT, DipCOT
Head Occupational Therapist, Hillingdon Mental
    Health Services and Occupational Therapy
    Professional Lead for Hillingdon Children's
    Therapy Service and Community Adult Physical
    Health Teams
Central and North West London NHS Foundation
    Trust
London, UK

ROSEMARIE STEVENS, BA, MA
Independent Researcher
Swindon, Wiltshire, UK

STEVE TAYLOR, BSc (HONS) OCCUPATIONAL
    THERAPY
Bristol Secure Services, Avon and Wiltshire Mental
    Health Partnership NHS Trust
Swindon, UK

HANNAH SPREADBURY-TROY, BSc (HONS)
Occupational Therapist – Bluebell Ward, National
    Deaf Mental Health Services
Springfield Hospital
London, UK

JULIE WALTERS, BA (HONS), PGDip, UnivDipOT,
PGDip (TLHE)
Senior Lecturer in Occupational Therapy, Faculty of
    Health and Wellbeing, Sheffield Hallam University
Sheffield, UK

JENNIFER WENBORN, DipCOT, MSc, PhD,
FRCOT
Honorary Senior Research Fellow – Occupational
    Therapist, UCL Division of Psychiatry
University College London
London, UK

Section 1

INFORMING PHILOSOPHY AND THEORY

SECTION OUTLINE

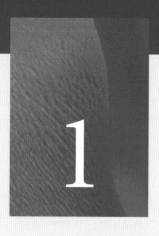

1

A HISTORY OF OCCUPATIONAL THERAPY AND PSYCHIATRY IN IRELAND

JUDITH PETTIGREW ■ BRID DUNNE ■ KATIE ROBINSON

INTRODUCTION

With the Republic of Ireland as a primary focus, this chapter provides an overview of the development of occupational therapy and psychiatry. The term psychiatry is used here to cover professionally-led systems and services to address mental distress and ill-health, including mental health services (Rose 2019; Beresford 2010). Writing about the history of psychiatry, Kelly points out,

> "there are as many versions of the history of psychiatry as there are historians, each presenting varying often competing narratives about the development of psychiatric practice, psychiatric institutions and psychiatrists"
>
> *(Kelly 2016, p. 2).*

The same is also true for occupational therapy. In this chapter some general histories of the profession's development are explored, along with a specific focus on Ireland, where professional occupational therapists did not begin to practice until the late 1940s, more than 20 years later than the pioneers in the United States and the United Kingdom. The Irish experience offers insights into similarities and differences with earlier accounts of the history of occupational therapy.

Beginning with the advent of moral treatment in the late 18th century as the first well-documented use of occupation as therapy, this chapter outlines significant trends and factors shaping the development of occupational therapy and psychiatry. One significant trend is the increasing attention given to the histories of people using services to address their mental health issues. The final section considers the historical origins of the user/survivor movement and its impact on mental health services.

BACKGROUND

Understanding the history of a profession offers insight into contemporary practice and continuing development (Higgs, Andresen and Fish 2004). Historical research can:

- demonstrate how key ideas have developed over time (Hocking 2008)
- strengthen understandings of contemporary practice (Pettigrew et al. 2017)
- celebrate the contributions of key individuals (Mahoney et al. 2017)
- and inform future professional directions (Wilcock 2002)

The opportunities afforded by historical analysis have not been fully realized in occupational therapy. Analysing histories can raise questions about shared assumptions as part of a process of critiquing professional knowledge and practice (Pettigrew et al. 2017). Much of the history of the profession is undocumented, and few studies analysing the history of the profession are available (Dunne et al. 2016). A small number of studies have drawn on analytical approaches, including interpretivism and feminism. However, there has been little historical analysis of occupational therapy informed by decolonisation, which involves asserting indigenous and local knowledge, histories and practices to challenge historical and powerful colonial explanations (Hammell 2019; Lokugamage et al. 2020).

Using a history of ideas approach to research, Ann Wilcock (1940-2019) investigated a range of historical documentary sources to understand how occupation was used as therapy, observing that it has long been associated with medicine as well as being used locally and informally to address health problems (Wilcock 2001). For example, in the pre-modern era, in Galen's humours of pathology, Graeco-Roman scholars identified exercise or activity as one of six "non-natural" features external to the body, which a person had some control over. The five other constellations that needed to be balanced and used moderately were:

- atmosphere and environment
- food and drink
- sleep and wakefulness
- retention and evacuation
- and passions of the mind (Ernst 2018)

Bynum (1994) points out that humouralism in some form continued to be in use in Western Europe at least up until the 19th century. Wilcock (2001) suggested that ideas such as this were the origins of the contemporary idea of work-life or occupational balance.

Moral Treatment

Moral treatment was an approach that emerged in the late 18th century, particularly in Europe, to improve the lives of people who were detained in psychiatric institutions. It was not a complete departure from earlier treatments such as routine confinement, bloodletting and restraint, but those in charge began to provide work and other activities, to improve care and to promote social and occupational engagement (Kelly 2016; Peloquin 1994; Peloquin 1989; Schwartz 2003). Moral treatment was based on humanistic values and marked the formal emergence of occupation as therapy for people and their mental health, creating the way for the later development of occupational therapy as a profession (Wilcock 2001; Peloquin 1989; Pettigrew et al. 2017).

An early proponent of moral treatment in Ireland was Dr. William Saunders Hallaran (1865-1825), the most prominent Irish psychiatrist of the 19th century. In 1810 he wrote the first Irish textbook on psychiatry and was considered progressive because of his concerns about the detrimental impact of living in institutions on patients who were obliged "to loiter away the day in listless apathy." He advocated exercise and productive activities such as horticulture, husbandry and farming, stating that such activity "seldom fails to confirm and to accelerate the prospect of recovery" and gave an early account of occupation as therapy (Box 1.1) (Hallaran 1810, p. 101).

BOX 1.1

WILLIAM HALLARAN DESCRIBES THERAPEUTIC OCCUPATION (1810)

In the first known published account of the use of therapeutic occupation, Hallaran (1810) wrote about a young man admitted to the asylum in a state of acute mania. Attempts to encourage the man to engage in light work failed. Later, he was discovered amusing himself by colouring on the walls of his room. He was promised better colours to work with, which lifted his mood, giving "immediate cheerfulness to his countenance" (*ibid*, p. 105). Hallaran describes how, after being provided with the "necessary apparatus" and beginning to paint, the young man "soon became elated with the approbation he had met with, and continued to employ himself in this manner for nearly two months after, with progressive improvement as to his mental faculties, when he was dismissed cured" (*ibid*, p. 105).

In the early decades of the 1800s in Ireland, there were private asylums, but many people were accommodated in Houses of Industry across the country along with other vulnerable people and criminals (Williamson 1970). The combination of poverty and mental ill-health created particular challenges. A select committee was appointed in 1817 by the British government to address these challenges, aiming for better public provision than the poor conditions of the Houses of Industry (Williamson 1970). The committee's report, and subsequent legislation over a number of years, led to a network of district asylums being established between 1825 and 1835 (Williamson 1970). Elizabeth Fry (1780-1845), an English prison reformer, reported appalling conditions following a three-month tour of prisons, lunatic asylums, Houses of Industry and infirmaries in Ireland in 1827 (Isba 2010). However, she also observed good practice in asylums at Limerick, Armagh and the Richmond (Dublin), where enlightened governors were engaging large numbers of patients in occupations including knitting, cleaning, spinning or needlework for women and gardening or weaving for men (Williamson 1970). The legislation supported a new inspection regime, and the Inspectors' annual reports from 1850-1880 describe extensive use of work or occupation for curative purposes, revealing a view of work as vital to health and well-being (Conway 2014):

> "They [in reference to the farms] afford outdoor occupation and if there be one curative or tranquillising accessory better than another it will be found in exercise and the healthful employment of the insane out of doors. The main deficiency in hospitals for the insane is referable in great measure to the absence of means for the continual occupation of their inmates, to whom nothing can be more injurious than a monotonous, do-nothing existence within the precincts of a lunatic institution."
>
> *Inspectors of Lunatics 1865, p.12*

At the Connaught Asylum in Ballinasloe, Co Galway, flexibility in women's work roles had a beneficial impact on their mental states and resulted in swifter discharge from hospital than the men (Walsh 2016). Women's occupations included cleaning, tidying, changing bed linen, working in the laundry, setting and clearing refectories, sewing, darning, helping patients to eat, weaving, waxing and polishing in contrast to the men who mainly participated in agricultural work. While there was broad agreement about the curative value of work from the asylum authorities' perspective, there were practical challenges in organizing and controlling the large numbers of people involved (Walsh 2016, p. 300). Hall (2016, p. 314) notes:

> "a pattern of regular daily activity was seen as conducive to less disturbed behaviour (not necessarily as therapeutic); and... the use of patient work in utility departments kept hospital costs down."

Working conditions were often poor. Referring to the Limerick Asylum, the Inspectors stated:

> "I regret to observe on the wretched condition of the laundry, in which I see no less than twenty three females actually jammed against each other at tubs, for want of space: as the laundry was before it is now much worse."
>
> *Inspectors of Lunatics 1864, p.30*

Decline of Moral Treatment

Moral treatment declined during the latter half of the 19th century for several reasons, including:

- dwindling optimism about recovery or cure
- increasing patient numbers, which defied treatment on moral principles
- challenges attracting enough skilled attendants (Paterson 2014; Scull 1993)
- overcrowding, requiring more staff, often untrained and adversely influencing the standard of care (Williamson 1970)
- financial pressures creating increased reliance on income from patient labour

From the second half of the 19th century onwards, the use of physically fit patients for work as much for economic benefits as therapeutic benefits became widespread (for example, work in hospital kitchens and laundries) (Paterson 2014). People incarcerated in the district asylums had little or no choice as to what occupations they could participate in. Ernst (2018), a historian, has commented that there was often contradictory use of occupation:

> "the historical role of patient work in psychiatry is subject to vacillation between therapy and empowerment on the one hand and coercion and punishment on the other hand"
>
> *(Ernst 2018, p. 248)*

Well known locations for pioneering moral treatment were the York Retreat in England and the Salpêtrière in Paris. Historians have been divided on the use of occupation in moral treatment. Foucault believed the Retreat's use of work was a way of imposing "*a moral rule, a limitation of liberty, a submission to order, an engagement of responsibility in order to disalienate the mind*" (Scull (1993), p102 Others consider that Foucault over emphasized the repressive nature of occupation, drawing attention to the importance of developing habits in preparation for life outside the institution *(ibid)*. This second perspective led to the formalization of occupational therapy, combined with influences of the movements in the late 19th and early 20th century to promote mental hygiene, arts and crafts, settlement houses and rehabilitation of injured World War I soldiers (Wilcock 2002). It is important to note that in the historical accounts of these movements, including moral treatment, the voices of people doing the work as a cure for their mental health problems are absent. It is therefore not possible to know about their experiences and perceptions of the therapeutic (or non-therapeutic) nature of this use of occupation.

THERAPEUTIC ENTHUSIASM AND OCCUPATIONAL THERAPY

The 20th century was characterized by tensions between social and psychopharmacological approaches to mental health problems, driven by enthusiasm for various treatments based on psychological, social and biological theories (Hess and Majerus 2011; Kelly 2016). In this section the main historical influences on occupational therapy are traced through psychoanalysis, the work of Adolf Meyer, biological therapies, community care and behaviourism.

Psychoanalysis

Sigmund Freud (1856-1939) established psychoanalysis in the final decade of the 19th century and through the early 20th century (Kenny 2016). Freudian psychoanalysis proposed that the unconscious mind contains memories of infantile sexuality and trauma that the person's conscious mind has repressed (Kenny 2016). Psychoanalysis as therapy involved guiding the person through various techniques to uncover and express these repressed memories. In the early to mid-20th century, psychoanalytical perspectives often dominated psychiatric treatment, particularly in the United States. Fidler and Fidler's 1963 book on occupational therapy in mental health reflects psychoanalytical theories, particularly emphasising the relationship between the occupational therapist and the person in therapy (Nicholls et al. 2012; see also Chapters 2 and 3).

Adolf Meyer

As well as perspectives that focused on a person's thoughts, feelings and inner struggles, the first half of the 20th century saw increasing attention on how biological, social and psychological factors converged to impact mental health. Psychiatrist Adolf Meyer (1866-1950) was a significant early proponent of this perspective, as well as being one of the earliest supporters of occupational therapy (Wilcock 2002). He was a strong advocate of social perspectives on psychiatry, identifying environmental causes for ill-health (Paterson 2014). As a passionate advocate for the use of occupation for therapeutic purposes, Meyer is considered to have influenced the core beliefs of occupational therapy (Hooper and Wood 2002).

Biological Therapies and Community Care

Other therapeutic approaches, informed by biological perspectives, were explored by psychiatrists in the early 20th century. Those most used were insulin coma therapy, electroconvulsive therapy and lobotomy, with varying degrees of success (Kelly 2016). Martin (1968) observed that these treatments served a punitive and therapeutic purpose, as fear of them served to control behaviour, ensuring compliance and the smooth running of institutions. Despite enthusiasm for new therapeutic techniques, the location of psychiatric care remained unchanged in the early 20th century

(Paterson 2014). People continued to be admitted to large psychiatric asylums, although there was increasing criticism of the conditions (Wilcock 2002; Beers 1908).

Internationally, where institutionalisation had been dominant, services began to be organized in community settings by the mid-20th century (Kelly 2016; Rosenbloom 2002). One of the major drivers of community care was the introduction of the first antipsychotic medications. These triggered a significant change in psychiatry, which seemed revolutionary at the time (López-Muñoz et al. 2005; Kelly 2016). This began with the chance discovery in 1952 of the first major tranquilizer, chlorpromazine. This could relieve symptoms of psychosis, reduce agitation and the frequency of hallucinations and partially restore disordered thinking (Duffin 2010). This discovery led to the development of other types of medication, including the first anti-depressant medications.

There was a broader therapeutic enthusiasm at this time in medicine, as apparently miraculous cures were discovered for various diseases and illnesses with increasing regularity (Majerus 2016). Medical science was no longer singularly focused on diagnosis but now also on curing serious physical illnesses by prescribing new drug therapies. For example, the introduction in 1943 of streptomycin, the first antibiotic, offered an effective treatment for tuberculosis. There was enthusiasm that psychiatry would be able to cure severe mental health problems in the same way (Majerus 2016). However, this hope has thus far failed to materialize, so while psychotropic medication continues to be a key element of psychiatric treatment, it is not a panacea (Fisher and Greenberg 2013).

Rosenbloom (2002) claims that the psychopharmacological revolution was the primary factor that led to the introduction of community care. From a medical perspective, the symptoms of schizophrenia made it challenging for people to live safely in the community prior to the widespread use of chlorpromazine. The decreasing number of people in inpatient psychiatric settings in the United States between 1953 and 1975 could have been because of the availability of antipsychotic drug therapies (Rosenbloom 2002). However, this was not the only factor as social change and pressure from the media also supported the steady decrease in the numbers of people in institutions (Kelly 2016).

With the end of World War II in 1945, the effectiveness of institutionalisation was increasingly questioned (Barton 1959; Goffman 1961). Social psychologists argued that improving the social environment could positively impact mental health, providing further support for closing large institutions, often characterized by deplorable conditions (Kritsotaki et al. 2016). By the end of the 20th century, much of mental health service provision was relocating from large institutions to the community.

Behaviourism

Behaviourism is a psychological theory and approach based on observing, measuring and learning new ways of doing things by rewarding and inhibiting actions in contrast to psychoanalysis and its focus on understanding the past (Cherry 2019). It emerged because psychologists had become increasingly involved in debates about how to treat mental health problems (Hall 2007; Murray 2018). The influence of behaviourism on psychiatry grew but later declined, influencing occupational therapy practice, particularly in the 1960s and 1970s (Braat et al. 2020; Kielhofner 1983).

External influences on occupational therapy such as behaviourism were dominant until the emergence of occupational science later in the 20th century. These influences overshadowed deep understandings of occupation and restricted practice. McKay (2008) identifies how the particular influences of behaviourism and psychoanalysis on occupational therapy in psychiatry contributed to a time of crisis and loss of commitment to the use of occupation for therapeutic purposes.

Formalizing Occupational Therapy

Occupational therapy was formalized in the early 20th century, and the term was officially adopted in 1917 in Clifton Springs, United States. The National Society for the Promotion of Occupational Therapy was formed, later becoming the American Occupational Therapy Association in 1923 (Quiroga 1995). In the United Kingdom occupational therapy was established by individuals who trained in the United States and Canada, supported by advocates from the medical profession (Wilcock 2002). Margaret Barr Fulton (1900-1989) was the first professionally qualified occupational therapist to work in the United Kingdom, having studied at the Philadelphia School of Occupational Therapy, United States (Paterson 2014). Initially, she found it difficult to secure work on her qualification and return to Scotland, but gained the support of Dr. David Henderson (1884-1965). He was a psychiatrist and occupational therapy advocate who founded the first United Kingdom occupational therapy department at Gartnavel Royal Hospital in Glasgow in 1922. Dr. Henderson introduced Fulton to a colleague at Aberdeen Royal Mental Hospital, where she worked from 1925 until her retirement, setting up a successful occupational therapy department (Paterson 2014).

The first United Kingdom education programme to offer professional training for occupational therapists was founded by Dr. Elizabeth Casson (1881-1954) in 1930 at Dorset House, Clifton Down, Bristol. The school moved to Barnsley Hall, Bromsgrove in 1941 and to Oxford in 1946 (Wilcock 2002). Casson was the first female graduate of medicine from Bristol University in 1919 and went on to practice in psychiatry (Wilcock 2002). She established Dorset House following a trip to the United States in 1925, where she observed occupational therapy education and practice. Dorset House was supported by the Association of Occupational Therapists (AOT) and the Scottish Association of Occupational Therapists. These associations set educational standards and promoted the profession with further schools of occupational therapy (Wilcock 2002).

Dr. Eamon O'Sullivan (1897-1966)

As a profession, occupational therapy did not become established in Ireland until the late 1940s, although therapeutic occupation was used long before. The first use of the term occupational therapy in Irish media was in a newspaper article about Peamount Sanatorium, Dublin, in 1930 (*Irish Times* 1930; Pettigrew et al. 2017). Early departments were staffed by occupational therapy workers, including nurses, attendants and/or craft teachers (Pettigrew et al. 2017). Psychiatrists advocated for occupational therapy, such as Dr. Eamon O'Sullivan (1897-1966). He was a psychiatrist who was appointed Resident Medical Superintendent at Killarney Mental Hospital (subsequently St. Finan's Hospital) in 1933, a post he held until his retirement in 1962 (Pettigrew et al. 2017).

On his arrival at the hospital, O'Sullivan established an occupational therapy department, which continued to develop during his career. He was influenced by the Simon method in use at Gütersloh Hospital, Westphalia in Germany (O'Sullivan 1955). Hermann Simon (1867-1947) was also a psychiatrist who proposed the concept of active therapy in 1923 to overcome the detrimental consequences of living in an asylum. Occupational therapy involved ensuring patients at the hospital were responsible for the results of their work and activities. He suggested that this enhanced their energy and capacities for resistance, tenacity, attention, self-esteem and responsibility (Schmiedebach and Priebe 2004). Simon's approach at Gütersloh was considered to be reforming. However, from the late 1920s onwards he began to reflect on the wider implications of his approach and increasingly approved of eugenic measures (Freis 2015).

While O'Sullivan was Resident Medical Superintendent at Killarney, the patients engaged in a wide range of activities. Men were mostly employed on the hospital farm and sold their produce to the local area. Women's occupations included weaving and making carpets and baskets. Other examples of handicrafts included leathercraft, toy making and painting. Socialisation activities for the patients included outdoor activities and film showings, organized under O'Sullivan's guidance. A hospital dance orchestra comprised of staff and patients performed at fortnightly dances (O'Sullivan 2007; Kerryman 1936; Kerryman 1940; Fogarty 2007). In 1932 an inspector, Dr. Kelly, stated in his report to the hospital committee that he was very pleased with occupational therapy, describing the department as a "hive of industry" and complimenting the "magnificently" made carpets and other products such as baskets, toys, leather-work, matting and tweeds (Mental Health Inspectors Report 1932).

One major project was the construction of Fitzgerald Stadium, Killarney, completed by patients in the 1930s. This involved hard physical labour, including levelling the pitch (Fogarty 2007). The project provoked public controversy because of concern about the potential exploitation of patients as labourers (Cronin 2015; Moran 2011; Pettigrew et al. 2020). However, interviews with former staff members from St. Finan's refuted these claims, and no records of patients' perspectives on this have been found. In the 1950s there was generally a greater concern for welfare, so practices such as patients working outside the hospital in nurses' homes or farms were more likely to attract attention.

Kerry County Council suggested this could be forced labour (*Kerry Champion* 19 January 1952). However, the view of the doctors was that "this work was occupational therapy and was as good outside as inside the institution" (*Kerry Champion* 19 January 1952). In this article some patients were interviewed, although the transcripts have not been found. Their views were summarized as "the minority of the patients said they wanted to go out [to work] and the majority said they wanted to stay in" (Kerry Champion 19 January 1952). However, the article is unclear as it states elsewhere that patients said they "wanted to be left out" *(ibid)*.

The *Irish Times* raised similar concerns in 1953, arguing that work outside the hospital could lead to "grave abuses" but also noting the therapeutic value of such a venture if it was adopted on a very "limited scale" with the exercise of "wise discretion" (*Irish Times,* 6 June 1953). Later that year, the *Kerryman* published an article outlining the prohibition of the practice of allowing patients to work with nurses outside the mental hospital, citing "the risk of liability for damages in case of an accident" (Kerryman, 12 December 1953). O'Sullivan was not alone in getting patients to construct buildings. The male occupational therapy department at Shenley Hospital in Hertfordshire, England, was completely built by patients in 1955 from digging the foundations to making the building blocks and completing the painting (Henson 1955).

The longstanding tension between encouragement and coercion was addressed in one of the first psychosocial textbooks of occupational therapy, which O'Sullivan published in 1955. The foreword was written by Dr. William Rush Dunton, Jr (1868-1966), an American psychiatrist and founding member of the American Occupational Therapy Association (Peloquin 1991) who stated, "It is pleasant to be able to say that I know of no other work on the subject, hitherto seen, which is so complete and specific." He also praised the emphasis on "the importance of consideration of the individual in prescribing occupational therapy for mental patients" (Peloquin 1991, pp. vi-viii) but noted that the lists for equipment and materials were "utopian in scope" (O'Sullivan 1955, pp. vii-viii).

In his textbook O'Sullivan advised that coercion or compulsion of any kind must not be used to convince patients of the value of treatment. Given that the power differential between patients and staff (and especially O'Sullivan) was considerable and rarely questioned, it would have been hard to resist an authoritative medical voice that consistently emphasized the relationship between work and mental health. It was not until 1959, when Russell Barton's *Institutional Neurosis* was published, that rehabilitation was advocated, which took account of patients' own wishes and concerns (Hall 2016). Formalizing these concerns, in 1961 new Mental Treatment Regulations specified that work allocated to patients in mental hospitals must serve a clear therapeutic purpose (Kelly 2016, p. 181).

O'Sullivan's enduring aim for recovery and his belief that, regardless of condition, each person could make a significant improvement resonates with current mental health policy and occupational therapy values. However, while much of O'Sullivan's practice can be explained by the historical context, key questions remain regarding his approach to work in the hospital. Like his counterparts in other hospitals, O'Sullivan's decision not to employ occupational therapists but rather to employ "more skilled members of the nursing staff" to deliver occupational therapy (O'Sullivan 1955, p. 17) may have contributed to the late development of professional occupational therapy in Ireland. However, there was also a practical element to this, as in the 1940s the only occupational therapists in Ireland were based in Dublin.

St. Patrick's Hospital, Dublin

Jonathan Swift (1667-1745), the Dean of St. Patrick's Cathedral and author of Gulliver's Travels, left the majority of his estate to institute a hospital for people with mental health problems (Malcolm 1989). St. Patrick's Hospital was the first psychiatric hospital in Ireland and is one of the oldest private psychiatric hospitals globally (Clare 1998). From 1899-1942 there was a period of development that included providing work and leisure activities for the patients and improving the hospital environment led by Dr. Richard Leeper (1864-1942) (Kelly 2016; Malcolm 1989). Following Dr. Leeper in 1946, Dr. Norman Moore (1911-1992) was employed as Resident Medical Superintendent. He had been working at the Crichton Royal Hospital, Dumfries, Scotland, for the previous six years and was inspired by the system of psychiatric care there, which included an occupational therapy department established by Rhonda Begg (Paterson 2010). While working there, he met an occupational therapy student on placement, Olga Gale (1926-2014). She was an Irish-woman who had been enrolled at Dorset House School of Occupational Therapy, Oxford, in 1944. When Dr. Moore returned to Ireland in 1946, he aimed to develop the hospital's services and invited her to set up the occupational therapy department (Dunne et al. 2018).

Olga Gale had attended two years of the occupational therapy course but did not finish because of ill-health, although the Dorset House archive records differ from Gale's recollections, as their records indicate that she completed the course in 1947 (Dunne et al. 2018; Dorset House archive 1947). However, it is clear that Gale never registered as a member of the AOT in the United Kingdom (BAOT/COT archives, Wellcome Trust, n.d.). On arriving at St. Patrick's, she was "horrified" having observed people sitting in corridors in chains, making her feel "petrified" (Dunne et al. 2018). However, she went on to set up the occupational therapy department and was given a "lovely room" called the solarium. She organized activities on an individual basis, including basketry, sewing, drawing, glove making and embroidery. She arranged for woodwork classes with a male nurse. Gale reported that the patients "treasured" the products that they made (ibid).

In occupational therapy at the time, craft was a significant aspect of occupational therapy education (Paterson 2010). Exam papers from the 1940s demonstrate that activities were commonly used as treatment (Dorset House Exam Papers 1946). Student occupational therapists were examined on psychology, psychiatry and how to use activities (including crafts) to treat physical and psychiatric conditions. The use of activities was based on a complex understanding of psychiatry and participation. For example, the applied psychology exam paper in June 1946 included questions on how patient attitude, interests, capacity and participation in groups would inform and constitute occupational therapy.

Gale also held dances and invited her friends to St. Patrick's Hospital, where they and the patients danced together. These dances were very popular. She held them with the aim of reducing stigma and increasing self-esteem and to give the patients an "opportunity for liberation." She met with Dr. Moore each month to discuss progress (Dunne et al. 2018). During this time there was greater access to resources and funding than public hospitals because St. Patrick's was privately funded. Gale described how patients mostly participated in social and craft occupations. In comparison, patients in public hospitals such as the Grangegorman Hospital, Dublin, were more often tasked with domestic and work-based activities that "kept hospital costs down" (Hall 2016, p. 314; Cahill and Pettigrew 2020).

By the mid-1950s, Ireland had the highest number of psychiatric inpatients worldwide per head of the population, with approximately 20,000 people detained in psychiatric institutions (Browne 1963; Brennan 2014). There were a number of social, medical, legal, economic and political factors for this, including an Irish tendency to institutionalise people as these were widely used to "serve various vulnerable, troubled or troubling populations of all ages" (Gilligan 2012; p. 129, Brennan 2014; Kelly 2016). Legislation to ensure legitimate admissions to asylums was frequently misused to manage social deprivation, poverty and ill-health (Kelly 2016; Brennan 2014). Institutions were also an important source of employment in small Irish communities, so local economic and social dependency contributed to a lack of political will to close them (O'Shea and Kennelly 2008). During this time, people admitted to psychiatric hospitals describe deplorable physical conditions, overcrowding, abuse, inappropriate admission and long-term incarceration (Kelly 2016; Prior 2012; Rafferty 2011; Greally 1971).

Development of Professional Occupational Therapy in Ireland

The need for occupational therapy services during the second World War led to an increased number of educational programmes in the United Kingdom (Wilcock 2002). The first professional occupational therapists also began to work in Ireland, having trained in the United Kingdom. Ann Beckett (1927-2002) was the first professionally qualified occupational therapist to practice in Ireland, having studied at Dorset House School of Occupational Therapy from 1945 to 1948. On her return to Ireland, she had an interview with the Minister for Health to discuss employment opportunities in the health service. However, he could not see any possibilities for professionally qualified therapists because of the already established personnel working in the role (Patterson 1992). Beckett was subsequently employed by the Irish branch of the British Red Cross and spent 16 years developing occupational therapy at the Central Remedial Clinic, Dublin, before moving to teach at St. Joseph's College of Occupational Therapy, Dublin (O'Mahoney 2015). The first professionally qualified occupational therapist in mental health was Margaret Sinclair (1930-1984), who worked at St. Patrick's Hospital for six months in 1953. Another influential and pioneering occupational therapist, Anna King, started working at St. John of God's Psychiatric Hospital, Dublin, later in the 1950s (Boland and Boyle 1997; Ring 2013).

The first professional occupational therapy education programme in the Republic of Ireland started in 1963 at St. Joseph's College of Occupational Therapy, Dún Laoghaire, Co Dublin. Graduates of this college were the only ones outside the United Kingdom awarded the Diploma of the AOT, and the original educators had trained as occupational therapists in the United Kingdom (Wilcock 2002; Pettigrew et al. 2017). The first cohort of students at St. Joseph's included a number of psychiatric nurses whom their hospitals had supported to become professionally qualified occupational therapists, including three from St. Finan's Hospital, Killarney. The programme eventually joined the Faculty of Health Sciences, Trinity College Dublin, University of Dublin in 1986.

The history and culture of Irish institutions shaped occupational therapy from the 1950s onwards until the numbers of occupational therapists trained and employed increased significantly in the late 20th century. Nurses or craft workers often delivered craft-based programmes to patients, which meant that professional colleagues such as doctors and nurses commonly believed (especially in psychiatric hospitals) that occupational therapy consisted entirely of craftwork. In oral history interviews, occupational therapists described how, at that time, their professional status had to be achieved by distancing themselves from unqualified occupational therapy workers and avoiding the use of crafts or using them only for clearly articulated goal-orientated reasons while also incorporating other types of treatment (Dunne et al. 2018; Williams et al. 1987).

Occupational therapy was a new, emergent health profession in 1950s Ireland, dependent on other professional groups for support to develop. The prevailing socio-political culture of the 1950s, combined with the profession's minority status, meant that professionalisation was the priority for early practitioners (Clouston and Whitcombe 2008; Brennan 2014; Saks 2009).

Occupational therapists attempting to initiate change reported issues with power and politics, increasing the challenge of reconciling the interests of staff and service user groups. This echoes a contemporary emphasis on ethical approaches to service provision, aiming to balance the work needed to meet the needs of service users while sustaining processes needed to keep services going (Cook 1995; Kronenberg and Pollard 2005). These approaches have been widely explored within occupational therapy in recent years in the context of occupational rights and occupational justice (Hammell and Iwama 2012; Galheigo 2011; Whiteford and Hocking 2011).

The system of institutional care continues to influence mental health services in Ireland despite a move to community care in recent decades (Barry 2015). Kelly (2016) argues that mental health care reforms in Ireland historically tended towards increased institutional care. He cautions that history must inform present-day decision-making, policy and practice to avoid repeating this pattern in the future. Occupational therapy, along with healthcare policies and practices, continues to face the challenge of transferring power from institutions to service users (Barry 2015; Lloyd and Williams 2009).

SERVICE USER ACTIVISM, CAMPAIGNING AND SCHOLARSHIP

This section gives an overview of the historical movements to change and improve psychiatry by the people treated and cared for within mental health services. While it is important to know how occupational therapy has emerged in these services, it is equally important to understand how contemporary and collaborative efforts to shape services have arisen from a long history of user activism, which is still unfolding (Social Care Institute for Excellence 2015). Presenting a comprehensive account of this history is challenging as there is variability in records and the use of terminology.

User activism emerged as a social movement in the 1960s and 1970s, but this was not the first criticism of psychiatry by service users that had been voiced. Campbell (2005) notes that protests have occurred ever since the creation of asylums, although before the 1970s this was more often than not by individuals rather than organized groups. The Survivor History Group, a network across the United Kingdom and Ireland, has created an openly accessible timeline and website. This covers:

- phases of the survivor movement, significant events and the establishment of survivor groups across the country
- celebration of the contributions of individuals
- aims to provide a permanent record of the politics and achievements of the survivor movement (https://www.nsun.org.uk/faqs/survivors-history-group) (Campbell and Roberts 2009)

For this chapter, we have started in the mid-19th century with the general movement for social reform that fostered the beginning of occupational therapy as well as user-led organizations and other initiatives to improve psychiatry.

Elizabeth Packard (1816-1897) was a campaigner for asylum reform in the United States, having spent three years in the Illinois State Hospital as a patient. She had been forcibly removed from her home and committed by her husband, having disagreed with him about many aspects of their shared life. Following her release from the hospital, she campaigned for better insanity laws (Himelhoch and Shaffer 1979). Clifford W. Beers (1876-1943) aimed to improving care following his psychiatric hospital admissions. Between 1900 and 1904 he had been hospitalized in Stamford Hall, the Hartford Retreat and the Connecticut State Hospital where he experienced degrading treatment and physical abuse. He subsequently wrote about his treatment and recovery (Ziegler 1931). In 1908 together with the psychiatrist Adolf Meyer, physician William H. Welch and philosopher William James, Beers organized the Connecticut Society for Mental Hygiene. In 1909, Beers launched the National Committee for Mental Hygiene (Parry 2010). However, it was not until the 1960s, when civil rights became a widespread concern, that social movements formed to campaign for better services (Crossley 1998).

The mental health user/survivor movement emerged from antipsychiatry when changes in social and governmental practices were resisted with action by patients and independent user-led groups (Campbell 2005; Gallagher 2017). Antipsychiatry is a term used to describe the critique of psychiatry that

emerged in the 1960s and 1970s, led by psychiatrists Thomas Szasz, RD Laing, David Cooper and Joseph Berk. Crossley (1998) suggests that antipsychiatry moved away from criticising or calling for improvements to a fundamental questioning of the very basis of psychiatry. It challenged the purpose of psychiatry, its foundational conception of mental illness and the distinction between sanity and mental illness while simultaneously exposing the social control function that psychiatry serves in society (Crossley 1998; Williams and Caplan 2012).

Antipsychiatry influenced user-led movements to change mental health services, along with deinstitutionalisation and new drug treatments (Tomes 2006). The term survivor was adopted to describe people who have survived mental health difficulties and the experience of mental health services and/or the associated social exclusion (Pilgrim 2005). In the United States the Oregon Insane Liberation Front, founded in 1970, has been frequently identified as the first user-led rights group there (Chamberlin 1990). In 1972 the newsletter *Madness Network News* was published for the first time, reflecting the emergence of a broader movement with common goals (Hirsch 1974). Tomes (2006) suggested that the survivor movement has had significant impacts on the American mental health policy-making climate, with the concept now widely accepted that users and survivors should be actively involved in decision-making in both therapeutic and policy domains.

Similarly, in the United Kingdom, service users now influence extensive aspects of mental health services, especially via co-production, which is discussed further in Chapter 12 (Momori and Richards 2017). This influence includes:

- consultation and monitoring of existing services
- providing input into the development of new services
- provision of training to mental health service providers
- involvement in employee recruitment
- participation in service user-led research
- developing and running service user-controlled services and artistic activities
- delivering greater mental health awareness and education (Campbell 2005; Momori and Richards 2017)

In the United Kingdom the history of collective action by mental health service users can also be traced to the early 1970s with the establishment of groups like The Mental Patients' Union (1973), PROMPT (1976) (later named Campaign Against Psychiatric Oppression) and the British Network for Alternatives to Psychiatry. These groups had varied functions and ambitions, including self-help, advocacy, media representation and campaigning. By the 1990s user-led groups had proliferated, and many networks developed, for example, Mindlink and Voices. Common to these political user-led groups were a rights-based orientation and recognition of the politically oppressive psychiatric system (Jackson 2008).

Within mental health services, efforts to develop leadership roles for users have been made over many years, especially within mental health day services in the United Kingdom, where Bryant (2011) notes the enduring difficulty in finding a balance between user-led services and services organized by staff. Bryant describes the growing attention to service user involvement in day services from the 1990s, such as the Community Group Network in southwest London, where sessional groups for service users were co-facilitated in a wide range of community settings, such as sports halls, to develop social networks and community integration (Brewer et al. 1994). Service users could take on specific roles such as helping others to attend or liaising with staff from the venue.

More recently, with the emergence of Mad Studies as an international academic movement, Beresford and Russo (2016) identify the user/survivor movement as the origin for this new field of study and the concepts of recovery and peer support. These concepts and Mad Studies challenge traditional professional authority and longstanding assumptions in psychiatry. Mad Studies attempts to reclaim madness as a political identity (Cresswell and Spandler 2016) and is a field of study that is:

"a project of inquiry, knowledge production, and political action devoted to the critique and transcendence of psy-centred ways of thinking, behaving, relating, and being."

LeFrançois et al. 2013, p. 13

Mad Studies did not emerge in isolation. It has connections with other radical mental health and user/survivor-led initiatives, including the international Mad Pride movement. Menzies et al. (2013) identified the theoretical and practical purposes for Mad Studies, combining critique of psychiatry with a focus on alternative means of helping people which are informed by:

"humanitarian, holistic perspectives where people are not reduced to symptoms but understood within the social and economic context of the society in which they live."

Menzies et al. 2013, p. 2

In contrast, mental health service user involvement in Irish policy, service development and service delivery remains a relatively new phenomenon (McDaid 2006; Deane 2011). Speed (2002) observed that there had been a lack of any concerted mental health user/survivor movement in the Republic of Ireland in contrast to other countries where user groups with a marked orientation towards strategies of empowerment and the provision of peer support and advocacy were evident. More recently, Kelly (2016) notes that the early years of the 21st century have seen the emergence and expansion of service user groups in Ireland.

Internationally, the extent to which occupational therapists have engaged with service user involvement in service delivery has been questioned. It is widely acknowledged that challenges to service user involvement in mental health services persist (Laitila et al. 2018). This is reflected in findings of a survey of mental health professionals, including occupational therapists, which highlighted slow changes in professionals' attitudes towards service user involvement (Kortteisto et al. 2018). Occupational therapists Wright and Rowe (2005) argued that enduring challenges of professional insecurity and role uncertainty inhibited the development of advocacy and genuine involvement of service users in the profession. Only time will tell if future occupational therapists can overcome the legacy of professional uncertainty and engage vigorously to realize the ambition of meaningful service user involvement in mental health services.

SUMMARY

Focusing on the Republic of Ireland, this chapter has presented an overview of histories of occupational therapy and mental health, highlighting some of the commonalities and differences of the development of the profession in Ireland and other countries. Occupation was used for therapeutic purposes before occupational therapy was established with the patronage of leading psychiatrists in institutions in the early decades of the 20th century. In Ireland there was a long transition from the pre-professional era to the employment of professional qualified occupational therapists. Early occupational therapists faced many challenges. This chapter ends with the history of the user/survivor movement and identifies that occupational therapists need to transcend professional status concerns and focus on real, meaningful participation of service users.

QUESTIONS FOR CONSIDERATION

1. How might historical research inform your professional development? Use the four themes identified at the beginning of the background section.
2. What was the aim of moral treatment, and how did it change the approach of those in charge of psychiatric institutions?
3. In relation to Box 1.1. explain the reasons why painting can be used as a therapeutic activity, referring to Hallaran's patient.
4. Consider the reasons for the decline of moral treatment: how might they have affected the people working and living in the institutions?
5. How did the biological perspective contribute to the development of mental health services in the mid-20th century?
6. Identify one of the three psychiatrists who contributed to the early development of occupational therapy in the United Kingdom and Ireland, giving details of their contribution.
7. Reflect on how work can appear to be coercive rather than therapeutic, and consider the approaches used by staff to prevent this.
8. What are the similarities and differences of Olga Gale's experience of occupational therapy to your own?
9. Why did occupational therapists focus on professionalization in the 1950s in Ireland, and how does this relate to the use of craftwork?
10. Summarize three ways in which the history of service user activism, campaigning and scholarship differ from the history of occupational therapy.

SERVICE USER COMMENTARY

This chapter grapples with the issue of how real work being done by patients is potentially exploitative. It also explores how the profession was in danger of being undermined by being over identified with craft (which could be done with unqualified people). The important issue of how the professional standing of occupational therapists relates to the autonomy of patients is not directly addressed, but the rise of the user/survivor movement and the academic field of "Mad Studies" are noted.

I have had mixed personal experiences with occupational therapy as a service user, a worker in a mental health service and more recently running an autistic Community Interest Company. Therefore my experience of occupational therapy comes from different perspectives, so I wonder about the inclusion of other histories relevant to occupational therapy. For example, the history of interoception which is the perception of the meaning of our internal senses. Knowledge of this is helpful to occupational therapists working with autistic people and/or people with mental ill-health.

I first found myself in a psychiatric hospital receiving occupational therapy services about 50 years ago. It turned out the occupational therapist had gone to the same

(Continued)

SERVICE USER COMMENTARY—cont'd

university as me (admittedly she had got a qualification whereas I would leave after a year, intending to transfer to art school but instead ended up in a psychiatric hospital). She gave me exercises such as fitting pegs into the correct size holes. I was unconvinced about the relevance of this to any life I might want.

The chapter discusses the controversy in the 1950s about the possible exploitation of patients doing work as therapy. I have relatively recent experience with this dilemma. In the 2000s I worked as a consumer adviser in a psychiatric department of a hospital serving a large area in New Zealand. One of the services had several workshops, a beautiful large market garden and a café where service users worked. When a law change made it illegal to pay anyone below the minimum wage for work, these services were shut down. I saw first-hand how people were devastated when their occupation was taken from them. They wanted to work, but their output made it economically unviable to pay the minimum wage. Production was not the point of their

work anyway. Many of these service users, whose only trips outside the home and connection with others was in these jobs, returned to the service in great distress as inpatients to the psychiatric ward. Of course, there are dangers of exploitation, but I believe there is a greater danger in being so rule bound that it is impossible to find a way to help individuals fulfil their unique potential.

There is discussion in the chapter about service user involvement, but it does not seem to get to grips with how that would connect with the actual practice of occupational therapy. One of the most useful interventions I saw working in the psychiatric service was the creation of sensory diets by occupational therapists done in genuine collaboration with individual patients. The way the chapter describes the move to service user involvement suggests that, in Ireland, it is hard for occupational therapists to juggle the need for professional recognition with the ability to integrate the perspective of service users.

Caroline Hearst

REFERENCES

Barry, O. (2015). Editorial. Irish. *Journal of Occupational Therapy, 43*(1), 2.

Beers, C. W. (1908). *A mind that found itself: An autobiography.* New York, NY: Longmans Green.

Beresford, P. (2010). *A straight talking introduction to being a mental health service user.* Ross-on-Wye: PCCS Books Ltc.

Beresford, P., & Russo, J. (2016). Supporting the sustainability of mad studies and preventing its co-option. *Disability & Society, 31*(2), 270–274.

Boland, L., & Boyle, B. (1997). Interview with Anna King on her retirement as director of the school of occupational therapy, T.C.D. Ir. *Journal of Occupational Therapy, 27*(2), 29–30.

Braat, M., Engelen, J., van Gemert, T., & Verhaegh, S. (2020). The rise and fall of behaviorism: The narrative and the numbers. *History of Psychology.*

Brennan, D. (2014). *Irish insanity 1800-2000.* United Kingdom: Routledge: Abingdon-on-Thames.

Brewer, P., Gadsden, V., & Scrimshaw, K. (1994). The community group network in mental health: A model for social support and community integration. *British Journal of Occupational Therapy, 57*(12), 467–470.

Browne, I. (1963). Psychiatry in Ireland. *The American Journal of Psychiatry, 119*(9), 816–819.

Bryant, W. (2011). Mental health day services in the United Kingdom from 1946 to 1995: An 'untidy set of services. *British Journal of Occupational Therapy, 74*(12), 554–561.

Bynum, W. F. (1994). *Science and the practice of medicine in the nineteenth century, Cambridge history of science.* Cambridge: Cambridge University Press.

Cahill, R., & Pettigrew, J. (2020). The development of occupational therapy in Grangegorman hospital, Dublin: 1934-1954. Ir. *Journal of Occupational Therapy, 48*(1), 69–87.

Campbell, P. (2005). From little acorns– the mental health service user movement. Beyond the water towers. In Sainsbury Centre for Mental Health (Ed.), Beyond the water towers. *The unfinished revolution in mental health services* (p. 73). London, UK.

Campbell, P., & Roberts, A. (2009). Survivors history. Life. *The Day, 13*(3), 33–36.

Chamberlin, J. (1990). The ex-patients' movement: Where we've been and where we're going. *The Journal of Mind and Behavior,* 323–336.

Cherry, K. (2019). *History and key concepts of behavioral psychology.* Available at: www.verywellmind.com/behavioral-psychology-4157183.

Clare, A. W. (1998). Images in psychiatry: St. Patrick's hospital. *The American Journal of Psychiatry, 155*(11), 1599.

Clouston, T. J., & Whitcombe, S. W. (2008). The professionalisation of occupational therapy: A continuing challenge. *British Journal of Occupational Therapy, 71*(8), 314–320.

Conway, F. (2014). *Work as therapy in Irish district asylums: 1850-1880.* Limerick: University of Limerick (Unpublished Masters dissertation).

Cook, J. V. (1995). Innovation and leadership in a mental health facility. *American Journal of Occupational Therapy, 49*(7), 595–606.

Cresswell, M., & Spandler, H. (2016). Solidarities and tensions in mental health politics: Mad studies and psychopolitics. *Radical and Critical Social Work, 4*(3), 357–373.

Crossley, N. (1998). RD laing and the British antipsychiatry movement: A socio–historical analysis. *Social Science & Medicine, 47*(7), 877–889.

Deane, L. (2011). Service user participation: Contemporary issues and obstacles for the national service users executive and service user participation. In *Critical social thinking: Policy and practice* (Vol. 3). Available at: www.ucc.ie/en/media/academic/appliedsocialstudies/docs/LauraDeane.pdf.

Dorset House Archive. (1946). *Applied psychology exam.* Oxford: Oxford Brookes Library.

Dorset House Archive. (1947). *Student records.* Oxford: Oxford Brookes Library.

Duffin, J. (2010). *History of medicine: A scandalously short introduction.* Toronto: University of Toronto Press.

Dunne, B., Pettigrew, J., & Robinson, K. (2016). Using historical documentary methods to explore the history of occupational therapy. *British Journal of Occupational Therapy, 79*(6), 376–384.

Dunne, B., Robinson, K., & Pettigrew, J. (2018). A case study of the development of occupational therapy at St. Patrick's Hospital Dublin, 1935-1969. Ir. *Journal of Occupational Therapy 45*(1), 31–45.

Ernst, W. (Ed.). (2018). *Work, society and psychiatry, c1750-2010.* Manchester: Manchester University Press.

Ernst W. (2018). The role of work in psychiatry: Historical reflections. *Indian Journal of Psychiatry, 60*(2), 248–252.

Fisher, S., & Greenberg, R. P. (Eds.). (2013). *The limits of biological treatments for psychological distress: Comparisons with psychotherapy and placebo.* Routledge: Abingdon-on-Thames.

Freis D (2015). *Curing the soul of the nation psychiatry, society, and psycho-politics in the German-speaking countries, 1918–1939.* PhD dissertation, European University Institute, Florence.

Galheigo, M. S. (2011). What needs to be done? Occupational therapy responsibilities and challenges regarding human rights. *Occupational Therapy Australia, 58*(2), 60–66.

Gallagher, M. (2017). *From mental patient to service user: Deinstitutionalisation and the emergence of the mental health service user movement in Scotland, 1971-2006.* PhD thesis. Glasgow: University of Glasgow.

Gilligan, R. (2012). De-institutionalisation of services for children in state care in Ireland – a case study of international relevance. *Ročenka textů zahraničních profesorů /The Annual of Texts by Foreign Guest Professors*, 129–141. Available at www.tara.tcd.ie/handle/2262/73789.

Goffman, E. (1961). *Essays on the social situation of mental patients and other inmates.* Doubleday NY: New York.

Grealy, H. (1971). *Bird's nest soup.* Dublin: Attic Press.

Hall, J. (2007). The emergence of clinical psychology in Britain from 1948 to 1958. Part II: Practice and research traditions. *History and Philosophy of the Life Sciences, 9*(2), 1–33.

Hall, J. (2016). From work and occupation to occupational therapy: The policies of professionalization in English mental hospitals from 1919 to 1959. In W. Ernst (Ed.), *Work, society and psychiatry, c1750-2010.* Manchester: Manchester University Press.

Hallaran, W. S. (1810). *An enquiry into the causes producing the extraordinary addition to the number of insane: Together with extended observations on the cure of insanity; with hints as to the better management of public asylums for insane persons.* Cork: Edwards and Savage.

Hammell, K., & Iwama, M. (2012). Wellbeing and occupational rights: An imperative for critical occupational therapy. *Scandinavian Journal of Occupational Therapy, 19*(5), 385–394.

Hess, V., & Majerus, B. (2011). Writing the history of psychiatry in the 20th century. *History of Psychiatry, 22*(2), 139–145.

Higgs, J., Andresen, L., & Fish, D. (2004). Practice knowledge—its nature, sources and contexts. In *Developing practice knowledge for health professionals* (pp. 51–69). Butterworth-Heinemann Oxford, UK.

Himelhoch, M. S., & Shaffer, A. H. (1979). Elizabeth Packard: Nineteenth-century crusader for the rights of mental patients. *Journal of American Studies, 13*(3), 343–375.

Hirsch, S. E. (1974). *Madness network news reader.* Glide.

Hocking, C. (2008). The way we were: Thinking rationally. *British Journal of Occupational Therapy, 71*(5), 185–195.

Hooper, B., & Wood, W. (2002). Pragmatism and structuralism in occupational therapy: The long conversation. *American Journal of Occupational Therapy, 56*(1), 40–50.

Inspectors of Lunacy. (1864). *The thirteenth report on the district, criminal and private lunatic asylums in Ireland, with appendices.* Dublin: Her Majesty's Stationary Office.

Inspectors of Lunacy. (1865). *The fourteenth report on the district, criminal and private lunatic asylums in Ireland, with appendices.* Dublin: Her Majesty's Stationary Office.

Isba, A. (2010). *The excellent Mrs Fry: Unlikely heroine.* New York, NY: Continuum International Publishing Group.

Jackson, C. (2008). Mad pride and prejudices. The Guardian. September 2018. Available at: www.theguardian.com/society/2008/sep/03/mentalhealth.

Kelly, B. D. (2016). Searching for the patient's voice in the Irish asylums. *Medical Humanities, 42*(2), 87–91.

Kenny, D. T. (2016). *A brief history of psychoanalysis: From Freud to fantasy to folly.* Victoria: Psychotherapy and Counselling Journal of Australia Fitzroy North.

Kielhofner, G. (1983). *Health through occupation: Theory and practice in occupational therapy.* FA Davis Company Philadelphia.

Kortteisto, T., Laitila, M., & Pitkänen, A. (2018). Attitudes of mental health professionals towards service user involvement. *Scandinavian Journal of Caring Sciences, 32*(2), 681–689.

Kritsotaki, D., Long, V., & Smith, M. (2016). Introduction: Deinstitutionalisation and the pathways of post-war psychiatry in the western world. In D. Kritsotaki, V. Long, & M. Smith (Eds.), *Deinstitutionalisation and after. Post-war psychiatry* (pp. 1–36). Cham: Palgrave Macmillan.

Kronenberg, F., & Pollard, N. (2005). Overcoming occupational apartheid: A preliminary exploration of the political nature of occupational therapy. In F. Kronenberg, S. S. Algado, & N. Pollard (Eds.), *Occupational therapy without borders: Learning from the spirit of survivors* (pp. 58–86). London: Elsevier.

Laitila, M., Nummelin, J., Kortteisto, T., & Pitkänen, A. (2018). Service users' views regarding user involvement in mental health services: A qualitative study. *Archives of Psychiatric Nursing,* *32*(5), 695–701.

Le François, B. A., Menzies, R., & Reaume, G. (Eds.). (2013). *Mad matters: A critical reader in Canadian mad studies.* Canadian Scholars' Press.

Lloyd, C., & Williams, P. L. (2009). The future of occupational therapy in mental health in Ireland. *British Journal of Occupational Therapy, 72*(12), 539–542 Toronto, Canada.

Lokugamage, A. U., Ahillan, T., & Pathberiya, S. D. C. (2020). Decolonising ideas of healing in medical education. *Journal of Medical Ethics, 46*(4), 265–272.

López-Muñoz, F., Alamo, C., Cuenca, E., Shen, W. W., Clervoy, P., & Rubio, G. (2005). History of the discovery and clinical introduction of chlorpromazine. *Archives of Psychiatric Nursing, 17*(3), 113–135.

Majerus, B. (2016). Making sense of the 'chemical revolution'. Patients' voices on the introduction of neuroleptics in the 1950s. *Medical History, 60*(1), 54–66.

Malcolm, E. (1989). *Swift's hospital: A history of St. Patrick's hospital, Dublin, 1746–1989.* Dublin: Gill and MacMillan Ltd.

Martin, D. V. (1968). *Adventure in psychiatry. Social change in a mental hospital.* Oxford: Bruno Cassire. [1962].

McDaid, S. (2006). *Equal and inclusive user involvement in the mental health services in Ireland: Results from participatory action research.* Dublin: University College Dublin.

McKay, E. (2008). What have we been doing? A historical review of occupational therapy. In E. A. McKay, C. Craik, K. H. Lim, & G. Richards (Eds.), *Advancing occupational therapy in mental health practice.* Blackwell Oxford.

Menzies, R., Le François, B. A., & Reaume, G. (2013). Introducing mad studies. In B. A. Le François, R. Menzies, & G. Reaume (Eds.), *Mad matters: A critical reader in Canadian mad studies* (pp. 1–22). Canadian Scholars' Press Toronto.

Momori, N., & Richards, G. (2017). Service user and carer involvement: Co-production. In C. Long, J. Cronin-Davis, & D. Cotterill (Eds.), *Occupational therapy evidence in practice for mental health.* Chichester: John Wiley and Sons.

Murray, M. (2018). The pre-history of health psychology in the United Kingdom: From natural science and psychoanalysis to social science, social cognition and beyond. *Journal of Health Psychology, 23*(3), 472–491.

Neve, M., & Turner, T. (1995). What the doctor thought and did: Sir James Crichton-Browne (1840–1938). *Medical History, 39*(4), 399–432.

Nicholls, L., Cunningham-Piergrossi, J., de Sena-Gibertoni, C., & Daniel, M. (2012). *Psychoanalytic thinking in occupational therapy: Symbolic, relational and transformative.* Chichester: John Wiley and Sons.

O'Mahoney, J. (2015). *Ann Beckett- 'a passion for people'. An analysis of the contribution of an occupational therapy pioneer.* Limerick: University of Limerick. (Unpublished Masters dissertation).

O'Shea, E., & Kennelly, B. (2008). The economics of mental health care in Ireland. Mental Health Commission, Dublin. Available at: www.mhcirl.ie/File/ecommhceire.pdf.

O'Sullivan, E. (1955). *Textbook of occupational therapy with chief reference to psychological medicine.* London: H.K. Lewis.

Parry, M. (2010). From a patient's perspective: Clifford Whittingham Beers' work to reform mental health services. *American Journal of Public Health, 100*(12), 2356.

Paterson, C. F. (2008). A short history of occupational therapy in psychiatry. *Occupational Therapy in Mental Health, 4,* 2–14.

Paterson, C. F. (2014). *Opportunities not prescriptions: The development of occupational therapy in Scotland: 1900-1960.* Aberdeen: Aberdeen History of Medicine Publications.

Patterson, M. (1992). Ann Beckett interview. Ir. *Journal of Occupational Therapy, 22*(1), 31–33.

Peloquin, S. M. (1989). Moral treatment: Contexts considered. *American Journal of Occupational Therapy, 43*(8), 537–544.

Peloquin, S. M. (1994). Moral treatment: How a caring practice lost its rationale. *American Journal of Occupational Therapy, 48*(2), 167–173.

Pettigrew, J., Robinson, K., Dunne, B., & O'Mahoney, J. (2017). Major trends in the use of occupation as therapy in Ireland 1863-1963. Ir. *Journal of Occupational Therapy, 45*(1), 4–14.

Pettigrew, J., Shalvey, A., Dunne, B., & Robinson, K. (2020). Eamon O'Sullivan: 20th-century Irish psychiatrist and occupational therapy patron. *History Psychiatry, 31*(4), 470–482.

Pilgrim, D. (2005). Protest and co-option – the voice of mental health service users. In A. Bell, & P. Lindley (Eds.), *Beyond the water towers: The unfinished revolution in mental health services 1985–2005* (pp. 17–26). London: The Sainsbury Centre for Mental Health.

Prior, P. (2012). Overseeing the Irish asylums: The inspectorate in lunacy, 1845-1921. In P. Prior (Ed.), *Asylums, mental health care and the Irish: Historical studies, 1800-2010* (pp. 221–245). Dublin: Irish Academic Press.

Rafferty, M. (2011). Behind the walls: Part 1. RTE, 1 05/09/2011, 21h30 Available at http://www.iftn.ie/news/?act1=record&aid=73&rid=4284169&tpl=archnews&only=1 (accessed March 13th 2022).

Rose, N. (2019). *Our psychiatric future.* Cambridge: Polity Press.

Rosenbloom, M. (2002). Chlorpromazine and the psychopharmacologic revolution. *JAMA, 287*(14), 1860–1861.

Saks, M. (2009). Leadership challenges: Professional power and dominance in healthcare. In V. Bishop (Ed.), *Leadership in the healthcare professions* (pp. 52–74). Maidenhead, Berkshire: OPU/McGraw-Hill.

Schwartz, K. B. (2003). History of occupation. In P. Kramer, J. Hinojosa, & C. B. Royeen (Eds.), *Perspective in human occupation: Participation in life* (pp. 18–31). Philadelphia: Lippincott Williams and Wilkins.

Scull, A. (1993). *The most solitary of afflictions: Madness and society in Britain, 1700–1900.* New Haven: Yale University Press.

Smith, L. (2008). "Your very thankful inmate": Discovering the patients of an early county lunatic asylum. *Social History of Medicine, 21*(2), 237–252. New Brunswick, NJ.

Social Care Institute for Excellence (SCIE). (2015). *Co-production in social care. Guide 51.* Available at: www.scie.org.uk/publications/guides/guide51/.

Speed, E. (2002). Irish mental health social movements: A consideration of movement habitus. *Irish Journal of Sociology, 11*(1), 62–80.

Survivors History Group. Research and resources. Available at: www.nsun.org.uk/faqs/survivors-history-group.

Tomes, N. (2006). The patient as a policy factor: A historical case study of the consumer/survivor movement in mental health. *Health Affair, 25*(3), 720–729.

Tourney, G. (1967). A history of therapeutic fashions in psychiatry, 1800-1966. *The American Journal of Psychiatry, 124*(6), 784–796.

Whalley Hammell, K. (2019). Building globally relevant occupational therapy from the strength of our diversity. *World Federation of Occupational Therapists Bulletin, 75*(1), 13–26.

Whiteford, G. E., & Hocking, C. (Eds.). (2011). *Occupational science: Society, inclusion and participation.* United Kingdom: Wiley Blackwell.

Wilcock, A. A. (2002). *Occupation for health: A journey from prescription to self-health* (Vol. 2). College of Occupational Therapists.

Williams, A., & Caplan, A. (2012). Thomas Szasz: Rebel with a questionable cause. *Lancet, 380*(9851), 1378–1379. London, UK.

Williamson, A. (1970). The beginnings of state care for the mentally ill in Ireland. *Economic Society Review, 10*(1), 280–291.

Wright, C., & Rowe, N. (2005). Protecting professional identities: Service user involvement and occupational therapy. *British Journal of Occupational Therapy, 68*(1), 45–47.

Ziegler, L. H. (1931). Mental hygiene and its relationship to the medical profession. *Journal of the American Medical Association, 97*(16), 1119–1122.

2

THE GROUNDS FOR OCCUPATIONAL THERAPY

WENDY BRYANT ■ NICOLA PLASTOW

INTRODUCTION

Occupational therapy focuses on what people, including those with mental health problems, do in everyday life. Changes in people, their environments and their occupations are the aims of occupational therapy. When occupational therapy is grounded in knowledge about occupation and mental health, the therapist can explain the benefits, challenges and opportunities. The grounds for occupational therapy require many different types and areas of knowledge about people with mental health problems, their environments and occupations. This chapter is concerned with the accessible knowledge that has been discussed and shared within the profession as a resource for knowing what to do and why (Fish and Boniface 2012).

As occupational therapists learn from their own experience and the experience of others, they draw on multiple, evolving sources. For example, Wilcock (1993) analysed human history and evolution to indicate how people use occupation to adapt to, change and respond to their physical and social environments, shifting the grounds for occupational therapy. Her work was an early influence on the growth of occupational science as a discipline, showing how researching and theorising about occupation could support occupational therapy to address public health. There are opportunities for cooperation and conflict as knowledge is constructed and negotiated within the profession (Paganizzi 2017). Therefore knowledge has practical, social, cultural, historical and political dimensions, like different terrains in a landscape. This view contrasts with the idea of a single reliable source of knowledge that can be learned and applied in practice. Students learn how to be a therapist and how to structure the therapy they provide, covering the grounds for the profession in terms of the extensive knowledge required.

When students shift their learning to the practice setting, a gap between theory and practice could be revealed. Many strategies aim to bridge the gap, such as those involving service users and practitioners in providing education (Lim and Lim 2016). With

experience, occupational therapists can see how theories are not separate from practice but that they evolve together (Fish and Boniface 2012).

Three components (people, environment and occupation) form the basic structure for the greater part of this chapter, with particular reference to the European Conceptual Framework, which is illustrated in Fig. 2.1 (Creek 2010). In the framework, multiple connections are made between three distinct areas: a personal inner world or phenomenological self, the nature of occupation and the external world or environment (Creek 2010). When people have mental health problems, how they choose to do things engages both inner and outer worlds (Creek 2010).

In this chapter, the first section focuses on people, including the terms used to describe people who engage with occupational therapy to address their

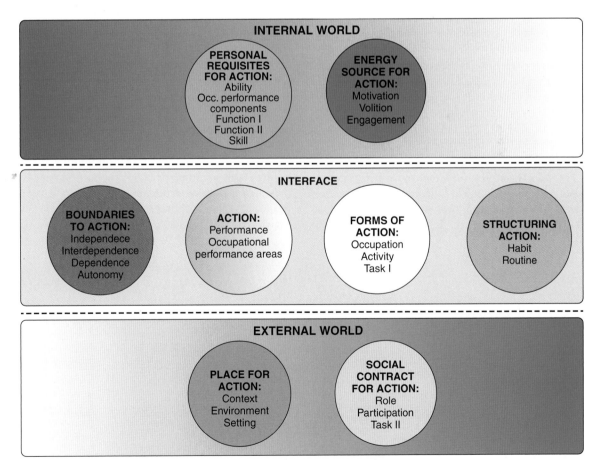

Fig. 2.1 ■ **European Conceptual Framework.** (Creek 2010. Reproduced with permission.).

mental health needs. Spirituality is explored as an important source of knowledge and beliefs about people, their occupations and mental health. Next terms and ideas associated with the environment are discussed. An overview of occupation covers definitions and predominant theories. Complexity is introduced to bring these different areas of knowledge together. The final section of the chapter considers how knowledge is advanced, relating to professional development, scholarship and research.

PEOPLE ENGAGING WITH OCCUPATIONAL THERAPY

The terms used to refer to people experiencing mental health problems vary, reflecting and revealing challenges within person-centred practice (Health Foundation 2016; also see Chapter 4). Awareness of these terms is critically important, as some are stigmatising and make it hard to remember the person behind them (Beresford 2010; Subramaniam et al. 2017; see also Chapters 11 and 12). Other terms, such as 'user' or 'survivor' help people using the service and health professionals to decide how to act and address the situation. Referring to a person or oneself as 'OCD' (i.e., living with obsessive compulsive disorder) or a 'nutter' is different than describing them as 'a person with mental health problems.'

Fig. 2.2 presents four different terms used to refer to people (middle rows) in different areas of practice (bottom row). The top row suggests the theoretical origins for these terms. There are other terms not included, such as when people are called 'residents,' where it also would be useful to consider underlying assumptions about the nature of their lives and how services can help.

In Fig. 2.2 'patient' is used to describe people who consult a doctor or other health professional in a healthcare setting (Health Foundation 2020). People who are seriously unwell and need to be treated in a secure place are known as 'patients' for legal purposes (MIND 2018). Being a patient means being given a diagnosis and treatment in a formal process. Medical and legal thinking require systematic processes to minimize harm.

The power given to professionals when people are called 'patients' is criticized by activists (Beresford 2010), who question the use of formal diagnosis to inform decisions and organize services. The terms 'user' and 'survivor' are used to describe people involved in research and service development, addressing potential power imbalances. User/survivor indicates the importance of knowledge gained from using mental health services, as well as surviving them. Sociopolitical theories inform this way of working together. Some people are critical of the term 'user' because of the implied passive role and its association with drug addiction (Beresford 2010).

Many health professionals use the term 'client.' This term was adopted by emerging community mental health teams wanting to highlight the difference in their approach from inpatient work (Costa et al. 2019). Work with clients is understood as a joint process of drawing on human qualities and strengths, informed

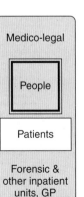
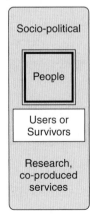
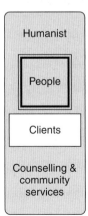
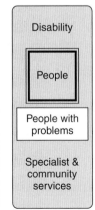

Medico-legal	Socio-political	Humanist	Disability
People	People	People	People
Patients	Users or Survivors	Clients	People with problems
Forensic & other inpatient units, GP surgery	Research, co-produced services	Counselling & community services	Specialist & community services

Fig. 2.2 ■ **Terms used to describe people who are in contact with mental health services.**

by humanism. However, the dictionary definition of client suggests payment and choice of providers, which may not be the case with publicly funded mental health services (Collins English Dictionary 2020).

Mental health is affected by many different factors and therefore the use of the term 'people with problems' (such as people with depression) separates a person from their mental health issue (Goodley 2017). Disability theorists and activists have stressed the importance of putting the person before the problem, making it unacceptable to describe people as 'schizophrenics' or 'anorexics', for example. The label schizophrenic consumes the whole person into the problem, in contrast to a person with schizophrenia (Beresford 2010). However, other activists point out that the problem seems to tag along, like an unwelcome burden, and they would rather be called by their names, or just 'people' (Goodley 2017).

Fig. 2.2 is simplified to encourage further investigation. For example, the self-advocacy movement urges us to 'label jars, not people,' reflecting disability activism, a social and political movement (Goodley 2017). Reflection on terminology can reveal how we think about the people we are working with. For example, recognizing people as fellow human beings is central to humanism (a philosophy) and to human rights (a set of moral principles and a political movement) (Bacha et al. 2019). An occupational therapist using the term 'older people' rather than 'the elderly' does so to reflect a belief that the latter term is dehumanising, as it could be applied to any object.

It is not necessary to be a philosopher or activist to hold beliefs about people: across all cultures, spiritual beliefs express how people understand the purpose and meaning of life. Mental health problems, disrupting lives and threatening life itself, challenge these beliefs. Spirituality is therefore another area of knowledge about people which is important for occupational therapy and mental health.

Spirituality

Spirituality is the aspect of life through which people look for meaning, purpose and integrity or transcendence. Through spirituality significant and sacred relationships are experienced with the self, family, community and nature (Soomar et al. 2018). Spirituality is expressed in beliefs, values, cultural or family traditions and in spiritual or religious practices. These expressions of meaning and purpose may therefore involve specific occupations, alone and together, often to address difficulties in life (Jones et al. 2016). Most people who wish to discuss concerns about their mental health go first to a trusted friend, family member, religious leader or traditional healer before accessing helplines and mental health services (Small 2017; Slewa-Younan et al. 2020; Filiatreau et al. 2021; Kim and Lee 2021). For people taking prescribed medication alongside remedies recommended by their traditional healers, there may be unknown risks (Zingela et al 2019). The World Health Organization (WHO 2019) therefore recommends attention to traditional and alternative healing practices, as many are associated with spiritual and cultural practices.

Serious mental health problems can disrupt a person's sense of self and their connections with supportive communities, affecting how they express and explore their spirituality. Being anxious and agitated makes it difficult to reflect on the meanings of experiences. For some people, religious or other important beliefs may be distorted by psychosis, affecting the way in which they see themselves and others. Depression or a diagnosis of dementia may lead to a loss of hope, meaning and connectedness with others. Receiving inpatient care may restrict participation in occupations that are important to people. Despite these problems, a person's spirituality may be an important resource for enhancing personal agency and hopefulness, enabling them to benefit from occupational therapy (Soomar et al. 2018).

Reflecting on their own spirituality may enable occupational therapists to take a non-judgemental and culturally sensitive approach to individuals and communities they are working with (Jones et al. 2016). This is particularly important to avoid unintentionally causing offence or missing opportunities to engage with a source of personal agency and hope.

Beliefs About Mental Ill-Health

Alongside spiritual beliefs, people have personal beliefs about mental ill-health. In the same way that there are different terms for people who use occupational therapy services (see earlier in this chapter), there are different terms that represent different beliefs about mental health. 'Mental health problem' emphasizes the link between mental health and ability or function. 'Mental disorder or illness' refers to diagnosis and emphasizes a medical approach. In this section, 'Mental Ill-Health' is an umbrella term that reflects mental health problems, mental illness and other ways of thinking about the ways in which people experience mental health. These personal beliefs, regardless of who holds them, are likely to be different to professional beliefs, so occupational therapists carefully negotiate interactions in therapy, as they are often working with people with different beliefs to their own. The differences may be in the way people are viewed in the context of a particular service in comparison to how people see themselves (e.g., patient vs. survivor); differences in spirituality or cultural and ethnic background; or differences in life experience.

An occupational therapist's perspective on a condition or diagnosis will often be substantially different to how the person directly affected understands and experiences it. For example, some developmental conditions, such as autism and attention deficit and hyperactivity disorder, may not be viewed as mental health conditions by the people experiencing them. This is illustrated by a survey of people in the autism community in the United Kingdom who said 'autism is not a disability, disorder or syndrome, more a different way of perceiving the world' and 'autism is just another way of thinking, not some sort of disease that one can catch' (Kenny et al. 2016, p. 448).

Similarly, while hearing voices may be a symptom of psychosis, there are many people who experience this but never access mental health services and regard the experience as affirming and positive (Dillon and Hornstein 2013; Ghana et al. 2015). Likewise, behavioural disturbances may be interpreted in different ways depending on the cultural context. For example, in isiXhosa culture (in South Africa and Zimbabwe), experiences of agitation, aggression and persecutory delusions may be the first indication of a calling to become a traditional healer, a new occupational identity (Edwards et al. 2014; Van der Watt et al. 2019).

Separating problems of the body from those of the mind has influenced Western approaches to health in contrast with other health traditions like traditional Chinese medicine and Ayurveda in which the person is treated as a whole in the context of their environment (Gopalkrishnan 2018). Accordingly, the origins of mental health problems may also be understood differently. For example, the cause of depression may be understood as an imbalance of neurotransmitters (biological origin); the result of disordered patterns of thinking (cognitive origin); possession by spirits or black magic (spiritual origin); or the result of dispossession, oppression and trauma resulting from societal/systemic racism (historical origin).

A person's beliefs about the origin and nature of their mental health problems influence where and from whom they seek support and what forms of intervention they find acceptable and likely to work. Beliefs can change as new ideas emerge. For example, in the last 15 years mindfulness, defined as 'awareness that emerges through paying attention on purpose, in the present moment, and non-judgementally to things as they are' (Williams et al. 2007, p. 47), has emerged as a popular way to promote mental health. More recently, medical treatments have been developed from new insights into the link between the inflammatory response, gut health and mental health (Bullmore 2018). Systematic reviews have indicated significant differences in the ecology of microorganisms living in the gut, between healthy participants in control groups and people with autism, schizophrenia and bipolar mood disorder and depression (Nguyen et al. 2018; Liu et al. 2019).

If a person believes that healing happens collectively, then a group intervention may be more effective than individual sessions. Agner (2020) advocates for cultural humility, that is, occupational therapists should be flexible, be aware of their own biases, be committed to a learning-oriented approach and recognize the power in their interactions with others. This can develop from cultural competence, defined by Awaad (2003) as having these components:

1. Understanding what culture is and how it is lived at different levels (e.g., individual, family, community, nation)
2. Self-reflection on one's own culture, including the culture of occupational therapy
3. Being able to use knowledge and specific cultural information to interact successfully with service users.

When people are active participants in occupational therapy, a cultural partnership can be established between them and their therapist (Gopalkrishnan 2018). This could involve carefully exploring beliefs about mental ill-health, recognizing the impact of the environment and being open to different ways of defining occupation and its significance.

Motivation and Volition

Motivation and volition are qualities which shape what people do and are therefore important to occupational therapists. Many academic disciplines are interested in these qualities, too. Like other mental health professionals, occupational therapists frequently draw on psychological theories, applying them to practice situations such as when people refuse or struggle to engage with therapy. The difference between motivation and volition is discussed here, using the example of washing and drying clothes, with more details in Box 2.1.

Motivation is 'a drive that directs a person's actions towards meeting needs' (Creek 2010, p. 25). A drive is experienced as energy or impulse to action. The need for clean clothes could generate the energy for a person to wash them as described in Box 2.1. Conversely, if the person does not feel the need for clean clothes, they may not be motivated to do the washing.

Volition is the 'ability to choose to do or continue to do something, together with awareness that the performance of the activity is voluntary' (Creek 2010, p. 26). The example given in Box 2.1 illustrates the dynamism of volition when someone is deciding whether or not to do something. Making a choice is an ability which can be compromised in different ways (Table 2.1).

Motivation and volition often overlap but it is helpful to distinguish between the two, as indicated in Table 2.1. A clear distinction enables the therapist to respond in a helpful way when people are reluctant to engage with occupational therapy. Factors other than motivation and volition are often external, which is broadly understood as the environment, discussed next.

BOX 2.1
VOLITION IN ACTION

Volition is indicated when people make choices. People often have favourite clothes they choose to wear for different situations, such as a particular outfit for a family celebration. If the outfit is not clean enough to wear, the individual may choose to wash it in time for the celebration. If, conversely, they choose not to go to the celebration, they may decide not to wash those particular clothes. The choice of whether or not to attend the celebration also depends on other factors. For example, the person may feel it is more important to work that day and earn money. Alternatively, they may be experiencing an episode of depression and feel unable to decide, lacking energy for anything about the family celebration.

TABLE 2.1		
When People are Reluctant to Engage with Occupational Therapy		
Motivation	They do not have the energy for occupational therapy today, because their mental health problems or other interventions affect their energy levels or because their energy is taken up with other basic drives such as hunger or thirst.	The therapist responds by carefully assessing the situation, addressing other needs if appropriate and addressing the demands involved in occupational therapy, adapting activities to engage the person (see Chapters 5 and 6).
Volition	They do not know enough to make a choice about occupational therapy or struggle to make decisions and initiate action for other reasons, for example, anxiety or obsessive thinking.	The therapist responds by carefully assessing the situation, offering relevant information if required. Activities are selected and designed at an appropriate level, and steps are negotiated to increase the person's decision-making ability (see Chapters 3, 5 and 6).
Other Factors	Autonomy is another consideration: external factors, such as other people, or internal factors, such as hearing voices may interfere with perceptions of occupational therapy. A person may have also investigated occupational therapy and decided it is not for them.	The therapist reflects in the situation, considering other factors and possible responses (see Chapter 3).

(Adapted from Creek 2007).

ENVIRONMENT

The environment can be understood in a number of ways. For example, as the external world (see Fig. 2.1), the environment affects and is affected by people's inner world, that is, their thoughts and. By changing what they do and how they do it, people respond to the environment and have impacts on it. (Creek 2010). In occupational therapy, the term 'environment' is often used to refer to the impact of external factors on people and their occupations. Environment is defined by Creek (2010, p. 25) as the 'external physical, socio-cultural and temporal factors that demand and shape occupational performance.' For example, for people with alcohol problems there could be several environmental factors to consider (see also Chapter 27):

- physical access to suppliers and personal stores to meet the need for alcohol and safe access to other physical facilities, such as water, food and a bathroom for self-care activities;
- sociocultural demands to drink with others, shaped by legislation to restrict public drinking (Thomas et al. 2017);
- temporal factors in overcoming alcohol problems, which could involve taking time to allow the body to adjust. Alcohol shapes time use, such as when particular times are associated with the demand for alcohol (Creek 2010; see Chapter 27).

Environment can also be understood as part of the 'place for action' (see Fig. 2.1) (Creek 2010, p. 189). To illustrate these understandings of the environment, Box 2.2 offers the experiences of Craig, who experienced occupational therapy for his mental health problems (Combat Stress 2022). Craig's experience of occupational therapy can be understood by seeing the residential course as a place for action where he learned about pottery. The therapeutic context shaped his engagement with pottery as an occupation. Creek (2010, p. 198) suggests that context is 'the relationships between the environment, personal factors and events that influence the meaning of a task, activity or occupation for the performer.' Not many people who encounter pottery in occupational therapy go on to set up their own studio: the therapeutic context is what makes the difference for each individual. Different ways in which the environment may be analysed

---

BOX 2.2
ENVIRONMENT, POTTERY AND THE SOLDIER

Craig Mealing is a potter who discovered his art through occupational therapy at Combat Stress, an organization in the United Kingdom that addresses the mental health needs of veterans of the armed forces (Mealing 2021). After leaving the Army in 2013 his use of alcohol to help self-medicate and to cover up mental health issues escalated until, after being told he had post-traumatic stress disorder, he became homeless when his relationship ended. He was introduced to working with clay by an occupational therapy technician during a residential course.

Craig's story can illustrate two general understandings of the environment:

- Environment as a social determinant for causing and/or sustaining mental health problems, such as when people are homeless (see Chapters 12 and 29).
- Environment as a space and place (Tuan 1977). As a space, there are possibilities for action. When those possibilities are realised, the space becomes a place. When Craig started working with clay, the environment changed for him. He got lost in the clay yet felt connected.

---

and adapted in occupational therapy are discussed in Chapter 6.

As a lens for understanding the environment, occupation therefore forms a key part of knowing the grounds for occupational therapy. The next part of this chapter explores occupation in theory.

OCCUPATION

Understandings of occupation emerge from professional practice, research and scholarship and from occupational science, an academic discipline (Zemke and Clark 1996). In this section occupation is defined first, before discussing how knowledge about it ranges from isolated concepts to a worldview. Theories about occupation are explored, starting with people as occupational beings. Finally, occupational justice and related ideas are briefly discussed.

In everyday conversation 'occupation' often refers to a person's job or employment or an activity or hobby they enjoy. Occupational therapists extend this definition to include all activities that are necessary for survival and human flourishing (Wilcock 1993). By thinking about occupation in this way, its therapeutic potential can be analysed and realized. Occupational therapists organize their thinking about a person's occupations into different theoretical levels. These are illustrated in Fig. 2.3 as concepts, theories and constructs, frames of reference and worldviews.

There is a highly simplified view through a window in Fig. 2.3, imagining an occupational therapist taking in and considering a situation from the details to a broad perspective. The brick wall is a metaphor to signal how, when a person thinks about a situation, they can focus on the details (or bricks) and on how the details fit together as a structure. This wall could be part of a structure, such as a building or could mark the boundaries of a plot. In professional practice, structures could be models of practice and practice frameworks, which are introduced in Chapter 4 as part of the occupational therapy neighbourhood. In Fig. 2.3 the brick wall is situated in the world (the clouds in the sky) and is framed by a particular perspective (the frame around the scene). Working through Fig. 2.3, each element represents a different level of thinking about occupation:

- A concept is an idea about something. The bricks in the wall represent the many concepts associated with occupation.
- A construct links different concepts together, like mortar joining the bricks.

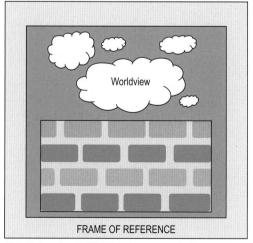

Fig. 2.3 ■ **Levels of thinking about occupation: concept, construct, theory, worldview, frame of reference.**

- A theory emerges when concepts and constructs are organized into a logical whole, like the wall. The strength and relevance of a theory is decided not just by which concepts are linked together, but also by how the theory looks and works from a distance in relation to other features of the grounds of occupational therapy.
- This distance is suggested by the clouds as a vantage point for a worldview, which describes how people think about life and the world in general. In a particular community such as the occupational therapy profession, this might be described as a paradigm.
- Another way to take a distinct view on occupation is to look through a metaphorical window. In Fig. 2.3, a frame cuts around what can be seen, focusing the view. A frame of reference draws on a particular worldview, often from another discipline with its associated terminology and theories, to apply to practice (Hinojosa 2017; see Chapter 4).

Bringing these different levels together, an occupational therapist considers a situation, thinking through different options for action. For example, Aisling, an occupational therapist working in a community mental health team, has contact with Shauna, a woman who is reluctant to leave her home because she feels life is hopeless. Aisling thinks about the concept of agency, which is the power a person has to act for themselves (Lindstrom et al. 2013), perhaps in connection with the construct of self-care, which involves many daily activities. Shauna feels she is barely managing the basics of self-care to survive. Connecting survival with agency and self-care, Aisling starts to bring concepts and constructs together, theorising about Shauna's self-care occupations and how they affect her health and wellbeing (Wilcock 1993). She knows that she is theorising about occupation as much as survival because of the worldview she takes as an occupational therapist.

Coming back to the situation, Aisling recalls that Shauna described difficulties in distracting herself from her feeling of despair. These difficulties could be interpreted and addressed using contrasting frames of reference (see Chapter 4), for example, pinpointing and challenging thoughts preceding feelings is suggested by a cognitive-behavioural frame of reference

(Ikiugu 2007). However, Aisling explains that occupational therapy could proceed by focusing on an activity which is full of positive meaning for Shauna, who suggests attending to her houseplants. This approach draws on a positive psychology frame of reference (Robinson et al. 2012). From this starting point, which is occupation-centred, Aisling can continue to think about the links between the activity and Shauna's self-care occupations. These links can be traced in a practice framework, which is a bigger structure to support Aisling's practice (see Fig. 2.1 and Chapter 4).

Occupational Beings

Within their professional worldview for understanding people, occupational therapists use the term 'occupational being' which emphasizes people's fundamental need for occupation to survive and thrive (Wilcock 1993; Clark 1997). Fig. 2.4 draws together relevant concepts, constructs and theories to explain the term, with people as occupational beings at the centre. By connecting doing-being-becoming-belonging, Wilcock (2006) suggests different aspects of occupational beings (Hitch et al. 2014).

The doing-being-becoming-belonging framework has been used to structure discussions about how and why people engage in occupation (Hitch et al. 2014; Hitch and Pepin 2020). Newport and Clarke (2020) used it to interpret the findings of their study of people with severe mental health problems participating in an occupational therapy programme. What people do expresses their identity (being), their future and capacity for self-transformation (becoming) and their context (belonging).

In Fig. 2.4, the framework has been expanded to include other terms used in occupational therapy. Doing is connected with performance, being with engagement, becoming with development and belonging with context.

- When occupational therapists observe what people are doing, they are thinking about occupational performance (Creek 2010).
- Engagement is the commitment or energy an individual puts into being occupied: a 'sense of involvement, choice, positive meaning and commitment while performing an occupation or activity' (Creek 2010, p. 166).

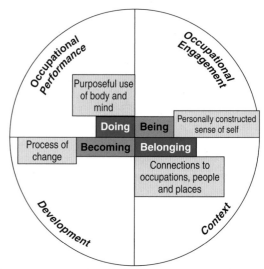

Fig. 2.4 ■ **Occupational beings.**

- Development refers to processes of growth and change, which occur during engagement and influence becoming (Hitch et al. 2014).
- Putting an occupation in context means considering belonging: where and how it belongs to the current situation, the social environment, and personal and historical factors (Creek 2010).

In Fig. 2.4, the four different aspects of an occupational being are closely connected. For example, if someone is struggling to engage and seems distant, it will be reflected in what they do, how they develop and their sense of ownership over what is happening. In Newton and Clarke's study (2020), as participants progressed through the programme, their sense of being and belonging strengthened and they could do more, taking risks they had avoided before.

In Fig. 2.4, doing and becoming are often associated with occupational therapy for individuals, reflecting the many dominant individualist ideas about occupation and mental health, which can sideline family, community and collective occupation (Ramugondo and Kronenberg 2013). Belonging was added to the framework in 2006, for balance, as previously, social aspects had been implied (Wilcock 2006; Hitch et al. 2014).

Theories Used in Occupational Therapy

As structures for practice, which are discussed in more depth in Chapter 4, models and practice frameworks are built on common theoretical grounds about occupation. To cover some of this ground, in this section some theories used in occupational therapy are briefly introduced. Each theory is connected with the case study in Box 2.3, suggesting ways of understanding Nomvula's situation.

Person, Environment and Occupation

This theory is concerned with the relationships between person, environment and occupation when analyzing how occupational therapy works (Law et al. 1996). For example, Nomvula often could not manage the stairs. Her depression and breathing difficulties, as aspects of her person, were combined with aspects of her environment (a first-floor flat) and her occupations, such as getting food. An occupational therapist addresses these aspects together, remembering that sorting out one difficulty will impact the others (Law et al. 1996).

Occupation, Activity and Task

Occupational therapists distinguish between occupation, activity and task in theory, to refer to and define

---

BOX 2.3
NOMVULA

Nomvula was a retired professional singer. Retirement had happened slowly, as Nomvula's respiratory disease got worse, making her feel depressed. She spent more time sitting indoors, alone. Seeing the change in her habits, Nomvula's friend Andre had encouraged her to seek help from the council with the stairs to her rented flat. There were issues with shopping, meeting other friends and attending appointments, and Nomvula was not going out very often. She spent a lot of time in bed because her motivation was low, which also meant she mainly ate tinned soup.

Nomvula's occupational therapist, Thandi, initially arranged for a stairlift to be installed, but Nomvula was anxious about using it and began to feel another solution was to move home to live on the ground floor. In the meantime, Andre was also becoming increasing mentally unwell and, sadly, took his own life. Switching priorities, Thandi liaised with the local housing department to secure alternative ground floor accommodation near Nomvula's other friends, the GP surgery and shops. After moving, although still grieving for Andre, Nomvula started to recover and establish new forms of occupations.

---

the things people do (Creek 2010). Nomvula sought help with shopping (occupation). She messaged Andre, her friend (task) and shared her shopping list (task). Andre did the shopping. Later, they unpacked the shopping together (activity). Tasks and activities are often part of more than one occupation, so when messaging her friend, Nomvula might ask Andre to stay to chat when she visited with the shopping (Creek 2010).

Occupational Performance

How a person acts in the outer world to express their inner world is revealed by what they do and how they do it, or their occupational performance (Creek 2010). Law et al. (1996, p. 16) defined occupational performance as 'the dynamic experience of a person engaged in purposeful activities and tasks within an environment' that draws together the elements of person, environment and occupation. Occupational therapists analyse and interpret their observations of a person's occupational performance, to understand the impact of mental health problems. Nomvula told Thandi, her occupational therapist, that looking at her reflection in the bathroom mirror made her feel worse, so she returned to bed where there were less performance demands on her.

Performance, Engagement and Participation

Occupational therapists connect performance with engagement in activities and participation in life to explain the quality of people's involvement (Morris and Ward 2018). Nomvula was not engaged with food preparation, although she could perform the necessary tasks. With so much time spent in bed limiting her participation in life, Nomvula was not meeting her own needs effectively, with implications for her health and well-being (Holahan 2014).

Subjective Values

Occupations have different subjective values, categorised by Wilcock and Townsend (2014) into 'want to do,' 'need to do,' and 'have to do.' Nomvula felt she had to do the things she did to survive but needed to move away because she wanted to live somewhere where she could go out on her own.

Time Use

Theories about time use reveal the patterns of what people do, including habits and routines (Clark

1997). Nomvula's perception of time (temporality) changed, as the tempo (pace) of her life slowed when she retired.

Human Needs

Maslow's (1943) hierarchy is widely used to understand human needs, including occupations. However, as a hierarchy, assumptions are made about the relative importance of different needs, for example, indicating that physiological needs are fundamentally more important than the need to belong. Maslow's work has been extended by Chilean economist Max-Neef, who organized human needs into a matrix rather than a hierarchy, recognizing that needs could be divided into valued principles such as subsistence and affection, and experiences such as being, having, doing and interacting (1991, pp. 31–33). After she had moved, several of Nomvula's needs were satisfied: for example, the need for subsistence was satisfied by having a ground floor flat near to shops and her need for affection by interacting with more of her friends.

Transactional Perspective

Performing occupations changes people and their environments. This perspective theorises about a world that is continually changing because of what people do, both alone and together. Dickie et al. (2006) used the term 'transactional' to indicate that occupations have a function in conducting, or coordinating, these changes. If occupations are seen as 'functional coordinators' aiming to sustain life (Cutchin et al. 2017, p. 435), then people are pragmatic, doing what seems best at the time (see Chapter 3 for further discussion of pragmatism). The shift in Thandi's actions was a pragmatic response to the changes in Nomvula's life.

Form, Function and Meaning

Nelson's theory of therapeutic occupation brings together occupational performance, form, function and meaning (Nelson 1988; Nelson 1996).

- The occupational *form* is the way people do things shaped by physical and sociocultural factors. Nomvula chooses to wash, dry and style her hair in a particular way, shaped by the tools she uses and the times and places she does it (see Box 2.4). Her occupational performance is

---

BOX 2.4
THERAPEUTIC OCCUPATION

The occupational therapist, Thandi, observed Nomvula's difficulties in caring for her hair. Thandi considered occupational form, function (purpose) and meaning to be equally important and connected. Adapting the occupational form of hair care required insight into its meanings, such as the significance of hair care practices for Black women (Ndichu and Upadhyaya 2019). In Nelson's (1996) theory of therapeutic occupation, the core action of the therapist is described as adapting and redesigning occupational forms in collaboration with the service user. Because Nomvula's difficulties arose partly from low mood and breathlessness, working together to adapt and redesign the occupational form involved:

- Identifying small steps which felt achievable
- Adding rest breaks, locating somewhere to sit
- Engaging others for encouragement and assistance
- Practising helpful responses to anxiety and negative thoughts when looking in the mirror

Revisiting occupational form, Bryant (2016) proposed it as an important ally to the concept of occupational alienation, which is discussed further in this chapter. The actions of the therapist are also a focus in Chapters 3 and 4.

(Nelson 1996)

---

characterized by the form, but also changes it (Nelson 1988).

- The *functions* are the purposes of occupational performance. As Nomvula recovers, she changes what she wants to achieve from avoiding the bathroom mirror to preparing to go out, so she cares for her hair with more attention.
- The *meanings* are how people make sense of their occupational performance. This could include what Nomvula feels physically or emotionally about caring for her hair.

Forms, functions and meanings of occupational performance can influence how occupational therapists think and act in practice, as illustrated in Box 2.4 in which Nomvula's experience of occupational therapy is explained further.

The grounding belief for these theories is that occupation is as essential to health as food and drink and must be addressed when health problems occur (Wilcock 1993). Problems with occupation can threaten life itself (Stewart et al. 2016). A person with an eating disorder, which severely affects social and occupational engagement with food and exercise, faces an increased risk of premature death (Iwajomo et al. 2020). Anxiety may drive a person to check something obsessively before leaving home, making it harder to go out and participate in activities which might offer relief. As contexts change, occupational performance problems will vary, so a person with dementia may be able to brush their teeth at home but not in an assessment unit (Dunn et al. 1994). For groups of people, consequences of ongoing problems with occupation can be a justice issue.

Occupational Justice and Injustice

Justice, injustice and power are profoundly connected, with justice as an ideal, polluted by injustices and abuses of power. There are many dimensions to justice, such as social justice where equal rights are shared by all society (Collins English Dictionary 2020). The World Federation of Occupational Therapists (WFOT) position statement on human rights defined occupational justice as *'the fulfilment of the right for all people to engage in the occupations they need to survive, define as meaningful, and that contribute positively to their own well-being and the well-being of their communities.'*

WFOT 2019

Therefore occupational justice is a driver for population health and well-being, which can guide occupational therapists through the tensions between individual freedoms and justice for all. The humanist belief that people want to do the best for themselves and others is often challenged when working with people who have mental health issues (Humanists UK 2020). Engaging in harmful occupations can be directly associated with mental health problems, sometimes as a coping strategy to manage symptoms. Occupational science research has been criticized for ignoring unproductive, unhealthy and illegal occupations associated with self-harm, trauma and abuse (Twinley and Morris 2014; Kiepek et al. 2019).

Occupational injustices occur when external restrictions on necessary occupations apply for long periods (Whiteford et al. 2020). In society, controlling individual freedom to engage in potentially harmful occupations may be appropriate to protect public safety, such as restricting everyone's access to firearms to limit gun violence. However, occupational injustices have negative consequences for the mental health of individuals and communities. Their occupations may be restricted by those monitoring their health for safety and/or to punish them. This can happen in any place or relationship where choice and access are controlled by individuals on behalf of others. It could be at home when a caring relative is anxious, frightened and feeling unsupported.

The right to engage in occupation is also known as occupational rights (Hammell 2015). To protect rights, discussions and agreements informed by occupational justice can enable the fairest outcome (Hocking and Mace 2017). This process can be complex when working with situations in which there is a risk of harm because of mental health issues, but occupational justice offers a direction for improving people's lives by asserting their occupational rights (Hammell 2015; see also Chapters 9, 21 and 26).

Risk Factors for Occupational Injustice

Occupational injustice offers a focus on enduring external restrictions or determinants and indicates factors which impact on a person's inner world of mental health problems. Examples of external determinants are discriminatory legislation, illegal activities, poverty and conflict (WFOT 2019; see Chapter 12). A person who develops severe anxiety about leaving home because of experiences of conflict might be prevented from working and be forced to live in poverty. Wilcock (1998) originally named three risk factors as external determinants for occupational injustice:

- Occupational deprivation occurs when people are deprived of an occupation necessary for their health and survival (Whiteford et al. 2020);
- Occupational alienation occurs when people have to do something in a way that does not satisfy their needs (Bryant 2016);
- Occupational imbalance occurs when people have to spend too much time on some things (and not enough on others) and when opportunities for participating in occupations are unequal (Durocher 2017).

Other risk factors for occupational injustice have since been identified, including occupational apartheid and occupational marginalization (Durocher 2017; see Chapters 12 and 29).

Rather than separately addressing each occupational risk factor for an individual, addressing occupational injustice requires broader consideration of what people are doing. This includes what the occupational therapist is doing, as this, too, affects service users' freedom to shape and negotiate occupations. Occupational deprivation is sometimes used as a justification for occupational therapy in mental health services. Perceiving that people cannot do what they need to do, occupational therapists might respond by providing opportunities, such as weekly group occupational therapy sessions. However, this response does not take into account the other risk factors. Control of the resources for occupation is retained by the occupational therapists, who might restrict provision to weekly sessions and determine the occupational form and function. Some people might feel occupationally alienated by group activities, which could alter the balance of their daily occupations and feel unmanageable. Therefore, to address occupational injustice, all risk factors are considered in partnership with those experiencing them.

The Problem with Meaning

The definition of occupational justice includes a person's right to identify their valued occupations, but these occupations may have different values and meaning for other people (Kiepek et al. 2019; WFOT 2019). The subjective nature of meaning is challenging when negotiating the focus of occupational therapy in mental health settings. Understanding people's narratives can reveal the meanings of their occupations, but, if they are ashamed, they may conceal those meanings (Hasselkus 2011). For example, a newly rehoused man may give a vague explanation for why he is unable to shop for food, implying his general anxiety has been worsened by the move. Later, however, the real reason for his evasiveness may be revealed: an accusation of sexual assault, a pending trial and the fear that his new neighbours might attack him.

When people talk about meanings with their therapists, it is helpful to distinguish between these different senses (Crabtree 1998):

- Meaning as intention: those occupations people intend or mean to do as opposed to those they are forced to do by circumstance;

- Meaning as significance: those occupations that change life;
- Meaning-making: unfolding as people perform, engage and participate in chosen, significant occupations.

Occupations could be full of meaning in any of these senses, so occupational therapists might have to make assumptions because of the fleeting and vague nature of meaning (Brooks 2015). However, this is risky because assumptions may reflect social privilege (Hammell 2015), stereotyping of others (also a determinant of occupational injustice) or judgements as expressions of power (see Chapter 12).

Power

Different ways of understanding power are associated with energy, capacity and authority. Justice is concerned with capacity and authority. The use of power and how it is shared, can indicate injustice, through misuse of power (Hui and Stickley 2007). In a deliberative democracy (which values transparency of debate and decision-making) powerful people are urged to share their power, to give others a chance (Held 2016). This way of seeing power is like imagining voices in a discussion. If one person speaks all the time, others do not have a chance to be heard. However, if power is imagined as voices coming together to sing, the sound is much more powerful. Similarly, when people do things together, the impact of occupation can be more powerful. As a resource for action or energy source, power is neutral. However, the power of occupational engagement on individuals and communities is not necessarily positive, as indicated in experiences of trauma and abuse. Three different occupational perspectives on this are considered here.

The dark side of occupation is a construct developed by Twinley (2013; Rule and Twinley 2020) based on her research into woman-on-woman rape in prisons. When people engage in occupation and know or use the potential to harm health and well-being, they could be engaging in dark side occupations, such as violence, crime, smoking and over-working (Twinley 2013).

The shadow side of occupation is a theory developed by Nicholls and Elliot (2018) drawing on their separate research areas and psychoanalysis to explore racism and shame. The therapists' acknowledgment of their own feelings of shame was an important way of understanding the experiences of others. It was also a step towards becoming ethically reflexive professionals capable of learning from their own misunderstandings and errors. (see Chapter 9).

Sanctioned and non-sanctioned occupations, as described by Kiepek et al. (2019), are those that are acceptable or not, as defined by social norms. These norms can change over time so that all occupations could potentially be sanctioned or non-sanctioned, depending on the context. Smoking cigarettes is an example of an occupation which was initially promoted as being a good thing to do. As undesirable effects on health emerged, it is steadily becoming a non-sanctioned occupation in many, but not all, cultures.

These different understandings of occupation, people and their environments suggest there are many things to consider within the grounds for occupational therapy. Understanding complexity offers a way of bringing these considerations together and appreciating them as a whole.

A COMPLEX INTERVENTION

When defining occupational therapy as a complex intervention, Creek (2003) observed how occupation could be both the means and the outcome of therapy simultaneously (see Chapter 4). In other words, people have the capacity for renewal and development at the same time: while doing everyday activities and tasks that are essential for survival, the person also progresses towards important life goals. Similarly, the theoretical grounds for the profession are constantly renewing and developing, as therapists conduct and advance their everyday practice, revisiting areas of knowledge and gaining new understandings.

Understanding occupational therapy in this way is based on complexity theory. Pentland et al. (2018) used the term 'multiple, complex dynamic systems' to develop Creek's (2003) definition. As occupational therapy unfolds, multiple processes of renewal and development are taking place at the same time, involving separate but linked systems. The people involved are each a separate system, as is the therapy itself and the contexts in which it takes place. For example, visiting a person at home after discharge from hospital might bring the home context and the people present into occupational therapy as new, separate systems. Dynamics drive change and could be associated with any components in the systems, which are constantly interacting. To understand how occupational therapy drives change, Pentland et al. (2018, p. 9) identified components such as a 'shared understanding of the person-in-context.' In the example of a home visit, the occupational therapist develops and shares new understandings of the person from the other people present and the environment.

Identifying which component of occupational therapy has driven a change can be difficult, because there are many simultaneous interactions between the components. In theory it is possible to isolate specific components and design an occupational therapy intervention, creating a special form or shape of it for research and measuring outcomes. However, this does not address the goals of the intervention, which, in the real world for each individual are often varied and change over time. Some outcomes of occupational therapy can be observed, for example, changes in attention span, whereas others are dependent on interpreting what is reported or expressed. For example, a person may start crying in a relaxation session. The therapist's response has two initial purposes: to offer attention and to find out more. This reflects the dual nature of occupational therapy, which is discussed further in Chapter 3.

There are many implications from using complexity theory to understand occupational therapy, such as exploring multiple explanations for situations, which are often unpredictable (Whiteford 2005; see also Chapters 3 and 4). When people and their contexts are seen as complex systems, this challenges mechanistic perspectives which trace cause and effect to specific components. For example, rather than disputing whether mental health issues are socially determined or due to brain dysfunction (see Chapter 12), complex thinking allows both explanations to be accepted, recognizing how they interact.

In occupational therapy there could be simultaneous changes occurring at any time, in systems such as cells, body structures, people, groups, organizations, communities and globally. Physicist Fritjof Capra (2002) applied the terms 'structures,' 'networks' and 'organisms' to all these systems to show how complexity theory can be used to understand changes at different levels. For example, an organization such as a particular mental health service can be conceptualized as a machine or as a living organism, with formal structures and informal communication networks. Structures change and emerge in new forms as the organization develops, while informal networks maintain the organism in constant renewal. These changes are constant and often challenging features of occupational therapy practice and have implications for advancing knowledge.

ADVANCING KNOWLEDGE

When knowledge is understood as the grounds for occupational therapy, each working day or new phase of study could be considered as if entering a landscape; each person having their own starting point. Like using a map of an unknown place, exploring could involve digging deeper or across theories, constructs and concepts or into the structures of frameworks and models to know more (see Chapter 4) or both.

Knowledge, therefore, is not static but continuously evolving with experience (Arblaster et al. 2019). Individual perceptions can be discussed and shared to broaden and deepen understanding, giving knowledge a social dimension, as in professional discourse and debate. For example, in many training courses before covering areas of shared interest, participants are asked to identify their individual learning goals and reflect on them at the end. Advancing knowledge has sometimes been assumed to be the responsibility of scholars and researchers, but everyone can contribute to greater shared knowledge and understanding. Experience, practice, scholarship and research are ways of advancing knowledge, each involving different ways of knowing.

Ways of Knowing

There are many ways of categorising knowledge, with different forms reflecting their distinct nature and functions (Stevens 2018). Groups of people draw on each other's knowledge as well as on such sources as printed and online media (Marcolino et al. 2021). In Fig. 2.5, there are 10 people with different roles, connected to four contrasting forms of knowledge:

Embodied knowledge

Refers to our knowledge that is so familiar that we forget or are unaware of it. It is also referred to as 'tacit knowledge' (Polanyi 1966; Arntzen 2018; see Chapter 3). For example, the occupational therapist and mental health nurse in Fig. 2.5 may not be surprised by how many people struggle to find the energy to get dressed in the mornings but others, such as the auditor and the commissioner, may not have this knowledge.

Experiential knowledge

Comes from direct experiences that others might only know in theory (Faulkner 2017). A researcher cannot gain experiential knowledge about the impacts of living with psychosis or depression from hearing service users' or carers' experiences in interviews. Valuing experiential knowledge is the basis for coproduction and collaborative research (see Chapter 12; Faulkner 2017). Experiential knowledge is sometimes known as 'subjective knowledge' because the experiences are filtered by the individual (Franco 2013).

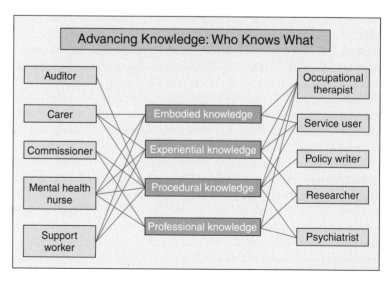

Fig. 2.5 ■ **Advancing knowledge: who knows what.**

Procedural knowledge

Involves knowing how something works and how to operate it, such as knowing how to wash and store clothes or how to use an assessment tool (Schell and Schell 2008; see also Chapter 3). Important in a new situation, procedural knowledge becomes embodied over time, differentiating novices from expert practitioners (see Chapter 3). In the community, support workers, carers and service users often have valuable procedural knowledge, which might be ignored in a hospital setting.

Professional knowledge

Is learned formally for a qualification and through continuing professional development (see Chapters 7 and 11; Kinsella 2009). Insights into practice can be broadened and deepened to make new connections between different knowledge sources, offering alternative understandings. Gaining such insights is dependent on reflective practice (Kinsella 2009; see Chapter 3).

In Fig. 2.5, the connections between people and the different forms of knowledge are simplified, as in reality each individual has multiple ways of knowing and engaging with multiple, dynamic, complex systems (see previous section). To use these systems and share knowledge, service delivery, developments and research are usually planned in partnerships (see Chapter 8). An example is given in Chapter 5 in which the collaborative process of creating a standardized assessment is described. Different forms of knowledge bring diverse perspectives on people's lives, but much depends on how knowledge is valued.

Valuing Knowledge

When people are advancing their knowledge, some sources are valued more than others, depending on how easy the source is to access, its perceived relevance and authority and how much it can be trusted. For example, a person in Fig. 2.5 asks one of the others about occupational therapy. The person might be a policy writer who approaches a researcher, commissioner or psychiatrist about a gap in their procedural knowledge about specific mental health professions, taking time to discover more about occupational therapy. A mental health nurse who has worked closely with occupational therapists has both embodied and experiential knowledge of the profession but will probably be aware of the limits of their procedural knowledge about how to do occupational therapy and their professional knowledge about why it works. A service user and carer might approach a support worker who has not come across occupational therapy and cannot help.

Valuing different ways of knowing was explored by Brazilian educator Paulo Freire (1921–1997), who saw that education could be used as a form of control if knowledge was seen as something that could be deposited in people, like putting money into a bank account (Freire 1970). In contrast, knowledge is powerful when people actively cooperate to share and question ideas, discovering more about their particular situation (Magalhães 2012). Imagine you are an occupational therapy student who has had a job in a hospital. Your knowledge is strong in certain situations but not all. This influences your approach to learning and to the other students. Freire (1970) suggested that naming areas of knowledge could address power imbalances and increase cooperation and dialogue. Therefore knowledge gained from working in a hospital is valued when named as 'prior learning' or 'experiential knowledge', with a defined place in the journey of becoming an occupational therapist.

Values affect who knows what and who shares their knowledge, especially what is considered to be legitimate knowledge (Kinsella 2009; Faulkner 2017). Reliability and validity are concepts discussed in Chapter 5, with particular reference to creating a standardized assessment, but are broadly relevant. When a knowledge source is reliable and valid, it is thought to be correct and sensible (Collins English Dictionary 2020). Sometimes, conflict arises when new knowledge is seen as irrelevant or threatening or potentially undermining people's experiences of occupational therapy.

When covering new ground for understanding occupational therapy and thinking critically, Bryant (2016) suggested that attending to assumptions, whoever holds them, can expose:

- values which focus and/or restrict what we know already,
- values about what we think we need to know, and
- values shaping the questions we pose to evaluate new knowledge.

For example, in trying to understand the experiences of bipolar disorder, a list of symptoms in a classification system such as the International Classification of Diseases (ICD-10; WHO 2016) might be assumed to give essential information. Yet this source is oriented to psychiatric diagnosis and may have limited relevance for planning occupational therapy. To evaluate sources

---

BOX 2.5
QUESTIONS FOR CRITICAL THINKING

When encountering new ideas and knowledge, asking questions like these reveals values and assumptions:

1. **When** did this knowledge emerge? Has it evolved since?
2. **What** is it about? Is it relevant to my current knowledge gap?
3. **Why** did this knowledge come about? Did it replace older ideas? Was it in response to external changes?
4. **Where** did it emerge from? What else do we know about this source?
5. **Who** was involved in shaping it?
6. **How** does it address my specific gaps in knowledge?

---

of knowledge, practice is guided by critical thinking, using questions such as those in Box 2.5. These questions form the basis for critical appraisal tools of the quality of research evidence (see Chapter 4). However, these questions could also be asked by a person experiencing occupational therapy for the first time.

Box 2.6 illustrates one way in which an occupational therapist advances their knowledge, reading published peer-reviewed articles as part of continuing professional development (see Chapter 7). If Alex wanted to propose a new community service to funders, then the articles by Sakornsatian (2009) and Franco (2013) are unlikely to be valued as strong evidence, being focused on personal experience rather than a scientific trial (see Chapter 4). However, Sakornsatian (2009) values indigenous or home-grown knowledge, and Franco (2013) is based on direct experience.

Coproduction and other collaborative approaches have grown to challenge the imbalance of power given to scientific and economic research and the discrimination which excludes many people with mental health problems from the research community and from key roles in society (see Chapter 12). Decolonization challenges the dominance of knowledge historically linked with Western Europe, overshadowing other ways of knowing about people, their environments and their occupations (Ramugondo 2018).

Mind the Gap

To advance knowledge is to start an enquiry, which is refined with awareness of different forms of knowledge and how they are valued by different stakeholders. The enquiry begins by defining a gap in knowledge which

---

BOX 2.6
USING CRITICAL QUESTIONS TO ADVANCE KNOWLEDGE

An occupational therapist, Alex, was working with a woman, Ella, whose mental health problems arose following experiences of violent sexual assault. A senior colleague recommended two accessible articles, Sakornsatian (2009) and Franco (2013) for continuing professional development.

Sakornsatian (2009) described the challenges for women of living in areas of ongoing armed conflict and how a community occupational therapist in Thailand worked with them to establish self-help groups. The scope of occupational therapy was suggested, with details of how one woman was helped to recover.

Franco (2013) explored two aspects of her life experiences of rape as a young woman in the 1970s and of paranoid schizophrenia. With each advance in knowledge, she was able to understand more about how to help herself, eventually finding a psychoanalytic frame of reference most helpful.

Alex read the articles and made notes on his initial thoughts. On reflection, he noticed the emphasis on self-help and questioned how useful the articles were for his professional practice. Then he used critical appraisal questions to identify that the articles addressed the gaps in his experiential and embodied knowledge. He could also identify strengths, limitations and further gaps to address.

BOX 2.7
MIND THE GAP

'Mind the gap' is an audio-recorded warning given on the London Underground railway at stations where there is a large gap between the train and the platform. To 'mind the gap' means to take care when getting on and off the train. As a metaphor for addressing knowledge gaps, it could suggest the dangers of jumping too far across the gap, potentially losing balance and control, colliding with unrelated areas of knowledge and missing details about the context. There are also dangers in being too cautious in minding the gap, perhaps avoiding it altogether, taking a detour and abandoning that route to advancing knowledge. If the warning is ignored, there is a risk of falling into the gap and having to stop the journey. Being mindful of the gap, you are aiming to address means taking care to keep focused, noticing details and continuing to make progress.

---

must be kept in mind to progress. In Box 2.7 the relationship between the enquiry and the knowledge gap is explored, using a metaphor of 'Mind the Gap.'

Minding the gap to progress an enquiry can have many benefits for developing practice locally and internationally. A starting point could be the experiential knowledge shared in the following quote from a blog which captures experiences of occupational therapy and activity groups in acute mental health units from a user perspective (Purplepersuasion 2018):

> When it ran, I went to "healthy snacks" [a group] which had somehow, much to everyone's delight, morphed into decorating cookies and making milkshakes. I did try to go to creative writing but it only happened once. All of these activities were organised by the tireless Activities Coordinator because the ward was "between" Occupational Therapists.'
>
> **Purplepersuasion 2018**

The context for an enquiry will determine who takes it forward and what knowledge is gained. For example:

- Locally, from a user perspective, some service users on the ward might try to find out why the healthy snacks group had changed focus, what was blocking the creative writing group from happening and when occupational therapists were likely to be offering a service again. As well as enabling access to helpful activities and occupational therapy, this would convey the importance of these being reviewed and reinstated.
- Locally, from the occupational therapist's perspective, the new member of staff might investigate the priority given to activities, while being mindful of work with individuals preparing to leave the unit. Enquiry into guidelines and evidence for different interventions would ensure relevant knowledge is developed and used.
- Nationally and internationally, staff on the unit might be involved in a research project, advancing professional knowledge about occupational therapy.

TABLE 2.2			
Knowledge and Practice			
	Practice Theory	**Practice Epistemology**	**Knowledge Transfer**
Main Perspective on Knowledge and Practice	There are many experiences and contexts that continually shape our everyday knowledge and practices.	There are many uncertainties and complexities of our practice, which is formed of our actions, knowledge and context.	There are clear and valid research findings which could inform our practice.
Discipline	Wide range of disciplines including philosophy, cultural theory and sociology	Applied philosophy, social and political sciences	Implementation science
Key Ideas	Everyday life is formed of practices which are simultaneously personal and social. Practice combines form and performance and is always context-bound.	Practice can be understood in terms of the action that can be taken now, ongoing business and the constantly evolving situation.	It is essential to know how to effectively translate innovative ideas and findings from research and scholarship into practice.
Nature of the Knowledge-Practice Gap	Not separate entities but bound together. Gaps occur in understanding of social and historical contexts.	Not knowing what to do could be due to gaps in understanding the situation or routine approaches to it. Dialogues about the situation shift as it unfolds.	Knowledge and practice are separate entities, with problems in practice arising because of insufficient knowledge. Evidence-based practice is enhanced by knowing about implementation.
Influence on Occupational Therapy	Enhances understanding of occupation, emphasizing social practice and an alternative perspective to dominant theories separating out person, environment, occupation and performance.	Offers fresh insights into how occupational therapists practice. Valuing different forms of knowledge enables more detailed and inclusive accounts of practice.	Ensures practice is effective and based on sound evidence rather than hunches, intuitions and expert knowledge.
References	Bukhave and Creek 2020	Cook and Wagenaar 2012; Cordingley 2015	Grol 2008; Bauer et al. 2015; Khalil 2016

Knowledge and Practice

Advancing knowledge about occupational therapy is to know more about how to practice. Equally, practice determines the knowledge we require in the present and future. Therefore to advance knowledge is also to advance practice. Three frameworks for understanding knowledge and practice are briefly summarized in Table 2.2.

For occupational therapists interested in mental health, knowledge and practice can be advanced through study, experience, reflection, supervision, listening to service users and systematic investigation, such as research. The starting points for occupational therapy research and scholarship could be orientated to:

1. Theories of occupation and occupational science, as described in this chapter.
2. The process of being and becoming a therapist, as explored in Chapter 3.
3. Structures for practice, such as evidence-based practice, which are discussed further in Chapter 4.
4. Coproduction and other collaborative approaches, which are discussed further in Chapters 10 and 12.

These starting points overlap but help to decide how a knowledge gap is defined and refined, including the question(s) for further enquiry. The points differ in how different forms of knowledge are valued but are oriented to issues of shared concern. The chapters in this textbook are all focused on knowledge and practice that are the grounds for occupational therapy and mental health, implying many possibilities and issues for advancing knowledge. Understanding the relationship between knowledge and practice can enable new and diverse approaches to enquiry, which are continually emerging.

SUMMARY

In this chapter the grounds for occupational therapy covered the broad areas of the person, their environments, occupation, complexity and advancing knowledge. Within each of these areas different perspectives on knowledge have been mapped out, referring to the other chapters in this textbook for more detail. While there are many sources of knowledge about occupational therapy, there are particular challenges and considerations associated with mental health issues. These have been explored using relevant literature and examples. These challenges and considerations will be developed further in Chapters 3 (Being a Therapist) and 4 (Structuring Practice).

SERVICE USER COMMENTARY

One of the main problems is service users feel that they are not listened to and that what they say is not important. Many feel undervalued and frustrated. In the hospital setting each person is one among maybe 20 service users vying for a health professional to listen to their needs and views. If they discuss (usually in passing) an issue affecting them with staff, this can be forgotten because there are so many others wanting attention. By the time staff get to the office, they might not remember all conversations apart from maybe the service users they are key working. I have personal experience of this happening continually on the ward, making me feel I am not important enough to be listened to. Needs are not met, and admission becomes a punitive approach in which the only continuum is being locked in.

Occupational therapists are the catalyst of ward activities, but they are also much more. Their amalgamated types of knowledge are used to inform, organize and assist in aiding service users make choices. For example, in a well-attended morning meeting, occupational therapists use lay language so that service users can relate and feel at ease relaying back information and their own knowledge. By using preferred names, service users feel their individual and specific issues are being addressed. The occupational therapist ensures even the quietest service users are given a voice. Empowering service users may mean that, at some stage during their time in occupational therapy, they open up about issues affecting them.

Occupational therapists can offer a therapeutic environment to discuss agency and ability and overcome occupational problems. This happened with me: in our morning meeting one service user decided we should bake. All ingredients were bought, but she never fulfilled that promise, so I stepped in to make garlic bread for the ward with the head occupational therapist. My only volition was not to tell him anything about my life, but he created the situation to make that possible. I still do not know how he did it. In fact, it was such a relief to talk. I was sectioned and no one had asked me how I was feeling during that time. The occupational therapist did, and I was more open about my feelings as a result.

New knowledge is possible within occupational therapy whether theoretical, professional, reflexive, experiential or when working with service users. Irrespective of sex, gender or cultural needs, this knowledge is transferable into skills and is passed down and learned from one generation of experienced occupational therapists to another.

Karan Essien

REFERENCES

Agner, J. (2020). Moving from cultural competence to cultural humility in occupational therapy: A paradigm shift. *American Journal of Occupational Therapy, 74*(4), 1–7.

Arblaster, K., Mackenzie, L., Gill, K., Willis, K., & Matthews, L. (2019). Capabilities for recovery-oriented practice in mental health occupational therapy: A thematic analysis of lived experience perspectives. *British Journal of Occupational Therapy, 82*(11), 675–684.

Awaad, J. (2003). Culture, cultural competency and occupational therapy: A review of the literature. *British Journal of Occupational Therapy, 66*, 356–362.

Bacha, K., Hanley, T., & Winter, L. A. (2019). *Like a human being, I was an equal, I wasn't just a patient: Service users' perspectives on their experiences of relationships with staff in mental health services. *Psychology and Psychotherapy: Theory, Research and Practice*. Available at https://onlinelibrary.wiley.com/doi/full/10.1111/papt.12218.

Bauer, M. S., et al. (2015). An introduction to implementation science for the non-specialist. *BioMed Central Psychology, 3*(1), 32. 16 Sep. Available at https://doi:10.1186/s40359-015-0089-9.

Beresford, P. (2010). *Being a Service User: Ross-on-Wye*. PCCS Books.

Brooks, D. (2015). *The problem with meaning*. The New York Times. Jan 5. Available at https://www.nytimes.com/2015/01/06/opinion/david-brooks-the-problem-with-meaning.html.

Bryant, W. (2016). The Dr Elizabeth Casson Memorial Lecture 2016: Occupational alienation – A concept for modelling participation in practice and research. *British Journal of Occupational Therapy, 79*(9), 521–529. Available at https://doi:10.1177/0308022616662282.

Bryant, W., Tibbs, A., & Clark, J. (2011). Visualising a safe space: The perspective of people using mental health day services. *Disability and Society, 26*(5), 611–628.

Bukhave, E. B., & Creek, J. (2020). Occupation through a practice theory lens. *Journal of Occupational Science*. Available at https://doi:10.1080/14427591.2020.1812105.

Bullmore, E. (2018). *The Inflamed Mind: A Radical New Approach to Depression*. London: Short Books.

Capra, F. (2002). *The Hidden Connections*. London: Flamingo.

Clark, F. (1997). Reflections on the human as an occupational being: Biological need, tempo and temporality. *Journal of Occupational Science, 4*(3), 86–92.

Collins English Dictionary. (2020). Available at https://www.collinsdictionary.com/dictionary/english.

Combat Stress. (2022). Craig's Case Study. https://combatstress.org.uk/craig-case-study.

Cook, S. D., Wagenaar, N., & Wagenaar, H. (2012). Navigating the eternally unfolding present: Toward an epistemology of practice. *The American Review of Public Administration, 42*(3). originally published online 22 June 2011.

Cordingley, K. (2015). *How do occupational therapists practising in forensic mental health know? A practice epistemology perspective*. Unpublished PhD. Available at http://bura.brunel.ac.uk/handle/2438/12205.

Costa, D. S. J., Mercieca-Bebber, R., Tesson, S., Seidler, Z., & Lopez, A.-L. (2019). Patient, client, consumer, survivor or other alternatives? A scoping review of preferred terms for labelling individuals who access healthcare across settings. *British Medical Journal Open, 9*(3). Available at https://bmjopen.bmj.com/content/9/3/e025166.

Crabtree, J. L. (1998). The end of occupational therapy. *American Journal of Occupational Therapy, 52*, 205–214.

Creek, J. (2003). *A Definition of Occupational Therapy as a Complex Intervention*. London: College of Occupational Therapists.

Creek, J. (2007). Engaging the reluctant client. In J. Creek, & A. Lawson-Porter (Eds.), *Contemporary Issues in Occupational Therapy* (pp. 127–142). Chichester: John Wiley & Sons.

Creek, J. (2010). *The Core Concepts of Occupational Therapy: A Dynamic Framework for Practice*. London: Jessica Kingsley.

Creek, J. (2014). The knowledge base of occupational therapy. In W. Bryant, J. Fieldhouse, & K. Bannigan (Eds.), *Creek's Occupational Therapy and Mental Health* (5th ed.). London: Elsevier.

Cutchin, M. P., Dickie, V. A., & Humphry, R. A. (2017). Foregrounding the transactional perspective's community orientation. *Journal of Occupational Science, 24*(4), 434–445.

Dickie, V., Cutchin, M. P., & Humphry, R. (2006). Occupation as transactional experience: A critique of individualism in occupational science. *Journal of Occupational Science, 13*(1), 83–93.

Durocher, E. (2017). Occupational justice: A fine balance for occupational therapists. In N. Pollard, & D. Sakalleriou (Eds.), *Occupational Therapies Without Borders* (2nd ed.). Oxford: Elsevier.

Faulkner, A. (2017). Survivor research and Mad Studies: The role and value of experiential knowledge in mental health research. *Disability & Society, 32*(4), 500–520.

Fish, D., & Boniface, G. (2012). Reconfiguring professional thinking and conduct: A challenge for occupational therapists in practice. In G. Boniface, & A. Seymour (Eds.), *Using Occupational Therapy Theory in Practice*. Chichester: Wiley-Blackwell.

Franco, L. (2013). The causes of one case of schizophrenia and its implications for other psychoses*Free Associations: Psychoanalysis and Culture, Media, Groups, Politics Number* (64). October.

Freire, P. (1970). *Pedagogy of the Oppressed*. London: Penguin Books.

Goodley, D. (2017). *Disability Studies: An Interdisciplinary Introduction* (2nd ed.). London: SAGE.

Grol, R. (2008). Knowledge transfer in mental health care: How do we bring evidence into day-to-day practice? *The Canadian Journal of Psychiatry, 53*(5), 275–276.

Hammell, K. W. (2015b). Occupational rights and critical occupational therapy: Rising to the challenge. *Australian Occupational Therapy Journal, 62*(6), 449–451.

Hasselkus, B. (2011). *The Meaning of Occupation* (2nd ed.). New Jersey: SLACK.

Health Foundation. (2016). *Person-Centred Care Made Simple: What Everyone Should Know About Person-Centred Care*. London: The Health Foundation.

Health Foundation. (2020). *Terms*. Available at https://www. mentalhealth.org.uk/a-to-z/t/terminology.

Held, D., & Recorded Books, I (2016). *Models of Democracy*. Cambridge: Polity.

Hitch, D., & Pepin, G. (2020). Doing, being, becoming and belonging at the heart of occupational therapy: An analysis of theoretical ways of knowing. *Scandinavian Journal of Occupational Therapy*. Available at https://doi:10.1080/1103812 8.2020.1726454.

Hitch, D., Pépin, G., & Stagnitti, K. (2014b). In the footsteps of Wilcock. Part Two. The interdependent nature of doing, being, becoming, and belonging. *Occupational Therapy in Health Care*, 28(3), 247–263.

Hitch, D., Pepin, G., & Stagnitti, K. (2018). The pan occupational paradigm: Development and key concepts. *Scandinavian Journal of Occupational Therapy*, 25(1), 27–34.

Hocking, C., & Mace, J. (2017). Occupational science informing practice for occupational justice. In N. Pollard, & D. Sakalleriou (Eds.), *Occupational Therapies Without Borders* (2nd ed.). Oxford: Elsevier.

Holahan, L. F. (2014). Quality-in-doing: Competence and occupation. *Journal of Occupational Science*, 21(4), 473–487. Available at https://doi:10.1080/14427591.2013.815683.

Hui, A., & Stickley, T. (2007). Mental health policy and mental health service user perspectives on involvement: A discourse analysis. *Journal of Advanced Nursing*, 59(4), 416–426.

Humanists, U. K. (2020). What makes something right or wrong? Animated video. Available at https://humanism.org.uk/thatshumanism/.

Iwajomo, T., Bondy, S. J., de Oliveira, C., Colton, P., Trottier, K., & Kurdyak, P. (2020). Excess mortality associated with eating disorders: Population-based cohort study. *The British Journal of Psychiatry*, 1-7. Available at https://doi:10.1192/bjp.2020.197.

Kenny, L., et al. (2016). Which terms should be used to describe autism? Perspectives from the UK autism community. *Autism*, 20(4), 442–462. Available at https://doi:10.1177/1362361315588200.

Khalil, H. (2016). AACPA knowledge translation and implementation science: What is the difference? *International Journal of Evidence-Based Healthcare*, June, 14(2), 39–40. Available at https://doi:10.1097/XEB.0000000000000086.

Kiepek, N. C., Beagan, B., Rudman, D. L., & Phelan, S. (2019). Silences around occupations framed as unhealthy, illegal, and deviant. *Journal of Occupational Science*, 26(3), 341–353. Available at https://doi:10.1080/14427591.2018.1499123.

Kinsella, E. A. (2009). Professional knowledge and the epistemology of reflective practice. *Nursing Philosophy: An International Journal for Healthcare Professionals*, 11(1), 3–14.

Lim, S. M., & Lim, H. B. (2016). Singapore's perspective on applied learning in occupational therapy: Beyond clinical practice education. *World Federation of Occupational Therapists Bulletin*, 72(1), 41–42.

Lindström, ., Sjöström, S., & Lindberg, M. (2013). Stories of rediscovering agency: Home-based occupational therapy for people with severe psychiatric disability. *Qualitative Health Research*, 23(6), 728–740. Jun.

Liu, F., Li, J., Wu, F., Zheng, H., Peng, Q., & Zhou, H. (2019). Altered composition and function of intestinal microbiota in autism spectrum disorders: A systematic review. *Translational Psychiatry*, 9(1), 1–13.

Magalhaes, L. (2012). What would Paulo Freire think of occupational science? In G. Whiteford, & C. Hocking (Eds.), *Occupational Science: Society, Inclusion, Participation*. Blackwell.

Marcolino, T. Q., Kinsella, E. A., Araujo, da S., et al. (2021). A community of practice of primary health care occupational therapists: Advancing practice-based knowledge. *Australian Occupational Therapy Journal*, 68(1), 3–11.

Maslow, A. H. (1943). A theory of human motivation. *Psychological Review*, 50(4), 370–396.

Max-Neef, M. (1991). *Human Scale Development: Conception, Application and Further Reflections*. New York: The Apex Press. Available at http://www.wtf.tw/ref/max-neef.pdf.

Mealing, C. (2021). Pots the Soldier Designed. Available at https://potsthesoldierdesigned.com/.

Mind. (2018). *Mental Health Act 1983*. Available at https://www.mind.org.uk/information-support/legal-rights/mental-health-act-1983/about-the-mha-1983/.

Morris, K., & Ward, K. (2018). The implementation of a new conceptual framework for occupational engagement in forensic settings: Feasibility and application to occupational therapy practice. *Mental Health Review Journal*, 23(4), 308–319.

Nelson, D. (1988). Occupation: form and performance. *American Journal of Occupational Therapy*, 42(10), 633–641.

Nelson, D. (1996). Therapeutic occupation: A definition. *American Journal of Occupational Therapy*, 50(10), 775–782.

Newport, A., & Clarke, C. (2020). The experiences of people with severe mental health conditions participating in the Occupation Matters Programme: An interpretative phenomenological analysis. *British Journal of Occupational Therapy*, 83(10), 620–630.

Nguyen, T. T., Kosciolek, T., Eyler, L. T., Knight, R., & Jeste, D. V. (2018). Overview and systematic review of studies of microbiome in schizophrenia and bipolar disorder. *Journal of Psychiatric Research*, 99, 50–61.

Nicholls, L., & Elliot, M. L. (2019). In the shadow of occupation: Racism, shame and grief. *Journal of Occupational Science*, 26(3), 354–365. Available at https://doihttps://doi:10.1080/14427591.2 018.1523021.

Paganizzi, L. (2017). Political activities in the classroom: Although difficult, change is possible. In N. Pollard, & D. Sakalleriou (Eds.), *Occupational Therapies Without Borders* (2nd ed.). Oxford: Elsevier.

Pentland, D., Kantartzis, S., Clausen, M. G., & Witemyre, K. (2018). *Occupational therapy and complexity: Defining and describing practice*. London: Royal College of Occupational Therapists.

Polanyi, M. (1966). *The Tacit dDimension*. Gloucester, MA: Peter Smith.

Purplepersuasion. (2018). Warehousing. Available at https://purplepersuasion.wordpress.com/2018/06/19/warehousing/.

Ramugondo, E. (2018). Healing work: Intersections for decoloniality. *World Federation of Occupational Therapists Bulletin*, 74(2), 83–91.

Ramugondo, E. L., & Kronenberg, F. (2015). Explaining collective occupations from a human relations perspective: Bridging the individual-collective dichotomy. *Journal of Occupational Science, 22*(1), 3–16.

Rule, R., & Twinley, R. (2020). Developing an occupational perspective of women involved in sex work: A discussion paper. *Journal of Occupational Science.* Available at https://doi:10.1080/14427591.2020.1739552.

Sakornsatian, S. (2009). Occupational therapy in post-conflict mental health in Thailand. *World Federation of Occupational Therapists Bulletin, 60*(1), 59–60.

Stevens, S. (2018). Ways of knowing and unknowing in psychotherapy and clinical practice. *Journal of Trauma and Treatment, 7*(1). Available at https://www.hilarispublisher.com/open-access/ways-of-knowing-and-unknowing-in-psychotherapy-and-clinical-practice-2167-1222-1000418.pdf.

Subramaniam, M., Abdin, E., Picco, L., et al. (2017). Continuum beliefs and stigmatising beliefs about mental illness: Results from an Asian community survey. *British Medical Journal Open, 7*(4). Available at https://bmjopen.bmj.com/content/7/4/e014993.

Thomas, Y., Gray, M. A., & McGinty, S. (2017). The occupational wellbeing of people experiencing homelessness. *Journal of Occupational Science, 24*(2), 181–192.

Tuan, Y. (1977). *Space and Place: The Perspective of Experience.* Minneapolis: University of Minnesota Press.

Twinley, R. (2013). The dark side of occupation: A concept for consideration. *Australian Occupational Therapy Journal, 60,* 301–303.

Twinley, R., & Morris, K. (2014). Are we achieving occupation-focused practice? *British Journal of Occupational Therapy, 77*(6), 275.

Whiteford, G., Klomp, N., Wright, -St, & Clair, V. (2005). Complexity theory: Understanding occupation, practice and context. In G. Whiteford, & V. Wright-St Clair (Eds.), *Occupation and Practice in Context* (pp. 3–15). Sydney: Elsevier.

Whiteford, G., Jones, K., Weekes, G., et al. (2020). Combatting occupational deprivation and advancing occupational justice in institutional settings: Using a practice-based enquiry approach for service transformation. *British Journal of Occupational Therapy, 83*(1), 52–61.

Wilcock, A. (1993). A theory of the human need for occupation. *Journal of Occupational Science, 1*(1), 17–24.

Wilcock, A. (1998). Occupation for health. *British Journal of Occupational Therapy, 61*(8), 340–345.

Wilcock, A. (1999). Reflections on doing, being and becoming. *Australian Occupational Therapy Journal, 46*(1), 1–11.

Wilcock, A. (2006). *An Occupational Perspective of Health* (2nd ed.). Thorofare, NJ: SLACK.

Wilcock, A., & Townsend, E. (2000). Occupational terminology interactive dialogue. *Journal of Occupational Science, 7*(2), 84–86.

Wilcock, A., & Townsend, E. A. (2014). Occupational justice. In B. A. Boyt Schell, G. Gillen, & M. Scaffa (Eds.), *Willard and Spackman's Occupational Therapy* (12th ed) (pp. 541–552). Philadelphia: Lippincott Williams & Wilkins.

World Federation of Occupational Therapists (WFOT). (2019). *Position Statement. Occupational therapy and human rights (revised).* Available at https://wfot.org/resources/occupational-therapy-and-human-rights.

World Health Organisation. (2016). *International Statistical Classification of Diseases and Related Health Problems, 10th Revision (ICD-10).* Available at https://icd.who.int/browse10/2016/en#/F30-F39.

Zemke, R., & Clarke, F. (1996). *Occupational Science: The Evolving Discipline.* Philadelphia: F. A. Davis.

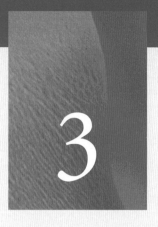

3

BEING A THERAPIST

WENDY BRYANT ■ NICOLA PLASTOW

CHAPTER OUTLINE

INTRODUCTION

Being an occupational therapist requires a person to think and act in particular ways. In this chapter, therapy in general is defined before exploring what is involved in these ways of thinking and acting in occupational therapy to address mental health problems. Those with expert knowledge in particular practices and processes could be understood as technologists and technicians, contrasted by Creek (2007) with a thinking therapist who 'does not see herself as an expert in her client's life, but recognizes that the client is the expert in his own life' (p. 12). Thoughtfulness, as a way of being a thinking therapist, can be described as three different things (Collins English Dictionary 2020). It might involve being quiet and serious; being kind and thinking carefully about other people before acting or thinking something through very carefully to inform what happens next. Being thoughtful prepares

the occupational therapist for sharing knowledge and understanding of people, their occupations and the context or environment of therapy.

Having defined therapy, the various aspects of being a therapist are explored, starting with reflection and professional reasoning. Students and occupational therapists in a new role actively consider each aspect of their practice before acting. When familiar with the setting, being a therapist becomes more automatic and part of professional identity. The varied ways of being a therapist are explored in a section on therapeutic use of self. Reflection, professional reasoning and therapeutic use of self mean that occupational therapy has been identified as a job least likely to be replaced by robots or artificial intelligence. This is because practice is as much an art as a science, a quality known as professional artistry. Recognizing the complexity of their practice, occupational therapists bring together

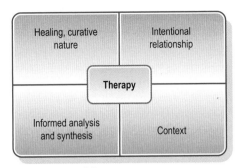

Fig. 3.1 ■ Features of therapy.

the various aspects of being a therapist, applying their knowledge and improvising approaches to ensure the therapy is relevant.

Defining Therapy

Therapy is defined as a specific intervention for a health problem (Collins English Dictionary 2020). Seeing a therapist to address mental health problems is often associated with fields such as psychotherapy in which talking therapies are used in contrast with drug treatment (Collins English Dictionary 2020). However, prescribed drugs are also therapy in medical terms. For an experience to be therapeutic, it simply has to have healing or curative intentions (Online Etymology Dictionary 2021). This healing feature of therapy along with three other features are shown in Fig. 3.1.

Healing processes and benefits are associated with spirituality by many people, because of their powerful transformative effects on life. The power to transform through healing or curing a health problem is also associated with medicine, sharing with occupational therapy the process of carefully identifying the problem before acting (see Chapter 4). Another important aspect of healing is the avoidance of harm (see Chapter 9).

Intentional relationship distinguishes a therapeutic relationship from others, signalling a formal agreement to address people's problems in a way that is beneficial to them (Taylor and VanPuymbrouck 2013) (see Chapters 7 and 9). This agreement could suggest a risk of paternalism but requires mutual trust to be effective.

Informed analysis and synthesis of the therapeutic media (occupations, words, behaviours or drugs) guides prediction about outcomes and, therefore, how therapeutic media are used in addressing the problem(s). For occupational therapists this means analysing, adapting and synthesizing occupations to create graded steps in performance and engagement (Creek 2014; see Chapter 6). A person receiving help for mental health problems might also experience analysis and synthesis of what they say in talking therapies and analysis of their response to medication to identify effectiveness and side effects.

Context describes the relationships between environment, people and events that influence the meanings of what people do (Creek 2010). For example, occupational therapy usually occurs in sessions with specific interventions. A mental health service has many different aspects, and not all of them have therapeutic purposes. For example, security concerns to keep people safe or other organizational priorities may require a pragmatic approach to therapy, influencing what can be done, who with, when and where (see Chapters 10, 21 and 26).

Being a therapist means simultaneously being aware of, thinking about, acting on and responding to the four different features of therapy shown in Fig. 3.1. There are recognized approaches to managing this, using the practices described in this chapter. However, some implications of being a therapist have been subject to recent discussions, as described in Box 3.1.

REFLECTIVE PRACTICE

To engage in reflective practice is to create space for thinking, as if taking more than a brief glance in a mirror when washing your hands (John 2017). Where reflection is encouraged, it can be empowering, challenging and enabling of deep learning. If a therapist stops learning from reflections, then their practice could become inflexible, undeveloped and possibly harmful. Reflection has been identified as a way of increasing awareness of diversity (Taff and Blash 2017) and, when part of collaborative learning (Noon 2018), an effective alternative to unconscious bias training sessions. Reflective practice is important for actively making links between knowledge and action in everyday practice, described by Schön (1983, p. 42) as a 'swampy lowland' where it is often hard to see a clear path ahead and each step benefits from careful consideration (Wong et al. 2016).

The World Federation of Occupational Therapists (WFOT 2016, p. 71) describes reflection as

At the 2018 World Federation of Occupational Therapists congress, a debate took place to examine whether being therapists, as opposed to workers or practitioners, was limiting occupational therapists' development (Sinclair 2018). Debating the therapeutic nature of occupational therapy helps build an understanding of what it currently means to be a professional at a time when there are wider challenges to professional claims of privilege, whether in knowledge, power and/or status (see Chapter 7). These challenges arise from people's perceptions of the potentially harmful nature of power, gained from professional knowledge, overshadowing the beneficial aspects of professional services. While access to knowledge has been transformed by the information technology revolution, access to power in terms of status and pay has not, leading some occupational therapists to question what is different about a professional.

This debate was shaped by understandings of the term 'therapy,' which are broadly suggested in Fig. 3.1 and influenced by Fisher's (2014, p. 98) core principles for occupation-centred therapy (see Chapter 2):

1) People are occupational beings;
2) Occupational challenges impact people's lives;
3) Occupation is powerful as a therapeutic change-producing agent.

Therapy for mental health problems takes on a particular focus when based on these principles. Working around Fig. 3.1, healing is suggested by therapeutic change, with benefits rather than harms and clearly focused on the challenges in life that arise from mental health problems. This focus confronts stigma and discrimination. The intentional relationship is expressed through occupation, with people preparing and engaging in doing things together in therapy, especially in groups (see Chapter 15). Analysis and synthesis involve attending to people as occupational beings, as well as the occupations that occur in therapy. The power of therapeutic occupation is enabled and restricted by the contexts, not just because others might not appreciate its beneficial power but because they might also perceive its potential to do harm in the wrong hands. In Chapter 1 this historical tension is discussed in relation to the use of work as therapy in asylums.

'systematically, routinely and critically thinking about your practice, to maximize learning from experience.' Learning from experience can be challenging; as if looking closely in a mirror to examine flaws in your appearance, as well as your attractive features. Reflection can reveal shortcomings as well as what is pleasing

and satisfying (Craig-Duchesne et al. 2018). Unexpected and unfamiliar situations require immediate and ongoing reflection, known as reflection-in-action (Priddis and Rogers 2018). One of the lay meanings of reflection is that a person's situation and/or their attitude shows in how they do things and relate to others (Collins English Dictionary 2020). A very anxious person may be extremely aware of how others react to them, making it important in therapy that an occupational therapist is immediately responsive, as well as reflecting later. The occupational therapist could take more time to listen to the person and reflect on what the person says, carefully considering how to respond in the moment.

Another way of understanding reflection emphasizes deep consideration after the event (reflection-on-action) (Priddis and Rogers 2018). Occupational therapists are encouraged to reflect on their experiences, draw conclusions and possibly decide to gain more relevant experience or knowledge (Wong et al. 2016). This is often the main purpose of reflection. However, it is also helpful to consider the nature of reflection and to foster it in practice: when people are quiet and thoughtful, reflection could be taking place. Wong et al. (2016) suggest that the challenge of reflection is to find the problem rather than to solve it. Group or team supervision can create space for shared reflections when the supervisor has relevant experience but is not in a position of power, as fear of being judged will affect the authenticity of reflections (Wong et al. 2016; Priddis and Rogers 2018). This power balance is particularly important for reflecting on incidents such as the suicide of a service user. The team's reflections are carefully facilitated before any decisions are made about future practice, if required.

Critical Reflection and Reflexivity

Critical reflection on assumptions, biases, and prejudices can enable personal and professional development. To critically reflect is not to focus on all the negatives of a situation but to open up to different ways of seeing, taking in issues of power and details of the context that are crucial in certain situations, such as when a person has not attended an appointment with a community team (Bassot 2016). Bailliard et al. (2020) suggest that occupational therapists critically reflecting together should consider that there is more scope for change if people from diverse perspectives are included. When mental health service users work with occupational therapists on service development and research, collaborative critical reflection can benefit the process and outcomes (Honey et al. 2019).

The term 'reflexivity' is also used to describe critical reflection. Originating in qualitative research in which it is essential to engage with multiple understandings of data, reflexivity has relevance to professional practice, describing 'how we think, feel and act and the assumptions we might be making' (Bassot 2016, p. 130). For example, Hammell (2019) highlights the importance of critically reflecting on the theories used by occupational therapists, which are often dominated by particular worldviews. Reflexivity extends reflection deeper into what lies behind a situation. Returning to the example of a person who did not attend an appointment, by questioning the grounds for this and the structured professional knowledge for understanding it, the therapist can find fresh insights into how to respond.

Recording and Sharing Reflections

Occupational therapists are required to engage in reflective practice and demonstrate their continuing professional development by recording and sharing their reflections for supervision and for their own records (Knightbridge 2019). Where as reflections are required to demonstrate continuing professional development, reflective models and frameworks are often used to structure and prompt reflections (Boud and Walker 1998; Wong et al. 2016; Knightbridge 2019). Reflective journals have been found to be effective as a basis for discussion in supervision (Craig-Duchesne et al. 2018). Not all occupational therapists keep reflective journals but Knightbridge (2019) suggested that reflection is increasingly valued with more experience in practice. At the end of a group session, reflection could involve the therapist and colleagues sifting through many experiences from the session and others in the past, allowing thoughts to weave around these experiences with perhaps one or two emerging as particularly important. Or it could be that something very striking happened in the group, focusing the shared reflections. It is not always obvious why a particular situation provokes reflection, so reflecting is sometimes a stage before analysis of professional reasoning, which is discussed next.

PROFESSIONAL REASONING

Reasoning is defined as 'the act or process of drawing conclusions from facts, evidence, etc.' (Collins English Dictionary 2020). It is necessary for the therapist to be able to explain and justify actions and decisions in different ways at different times, and these explanations should make sense in relation to:

- the person receiving occupational therapy;
- the setting;
- the information and evidence available from multiple sources, including observations and guidelines.

Reasoning involves different thinking skills, including 'applying rules, choosing, conceptualizing, evaluating, judging, justifying, knowing, perceiving and understanding' (Creek 2007, p. 9). It is like information processing in some ways (Marquez-Alvarez et al. 2019), but this frame of reference does not capture elements of reasoning such as 'intuition, embodiment, worldview and reflection,' described by Unsworth and Baker (2016, p. 10). The term 'professional reasoning' has replaced clinical reasoning because occupational therapy occurs in many places other than a clinical setting and engages with broader considerations beyond the person and their immediate presenting problem (Cole and Creek 2016).

Modes of Reasoning

Scholarly, professional dialogues about reasoning in occupational therapy began with Mattingly and Fleming (1994), who suggested that an occupational therapist's thoughts shift continuously between different modes. They used the term 'three-track reasoning' based on their mixed method research. The three different tracks or modes of reasoning are **procedural, interactive** and **conditional,** with narrative reasoning flowing through all three. Other modes have been described since (Coles and Creek 2016; Unsworth and Baker 2016; Marquez-Alvarez et al. 2019), suggesting different ways of reasoning. Naming modes can help experienced therapists explain their reasoning for others because, in practice, seamless switching between modes can make it difficult for them to identify and explain their reasoning.

Some modes of reasoning are briefly explained here, drawing on Mattingly and Fleming (1994) and Schell and Schell (2008). This explanation is illustrated with an example of a therapist, Mo, preparing to end her work with Hal, a person living with long-term mental health problems in the community. The reason for ending is that Mo is leaving to go and work elsewhere. The salient aspects of the situation are that Mo knows Hal well, the end of the therapeutic relationship is being planned and it is acknowledged that both feel sadness about this.

Procedural reasoning means thinking about guidelines, policies and agreed ways of doing things. This includes how to end the therapeutic relationship; for example, when to tell Hal that therapy is coming to an end. Usually this is done well before the last session, so there are opportunities for Hal to respond and discuss thoughts and feelings.

Interactive reasoning means drawing on the therapeutic relationship to think about the particular needs of the person or people receiving therapy. Mo and Hal think about how to say goodbye, depending on their way of working or interacting together. They might plan a final session together, or Mo may remind Hal that this is the last session.

Conditional reasoning means thinking about the wider context for occupational therapy. Conditional reasoning about how to end occupational therapy is shaped by several factors: Hal's situation, health issues and future (being offered occupational therapy from someone else or preparing to build new relationships with other mental health workers); Mo's situation (Mo may be moving away to another location and have many things to consider) and the conditions in which they are working together (some aspects of the service may stop with Mo's absence).

Narrative reasoning means thinking about the threads between this situation and others, using the idea of plot and actions. This might be the final chapter in the story of the therapeutic relationship between Hal and Mo but the beginning of new narratives for each of them. At the same time, there are ongoing narratives for Hal and his health problems and for Mo and her career and for the wider context with arrival of new staff who may have less or different prior experience.

Pragmatic reasoning means thinking about the practical aspects of occupational therapy that constitute resources and restrictions. Therapy sessions may have taken place in a particular room which is not always available, so the timing or occupational focus of the final sessions might have to be negotiated carefully to maintain continuity and ensure that therapeutic activities are finished.

Scientific reasoning means thinking systematically about a situation, using theories and evidence to understand its possible meanings. If Hal expresses anxiety about therapy coming to an end, Mo could draw on knowledge about relationships, such as attachment theory (Daniel 2013), and about anxiety, such as the stress response.

Deductive or diagnostic reasoning is a similar process to scientific reasoning but is aimed at reaching a conclusion, like a detective identifying who committed a crime by making deductions from clues. If Mo has anxiety about therapy coming to an end, discussing this in supervision is an opportunity to identify the causes. The anxiety may arise from cues coming from Hal, such as a tense facial expression, or Mo might be engaging in catastrophic thinking, predicting that Hal's situation will get worse without occupational therapy.

Ethical reasoning is informed by many factors, including codes of ethics, as discussed in Chapter 9. Mo might have to respond to a request from Hal to stay in touch using social media, considering the reasons for refusing the request and sharing them thoughtfully with Hal.

These eight modes of reasoning, like Mattingly and Fleming's three tracks, run in parallel, with Mo switching between them as the situation unfolds. If Hal brought a gift for Mo at the final session, several different modes of reasoning would be involved. Receiving gifts requires ethical reasoning: for example, if Hal offered Mo money, Mo would have to ensure Hal was aware of its value and refuse the gift to avoid exploiting Hal's potentially vulnerable situation. If the gift was small, like some flowers, interactive reasoning would help Mo think about how to respond in the context of this specific therapeutic relationship. Procedural reasoning would influence how Mo decided what to do with the gift, probably following employer guidelines. Pragmatic reasoning would also influence this decision; for example, if the gift was fruit that could be shared, it would be most practical to do this before the fruit perished. Acknowledging the gift might open up an opportunity to think about the occupational therapy as a reciprocal gift in the broader context of Hal's life, a form of narrative reasoning.

Many decisions in mental health services are made collaboratively by multidisciplinary teams. In the example used above in which occupational therapy is ending, it is likely that there are other people affected by this, as well as Hal. Team decisions will be focused on ensuring that ongoing support is available to those who need it. Mo could use interactive and conditional reasoning to think about specific individuals and to consider their future condition and needs.

Reasoning and Language

Creek (2016) pointed out the importance of language in reasoning and communicating, ensuring that what is thought, said and written matches the modes of reasoning: 'sometimes, changing the words we use to describe a situation can change how we see it and indicate alternative strategies' (p. 20). For example, Filippidou et al. (2014) investigated why people did not attend their appointments with community mental health teams, discovering that many had simply forgotten. Some team members had used interactive reasoning to draw conclusions about the therapeutic relationship whereas a more effective solution was to implement new procedures such as text reminders. One technique to explore professional reasoning is think-aloud, where the therapist speaks their thoughts out loud as they occur (Unsworth and Baker 2016). Recording, transcribing and analysing these thoughts can reveal the language used, the modes of reasoning and underlying assumptions (Creek 2016).

Novice and Expert Differences

Professional reasoning is learned and changes as expertise grows. Cartensen and Bonsaksen (2017) identified how this learning influenced the practice of novice and expert therapists, with collaborating and empathizing being more characteristic of the experienced occupational therapists. In contrast, students tended to prefer advocating or instructing. Experts and novices can learn from each other, using different approaches to suit the situation rather than following personal preferences. Differences between the reasoning styles of novice and expert are illustrated in the example in Box 3.2.

PROFESSIONAL IDENTITY

Being a therapist is an aspect of personal and social identity, which is a 'composite sense of self' (Plastow

BOX 3.2
NOVICES AND EXPERTS AT WORK

To understand how expertise influences reasoning, think of a complex building which is familiar to you; somewhere like a place of work, education or possibly a railway station. With regular journeys through the building it is easy to find your way without thinking about it. You can greet people you recognize, make diversions to avoid delays and think about something else other than your journey or your destination. But on your first visit to that building you may have noticed everything, including details like signs on doors that are not relevant to your journey or your destination. To avoid getting overwhelmed, distracted or lost, you had to concentrate hard on where you were going and what you were doing when you got there.

This is the difference between being a novice and being an expert. As a novice every new piece of information has to be filtered with constant reference to the principles that you have learned. This means reasoning is a slow but thorough process. As expertise grows there is a danger that relevant sources of information will be overlooked because they seem familiar and can therefore be disregarded. However, situations can also be appraised more efficiently because of their familiarity. Your depth of knowledge, and experience enables you to have a greater sense of the whole situation. Being an expert means that you might find it difficult to explain what you have done and why, because it was so automatic and your knowledge is now tacit. It is helpful to identify the areas of practice in which you have expertise to contrast with other areas in which you may feel like a novice, but know that more can be learned through experience.

et al. 2015, p. 668) acquired from experiences of engaging in occupation, as well as views of the self, self-concept and self-esteem (Christiansen 1999). For each occupational therapist, there will be many other social and occupational identities, such as cook, parent, sports player, sibling and/or gardener. A strong professional identity can be experienced when practice is consistent with the beliefs and values of the profession (Scanlan and Hazelton 2019; see Chapters 2 and 4). The way occupational therapists think and act is therefore central to professional identity.

During professional life many shifts in identity are experienced, such as when developing from a novice to an expert (see Box 3.2) or taking on new roles as community activist, advocate, manager, teacher or researcher. While developing new ways of being a therapist it is helpful to keep a stable and consistent sense of the composite self over time, a process known as identity maintenance (Plastow et al. 2015). The simultaneous processes of identity maintenance and development are complex (see sections on complexity in this chapter and Chapters 2 and 4).

Reflecting on what is not part of a professional role is part of identity maintenance (Binyamin 2021). Reflection could be helpful in situations such as service restructuring, where a job no longer feels like occupational therapy, the death (particularly suicide) of a service user being unable to provide occupational therapy to family and friends or exhaustion due to the pressures of service delivery. Challenges specific to mental health settings include the dominance of biomedical and psychological approaches (Devery et al. 2018) and disagreements with service leaders about the specialist nature of occupational therapy in generic settings (Horghagen et al. 2020). These challenges could change practice, further threatening professional identity. There are particular challenges for pre-registration occupational therapy students as they begin to develop their professional identity (see Chapter 11). Box 3.3 suggests examples of these challenges, which could be addressed with five strategies (Binyamin 2021). In addition, professional identity can be strengthened through effective team-working (Abendstern et al. 2017), occupation-centred practice (see Chapter 2) and developing ways of being a therapist as described elsewhere in this chapter, such as therapeutic use of self.

THERAPEUTIC USE OF SELF

Another focus for being a therapist is how to be with people. Evetts and Peloquin (2017) contrast therapeutic use of self with an individual reading a self-help book. Instead of reading the book alone, the individual works with the occupational therapist to influence what is happening, with both adapting responses to each other. For the therapist, developing therapeutic responses and thinking skills are integral parts of professional growth. The term 'therapeutic use of self' refers to how therapists work to ensure the shared experience is beneficial rather than harmful. They use their self-awareness, empathy, communication skills and reasoning to facilitate shifts in what is happening and exploring what those shifts mean

(Arntzen 2018). Therapists work verbally and non-verbally, exploring and holding what is being brought to therapy (Nicholls 2013). Like a dance, there are rhythms (or not), gestures, movements and mutual cooperation (or not).

When a person is in a crisis, the therapist can often be acutely aware of therapeutic use of self as different understandings and possible actions are explored. A mental health service user group, Recovery in the Bin (RitB), has summarized unhelpful examples, such as suggesting a person has a cup of tea, which could be appropriate but will rarely be sufficient to resolve the crisis (RitB 2017). They give other examples, which reflect experiences of crisis teams, although any setting could involve distressing and disorientating experiences. For the therapist, there are potential conflicts between being professional and being an individual who needs to monitor personal vulnerabilities and emotions (McAllister et al. 2019). Therapeutic use of self is an essential aspect of practice for managing these conflicts, achieving the best outcomes and modeling appropriate responses to others present (Mavindidze et al. 2019). In group work there are particular challenges for the therapist, which are discussed further in Chapter 15.

Good Intentions

To learn about therapeutic use of self, a therapist starts by exploring different ways of being; this exploration helps increase awareness of personal preferences. For example, the self-care activities occupational therapists recommend will be shaped by preferences from their personal experience. From a service user perspective, Edge (2019) says that watching survival films is her preferred activity for managing stress, rather than alternatives such as burning scented candles, having a bath or walking outside in a natural environment. After discussing possible activities, the occupational therapist could give practical support to watch a film. For example, if the person is in hospital, taking time to discuss the choice of film, planning how to obtain it and view it and negotiating access to the necessary equipment or devices with ward staff. The experience of exploring stress-reducing activities together involve different ways of responding, in contrast to simply advising a person to take a bath.

BOX 3.3

FIVE STRATEGIES FOR STRENGTHENING PROFESSIONAL IDENTITY

Binyamin (2021) studied the development of professional identity with occupational therapy students in Israel using a cognitive model. Focusing on situations where professional identity was threatened by dilemmas in therapeutic and working relationships, five strategies were identified, as shown below.

Overarching goal: When interactions appear personal and intrusive, professional identity can be reinforced in a helpful way by noticing what is happening and using it as a starting point to refocus on the goal of a session. For example, in a group session on using community resources, when a person asks the occupational therapy staff where they live, this could be widened to a group discussion about their knowledge of the local area.

Facts vs. interpretations: Situations are often interpreted before the facts are fully appreciated. Developing awareness of multiple perspectives through reflection can strengthen professional identity. For example, if a session is routinely interrupted by nurse colleagues, it could be because it is happening at the same time as a doctor's review, rather than constituting an attempt to undermine occupational therapy.

What is the person trying to tell me? Novice therapists are often focused on progressing a session. A service user may be seen as resistant if their response disrupts the plans for the session. To shift from feelings such as resentment to taking responsibility as a professional, interactive reasoning can inform adaptation of the session. Observing and listening carefully then sharing reflections can help slowly open up new possibilities for action.

Dialogue between inner voices: When situations get stuck, considering what is happening in deeper terms can increase the empathy and effectiveness of the therapist. Professional artistry brings together different ways of being a therapist in this process. A person who is feeling very paranoid may be absorbed with fear, which can make an occupational therapist feel like they cannot get through. Attending to how feelings are shaping and being shaped by inner dialogues can help a therapist start to connect.

Having, doing and being: Conflicts between personal and professional identities can be addressed with awareness of the salient identity in a situation, considering how what we have (experiences, tools, ideas, knowledge) and who we are (being) shape what we do. Being aware of how multiple identities, such as race, class and gender, shape who we are is also a feature of intersectionality (see Chapter 12).

Binyamin 2021

The intentional relationship model identifies different ways of being a therapist (Taylor and Vanpuymbrouck 2013), recognizing that being continuously aware of therapeutic intentions directs the therapist's choices for thinking and acting. This can transform the therapeutic relationship and everyday experiences for people receiving occupational therapy.

Challenges to Good Intentions

Therapeutic relationships are characterized by good intentions to facilitate change and transform lives (Townsend 1998). However, many challenges to good intentions occur, ranging from a disruption in a therapy session to broader contextual issues (see Chapters 4, 6 and 10). For example, an occupational therapist might have to respond to personal and possibly intrusive questions: managing self-disclosure appropriately requires self-awareness, empathy and reflexivity. In clinical settings it is usually recommended that personal information is not disclosed to service users so that the focus stays on their issues. However, self-disclosure can be the basis for successful peer mentorship, with peer workers learning how to disclose personal information appropriately and safely as part of their therapeutic use of self (Schwartz et al. 2020). Personal information is easily accessible in an online environment and could be brought into a therapeutic relationship. In response, occupational therapists can find themselves managing feelings such as surprise and anger, recognizing the potential for shame and avoidance (Dixon et al. 2020) and helping people learn the same skills.

Feelings about disclosure and shame are particularly significant when working within a psychoanalytical frame of reference, as its language of relationships, boundaries and containment can enhance the therapist's understanding of therapeutic use of self. Nicholls (2013) suggests that good intentions can come unstuck when 'the client may be either unwilling or unable to tell us what concerns them, and for our own inner reasons, we may not be able to hear them or respond with sensitivity and/or an acknowledgement of their hurt or shame' (Nicholls 2013, p. 20). If the occupational therapist does not seem to hear what a person is saying, this could be interpreted as reluctance to take on board or contain what is important to that person. Taking notice of difficult feelings and communications might raise two questions:

- To what extent do the difficult feelings belong to the therapist or to the person?
- Would it help the relationship to give voice to the feelings to clarify what is happening?

These questions could be considered during the interaction or on subsequent reflection. Engaging with these feelings within the session will help the person feel they are being heard and avoid the situation where 'all the while, [staff were] keeping genuine conversations about patients' experiences at bay' (RitB 2019).

Embodiment and Intersubjectivity

Arntzen (2018) observed that discussions about occupational therapy tend to centre on professional reasoning, the experiences the person shares with the therapist and the therapist's actions. Two further aspects are overlooked, which she described as embodiment and intersubjectivity. **Embodiment** is defined as 'my body as I experience it,' combining the physical body and our self-awareness (Arntzen 2018, p. 174). For example, liv1204 (Fighting to Liv 2019) describes her experiences of trying to avoid self-harm:

> 'I am calmer when I have something in my hand to hold and focus on... I was restrained by two officers when I tried to harm myself. An officer placed a bouncy ball in each of my hands and told me to squeeze, to focus on holding on. It meant I couldn't harm myself, and it relaxed me enough that they were able to stop restraining me'
>
> *Fighting to Liv 2019*

Self-harm reveals the strong connection and distinction between the physical body and the body we live in when one turns against the other. Holding the balls physically stopped liv1204 (Fighting to Liv 2019) and changed how she was living in her body.

Intersubjectivity refers to the shared intentions and meaning-making of everyone in occupational therapy sessions (Arntzen 2018). People might be asked to share experiences of occupation or complete a standardized assessment to elicit intentions and meanings. However, these can also be revealed by the therapist paying more attention and responding to what is happening during the session. The example from liv1204 (Fighting to Liv 2019) shows how the officer responded non-verbally by giving her two balls to hold. Simple instructions shifted the situation from being a crisis to a different way of engaging. These actions were intersubjective, being shared between the officer and liv1204. The shared actions involved a gesture and minimal verbal communication that changed the interaction from one of conflict and restraint to a shared intention to protect from harm.

Like Mattingly and Fleming (1994) conceptualizing occupational therapy as a two-body practice (see next section), Arntzen (2018) suggests that the body is ambiguous, with multiple ways of being that can be contradictory. Each of us might know what we are capable of, but we are not always able to realize our full capabilities. Understanding this ambiguity is important for occupational therapy. For example, a service user researcher suggested that attending a book group was helpful because:

> 'You don't have to read if you don't want to. You can just listen if you want. You don't have to speak and that was helpful as well, because at first I wasn't in my right state of mind. But as the weeks continued, I began to feel better and contribute more.'
>
> *Bryant et al. 2015 p. 19.*

It might seem contradictory to include people in a book group who do not participate in reading, apparently undermining the group's purpose. However, the purpose of the group was not only to share the experience of reading a book, but also to facilitate changes in how people participated. In explaining the group to potential participants, the occupational therapy staff were careful to ensure this dual purpose was understood.

Two-Body Practice: Pragmatism and Structuralism

Another way of understanding how to be a therapist is the idea of two-body practice, which originated with anthropologist Cheryl Mattingly. She observed therapists switching between two inter-related ways of knowing a person (Mattingly and Fleming 1994):

- As a living body, moving flexibly between different ways of knowing as the situation changes, which requires pragmatic thinking;
- As a machine, applying general rules to everyone, which requires structuralist understanding.

Pragmatic reasoning has already been discussed, as one of the different modes of professional reasoning. Mattingly and Fleming (1994) also identified a distinction between theoretical reasoning and clinical reasoning, which in some ways mirrors pragmatism and structuralism. However, two-body practice goes beyond reasoning, recognizing the embodied nature of occupational therapy (Arntzen 2019). For example, enabling people to participate in community sport could be a pragmatic decision by the occupational therapists to encourage physical activity with people in a small group in a leisure centre while working on their shared and individual challenges. At the same time the therapists could use structured knowledge of diagnosis, occupational injustice and the rules and culture of sport (Bullen and Clarke 2021).

Pragmatism means 'thinking of or dealing with problems in a practical way, rather than by using theory or abstract principles' (Collins English Dictionary 2020). Occupational therapists are being pragmatic when they are flexible, using the best available knowledge for a situation. However, if widely agreed principles are ignored, pragmatism risks becoming unethical, which is why structures for practice are established (Chapter 4) (Machan 2013). Pragmatism is integral to professional artistry (Schon 1983; see next section). For example, Daryl, an occupational therapist, is an accomplished actor; Kendra, a dramatherapist, works in the same service and needs a cotherapist. Daryl decides it is practical to take up the role. Together Kendra and Daryl develop effective and creative approaches, drawing on their shared understandings of performance in drama and therapy. However, each therapist also draws on their specific professional knowledge so that the group participants and the service benefit from both occupational therapy and dramatherapy. The scope of the situation is used while maintaining boundaries.

Pragmatism grows with experience, which makes practice difficult to fully explain at times. For example, placement educators may find it hard to explain to a student exactly how they build rapport with a person. There is often more scope to practice than initially appears to be the case. Only experience will enable the student to understand this (see Chapter 11). This is because pragmatism often relies on tacit knowledge, originally described by Polanyi (1966) as the knowledge we know so well that we are unaware of it.

Structuralism is based on the belief that there are underlying structures that can be unearthed and described, offering knowledge that can be widely applied (Hooper and Wood 2002). For example, when working with a person on managing anxiety, occupational therapists could draw on knowledge of the stress response and mindfulness techniques. One weakness of structuralism, however, is that it largely ignores context. The person receiving occupational therapy could be supported to learn this structural knowledge, but pragmatism is required to work out with the therapist how to apply it.

These two ways of understanding the scope of occupational therapy can conflict with each other (Creek 2010). Hooper and Wood (2002) suggest that the tension between pragmatism and structuralism underlies the enduring challenge of explaining occupational therapy. The ability to shift between pragmatism and structuralism characterizes two-body practice (Mattingly and Fleming 1994). For example, a person might be keen to start paid employment, but the occupational therapist might suggest attending community gardening sessions as a first step to develop work habits (see Chapter 20). This suggestion could be pragmatic, as the community gardening group is local and easily accessible, it is the busy season and the person could start straight away. Structuralist knowledge could also be used, as all activities can be analysed to facilitate a graded process of skill acquisition and there is evidence of effectiveness for the service in developing volunteers' pre-vocational skills (see Chapters 6 and 20). The occupational therapist could explain these suggestions to the person and the team, indicating the underlying assumptions and contextual understandings (Hooper and Wood 2002).

Therapeutic use of self, professional reasoning and reflection combine as elements of everyday occupational therapy practice, often unseen and unacknowledged. It is possible to learn these different elements step by step, as if working through a checklist. As professional artistry is developed, the different elements become familiar, both separately and in combination. Like moving from an outline drawing to mixed media artwork, professional artistry offers another way of understanding the complexity of practice.

PROFESSIONAL ARTISTRY

The concept of professional artistry was developed by Fish and Coles (1998) who saw the usefulness of contrasting artistry with technical and rational approaches to practice. They used the language of art to frame professional practice in health and education, echoed by medical humanities (Lake et al. 2015). Continuing professional development can be understood as learning professional artistry, using 'props and scaffolding to help the novice grow' (Dix 2010).

Definition

Professional artistry is a creative approach which synthesizes judgements, autonomy, reflection, risk monitoring and working with complex factors beyond the principles of practice (Fish and Coles 1998; Kinsella 2009; Wimpenny et al. 2014). Emphasizing artistic forms rather than scientific components, metaphors are used to express understandings of being a therapist (Pentland et al. 2018). For example, a student participant in Bazyk's et al.s study (2009, p. 182) described a moment of understanding:

> 'There really aren't words to describe the way it all made me feel, but I got goose bumps at one point during our session. All that talk about group process finally makes sense to me.'

Using metaphors such as 'goose bumps' brings artful aspects of practice to life. Drawing on reflections and experiences, professional artistry is evident when occupational therapy progresses in apparently effortless and mysterious ways.

In Box 3.4, there is an example of artful practice from a user perspective. A closer look at the story could suggest that the occupational therapist synthesised person-centred practice (see chapter 4), occupation-centred practice (see chapter 2), therapeutic use of self, embodiment and intersubjectivity. Returning to the story again at another time might reveal other aspects of occupational therapy.

Learning how to practice in this way can take time, but professional artistry is not restricted to people who have many years of experience. Bazyk et al. (2009) explored the development of artful practice on role-emerging placements, with student participants describing how understanding 'just clicked' (p. 184), enabling them to appreciate the wider context for their work. Often, this understanding developed after difficult experiences.

Origins

Kinsella (2009) traced how Dewey, an American pragmatist philosopher of education, found that artistry in everyday practice was associated with experiences of uncertainty. Schön (1983), who was influenced by Dewey, criticized technical and rational approaches, which focused practice on solving defined problems rather than exploring the unknown. Schön was the first to use the term professional artistry, describing it as 'improvization, thinking on your feet, pragmatism' (Smith 2001, 2011).

Using the Language of Art

Fish and Coles (1998) explored the language of art, finding how translating life experiences into art forms such as songs or paintings could bring previously overlooked aspects to attention. For example, the word 'performance' is associated with both the arts and occupational therapy. Lake et al. (2015) suggested that practice can be seen as a series of performances, with the 'patient as an audience member' (p. 769) bringing a new perspective to person-centred practice. Imagine Olivia (Box 3.4) in a theatre audience carefully observing Rachel's response to the revelation of suicidal feelings (Box 3.4). A live audience's response transforms the play, like in therapy sessions when people respond with pleasure, disappointment or tension and shape what happens next. This can also be observed in improvizations, such as visual minutes or playback theatre in which a troupe of players develop an experience from a member of the audience into a performance (More than Minutes n.d.; Rowe 2007). Other concerns of the arts are truth and beauty, which are explored in Box 3.5.

Developing Professional Artistry

Recognizing and developing professional artistry often starts with situations that are unfamiliar

BOX 3.4
ARTFUL PRACTICE

Olivia's community occupational therapist Rachel had many helpful approaches, subtly switching between them. For example, Rachel avoided giving psychiatric labels to Olivia's difficult feelings, thoughts and actions but was fully aware of their severity. Olivia thought people talking about "your depression" was depressing, like a heavy burden. Language was so important to her.

Rather than being told what to do, Olivia found herself discussing occupational therapy with Rachel at home and in the clinic. She appreciated how Rachel explained and varied the focus, respecting that different levels of privacy changed what was discussed. While they prepared a meal together at home, Olivia could share her thoughts and feelings about self-harming without worrying about who was listening in.

As she cleaned the vegetables, Rachel was calm and listened carefully, so Olivia felt she could share the details of her plans without fear of being dismissed or tipped into a crisis situation. Sharing these details was difficult, yet Rachel did not judge her. This meant that while the meal was cooking and Olivia put plates and cutlery on the table, they could discuss ways of managing everyday life as well as the difficult thoughts and feelings. Eating the meal together felt so normal. Olivia wondered how something so ordinary could happen alongside exploring her most difficult feelings.

BOX 3.5
TRUTH AND BEAUTY

Truth, or authenticity, involves judging an artwork to see if it is fake, derivative or truly original. Beauty, or aesthetics, appraises the capacity of the work to move and inspire the observer (Fish and Coles 1998). Dewey believed that aesthetics were particularly important for appreciating how everyday practice could be inspiring and satisfying (Kinsella 2009). Truth and beauty are also concerns of coproduction. In collaborative research by Bryant et al. (2012) the shared metaphor of a meeting in the mist illuminated how service users and professionals emerged from separate sides of a valley to meet in the mist, which slowly dispersed as they worked together. This metaphor captured the authenticity of the experience, coming from different perspectives and persisting when it was difficult to see the way ahead. Used in the group as a shared reference, it was followed by another metaphor (the Warp Factor) to describe the sense of breaking new ground. The process of searching for and agreeing metaphors is imaginative, creative and challenging, as authenticity and aesthetics are tested. In practice this could mean attending carefully, reflecting and expressing possible meanings of occupations as those meanings evolve in therapy.

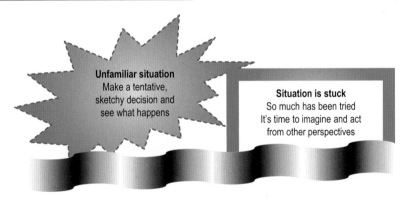

Unfamiliar situation
Make a tentative, sketchy decision and see what happens

Situation is stuck
So much has been tried
It's time to imagine and act from other perspectives

Situation is moving & changing now:
Choose and use resources in an intuitive way to keep it moving

Appraise: Critically examine what has happened and what the impression is now, by stepping back for a wider view and looking closely to notice the details

Fig. 3.2 ■ Developing professional artistry.

or stuck, as shown in Fig. 3.2. With imagination, sketchy steps forward and creative use of available resources, sustainable changes can be achieved (Bryant 2010). Fish and Coles (1998) emphasized that artistry includes appreciating the outcomes of practice,

like stepping back from work in progress to evaluate it. This might partly explain why dramas about healthcare settings are so popular in many cultures. Although the characters are flawed, their practice is usually engaging when it is imaginative and effective, containing moral and political messages. The characters survive the unexpected, encounter mysteries that are never completely solved and experience transformations, yet there remains a sense that they could develop further.

Direct experiences of occupational therapy on an inpatient unit are shared by Outdoor Prescription (2019) and summarized in Box 3.6. The therapy unfolded slowly so that the content and form of therapy were revealed in stages, rather than being clearly determined from the start (Fish 1998).

The occupational therapist perceived many dimensions of performance and acted to transform them, as if dancing steps in turn. The therapist's strategies to minimize distress and thereby avoid harm suggest that ethical reasoning was occurring (Lake et al. 2015). Sketching or suggesting structures and strategies for time use indicate an occupational focus and person-centred practice. These steps might appear logical in retrospect, but understanding professional artistry can reveal the ebbs and flows of the therapist's thoughts and actions. Recognizing complexity is another way of increasing appreciation of the details of practice.

RECOGNIZING COMPLEXITY

To recognize and think about complexity is to accept unpredictability and directly engage with the multidimensional, dynamic nature of life (Plsek and Greenhalgh 2001; Brown 2006). Explaining complexity theory, physicist Fritjof Capra (2002) suggested that inevitable but unpredictable outcomes emerge from two simultaneous processes: development and maintenance. Living organisms, ranging from individual cells to the global population, develop by adapting themselves and creating capacities. At the same time, they stay alive by renewing and replacing parts of themselves in a maintenance process, like nails or hair growing or people taking holidays from work. Applying this to occupational therapy, each new encounter offers the potential for both therapist and service user to develop and adapt knowledge, skills and understanding while also being engaged in the daily routines of living. This potential cannot be fully predicted: unexpected events like a fire alarm might interrupt it, or the encounter could be significant in hindsight after days or even years.

Box 3.7 illustrates how complexity theory can be used to understand occupational therapy in which Wendy creates, maintains and develops the therapeutic process of an assertiveness group by engaging in reflection in action and different modes of professional reasoning. At the same time, she facilitates opportunities for people to maintain, develop and adapt their capacities. Reflecting on these simultaneous processes in occupational therapy, Caulton and Dickson (2007, p. 95) suggested that 'knowing what to do is precisely the problem.' So much is happening at the same time, it is difficult to know fully what actions are possible and why. In their work with community programmes in New Zealand, they also observed that when possibilities were transformed into realities, the journey to create these possibilities was not always remembered, making it difficult to articulate the details in hindsight. Reflection is therefore important for absorbing complexities, with implications for the occupational therapy process. These are explored further in the next chapter. For the therapist who might feel daunted, it helps to see that complexity theory supports thoughtfulness to unpick and analyse multiple simultaneous processes, which make practice interesting and

BOX 3.7
USING COMPLEXITY THEORY TO UNDERSTAND PRACTICE

When Wendy worked on an acute unit, the unpredictable nature of the service meant it was important to work flexibly as, being acutely ill, people changed quickly and there was ongoing pressure to discharge them to minimize the disruption to their lives and enable others to be admitted. For two weeks an informal network of people in a similar situation formed on the unit. It was possible to create a group with them, focused on developing assertiveness skills. Wendy used a structure for the group, which she knew well from working in the community. In one session a participant was describing the difficulties of dealing with a receptionist in the GP surgery and Wendy recognized the surgery from her personal life. She considered how to use this unexpected insight within the session, deciding it would be helpful to adapt her approach to leading the session and share her recognition while maintaining her role as facilitator of the group.

Complexity theory has been used to emphasize certain aspects of Wendy's experience:

- Engaging with unpredictability;
- Working flexibly;
- Responding when people change quickly;
- Feeling the ongoing pressure to discharge people;
- Engaging with an informal network of patients;
- Creating a group;
- Developing assertiveness skills;
- Using a structure Wendy knew well;
- Reflecting on an unexpected insight during the session;
- Adapting her approach;
- Maintaining her role as facilitator.

These are familiar aspects of being a therapist and working in mental health settings; yet it is difficult to value and draw attention to them without seeing therapy as a living, rather than mechanistic, process.

constantly challenging, rather than mundane (Lazzarini 2016).

SUMMARY

Being an occupational therapist with an interest in mental health involves thinking and acting in particular ways. Understanding a person's mental health problems requires critical reflection and professional reasoning, thinking through possibilities for action. These thinking processes enable a therapist to explain

SERVICE USER COMMENTARY

The first thing my occupational therapist asked me was, 'What do you enjoy doing Hattie?'

I was 18 years old, detained against my will in a psychiatric hospital. I was feeling small, lost and trapped somewhere far away from any sense of who I was. I couldn't quite reach for the words to answer her question so I sat in silence until the words 'I don't know' fell out of my mouth. It's not that I didn't have anything I enjoyed or valued to talk about. I'd never stopped caring about the things that were important to me, but it is easy to forget who you are in a psychiatric hospital and my illness took up a lot of space at that time.

I thought about the question later, when I was sitting alone in my room on the uncomfortable plastic mattress with rip-proof sheets. The occupational therapist's question wasn't deep or emotional, but it felt significant. The question mattered less to me than the fact that the answer mattered to her; it wasn't just small talk to fill the silence. I'd become accustomed to the way the hospital staff would read my patient notes before meeting me and didn't have any more questions to ask me. I was used to not telling my own story.

So I went to find the occupational therapist to say that my favourite thing to do is sewing.

She found me a needle and thread, some soft fabric and a pair of real scissors. I held the items in my hands and we both looked at my arms with their patchwork of winding scars and scabs and sores, a souvenir of the harm that had caused so much pain but also kept me alive in its own way. The scissors were sharp and felt unfamiliar in the sterile environment of the psychiatric ward. I could sense she felt nervous, yet she afforded me the trust nobody else had as she knew that despite me being desperately suicidal and insistent on hurting myself in any way I could imagine, I still really loved sewing.

It was something about the way she trusted me enough to break the rigid ward rules so I could connect with something that mattered to me that stopped me from running off with the needles and scissors. Instead, I started sewing, which felt in a small but significant way like starting to stitch myself back together.

This chapter talks about being a therapist. To me this feels like something too big to fit neatly in the pages of a textbook and something which nobody can ever stop learning. I don't know if my therapist was consciously aware of everything the needle and thread meant to me, but she certainly knew that it meant more to me than I can express with words or with a needle and thread.

Harriet Porter

actions before, during and after occupational therapy. As well as studying occupation as a therapeutic medium, learning and gaining expertise in thinking and acting as a therapist are central aspects of developing a professional identity and therapeutic use of self. When working with mental health issues, therapeutic responses can be developed with awareness of embodiment and intersubjectivity. Being aware of ourselves and what is happening with others in an occupational therapy session enables pragmatic action to be taken at the same time as drawing on professional knowledge structures. Professional artistry offers a way of understanding how professional practice appears to effortlessly combine all these different ways of being a therapist using the language of art. Complexity theory could also be used to unpick and analyse practice challenges. Being a therapist is a continual process of learning how to think and act, using knowledge as the grounds for practice and professional structures as a guide (see Chapter 4).

REFERENCES

Abendstern, M., Tucker, S., Wilberforce, M., Jasper, R., & Challis, D. (2017). Occupational therapists in community mental health teams for older people in England: Findings from a five-year research programme. *British Journal of Occupational Therapy*, 80(1), 20–29.

Arntzen, C. (2018). An embodied and intersubjective practice of occupational therapy. *Occupational Therapy Journal of Research (Thorofare NJ)*, 38(3), 173–180.

Bailliard, A. L., Dallman, A. R., Carroll, A., Lee, B. D., & Szendrey, S. (2020). Doing occupational justice: A central dimension of everyday occupational therapy practice. *Canadian Journal of Occupational Therapy*, 87(2), 144–152. https://doi.org/10.1177/0008417419898930.

Bassot, B. (2016). *The reflective practice guide: An interdisciplinary approach to critical reflection*. Abingdon: Routledge.

Bazyk, S., et al. (2010). Service learning: The process of doing and becoming an occupational therapist. *Occupational Therapy in Health Care*, 24(2), 171–187.

Binyamin, G. (2021). Strategies for resolving relational dilemmas while developing therapists' professional identity. *Advances in health sciences education : Theory and practice*. https://doi.org/10.1007/s10459-020-10024-9.

Boud, D., & Walker, D. (1998). Promoting reflection in professional courses: The challenge of context. *Studies in Higher Education*, 23(2), 191–206.

Brown, C. (2006). The application of complex adaptive systems theory to clinical practice in rehabilitation. *Disability & Rehabilitation*, 28(9), 587–593.

Bryant, W. (2010). Unbelievable. Practice, theory and the work of Jennifer Creek. *British Journal of Occupational Therapy*, 73(10), 487–489.

Bryant, W., Andrews, C., Birken, M., Davidson, B., Gajoram, G., & Nicholson-Jones, D. (2015). You Know people Can Get Better. *Experiences of Occupational Therapy in an Acute Mental Health Unit, Through the Camera Lens*. University of Essex, Colchester. Available at: https://core.ac.uk/reader/74373624.

Bryant, W., Parsonage, J., Tibbs, A., Andrews, C., Clark, J., & Franco, L. (2012). Meeting in the mist: Key considerations in a collaborative research partnership with people with mental health issues. *Work*, 43(1), 23–31.

Bullen, D., & Clarke, C. (2021). Occupational therapists' experiences of enabling people to participate in sport. *British Journal of Occupational Therapy*, 84(11):703–712.

Capra, F. (2002). *The Hidden Connections*. London: Flamingo.

Carstensen, T., & Bonsaksen, T. (2017). Differences and similarities in therapeutic mode use between occupational therapists and occupational therapy students in Norway. *Scandinavian Journal of Occupational Therapy*, 24(6), 448–454.

Caulton, R., & Dickson, R. (2007). What's going on? Finding an explanation for what we do. In J. Creek, & A. Lawson-Porter (Eds.), *Contemporary Issues in Occupational Therapy* (pp. 87–114). Chichester: John Wiley & Sons Ltd.

Christiansen, C. H. (1999). Defining lives: Occupation as identity: An essay on competence, coherence, and the creation of meaning. *American Journal of Occupational Therapy*, 53(6), 547–558.

Cole, M. B., & Creek, J. (2016). *Global perspectives in professional reasoning*. Thorofare, NJ: SLACK Incorporated.

Collins English Dictionary. (2020). Available at: https://www.collinsdictionary.com/dictionary/english/reflection.

Craig-Duchesne, C., Rochette, A., Scurti, S., Beaulieu, J., & Vachon, B. (2018). Occupational therapy students' experience with using a journal in fieldwork and factors influencing its use. *Reflective Practice*, 19(5), 609–622.

Creek, J. (2007). The thinking therapist. In J. Creek, & A. Lawson-Porter (Eds.), *Contemporary issues in occupational therapy: Reasoning and reflecting*. Chichester: John Wiley and Sons Ltd.

Creek, J. (2014). The knowledge base of occupational therapy. In W. Bryant, J. Fieldhouse, & K. Bannigan (Eds.), *Occupational therapy and mental health* (5th ed.). London: Elsevier.

Creek, J. (2016). The language of professional reasoning. In M. B. Cole, & J. Creek (Eds.), *Global Perspectives in Professional Reasoning*. Thorofare, NJ: SLACK Incorporated.

Daniel, M. (2013). Beyond Bowlby: Exploring the dynamics of attachment. In L. Nicholls, P. J. Cunningham, G. C. de Sena, & M. Daniel (Eds.), *Psychoanalytic Thinking in Occupational Therapy: Symbolic, Relational and Transformative*. Chichester: John Wiley and Sons Ltd.

Devery, H., Scanlan, J. N., & Ross, J. (2018). Factors associated with professional identity, job satisfaction and burnout for occupational therapists working in eating disorders: A mixed methods study. *Australian Occupational Therapy Journal*, 65(6), 523–532.

Dix, A. (2010). *Reflection in practice: Schon and Science*. Available at: https://alandix.com/blog/2010/03/20/reflection-in-practice-schn-and-science/#:~:text=Sch%C3%B6n%20describes%20three%20main%20levels,rich%20background%20of%20past%20experiences.

Dixon, L. B., Adler, D. A., Berlant, J., et al. (2020). Managing our Public Selves. *Psychiatric Services*. Available at: https://ps.psychiatryonline.org/doi/full/10.1176/appi.ps.202000078.

Edge, J. (2019). *The Policing of 'Self-Care' - a Call to Repoliticise*. Available at: https://hagenilda.wordpress.com/2019/04/24/the-policing-of-self-care-a-call-to-repoliticise/.

Evetts, C., & Peloquin, S. (2017). *Mindful Crafts as Therapy*. Philadelphia: FA Davis Company.

Fighting to Liv. (2019). *Police Mental Health – Wellbeing Starts with the Organisation*. Available at: https://fightingtoliv.wordpress.com/.

Filippidou, M. S., & Lingwood, I. M. (2014). Reducing non-attendance rates in a community mental health team. *BMJ quality improvement reports*. https://doi.org/10.1136/bmjquality.u202228.w1114.

Fish, D., & Coles, C. (1998). *Developing Professional Judgement in Health Care*. Edinburgh: Butterworth Heinemann.

Fisher, A. G. (2014). Occupation-centred, occupation-based, occupation-focused: Same, same or different?. *Scandinavian Journal of Occupational Therapy*, 21, 96–107.

Hammell, K. W. (2019). Building globally relevant occupational therapy from the strength of our diversity. *World Federation of Occupational Therapists Bulletin*, 75(1), 13–26.

Honey, A., Berry, B., Hancock, N., Scanlan, J., Schweizer, R., & Waks, S. (2019). Using systematic collaborative reflection to enhance consumer-led mental health research. *British Journal of Occupational Therapy*, 82(11), 666–674.

Hooper, B., & Wood, W. (2002). Pragmatism and structuralism in occupational therapy: The long conversation. *American Journal of Occupational Therapy*, 56(1), 40–50.

Horghagen, S., Bonsaksen, T., Sveen, U., Dolva, A. S., & Arntzen, C. (2020). Generalist, specialist and generic positions experienced by occupational therapists in Norwegian municipalities. *Indian Journal of Occupational Therapy*, 48(2), 133–146.

John, C. (2017). *Becoming a reflective Practitioner* (5th ed.). Hoboken, NJ: Wiley-Blackwell.

Kinsella, E. A. (2010). Professional knowledge and the epistemology of reflective practice. *Nursing Philosophy*, 11(1), 3–14.

Knightbridge, L. (2019). Reflection–in–practice: A survey of Australian occupational therapists. *Australian Occupational Therapy Journal*, 66(3), 337–346.

Lake, J., Jackson, L., & Hardman, C. (2015). A fresh perspective on medical education: The lens of the arts. *Medical Education*, 49(8), 759–772. https://doi.org/10.1111/medu.12768.

Lazzarini, I. (2016). Nonlinear reasoning in cognition: Restoring the essence of the occupational therapy process. In M. B. Cole, & J. Creek (Eds.), *Global Perspectives in Professional Reasoning* (pp. 183–202). Thorofare, NJ: SLACK Incorporated.

Machan, T. (2013). Impractical pragmatism. *Philosophy Now*, 95, 30.

Márquez-Álvarez, L., Calvo-Arenillas, J., Talavera-Valverde, M., & Moruno-Millares, P. (2019). Professional reasoning in occupational therapy: A scoping review. *Occupational Therapy International*. https://doi.org/10.1155/2019/6238245. 2019, Article ID 6238245.

Mattingly, C., & Fleming, M. H. (1994). *Clinical reasoning: Forms of inquiry in a therapeutic practice*. Philadelphia: F.A. Davis Company.

Mavindidze, E., van Niekerk, L., & Cloete, L. (2019). Inter-sectoral work practice in Zimbabwe: Professional competencies required by occupational therapists to facilitate work participation of persons with disabilities. *Scandinavian Journal of Occupational Therapy*. https://doi.org/10.1080/11038128.2019.1684557.

McAllister, S., Robert, G., Tsianakas, V., & McCrae, N. (2019). Conceptualising nurse-patient therapeutic engagement on acute mental health wards: An integrative review. *International Journal of Nursing Studies*, 93, 106–118.

More than Minutes (n.d.). Visual Minutes. Available at: https://www.morethanminutes.co.uk/visual-minutes.

Nicholls, L., Cunningham, P. J., de Sena, G. C., & Daniel, M. (2013). *Psychoanalytic Thinking in Occupational Therapy: Symbolic, Relational and Transformative*. Chichester: John Wiley and Sons Ltd.

Noon, M. (2018). Pointless diversity training: Unconscious bias, new racism and agency. *Work, Employment & Society*, 32(1), 198–209.

Online Etymology Dictionary, 2021. Available at: https://www.etymonline.com/word/therapy#etymonline_v_10737.

Outdoor Prescription. (2019). Occupational therapy in mental health Treatment. Available at: https://outdoorprescription.wordpress.com/2019/07/11/occupational-therapy/.

Pentland, D., Kantartzis, S., Clausen, M. G., & Witemyre, K. (2018). *Occupational Therapy and Complexity: Defining and Describing practice*. London: Royal College of Occupational Therapists.

Plastow, N. A., Atwal, A., & Gilhooly, M. (2015). Food activities and identity maintenance among community-living older adults: A grounded theory study. *American Journal of Occupational Therapy*, 69(6). https://doi.org/10.5014/ajot.2015.016139.

Plsek, P. E., & Greenhalgh, T. (2001). Complexity science: The challenge of complexity in health care. *British Medical Journal*, 323(7313), 625–628.

Polanyi, M. (1966). *The Tacit Dimension*. Gloucester, Massachusetts: Peter Smith.

Priddis, L., & Rogers, S. L. (2018). Development of the reflective practice questionnaire: Preliminary findings. *Reflective Practice*, 19(1), 89–104. https://doi.org/10.1080/14623943.2017.1379384.

Recovery in the Bin (RitB). (2017). *Handy guide for Crisis Team Workers*. Available at: www.recoveryinthebin.org.

Recovery in the Bin (RitB). (2019). *I Have Never Been in a Place More Indifferent to Suffering than a Psychiatric Ward*. Available at https://recoveryinthebin.org/2019/03/18/i-have-never-been-in-a-place-more-indifferent-to-suffering-than-a-psychiatric-ward/.

Rowe, N. (2007). *Playing the Other: Dramatizing Personal Narratives in Playback Theatre*. London: Jessica Kingsley.

Scanlan, J. N., & Hazelton, T. (2019). Relationships between job satisfaction, burnout, professional identity and meaningfulness of work activities for occupational therapists working in mental health. *Australian Occupational Therapy Journal, 66*(5), 581–590.

Schell, B., & Schell, J. (Eds.). (2008). *Clinical and Professional Reasoning in Occupational Therapy*. Baltimore: Lippincott Williams and Wilkins.

Schön, D. (1983). *The reflective Practitioner: How Professionals Think in Action*. New York, NY: Basic Books.

Schwartz, A. E., Kramer, J. M., Rogers, E. S., McDonald, K. E., & Cohn, E. S. (2020). Stakeholder-driven approach to developing a peer-mentoring intervention for young adults with intellectual/developmental disabilities and co-occurring mental health conditions. *Journal of Applied Research in Intellectual Disabilities* (Online early view).

Sinclair, K. (2018). Connected in diversity; positioned for impact. *World Federation of Occupational Therapists Bulletin, 74*(2), 71–72. https://doi.org/10.1080/14473828.2018.1520031.

Smith, M. K. (2001). *Donald Schön: Learning, reflection and change*. The Encyclopedia of Pedagogy and Informal Education, 2011. Available at: www.infed.org/thinkers/et-schon.htm.

Taff, S. D., & Blash, D. (2017). *Diversity and Inclusion in Occupational*.

Taylor, R. R., & VanPuymbrouck, L. (2013). Therapeutic use of self: Applying the intentional relationship model in group therapy. In J. C. O'Brien, & J. Solomon (Eds.), *Occupational Analysis and Group Process*. St. Louis, Mo: Elsevier/Mosby.

Therapy: Where We Are, where We Must Go. *Occupational Therapy in Health Care, 31* (1), 72–83. https://doi.org/10.1080/07380577.2016.1270479.

Unsworth, C., & Baker, A. (2016). A systematic review of professional reasoning literature in occupational therapy. *British Journal of Occupational Therapy, 79*(1), 5–16. https://doi.org/10.1177/0308022615599994.

Wimpenny, K., Savin-Baden, M., & Cook, C. (2014). A qualitative research synthesis examining the effectiveness of interventions used by occupational therapists in mental health. *British Journal of Occupational Therapy, 77*(6), 276–288. https://doi.org/10.4276/030802214X14018723137959.

Wong, K., Whitcombe, S. W., & Boniface, G. (2016). Teaching and learning the esoteric: An insight into how reflection may be internalised with reference to the occupational therapy profession. *Reflective Practice, 17*(4), 472–482. https://doi.org/10.1080/14623943.2016.1175341.

World Federation of Occupational Therapists (WFOT). (2016). *Minimum Standards for the Education of Occupational Therapists Revised 2016*. Available at: www.wfot.org/ResourcesCentre.

Section 2

THE OCCUPATIONAL THERAPY PROCESS

4

STRUCTURING PRACTICE

NICOLA PLASTOW ■ WENDY BRYANT

CHAPTER OUTLINE

INTRODUCTION

In any landscape, we know where we are by observing the features of the natural and man-made environments. These features help us to understand which direction we should travel in. The occupational therapy landscape was introduced in Chapter 2 as the grounds for knowing and understanding practice. In this chapter, we introduce the features which structure occupational therapy. The first feature discussed is person-centred practice, followed by the occupational therapy process. Practice models, frames of reference and practice frameworks are explored as structures which are like buildings, with particular layouts and purposes. Exploring the landscape for

occupational therapy also involves discovering boundaries, which determine the scope of practice. Often practice follows pathways which are mapped out, to guide the therapist. There are different ways of considering whether the journey has been effective, which are discussed in the final section. The chapter is illustrated with service user perspectives on occupational therapy and examples of practice.

PERSON-CENTRED PRACTICE

Person-centred practice is an approach which puts people first, over and above service priorities, protocols and needs (Health Foundation 2016). Structuring practice

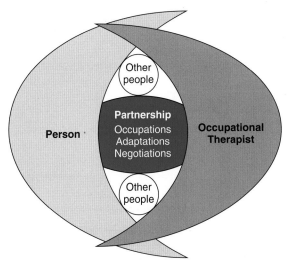

Fig. 4.1 ▪ **Person-centred practice.**

in this way occurs when there is joint work taking place, involving both the person engaging with occupational therapy and the person providing it (Fig. 4.1). In the United Kingdom the NHS Constitution sets out shared values for putting people first (Health Education England 2017), recognizing that families, groups and communities have a central place in the safe and effective delivery of health services. However, person-centred practice is an ideal, often being compromised in everyday practice. For example, sometimes an occupational therapist may need to sidestep some of a person's concerns, especially if they are acutely unwell and lack insight. While the occupational therapist centres their attention on the service user, person-centred practice also requires the service user to focus on how occupational therapy can help them.

Person-centred practice has other challenges. Once people have successfully accessed a service, it may be assumed that they will accept the help offered and follow any advice or plan suggested if they are given reassurance, information and support. Help and advice are important, as mental health problems can be bewildering and frightening. However, some people may struggle to engage with a service, to share their problems, to act on advice or to follow a plan. If a person struggles to engage, for example, when they appear non-adherent with an agreed plan, it is important to find out why by attending to the outcomes the person values most (see Chapter 22; Fulford 2020).

Fig. 4.1 shows that several people can be involved in person-centred practice at any one moment, such

as other members in a group session, a carer or a colleague. Person-centred practice is a partnership that brings people together to negotiate and adapt occupations for particular purposes (Sumsion 1999). The occupational therapist engages with each person to bring their perspective into the therapeutic process.

People's fears, aspirations and understanding influence how they approach occupational therapy. Person-centred practice involves attending carefully to these influences. For example, a person's approach can be sensed at the beginning of a group session with a warm up led by therapists. Greeting each person in turn brings them to the attention of the group and gives them an opportunity to express their fears, hopes and meanings, verbally and non-verbally. These greetings also enable the therapists to express their approach to the group and offer respect to everyone present. Some group members may seize the opportunity to engage, but others may find it is difficult to bring themselves into the centre of the group's attention. This difficulty could arise for many reasons, including not understanding occupational therapy, fear, distrust or feeling sleepy due to medication side effects. A person may not be able to clearly state their difficulties but could express them in response to what happens in the group or when sharing their experiences in stories (Arblaster et al. 2019). The occupational therapist uses reflection and reasoning to interpret these stories (see Chapter 3).

Keeping a person at the centre of practice involves much more than finding out what the person wants. This approach is significant in mental health settings where, to protect safety, procedures can override personal preferences, for example, by the way the Mental Health Act is used in the United Kingdom (Rethink Mental Illness 2011; see Chapters 21 and 26). Routine procedures can centre on people or marginalize them. Alternative possibilities can be considered and balanced as part of two-body practice (see Chapter 3): moving between being pragmatic and taking the most practical approach at the time to being structural and sticking to procedures and plans. Person-centred practice requires therapists and service users work together:

- by focusing together on the service users as occupational beings (see Chapter 2);
- with therapists, enabling therapeutic relationships to evolve, moving between different modes of reasoning and attending to embodied feelings (see Chapter 3);

■ discussing the structure for the joint work, usually in the form of the occupational therapy process, which is explained in the next section.

OCCUPATIONAL THERAPY PROCESS

Occupational therapy addresses people's problems in a relevant and effective way by working through a series of stages that are known collectively as the occupational therapy process. This term suggests a logical progression, as if reading a handbook from start to end. However, in practice, the process is more complex, progressing in a non-linear way as if revisiting certain sections in a book many times before reaching the end. Each of the stages of the occupational therapy process is described here, and then the complexity of applying the process in practice is explored in more depth.

Combining person-centred practice with this structured process enables people engaging with occupational therapy to decide their own priorities and evaluate how effective it has been for them. To achieve this partnership the occupational therapist shares their thinking with the person as far as is possible and appropriate.

Referral

People may come into contact with an occupational therapy service in different ways. A person may be referred by another health or social care professional or may decide themselves to seek the services of an occupational therapist (self-referral). The person making the referral will often have identified needs that they think will best be addressed by an occupational therapist. In some settings the occupational therapist works with a community so there are no individual referrals. At the point of referral the occupational therapist reviews the available information to decide whether or not the referral is appropriate. If not, the occupational therapist communicates with the referring agent to explain why occupational therapy is not recommended.

Information Gathering and First Contact

If the referral does not contain enough information, the occupational therapist may consult with the referring agent or access the person's health records to gain background information. The occupational therapist then contacts the person to arrange an initial meeting. This contact may be by telephone, face-to-face or in a written format such as a letter or email, depending on where the person is staying. During this initial contact the therapist begins to establish rapport with the person and explains how occupational therapy might be of benefit to them. The occupational therapist also gains an initial idea of the most significant problems with occupational performance the person is experiencing and what they hope to achieve with occupational therapy. Information from this initial contact and the referral, as well as the therapist's professional expertise, is used to reason through:

■ the most likely problems with occupational performance and possible goals;
■ the ways of approaching practice (see later section);
■ the most important assessments to select (see Chapter 5);
■ the possible scope and focus of therapy (see later sections).

This initial contact may also alert the therapist to potential precautionary measures to take, which are actions the occupational therapist takes to ensure the safety and well-being of the person and themselves (see Chapters 7, 21, 22 and 26).

Assessment

Assessment of a person's abilities and needs provides a performance baseline before starting occupational therapy and highlights where the intervention will be focused. Repeat assessments are used to track the person's progress towards meeting their goals and as outcome measures (see Chapter 5). For some people, assessment is structured to include all relevant aspects of their life. For others, assessment may focus on a discrete area, such as return to work (see Chapter 20).

Assessment is discussed in depth in Chapter 5 but is introduced here as an integral part of the occupational therapy process. Key points from Chapter 5 include:

■ assessment occurs in stages, from initial information gathering onwards;
■ the choice of method and focus of assessments are influenced by the person being assessed, the therapist's knowledge and skills and the context;

- assessment findings can be reported in different ways, with varied implications depending on who the findings are being reported to and how well they understand them. Discussing them with the service user in collaborative goal setting may require understanding of more details than a report to the multidisciplinary team for discharge planning.
- Standardized assessment tools and outcome measures can offer results which can be compared either with population norms or with previous assessments completed with the person but only if the guidelines are followed carefully.

Assessment begins informally by asking the person about the occupations which are affected by their mental health problems. If they cannot express their needs or have difficulty evaluating their occupational performance themselves, then the occupational therapist will seek perspectives from people who know the person well, such as family members or caregivers. At this stage of assessment the accuracy of the self-report is much less important than understanding what is really important to the person.

In Chapter 5 a distinction is drawn between assessment of occupational performance components or skills and broader assessment of the person as an occupational being (see Chapter 2). Negotiating what to assess will also impact on other stages of the occupational therapy process, for example, building rapport and planning interventions. If a practice model is being used, this will influence choice of assessment tools such as the model of human occupation screening tool. Assessment does not happen only once during the occupational therapy process. Instead, it may occur during every contact with the person, especially if the occupational therapist notices changes in the person, their environment or their occupational performance. New insights into strengths and limitations are often gained as the occupational therapist gets to know the person better performance. New insights into strengths and limitations are often gained as the occupational therapist gets to know the person better. These repeated assessments may be done through observation or the use of a particular assessment or outcome measure.

Formulation and Expected Outcomes

At the end of a detailed assessment process, the occupational therapist and the person will, together, summarize the assessment findings in a way that informs goal setting and intervention. Practice models may guide the terminology used in a formulation. Collaboratively agreeing the expected outcomes enables further discussion between the therapist and person about the assessment findings. The time taken to think through a formulation together is therefore valuable, to promote awareness and understanding. Formulation is always a collaborative process not only between the occupational therapist and the person, but also with others who may want to explore the relevance and importance of any ideas or discuss possible goals. A clear formulation will enable the occupational therapist and person to explain what has been agreed to others involved.

Goal Setting

Following the collaborative process of formulation, the occupational therapist and the person negotiate their anticipated outcomes, agreeing on goals which the person wants to achieve. Goal setting might take place individually or in a group session. While individual goal setting will always focus on the goals of the person, group goal setting may include what each group member hopes to achieve individually by participating in a group and/or what the group aims to achieve together. Details of the goal-setting process and different types of goals are found in Chapter 6. People in contact with mental health services are not always able to fully participate in the goal setting process because they may be experiencing psychosis, are disorientated or are unable to communicate their needs. In these cases the occupational therapist consults with a caregiver to ensure that the goals remain firmly centred on the person's needs. The process of goal setting may happen more than once during occupational therapy, especially if goals are achieved earlier than expected or if it becomes evident that goals need to be broken down into more achievable steps.

Intervention Plan

The plan provides an individualized blueprint for occupational therapy that is negotiated with the person and/or their carers. It includes:

- when sessions will start;
- how many sessions will be carried out before the next assessment;
- the focus of therapy, based on the goals set;

- how the goals will be met;
- how the therapist and person will know when the goals have been met.

The occupational therapist considers a number of factors when deciding how best to meet goals. These factors include the most appropriate frame of reference or approach (see later in this chapter) and which treatment modalities or occupations will both suit the person and help them achieve their goals. Treatment modalities are specific techniques, such as sensory approaches, relaxation techniques, psychoeducation or motivational interviewing.

Implementing the Plan

At this stage the person engages in occupation-centred sessions guided by their occupational therapist to meet their goals and influence their health, well-being and participation. Other people may also be involved, including occupational therapy technicians or assistants, other professionals, carers, peers, community support workers and volunteers. Examples of occupations that may form part of this stage are explained in Chapters 13 to 20. The occupational therapist carefully analyses the activity to be used and adapts it to provide the just-right challenge or best fit (see Chapter 6). There is often an element of positive risk-taking at this stage, because a degree of challenge is required if people are to achieve their goals. The occupational therapist carefully assesses the risks inherent in activities and the potential harms that may result (see Chapter 9 and 22) and takes steps to mitigate those risks. In occupational therapy groups, the activities used to implement the plan or interventions are characterized by:

- their focus on occupational performance;
- the clear goals of the group being matched to the individual goals of each group member;
- the inclusion of an activity or occupation; and
- the specific and intentional use of questions during the group to prompt reflection and facilitate growth (Occupational Therapy Association of South Africa (OTASA) 2015; see also Chapter 15).

Many occupational therapists identify the implementation stage of the process as the intervention, although seeing all stages of occupational therapy as intervention is important for research, scholarship and planning services (Pentland et al. 2018). However, the word 'intervention' is used in different ways in the occupational therapy literature. The American Occupational Therapy Association (AOTA) practice framework uses intervention to categorize the skilled services an occupational therapist provides that facilitate engagement in occupation (AOTA 2020). In contrast, the Royal College of Occupational Therapists in the United Kingdom use the term 'complex intervention' to refer to all components of the occupational therapy process (Pentland et al. 2018; AOTA 2020). Furthermore, the word 'intervention' has gradually replaced 'treatment', as occupational therapists have moved away from using medical frames of reference to explain their work. Some occupational therapists choose not to use the word 'intervention', feeling that it implies a passive role for the person engaging with occupational therapy and an active role for the occupational therapist who is intervening. The word 'therapy' is said to cover both treatment and intervention. However, it is important to realize that the occupational therapy process covers other stages and that it is important to describe the stage in which people and occupational therapists are engaged in actively addressing the goals that have been agreed.

Evaluation

Evaluation involves interpreting and appraising the evidence to identify if the occupational therapy intervention is effective and relevant. Evaluation at the end of a session indicates whether the goals of that session were met. Evaluation of the person's progress towards their objectives (short-term), aims (medium-term) and goals (longer term) is a collaborative process taking place between the occupational therapist and the person throughout the intervention. Evaluation includes using outcome measures (see Chapter 5) and discussion with the person.

Conclusion of Occupational Therapy

The conclusion of occupational therapy is reached by agreement between the person, their carer or significant others and the occupational therapist. It may be useful to provide a report to the person who made the initial referral to occupational therapy, indicating the goals, assessment findings, a summary of progress and any residual limitations that the referring person needs to be aware of. The therapist ensures that the service user is aware of any

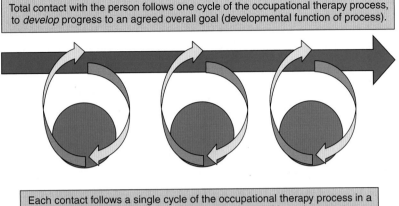

Total contact with the person follows one cycle of the occupational therapy process, to *develop* progress to an agreed overall goal (developmental function of process).

Each contact follows a single cycle of the occupational therapy process in a person-centred approach, to *maintain* the relationship and momentum of therapy (maintenance function of of process).

Fig. 4.2 ■ **A complex process.**

recommendations for the future, including further occupational therapy, suggestions about specific occupations or other services the person could access to maintain their mental health. These recommendations should be as specific as possible and should include how the person can access other services and when and where these services are available.

A Complex Process

Complexity theory has enabled understanding of occupational therapy as a complex intervention (Pentland et al. 2018; see Chapter 2) and the interdependent thinking and acting processes of being a therapist (see Chapter 3). Fig. 4.2 illustrates how the occupational therapy process develops over time (developmental function) and is sustained by micro cycles (maintenance function), drawing on Capra (2002) (see Chapter 2). These two functions of the occupational therapy process connect with each other in different ways at different times, changing multiple aspects of life in unexpected ways.

Complexity theory shifts thinking from seeing people as systems or machines to seeing them as living organisms (Capra 2002). If the occupational therapy process is seen as a procedure to impose on people, then they may be viewed as passive or even resistive at times. However, if the occupational therapy process is seen as a structure for communicating and engaging with people and the things they do, opportunities

BOX 4.1
MACRO AND MICRO PROCESSES DURING INTERVENTION

Al has been living for many months in a rehabilitation unit, working towards his long-term goal of living independently. Multiple micro cycles of the occupational therapy process occur as he gains and practises relevant occupations. As time unfolds, setbacks and unexpected new situations arise, such as a change of staff in the unit or an opportunity for Al to be a part-time volunteer in a local organization. When Al agrees to get up earlier for breakfast every morning, this enables several new developments to occur. At the same time, the establishment of this new habit is a step towards his long-term goal of independence. During this time, an occupational therapy student, Em, works with Al, planning sessions that enable him to work towards agreed goals. There are micro occupational therapy processes in every session: building the relationship, assessing specific challenges, agreeing which strategies to try, trying them and evaluating the outcomes.

emerge to draw on their energy and creativity, as illustrated in Box 4.1. If Al did not get up one morning, this would be the time for him to explore with Em what was happening, possibly revisiting his long-term goal, taking a break or finding another focus for the day's session. This flexible and open approach is part of person-centred practice but can be difficult to fit with organizational priorities that are designed to monitor progress through services. The complexity of the occupational therapy process allows for both structural and pragmatic thinking (see Chapter 3) and for finding a balance between a person-centred approach and a therapist- or service-led approach to practice.

Lazzarini (2016) takes complex thinking further, with occupational therapy changing habits to create new patterns of occupational performance, using the word 'perturbation' to specify the quality of the change. In complexity theory, a perturbation is a 'small change in the movement, quality, or behaviour of something' (Collins English Dictionary 2020). Although the change might be small, the impact can be significant. Lazzarini (2016) stresses the importance of the occupational therapist engaging in reflection during sessions and afterwards to be alert for all changes (see Chapter 3). When the occupational therapy process is seen as non-linear, there is space for reflection so that approaches can shift during therapy and between sessions. For example, on the morning that Al does not get up in time for breakfast, an old-established habit could be re-emerging. In response, Em might look for and suggest signs to reinforce the new habit, which could involve setting a bedside alarm or laying out clothes for the day ahead. Distinguishing established habits and new intentions is part of non-linear thinking, connecting different components of occupational performance. The European Conceptual Framework (Creek 2010) introduced in Chapter 2 offers multiple ways of tracing new connections between different components of occupational performance and the internal/external worlds of the performer. This means there are different ways of approaching practice, which are discussed next.

STRUCTURES FOR PRACTICE

In Chapter 2 we introduced the idea of a wall made of bricks (concepts) that are joined with mortar (concepts) to form a wall (theory) that can be part of either a structure on the ground or a boundary wall. We also introduced the idea that theories can be viewed from different perspectives. This part of the chapter develops the knowledge landscape by using an analogy of an occupational therapy neighbourhood for professional knowledge, such as practice models, frames of reference and practice frameworks. This analogy was initially proposed by Plastow and Bester (2015, Private communication) and further developed by the authors of this chapter. An analogy explains something complex using something simpler, showing how the two situations are similar (Collins English Dictionary 2020). Here, the features of a simple neighbourhood provide orientation in an occupational therapy landscape to structure practice.

A Neighbourhood Analogy

From above, a neighbourhood view reveals defining features or landmarks such as buildings, pavements, roads, people, rivers and trees (Fig. 4.3). For an occupational therapy landscape, this is like taking a world-view which helps to unify the profession and define its nature and purpose, aiming to reach a 'consensus regarding the most fundamental beliefs of the profession (e.g., occupation, purposeful activity, function)' (Kielhofner 2009). A worldview is also known as a paradigm (see Chapter 2), so as paradigms shift so do worldviews. For example, Hitch et al. (2018) proposed a Pan Occupation Paradigm using the framework of doing-being-becoming-belonging as a central focus.

An aerial view of a neighbourhood shows buildings of varying sizes and different architectural styles. Similarly, there are practice models, frames of reference and practice frameworks which are structures for occupational therapy and serve different purposes. Using the analogy of a theory as a wall, we understand that these structures develop at different times in different places and are constructed by connecting theories which are often shared or similar. Gradually, core theories, developed in the 1950s and 1970s, have been organized into models of practice in the 1980s and 1990s and then into practice frameworks over the past two decades.

An aerial view of the neighbourhood also implies having a vantage point from which different features exist in relation to each other. For example, some models of practice may be next-door neighbours, that is, closely related to each other; while others may be distant neighbours. Occupational therapists familiar with their area of the neighbourhood often have a sense of community and cohesion with others who are there. Service users who are new to the neighbourhood may feel differently about being there.

Finding ways around practice involves using principles. Like a highway code or signposted pathway that links the environment in a pragmatic way, principles for practice are guidelines for action and become tacit with time. They are visible in application and directly related

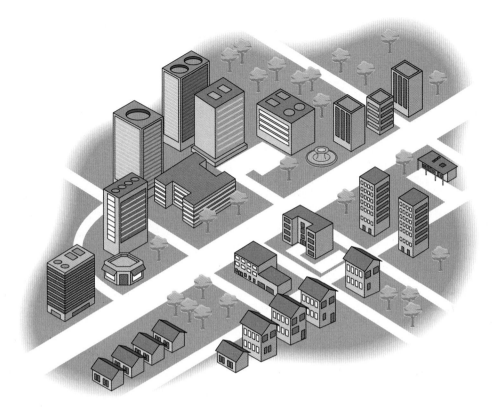

Fig. 4.3 ■ **A view of a neighbourhood to understand occupational therapy's world view.**

to reasoning. The therapist chooses the principles for action depending on their agreed destination with the service user. Their safe and timely arrival depends on the chosen principles. Frames of practice often influence principles, discussed further later in this chapter.

Professional reasoning guides choices in how practice is structured, because it is not possible to be completely certain what will work best for each individual (see Chapter 3). The distinction between models and frameworks is best understood by their nature and purpose, and is not always indicated by their names. For example, the ecology of human performance framework (Dunn et al. 1994) is called a framework. However, using ecological theories, it models the interdependence between the person and their environment and the impact on occupational performance.

Practice Models

When a person accesses a building, they do not routinely consider construction materials such as bricks and mortar. Similarly, practice models are visual images, constructed from theories, to explain processes and predict outcomes (Creek 2014). As models *of* practice, they can offer an ideal, like houses in a model neighbourhood. As models *for* practice, they can be a visual guide to how different elements and details work together, like an architectural model (Fish and Boniface 2012).

Occupational therapists use practice models to maintain an occupational focus, distinguish their practice from other mental health professions and promote consistency across an organization. The focus on occupation is facilitated by using practice models in three ways:

1. By presenting the nature of people, occupations and their environments and the relationships between these different elements;
2. By indicating what happens when problems in occupational performance occur;
3. By explaining how occupational therapy works.

An effective practice model specifies the scope, process and outcomes of occupational therapy and makes therapists more accountable to themselves, to their service users and employers and to society (see Chapter 7). As do different homes in the occupational therapy neighbourhood, models have defining features, illustrated in the examples below:

- The Model of Human Occupation is based on a system with a central, dynamic interaction between the person (volition, habituation and performance capacity), their occupations and their environment (Taylor 2017). Change in one part of the system (such as establishing a morning self-care routine) can lead to changes in another part of the system (such as motivation to get out of bed and a sense of competence).
- The context for occupational performance and engagement signals the importance of human interdependence in the Kawa (river) model (Paxson et al. 2012).
- The Vona du Toit model of creative ability (de Witt 2014) draws together theories about the ability to engage in occupations freely and without any inhibitions, limitations or anxiety at the maximum level of competence. Levels of creative ability are indicated by the interaction between motivation and action. A person moves from one level of creative ability to the next until they have reached their creative potential.
- Being client-centred is central to the Canadian Model of Occupational Performance and Engagement (Warren 2002; Law and Laver-Fawcett 2013), which focuses on occupational performance as the dynamic interaction between the person (physical, mental and affective components), their occupations (self-care, productivity and leisure) and their environment.

Each model has its own terminology and limitations: none covers every aspect of occupational therapy. Multiple models could be used, with one as an organizing model of practice and the other(s) as complementary (Ikiugu et al. 2019). At other times therapists use models developed in other professions or develop personal practice models.

Frames of Reference

In the occupational therapy neighbourhood, frames of reference are like rooms in a house:. Mosey (1989) defined them as 'structure[s] used to transform theory into applicable information - to link theory to practice' (Mosey 1989, p. 196). Anne Cronin-Mosey (1938–2017) was an American occupational therapist and scholar who influenced professional understanding of the use of theory in practice, presenting her original ideas from the 1970s onwards (Hinojosa 2017). She introduced frames of reference, suggesting they were used by occupational therapists to translate theories into 'concepts, definitions and postulates', with postulates being the 'principles to guide intervention' (Mosey 1989, p. 196).

All mental health professionals refer to theories which have been developed by various disciplines. Framing the theories they refer to makes the details more accessible for understanding practice situations. For example, the use of weighted blankets to regulate emotions when people are in acute distress is informed by a frame of reference for trauma-informed care. In turn, this frame of reference draws on knowledge of sensory processing to create one of several principles for practice, which are guidelines for action (Eron et al. 2020). In the same way that a person may have instructions on their phone or on paper to find their way around a new place, principles of a frame of reference guide a therapist on how to structure an intervention to achieve the desired outcome.

In the occupational therapy neighbourhood, a practice model, as a house, might contain several frames of reference, or rooms, each having a particular purpose and containing specific tools or equipment like a kitchen or bedroom. Along with principles to guide practice, frames of reference provide specific terminology. Returning to the example of weighted blankets, Eron et al. (2020, p. 1) used the terms 'sensory modulation' and 'deep pressure stimulation' to explain more about their use. It would be inconsistent and unclear for an occupational therapist to speak about 'social inclusion' in this context, as this term draws on a different frame of reference drawing on knowledge about citizenship (Table 4.1; Lopes and Malfitano 2017). The terms 'sensory modulation' and 'deep pressure stimulation' reveal particular epistemologies or ways of knowing about people who are stressed or distressed: in this situation

TABLE 4.1
Using Frames of Reference in Practice

Practice example: Jo arrives late, fifteen minutes after today's session was scheduled to start

Key Principles	Questions for Reflection in and on Action
Common to all frames of reference	
Jo's late arrival may or may not be significant. It can be understood in different ways, which are not necessarily mutually exclusive. How the event is framed will influence what happens next in occupational therapy. Knowing which frames of references are being used helps the therapist to communicate with Jo and others involved.	How can Jo's late arrival be understood? Is it appropriate to focus on it in therapy or to acknowledge it and then return to the activities as planned?
Citizenship (Lopes and Malfitanio 2017)	
Taking part in occupational therapy involves a formal social contract, with rights and obligations, which is different to a negotiated informal relationship. Being a citizen means being included in overlapping groups in society, such as those related to gender and race (see Chapter 12). Being excluded from society can impact on occupational performance in multiple ways.	Which aspects of Jo's life have contributed to their late arrival? Do these aspects reflect a conflict between different social roles, generating a struggle to belong and be included in occupational therapy? When and how could these aspects, conflicts and struggles become a focus for dialogue in occupational therapy?
Cognitive-behaviourism (Ikiugu 2007; see also Chapter 14)	
Behaviours have consequences, establishing feedback loops. The person learns to repeat a behaviour, so it becomes reinforced as a habit, even if it is dysfunctional. Thoughts are also part of the feedback loop and cognitive dysfunction can be caused by thinking errors. Behavioural and cognitive dysfunctions can be challenged by learning and rehearsing specific strategies.	Is Jo's late arrival indicative of cognitive and/or behavioural dysfunction? If so, how could the situation be used to review what happened and explore Jo's thoughts about it? Does Jo need more opportunities to rehearse new habits? Which strategies would be most helpful to learn now?
Positive psychology (Robinson et al. 2012)	
Activities that are engaging and highly valued will enable people to feel fulfilled and to flourish. Such activities or occupations are seen as full of positive meaning or meaningful. Happiness and subjective well-being can be encouraged by optimal experiences or flow. Occupational engagement is shaped by balance, wisdom, hope, resilience and happiness.	How does Jo feel? In the reduced time available, is there still scope to create opportunities for occupational engagement which are full of positive meaning? How can the session/therapy be refocused on positive feelings and activities? Where does this session fit with Jo's goals to feel better, more fulfilled and happier?
Psychodynamic (Nicholls et al. 2013; Creek 2014)	
The things we do hold many meanings, which are often unconscious. These meanings are influenced by how we feel, how we see ourselves and how we relate to other people. Activities can reveal different meanings symbolically, including those that make us feel unsure or uncomfortable. The occupational therapist perceives difficult meanings and waits, or contains them, until the person feels safe enough to express and explore them. Feeling safe depends on the therapist protecting the boundaries of therapy by responding carefully to feelings, thoughts and actions.	What are the possible meanings of Jo's late arrival? How can these meanings be observed and explored within the session? Could Jo's choices reveal difficult/ambivalent feelings, resistance to change and/or new understandings? What are my feelings as a therapist? How do they reflect Jo's feelings and broader reasons for engaging in occupational therapy? How does arriving late challenge the boundaries of the session and what do I need to say/do in response?

Continued on following page

TABLE 4.1	
Using Frames of Reference in Practice (Continued)	
Relational security (Royal College of Psychiatrists 2015)	
Keeping everyone as safe as possible involves being alert to how people are shaping relationships so that boundaries and approaches to boundary testing are consistent. It is important for the therapist to act but also maintain a balance between restrictions and growth. Boundaries can be categorized into non-negotiable or flexible, with emphasis placed on the decision-making process for each new situation.	Did we all arrive on time? What has been agreed about late arrivals? How does this situation relate to Jo's overall goal in occupational therapy? Is Jo's late arrival the most relevant aspect of the situation? Is Jo testing a non-negotiable boundary? Or are the rules about punctuality flexible, making it essential to explain my decision this time? How can I access support from my team?
Sensory processing and integration (Mori et al. 2017)	
Occupational performance problems, such as being in the right place at the right time, could be issues with sensory modulation, processing and integration. These problems can be addressed by using remedial activities, adaptations such as noise-cancelling headphones, sensory diet programmes, modifications to the built environment to increase or decrease sensory input and education on how to manage sensory functions.	Have there been sensory processing problems in Jo's preparations for the session? Is Jo avoiding occupational therapy because it is over-or under-stimulating in a somatosensory, vestibular or auditory way? Are there changes in Jo's motor performance, social performance or emotional regulation skills? Does this situation indicate that the remedial activities planned need to be changed?
Trauma-informed care (Machtinger et al. 2018)	
Persistent health and performance problems can be a response to current or past trauma. Disclosure is complex and not necessarily required in detail for a helpful response. The therapist seeks to create a calm, empathetic and safe place, for example, by asking what happened rather than what is wrong.	How does Jo seem? Has something awful happened? What is the priority for this session and how can I facilitate safety, empathy and empowerment? What resources could be helpful? How can I draw attention to Jo's strengths and draw on my own? Who needs to know about this situation and the outcomes of the session?

emphasizing the significance of the autonomic nervous system. The words used by an occupational therapist to explain how a weighted blanket could help a person feel calmer would reveal the frames of reference guiding their actions. This is because different frames of reference adopt distinct and diverse terminologies. Similarly, the words that people use to talk about their direct experience of mental health problems would reveal their expertise and/or lay knowledge (Rogers and Pilgrim 2014; Rose 2017). In Chapter 2 there is further discussion about different forms of knowledge, how they are valued and the implications for advancing knowledge (see also Chapter 11).

Ashby et al. (2017) suggested that most frames of reference are not exclusive to one profession and that their influence can be revealed through discussion in team meetings and supervision sessions. Identifying the frames of reference used in a team can help bridge conflicting views for the benefit of the people using services. When frames of reference are shared with people engaging with occupational therapy, the therapist's

thinking is revealed to inform and broaden the process of goal setting. For example, Charlie is struggling with the prospect of returning to work and agrees to try a staged approach with a cognitive-behavioural frame of reference (Ikiugu 2007). The occupational therapist, Tai, could explain how learning new thinking skills (cognition) could support Charlie's efforts to gradually regain work habits (behaviours), with careful professional reasoning and therapeutic use of self (see Chapter 3).

Table 4.1 has been developed using a practice example and seven alternative frames of reference (other frames of reference used by occupational therapists are discussed in relevant chapters). Principles, as guidelines for practice, are summarized briefly, alongside suggested questions about the example for reflection in and on action (see Chapter 3).

Some of these frames of reference draw on psychological theories and concepts (see Chapter 2). Ashby et al. (2017) suggested there was team pressure for occupational therapists to align with service aims by delivering psychological therapies. It is helpful to recognize that these therapies share frames of reference, such as cognitive-behaviourism, which can be used in occupational therapy without compromising occupation-centred practice, which is discussed later in this chapter (Ashby et al. 2017). When an occupational therapist is able to recognize different frames of reference, they can also think about how therapeutic activities can be used in different ways to achieve the same outcome (see Chapter 6). For example, relaxation training is often understood within a cognitive-behavioural frame of reference but African drumming, using a sensory-motor frame of reference, can be used as an alternative to progressive muscle relaxation or visual techniques with similar positive effects (Plastow et al. 2018).

Practice Frameworks

Like a retail or business district in a neighbourhood, practice frameworks define the nature and scope of occupational therapy. They are used to explain what occupational therapists do for those funding and approving services and for pre-registration education. Models are sometimes used within the frameworks as visual explanations. Practice frameworks that detail the principles, theories and procedures of occupational therapy include:

- AOTA's Occupational Therapy Practice Framework (OTPF) (American Occupational Therapy Association 2020)
- Canadian Association of Occupational Therapist's (CAOT 2012) profile of practice of occupational therapists in Canada (https://caot.ca/document/3653/2012otprofile.pdf).

The terms models and frameworks are sometimes used interchangeably. For example, the multi-professional International Classification of Function (World Health Organization (WHO) 2018) is described as both a model and a framework (https://www.cdc.gov/nchs/data/icd/icfoverview_finalforwho10sept.pdf). The Do Live Well Framework (Moll et al. 2015) has a diagram modelling the dynamic relations between key components of the framework. While there is not an international practice framework for occupational therapy, the World Federation of Occupational Therapists (WFOT; 2017) sets out minimum standards for pre-registration education, suggesting a common purpose, direction and scope for occupational therapy.

Not all frameworks are primarily practice frameworks: the European Conceptual Framework (Creek 2010) is a descriptive theory used by occupational therapists to understand the precise meanings and relationships of the terms applied in practice (see Chapter 2).

SCOPE OF OCCUPATIONAL THERAPY

Exploring boundaries for occupational therapy indicates the scope and limits for practice. Boundaries, like fences in a neighbourhood, can be points of contact and dialogue with different structures and grounds for practice. In this section the scope of occupational therapy is discussed in relation to occupation-centred practice, recovery-oriented practice, generic and specialist practice and dimensions of occupational therapy

Occupation-Centred Practice

Occupation-centred practice involves thinking and reasoning about occupation throughout the therapeutic process. Taking this worldview is a powerful means of orientating practice, like a compass always pointing north (Fisher 2013). Occupation-centred practice is focused on gathering information from people about their occupational performance: how it is shaped by their environments and their capacities to meet the demands of occupations (Hocking 2009). For example, the occupational forms and functions of shopping suggest varied environments and demands; between ordering online, driving to a large supermarket or walking to a smaller shop. Assessing capacities to meet the demands of shopping could consider different activities, such as making a shopping list, choosing items or paying for them. Or it could involve assessment of occupational performance components, such as motivation or cognition; for example, being able to locate and recognize items in shops.

Distinguishing between occupation-as-ends and occupation-as-means is another aspect of occupation-centred practice:

- occupation-as-ends refers to when the goal of therapy is to perform a specific occupation relevant to a person's situation and life roles (Trombly 1995);
- occupation-as-means refers to the use of therapeutic occupations that are designed, adapted and practised to develop specific capacities and skills (Gray 1998).

Reaching goals does not always involve occupation-as-means. For example, a call alarm could be recommended to support independent living: some minor adaptation may be required to ensure the person can use, it but being able to summon help independently is the goal of therapy rather than the means (Trombly 1995). Choosing occupations-as-means takes into account an end goal but may not be overtly related to it. Outdoor prescription (2019) describes how an occupational therapist enabled a service user to engage in pottery by adapting the task, with immediate benefits, in contrast to other activities which seemed too difficult or pointless. Critical to using occupation-as-means is that the activities, tasks and skills have a point and are achievable, satisfying and relevant to the person (Gray 1998). Therefore occupation-centred practice is defined by a clear purpose for occupational engagement, signalling occupation as ends. The importance of occupation-as-means is indicated by how activities are not simply chosen for convenience because they are readily available (Box 4.2).

Csikszentmihalyi's (1997) concept of flow offers another way of understanding the purpose and benefits of occupation-as-means and is indicated when people are completely immersed in an activity for its own sake. Flow occurs when the level of challenge in the activity matches people's skill level, a just-right challenge, so they lose track of time and escape from other preoccupying thoughts and feelings. To create this just-right challenge, occupational therapists use a range of strategies including activity analysis and adaptation (Rebeiro and Polgar 1999; see also Chapter 6). Experiences of enjoyment, achievement and competence associated with flow can benefit people with mental health problems, as indicated in the study by Hollands et al. (2015) of the benefits of the Maori performing arts, Kapa Haka, and sensory modulation (see also Chapters 6, 16 and 19).

Recovery

Internationally, many mental health services focus on personal recovery in which people adapt to their mental health problems and focus on how they would like to live their lives in contrast to clinical recovery in which a person is cured (Leamy et al. 2018). Using a positive psychology frame of reference, recovery-oriented practice requires staff, including occupational therapists, to work in close partnership with people using mental health services, holding on to hope for

> **BOX 4.2**
> **SLEEP**
>
> For people with mental health problems, sleep is often an issue: difficulty in getting to sleep or staying asleep (Ho and Siu 2018). Medication may be offered by a doctor, working to a biomedical frame of reference. Strategies to challenge intrusive thoughts might be utilized by many professionals, working to a cognitive-behavioural frame of reference (see Table 4.1). Others might explore troubled dreams using a psychodynamic frame of reference. Sleep hygiene combines different environmental and behavioural strategies (Irish et al. 2015).
>
> Understanding the nature of sleep as an occupation offers direction for adapting routines and habits and giving coherence to strategies for sleep hygiene (Ho and Siu 2018). If good sleep habits are identified as both means and ends of therapy for a person, strategies and environmental changes are made more relevant with continual adaptation and interpretation (Creek 2010). For example, when discharge planning revealed concerns about sleep disturbance at home, an occupational therapist discovered that the person's upstairs bedroom was lit by lamp posts immediately outside the window, which had no curtains. Fixing up curtains to obscure the light was considered as much an integral part of discharge planning as food preparation and self-care, recognizing sleep as a necessary occupation for health and survival.

their future and focusing on how to improve the quality of diverse aspects of their lives (O'Hagan 2004). Many advocates of recovery describe it as an approach, rather than a model, to emphasize the required changes in thinking, doing and interacting for staff (Slade et al. 2008, 2014).

Recovery-oriented services can influence the focus of occupational therapy, especially as they have to prove their effectiveness by measuring outcomes. The CHIME framework was developed to define recovery processes for practice and research (Leamy et al. 2018, p. 449):

■ **C**onnectedness;
■ **H**ope and optimism about the future;
■ **I**dentity;
■ **M**eaning in life;
■ **E**mpowerment.

In the United Kingdom, Recovery Colleges have been widely established. These are services for people with mental health problems to learn about recovery using an educational approach. Instead of being patients or service users, they are students, and the people leading the recovery courses are known as tutors rather than therapists. This is important because the role of an educator is different to that of a therapist (Cameron et al. 2018; see Chapter 11 and 14). Direct experience of recovery is particularly valued as a resource for learning, therefore many tutors are peer workers.

The origins of the recovery movement are indicated in Fig. 4.4, where the shared historical roots with occupational therapy can be traced (Davidson et al. 2010; see Chapter 1). Recovery was initially proposed by a group of people in the United States with severe and enduring mental health problems. Many had observed that professionals could be more effective if they shifted their attention from symptoms to every aspect of living, because people became stuck in services that were not meeting their needs (O'Hagan 2004). This reorientation of staff and services is an ongoing challenge (Clarke et al. 2020; see Chapters 10 and 12).

Generic and Specialist Practice

In a multidisciplinary mental health team some aspects of the professional work are shared or generic. Other aspects are specialist and clearly defined, for example, some aspects of practice are statutory and can only be carried out by suitably qualified staff. Generic practice is based on knowledge about mental health, ill-health, procedures, approaches and other services. It is a pragmatic way of addressing the needs of service users efficiently. For occupational therapists working in statutory mental health services, generic roles such as care coordination in the United Kingdom could divert the profession away from occupation-centred practice (Pettican and Bryant 2007). Goh et al. (2019) took a broader view, recognizing opportunities, especially in non-statutory settings (see also Chapter 29).

While some distinctions can be drawn between generic and specialist practice by referring to what different staff do, the rationale behind what they do can reveal specialist knowledge: knowing how and why. Occupational therapists know how to optimize occupational performance through therapeutic occupation, so they do not address psychiatric symptoms with medication. However, they use knowledge of the effects of medication to understand the impact on occupational performance, such as knowing it can take weeks rather than hours for anti-depressant medication to have full benefits.

Occupations are often the focus of public health initiatives to promote mental health, such as Better Health in the United Kingdom (https://www.nhs.uk/better-health/) and WoW! (Western Cape on Wellness, https://www.westerncape.gov.za/westerncape-on-wellness/) in South Africa. Sports and arts organizations access public funding by indicating the benefits they bring for health and well-being but do not always specify what they achieve with marginalized groups such as people with severe mental health problems (Wilson et al. 2015; Long and Blanchini 2019).

From an occupational perspective, these public health initiatives originate in guidelines for living a healthy life, evidenced in the earliest written guides used by people in ancient societies, such as in Greece (Wilcock 2001). The initiatives recognize the

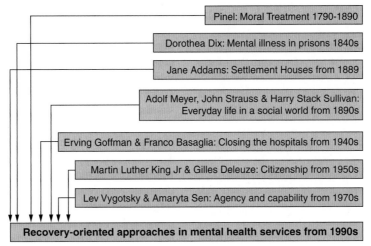

Fig. 4.4 ■ **The roots of recovery.**

significance of occupation for health but are not occupational therapy. The therapeutic nature of occupation can be appreciated by a person who feels better, calmer and transformed through occupational engagement. However the specialist knowledge providing direction for occupational therapy extends beyond this appreciation. Design and delivery of occupation-based therapeutic interventions are shaped by deep understanding and intentional use of occupation as means and ends (Health and Care Professions Council 2018). The example in Box 4.3 explores this in relation to yoga.

Knowing the scope of occupational therapy is part of professional accountability (see Chapter 7) and EBP (see later section). Smith and D'Amico (2019), for example, recommended that yoga could be used with people with Alzheimer's disease and other types of dementia, but it is significant that their review was based on sessions led by yoga teachers.

Dimensions of Occupational Therapy

Another way to understand the scope of occupational therapy is to consider the dimensions of the neighbourhood to map practice in different directions. Describing dimensions is to describe different aspects, or the size and scope, of something (Collins English Dictionary 2020).

For example, seeing a person as an occupational being was discussed in Chapter 2 using the dimensions of doing, being, becoming and belonging (Hitch and Pepin 2020). Similarly, investigating contexts at micro, meso and macro levels enables occupational therapists to step back for a wider perspective (Bailliard et al. 2020). Davis and Polatajko (2014) distinguished between the occupation (micro), the individual (meso) and the human race (macro), suggesting contexts for change in occupation over time. Alternatively, the experiences of children seeking asylum were explored by Trimboli (2017), who linked macro, micro and meso levels with the person-environment-occupation practice framework. Exploring dimensions of occupational therapy and occupation gives occupational therapists more choice about how to act as practitioners, researchers, scholars and educators. Dimensions indicate the scope of the grounds and structures for practice, like a map. While a clear map can guide occupational therapy as a journey, whether for a whole career or a person briefly engaging with it, the success of the journey depends on the effectiveness of practice.

THE ELEMENTS OF EFFECTIVE PRACTICE

This final section considers three elements of practice that ensure it is effective for the people who engage with occupational therapy and their families, carers and colleagues. These include EBP, use of the core skills of occupational therapy and how the therapist focuses the intervention to best meet the needs of the person.

Evidence-Based Practice

Evidence-based occupational therapy is a way of thinking and working in which decisions made during the occupational therapy process are based on the values and preferences of the person with the mental health problem, the expertise of the occupational therapist, and the best available research evidence. Each person has their own expertise in what it is like to live with their mental health problem, what services or techniques have worked well for them in the past and which approaches they have experienced as ineffective. They will also have a personal context for occupational participation, which will influence the decisions they make during the occupational therapy process. The occupational therapist has expertise based on their experience of working with this person and others with similar

---

BOX 4.3
SPECIALIST KNOWLEDGE AND YOGA

The specialist knowledge of occupational therapists overrides other areas of expertise they may have. For example, Lee may be a trained yoga teacher, but during time employed as an occupational therapist, the priority is to address occupational goals, not to teach the performance of yoga poses.

The therapy starts by identifying goals with Abi, who has multiple mental health issues associated with experiences of childhood abuse. Participation in yoga classes might be a goal or a means to achieving a different occupational goal, such as going back to college. Activities such as choosing appropriate clothing and planning the journey might be included. Lee draws on his specialist knowledge of motivational theory, cognitive processes, sensory processing and therapeutic use of self to build and maintain a relationship with Abi (D'Amico et al. 2018). Without identifying occupational goals, Abi's problems motivating or organizing herself mean she would struggle to establish the habit of attending a class and achieving her goals.

occupational performance issues. In healthcare, the emphasis in EBP is placed on research, including thinking critically about whether published research is valid, important and applicable to the person they are working with (see Chapters 2 and 5).

EBP is a process that is followed at different levels of service, from individual interventions to service design and review. It can be a collaborative process with a mental health service user when deciding on the best interventions to achieve the person's goals. An individual or a small group of occupational therapists may use evidence-based practice as a continuing professional development activity. At an organizational level, evidence-based practice can be used for staying up to date on the latest available evidence for assessments and treatments within regular service delivery, when planning a completely new service or when wanting to understand service user's experiences.

EBP has evolved across all health professions into a five-step process (Albarqouni et al. 2018).

Step 1: Developing a question. As a first step, the occupational therapist thinks about the details of the problem they want to address. When considering the effectiveness of an intervention, measured through specific outcomes, the thinking process could be structured by the acronym PICO:

- P - the person or people that engage with services;
- I - the assessment/intervention being considered;
- C – comparison with other assessments/interventions; and
- O - the desired outcome.

A more detailed acronym, PROGRESS-Plus, has been developed by the Cochrane Equity group to identify personal characteristics that may affect a person's opportunities for health and the outcomes of interventions (see https://methods.cochrane.org/equity/projects/evidence-equity/progress-plus). The occupational therapist uses each of the components in each acronym to develop a question that is specific to the needs of the particular person within their context.

For example, Na'ifah is a 55-year-old woman living in Cairo who developed depression after a stroke. One of the factors contributing to her high levels of stress is her perceived inability to prepare meals to the expected standard, so she would like to regain her cooking skills. The occupational therapist is unsure whether sessions would be more effective if done in her home or in the clinic. Table 4.2 presents how each of these elements is considered to develop a question for Na'ifah.

There are different approaches to developing an evidence-based question. A structure like PICO will

TABLE 4.2
Using PICO to Understand Na'ifah's Situation.

PICO Component	
Person	Place of residence - Cairo Race/ethnicity/culture/language - Egyptian Occupation - Homemaker Gender/Sex - Female Religion - Muslim Education - Primary school Socioeconomic status - Low income Social capital - Supportive husband Personal characteristics associated with discrimination - 55 years old, depression, stroke, moderate disability, being a woman Relationships - Lives with husband and parents-in-law
Intervention	Cooking at home
Comparison	Cooking in the clinic
Outcome	Cooking skill or other occupational performance measure
PICO Question	What is the effectiveness of a home-based cooking skills intervention in comparison to a clinic-based cooking skills intervention for a married Muslim woman aged 55 with low levels of education and low income with depression and stroke?

likely identify quantitative studies using a particular outcome measure. If a person's experiences, feelings or attitudes are of interest, an alternative acronym is SPIDER:

- S - Sample;
- P - Phenomenon of interest;
- D - Design;
- E - Evaluation; and
- R - Research type

Step 2: Gathering the best available evidence to answer the question. The three sources of evidence to consider when answering the question include the knowledge and experience of the person with the mental health problem, the occupational therapist's expertise and research evidence. To identify available research evidence, the therapist begins with the most recent clinical guidelines and then moves on to consider other sources of evidence in the hierarchy of research (Merlin et al. 2009). Clinical guidelines, which may or may not be occupational therapy specific, are available from a number of sources. Some sources that may be helpful for Na'fiah include:

- Government agencies, such as the UK National Institute for Health and Clinical Excellence (NICE); for example, NICE Guideline [CG 90] Depression in adults: recognition and management https://www.nice.org.uk/guidance/cg90;
- WHO; for example, the WHO Mental Health Gap Action Programme (MHGAP) provides guidelines for the development of mental health services in low resource settings using a task-shifting approach (see https://www.who.int/teams/mental-health-and-substance-use/mental-health-gap-action-programme);
- WFOT and national professional bodies, for example, the WFOT Position Statement: Occupational Therapy and Mental Health (file:///C:/Users/nap/Downloads/WFOT-Position-Statement-Occupational-Therapy-and-Mental-Health-2019.pdf).

Step 3: Systematic and critical appraisal of the evidence. Critical appraisal is not limited to assessing the quality of the research evidence. Occupational therapists also need to consider whether the evidence is contextually relevant, whether it will help the service user achieve their goals and how the evidence can be applied within the limits of available resources (see Chapter 2). For example, the occupational therapist working with Na'fiah may only be able to find evidence comparing home versus clinic interventions for developing skills with people with schizophrenia (Duncombe 2004) or the effectiveness of cooking interventions for people with psychosocial problems (Farmer et al. 2018).

Step 4: Applying the evidence to address the problem. Occupational therapists should summarize what they have found in response to their question and share this with the person, group or community. Then they work in partnership to decide on the best approach.

Step 5: Evaluation and revision of the prior steps in the process and identification of any areas of change for the future. This final step provides an opportunity for reflection (see Chapter 3) so that what has been learnt through this process becomes part of the therapists' best available evidence in similar situations.

Box 4.4 illustrates the ongoing process of EBP during the COVID-19 pandemic.

Core Skills

Effective practice is also dependent on occupational therapists being competent in using their core skills. The word 'skill' can be understood in two different ways (Collins English Dictionary 2020):

- An activity that is learned for a particular job, for example, how to write case records of occupational therapy. In a job application, a person might confirm they have skills in record-keeping, using particular tools;
- How well the job is done, for example, an occupational therapist could be skilled in listening and responding to people who are highly anxious and distracted. Being skilled in this situation means people feel heard, and that the session is occupation-centred and relevant to their goals.

Skills can be described by verbs, such as writing or listening, but need to be contextualized to be identified

BOX 4.4
EVIDENCE-BASED PRACTICE DURING COVID-19

The threat to survival from the COVID-19 pandemic has challenged health professionals and researchers to develop new guidance for evidence-based practice (EBP), covering issues such as rehabilitation for the effects of having been treated in intensive care (Cochrane Collaboration 2021). Kunzler et al. (2021) focused on the wider impact of the pandemic on mental health. They conducted a systematic review following the five steps of EBP (Albarqouni et al. 2018). This was a large-scale project involving a multidisciplinary team of 12 people, based in 7 different departments. However, the five steps were followed in the same way:

1. They asked about the impact on mental health for the general public, healthcare workers and people using health services, comparing it to how things were before the pandemic. They also aimed to identify protective factors and defined the impact in terms of psychological distress;
2. They decided to conduct a meta-analysis as well as a systematic review so that, in addition to gathering and appraising results from peer-reviewed papers, they also analysed all the data together to produce new results (Hanratty 2018);
3. Team members independently appraised each source to decide if it could be used. Then they used several methods of analysis to answer their questions;
4. They found that, in general, during the early stages people were more anxious and depressed by the COVID-19 pandemic than previous pandemics. Healthcare workers were less stressed than expected, which they suggested was due to being previously exposed to chronic stress. Protective factors were related to resilience, so they suggested public health measures should be focused not only on

resilience training, but also on understanding who should be targeted;
5. They identified that the majority of studies came from China and that experiences of older people were not fully investigated. Further research could reveal implications for particular groups of people and cultural considerations for public health interventions.

Before specific research findings about COVID-19 and mental health were published, the best available evidence came from first-hand accounts from the general public, healthcare workers and people using health services; relevant research into other health conditions or interventions (e.g., post-traumatic stress disorder (PTSD) is a recognized effect of being in intensive care); and the rapidly-developing expertise of frontline workers. Social media has played a critical role in the sharing of information internationally. At the same time, there was a resetting of research priorities, with funds being rapidly reallocated towards COVID-19 research and a significant push towards early publication of findings. New interventions emerged for different groups, for example:

- window therapy for older people living in care (https://hellocaremail.com.au/window-therapy-proving-laughter-best-medicine-lockdown/);
- digital resources to support mental health, including telerehabilitation (https://psycnet.apa.org/fulltext/2020-38975-001.pdf); and
- staff training in psychological personal protective equipment (Kitto and Bakhai 2020).

An ongoing concern during the pandemic has been to understand which interventions are effective and which are ineffective. Over time, further reviews will address this concern.

---

as core to occupational therapy. For example, writing case reports after therapy has ended or listening to vulnerable people explain their difficulties throughout the occupational therapy process. Creek (2014) described core skills as ways of thinking and acting which draw on techniques, knowledge and understanding that are specific to occupational therapy, regardless of the setting. These ways of thinking and acting are also influenced by professional beliefs and values (see Chapter 2).

Pre-registration occupational therapy programmes provide opportunities for students to learn core skills and then verify that they are competent to practice through assessment of their learning (Plastow and

Bester 2020; see Chapter 11). Competencies are 'behaviours, actions and abilities' which can be observed, giving insight into a therapist's skills and knowledge (Plastow and Bester 2020, p. 499). A distinction between skills and competencies is important when applying for posts, planning continuing professional development and managing feedback about performance. Gaps in skills and knowledge can be addressed with professional development activities, whereas a lack of competence may trigger a performance management process (Chapter 8).

Fig. 4.5 suggests four areas of core skills. It is informed by the findings of Wimpenny and Lewis's

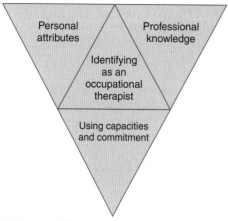

Fig. 4.5 ■ **Core skills.**

study (2015) from South African and UK occupational therapists who had recently graduated. They identified four areas of core skills in mental health settings:

- **Identifying as an occupational therapist** in two related senses: first, within an evolving individual relationship with the profession; second, while promoting an occupational therapy worldview on mental health in a multidisciplinary context;
- **Personal attributes and characteristics,** which influence career choice so that interest in the relationships between people, their occupations and their health is developed from the beginning of pre-registration education into professional beliefs and values (see Chapters 3 and 11). Plastow and Bester (2020) identified 10 graduate attributes important to occupational therapy including being culturally competent, occupation-based, and person-centred; valuing teamwork; understanding disability; and being clinically competent, able to advocate and work in diverse settings and committed to EBP.
- **Professional knowledge,** which Wimpenny and Lewis (2015) summarized as 'the principles of person-centred and holistic practice, the value of understanding mental health conditions, handling techniques, the contribution of occupational science and conceptual practice models, human development and equity and diversity studies' (p. 25). Continuing professional development can be focused on any of these areas to refine core skills for particular settings, for example, improving

---

BOX 4.5
CORE SKILLS IN PRACTICE

Dark (2019) explained how occupational therapy worked for her:

"But this particular occupational therapist took an interest in who I was and explored my future, passions and dreams. She noticed me as a person, not an illness, and invited me to take part in activities outside of the hospital walls. They included craft, dance, walking and going for coffee in town."

This extract offers a useful reference point for considering core skills. It could be assumed that anyone could have helped in this way, because the separate elements of Esther's experience do not suggest special techniques. However, the combination of these elements makes the difference, revealed here in Fig. 4.5. The occupational therapist's core skills, in actions, thoughts and communication, have been expressed with:

- *A distinct professional identity* enabling a competent and consistent focus on occupational performance, engagement and participation, building from when the occupational therapist 'noticed me as a person, not an illness'.
- *Being person-centred and occupation-based as personal attributes* means that people are valued as occupational beings (see Chapter 2), with Esther being invited to engage in occupations which enabled her personal recovery from mental health problems (see previous section).
- *Professional knowledge and understanding* that occupations can have many forms, functions and meanings (see Chapter 2) and that therapeutic activities can be used as an agent for change with thorough activity analysis and evidence-based practice (see Chapters 6, 13 and 19). In the blog, occupations ranged from being able to get out of bed to applying for an MSc.
- *Using capacity and commitment* to work alongside Esther to meet her goals beyond the hospital walls.

---

negotiation skills for working with people with learning disabilities and their carers.
- **Using capacities and commitment** to sustain practice and meet service demands. Core skills, such as being able to end a session (see Chapter 15) and communicate with team members concisely help occupational therapists to avoid becoming overwhelmed by the demand for their services.

In Box 4.5, these four areas of core skills are explored further, drawing on a blog by an occupational therapist with direct experience of engaging with services for her eating disorder (Dark 2019).

Although acquiring and refining core skills is important for developing from a novice to an expert occupational therapist (see Chapter 3), experts may feel their core skills are questioned or challenged in several different contexts:

- In collaborative approaches to providing services and advancing knowledge where diverse ways of knowing are valued, for example, in coproduction (see Chapter 2);
- In hierarchies of evidence where expert knowledge is seen as inferior to findings in published research, for example, in systematic reviews and randomized controlled trials (see Chapter 2);
- In political contexts where professional roles are devalued in preference to managerial roles, with downgrading of posts, increased surveillance, and monitoring through routine data collection (Clancy and Happell 2017; Worth 2018; Cain et al. 2020; Moth et al. 2020).

People engaging with services may also be marginalized by the second and third challenges, for example, when occupational therapy services are not commissioned because of an absence of randomized controlled trials or are reduced to balance the budget. Occupational therapists can respond by using their core skills to assert their professional knowledge and power. Focusing therapy is a key aspect of this response.

Approaches to Practice

Approaches to practice include the different ways occupational therapists think and act to ensure their work is effective. In Chapter 3 these different ways were discussed in detail and can be summarized as being shaped by:

- people's occupational performance, their needs and aspirations and their goals for therapy;
- the protocols, regulations and resources governing practice; and
- the occupational therapist's skills, knowledge and values.

Families, colleagues and others involved in occupational therapy also shape different approaches and are shaped by them. Earlier in this chapter, specific approaches were introduced (e.g., person-centred practice or recovery-oriented practice), and there are others in the remaining chapters of this book. This section covers four broad approaches which can enable people to achieve their goals in different ways.

Rehabilitative Approach

In a rehabilitative approach, the aim of occupational therapy is to restore skills or abilities that have been lost due to illness or injury (Molineux 2017). In mental health services, particularly in the United Kingdom, rehabilitation has been overshadowed by recovery-oriented approaches, although rehabilitation teams and units offer services to people with long-term mental health problems (Craig 2007; Dalton-Locke et al. 2021). An example of the rehabilitative approach is vocational rehabilitation in which there is a focus on skills for returning to paid employment (see Chapter 20).

Maintenance Approach

A maintenance approach aims to preserve occupational performance and/or quality of life for as long as possible, which includes skills and abilities gained with a rehabilitative approach (American Occupational Therapy Association 2020). Occupational therapists may work with people whose level of independence is expected to deteriorate as a result of their mental health condition to maintain their existing skills. For example, in dementia care, occupational therapists work with older people and their carers to maintain existing independent living skills for as long as possible (see Chapter 23).

Habilitative Approach

Habilitation is intervention to develop or attain age-appropriate skills for the first time. Some people have not had the opportunity or ability to develop age-appropriate skills needed for occupational performance. For example, a teenager with anxiety may not develop the skills needed to take the bus to school, because they are too anxious to travel alone. With such people, the occupational therapist might choose to adopt a habilitative approach.

Preventative Approach

For occupational therapists, a preventative approach aims 'to prevent the occurrence or evolution of barriers to performance in context' (American Occupational Therapy Association 2020, p. 64). People at risk of developing problems with occupational performance might include carers and those with existing health conditions (American Occupational Therapy Association 2020). For example, people with stroke have a significant risk of becoming depressed (approximately 30%) (Sarfo et al. 2017). The development of depression after stroke predicts greater levels of dependence and poorer rehabilitation outcomes. Similarly, occupational therapists working with children and young people with attention deficit hyperactivity disorder may offer interventions to prevent the development of secondary conduct, substance-related or addictive disorders.

Mental Health Promotion

Mental health promotion 'involves actions that support people to adopt and maintain healthy lifestyles and which create supportive living conditions or environments for health' (WHO 2004, p. 5). Increasing recognition of the impact of mental health and substance use problems on the global burden of disease (Rehm and Shield 2019) has enhanced opportunities for occupational therapists to work in mental health promotion. This approach focuses on promoting mental well-being through occupational participation. This is achieved by helping people develop their own strategies for well-being or by creating opportunities for participation in occupations that promote mental well-being in a specific population or group of people. Examples of these occupations include play (see Chapter 17), learning (see Chapter 14) and connecting with nature (see Chapter 19).

Occupational therapists working within mental health services need to think critically about the approach or approaches they use to ensure their services meet a range of needs. Although the main focus of a service may be on rehabilitation, maintenance or the development of new skills (habilitation), there may be also be opportunities for prevention and mental health promotion. Those occupational therapists who work outside of mental health services also have opportunities to prevent the development of mental health problems and/or promote positive mental health (McNulty 2021). For example, those working in care homes can help to prevent the development of depression by facilitating the transition of new residents into care (American Occupational Therapy Association 2020). Occupational therapists working with at-risk youth have a role to play in promoting the emotional resilience and coping skills that will help young people to thrive.

SUMMARY

In this chapter, structures for occupational therapy practice have been considered, with particular reference to people with occupational performance issues arising from mental health problems. All health and care professionals aim to put the person at the centre of their work, although occupational therapists bring multiple understandings of occupational performance to shape their approach to person-centred practice. Similarly, a logical process of engaging and working with people underpins much professional work, but effective occupational therapy practice starts with careful assessment and framing of occupational performance problems that guide the intervention. Gaining expertise in using a range of structures for practice includes learning and using terminology associated with different models, frames of reference and practice frameworks so that the occupational therapist can explain what is happening and why. Effectiveness is promoted by engaging with relevant and emerging evidence, maintaining core skills and being clear about the approach being used.

The process of understanding occupational therapy is continually changing; this is reflected in the statutory requirement to engage in continuing professional development, which ensures that occupational therapists structure their practice by maintaining and advancing professional, ethical and effective approaches to practice. These approaches are relevant to every aspect of occupation-centred practice to address mental health issues. Different contexts and settings shape approaches further and so the remaining chapters in this book offer further insight into specific areas of practice.

QUESTIONS FOR CONSIDERATION

1. Compare the characteristics of person-centred practice versus an occupation-centred approach.
2. How would you describe the way occupational therapy may be of benefit to a new service user?
3. Evaluate the practice model(s) used in your service by considering strengths and limitations. What other practice models would complement the model(s) that organizes your practice?
4. Choose two frames of reference from Table 4.1. Identify key principles for these frames of reference using the table and further reading.
5. Suggest a way in which the research project in Box 4.4 could be extended and how you might go about it.
6. Analyse your own core skills within each of the identifying areas from Figure 4.5. How might you develop these skills?

REFERENCES

Albarqouni, L., Hoffmann T., Straus S., et al. (2018). Core competencies in evidence-based practice for health professionals: Consensus statement based on a systematic review and delphi survey. *Journal of the American Medical Association Network Open*, 1(2). https://doi.org/10.1001/jamanetworkopen.2018.0281. e180281.

American Occupational Therapy Association. (2020). *Occupational Therapy Practice Framework: Domain and Process, 4th Edition*. [Bethesda, MD]: AOTA Press.

Arblaster, K., Mackenzie, L., Gill, K., Willis, K., & Matthews, L. (2019). Capabilities for recovery-oriented practice in mental health occupational therapy: A thematic analysis of lived experience perspectives. *British Journal of Occupational Therapy*, 82(11), 675–684.

Ashby, S., Gray, M., Ryan, S., & James, C. (2017). An exploratory study into the application of psychological theories and therapies in Australian mental health occupational therapy practice: Challenges to occupation–based practice. *Australian Occupational Therapy Journal*, 64(1), 24–32.

Bailliard, A. L., Aaron, R., Dallman, A. C., Ben, D. L., & Szendrey, S. (2020). Doing occupational justice: A central dimension of everyday occupational therapy practice. *Canadian Journal of Occupational Therapy*, 87(2), 144–152.

Cain, C. L., Taborda, C., & Frazer, M. (2020). Creating "risky" new roles in healthcare: Identities, boundary-making, and skilling under rationalization and consumer demand. *Work and Occupations*, 1. https://doi.org/10.1177/0730888420983396.

Cameron, J., Hart, A., Brooker, S., Neale, P., & Reardon, M. (2018). Collaboration in the design and delivery of a mental health recovery college course: Experiences of students and tutors. *Journal of Mental Health*, 27(4), 374–381.

Capra, F. (2002). *The Hidden Connections*. London: Flamingo.

Clancy, L., & Happell, B. (2017). Being accountable or filling in forms: Managers and clinicians' views about communicating risk. *Perspectives in Psychiatric Care*, 53(1), 38–46.

Clarke, E., Leamy, M., Bird, V., et al. (2020). Staff experiences of the REFOCUS intervention to support recovery in mental health: A qualitative study nested within a cluster randomized controlled trial. *Archives of Psychiatry and Mental Health*, 4, 024–032.

Cochrane Library. (2021). *Cochrane special collections*. Coronavirus (COVID-19): evidence relevant to clinical rehabilitation. Available at: https://www.cochranelibrary.com/collections/doi/SC000047/full.

Collins English Dictionary, 2020. Available at: https://www.collinsdictionary.com/dictionary/english/reflection.

Craig, T. (2007). What is psychiatric rehabilitation? In G. Roberts, S. Davenport, F. Holloway, & T. Tattan (Eds.), *Enabling recovery. The principles and practice of rehabilitation psychiatry*. 3–17. London: Royal College of Psychiatrists.

Creek, J. (2010). *The Core concepts of occupational therapy. A dynamic framework for practice*. London: Jessica Kingsley.

Creek, J. (2014). The knowledge base of occupational therapy. In W. Bryant, J. Fieldhouse, & K. Bannigan (Eds.), *Occupational therapy and mental health* (5th ed.). 27–48, London: Elsevier.

Csikszentmihalyi, M. (1997). *Flow and the psychology of discovery and invention*. New York: HarperPerennial.

Dalton-Locke, C., Marston, L., McPherson, P., & Killaspy, H. (2021). The effectiveness of mental health rehabilitation services: A systematic review and narrative synthesis. *Frontiers in Psychiatry*, 11 607933.

D'Amico, M. L., Jaffe, L. E., & Gardner, J. A. (2018). Evidence for interventions to improve and maintain occupational performance and participation for people with serious mental illness: A systematic review. *American Journal of Occupational Therapy*, 72 7205190020.

Dark, E. (2019). *My occupational therapist gave me hope when I had none. That's why I became one*. The Guardian. Thursday 7th November 2019. Available at: https://www.theguardian.com/society/2019/nov/07/occupational-therapist-gave-hope-mental-health.

Davidson, L., Rekfeldt, J., & Strauss, J. (2010). *The roots of the recovery movement in psychiatry. Lessons learned*. Oxford: Wiley Blackwell.

Davis, J., & Polatajko, H. (2014). Occupational development. In C. Christiansen, & E. Townsend (Eds.), *Introduction to occupation: The art of science and living* (2nd ed.). New York: Pearson Education.

Duncombe, L. W. (2004). Comparing learning of cooking in home and clinic for people with schizophrenia. *American Journal of Occupational Therapy*, 58(3), 272–278. https://doi.org/10.5014/ajot.58.3.272.

Dunn, W., Brown, C., & McGuigan, A. (1994). The ecology of human performance: A framework for considering the effect of context. *American Journal of Occupational Therapy*, 48(7), 595–607.

Eron, K., Kohnert, L., Watters, A., Logan, C., Weisner-Rose, M., & Mehler, P. S. (2020). Weighted blanket use: A systematic review. *American Journal of Occupational Therapy*, 74(2), 1–14.

Farmer, N., Touchton-Leonard, K., & Ross, A. (2018). Psychosocial benefits of cooking interventions: A systematic review. *Health Education & Behavior*, 167–180. https://doi.org/10.1177/1090198117736352.

Fish, D., & Boniface, G. (2012). Reconfiguring professional thinking and conduct: A challenge for occupational therapists in practice. In G. Boniface, & A. Seymour (Eds.), *Using occupational therapy theory in practice*. Chichester: Wiley-Blackwell.

Fisher, A. G. (2013). Occupation-focused: Same, same or different. *Scandinavian Journal of Occupational Therapy*, 20(3), 162–173. https://doi.org/10.3109/11038128.2012.754492.

Fulford, B. (2020). Values-based practice and patient engagement. Linking science with people. In A. Hadler, S. Sutton, & L. Osterberg (Eds.), *The wiley handbook of healthcare treatment engagement. Theory, research and clinical practice*. Chichester: Wiley Blackwell.

Goh, N. C. K., Hancock, N., Honey, A., & Scanlan, J. N. (2019). Thriving in an expanding service landscape: Experiences of occupational therapists working in generic mental health roles within non-government organisations in Australia. *Australian Occupational Therapy Journal*, 66(6), 753–762.

Gray, J. M. (1998). Putting occupation into practice: Occupation as ends, occupation as means. *American Journal of Occupational Therapy*, 52(5), 354–364. https://doi.org/10.5014/ajot.52.5.354.

Hanratty, J. (2018). *What is the difference between a systematic review and a meta-analysis? Campbell collaboration UK and Ireland*. Available at: http://meta-evidence.co.uk/difference-systematic-review-meta-analysis/.

Health Education England. (2017). *The NHS constitution*. Available at: https://www.hee.nhs.uk/about/our-values.

Health Foundation. (2016). *Person-centred care made simple. What everyone should know about person-centred care*. London: The Health Foundation.

Health and Care Professions Council. (2018). *Professions and protected titles*. Available at: https://www.hcpc-uk.org/about-us/who-we-regulate/the-professions/.

Hinojosa, J. (2017). How society's philosophy has shaped occupational therapy practice for the past 100 years. *Open Journal of Occupational Therapy*, 5(2).

Hitch, D., & Pepin, G. (2020). Doing, being, becoming and belonging at the heart of occupational therapy: An analysis of theoretical ways of knowing. *Scandinavian Journal of Occupational Therapy*. https://doi.org/10.1080/11038128.2020.1726454.

Hitch, D., Pepin, G., & Stagnitti, K. (2018). The pan occupational paradigm: Development and key concepts. *Scandinavian Journal of Occupational Therapy*, 25(1), 27–34.

Hocking, C. (2009). The challenge of occupation: Describing the things people do. *Journal of Occupational Science*, 16(3), 140–150.

Hollands, T., Sutton, D., Wright-St Clair, V., & Hall, R. (2015). Māori mental health consumers' sensory experience of Kapa Haka and its utility to occupational therapy practice. *New Zealand Journal of Occupational Therapy*, 62(1), 3–11.

Ho, E. C. M., & Siu, A. M. H. (2018). Occupational therapy practice in sleep management: A review of conceptual models and research evidence. *Occupational Therapy International*. https://doi.org/10.1155/2018/8637498. 2018 (8637498).

Ikiugu, M. (2007). *Psychosocial conceptual practice models in occupational therapy*. St Louis Missouri: Mosby Elsevier.

Ikiugu, M. N., Plastow, N. A., & van Niekerk, L. (2019). Eclectic application of theoretical models in occupational therapy: Impact on therapeutic reasoning. *Occupational Therapy in Health Care*, 33(3). https://doi.org/10.1080/07380577.2019.1630884.

Irish, L. A., Kline, C. E., Gunn, H. E., Buysse, D. J., & Hall, M. H. (2015). The role of sleep hygiene in promoting public health: A review of empirical evidence. *Sleep Medicine Reviews*, 22, 23–36. https://doi.org/10.1016/j.smrv.2014.10.001.

Kielhofner, G. (2009). *Conceptual foundations of occupational therapy practice* (4th ed.). Philadelphia: F.A. Davis Company.

Kitto, C., & Bakhai, K. (2020). Psychological PPE—the space between signposting and action. *British Medical Journal Opinion*. Available at: https://blogs.bmj.com/bmj/2020/08/14/psychological-ppe-the-space-between-signposting-and-action/?utm_source=feedburner&utm_medium=feed&utm_campaign=Feed%3A+bmj%2Fblogs+%28Latest+BMJ+blogs%29.

Kunzler, A. M., Röthke, N., Günthner, L., et al. (2021). Mental burden and its risk and protective factors during the early phase of the SARS-CoV-2 pandemic: Systematic review and meta-analyses. *Global Health*, 17(1), 34.

Law, M., & Laver-Fawcett, A. (2013). Canadian model of occupational performance: 30 years of impact!. *British Journal of Occupational Therapy*, 76(2). https://doi.org/10.4276/030802213X13861576675123. 519–519.

Lazzarini, I. (2016). Nonlinear reasoning in cognition: Restoring the essence of the occupational therapy process. In M. B. Cole, & J. Creek (Eds.), *Global perspectives in professional reasoning* (pp. 183–202). Thorofare, NJ: SLACK Incorporated.

Long, J., & Bianchini, F. (2019). New directions in the arts and sport? Critiquing national strategies. *Sport in Society*, 22(5), 734–753. https://doi.org/10.1080/17430437.2018.1430484.

Lopes, R. E., & Malfitano, A. P. S. (2017). Social occupational therapy, citizenship, rights, and policies: Connecting the voices of collectives and individuals. In D. Sakellariou, & N. Pollard (Eds.), *Occupational therapies without borders* (2nd ed.) (pp. 245–254). Edinburgh: Elsevier.

Machtinger, E. L., Davis, K. B., Kimberg, L. S., et al. (2019). From treatment to healing: Inquiry and response to recent and past trauma in adult health care. *Women's Health Issues*, 29(2), 97–102. Available at: https://www.whijournal.com/article/S1049-3867(18)30550-4/fulltext.

McNulty, C. (2021). *Being a feral occupational therapist*. World Federation of Occupational Therapists Bulletin. https://doi.org/10.1080/14473828.2021.1888405.

Merlin, T., Weston, A., & Tooher, R. (2009). Extending an evidence hierarchy to include topics other than treatment: Revising the Australian "levels of evidence". *BMC Medical Research Methodology*, 9(1), 1–8. https://doi.org/10.1186/1471-2288-9-34.

Molineux, M. (2017). *Oxford dictionary of occupational science and occupational therapy*. Oxford: Oxford University Press.

Moll, S.E., Gewurtz, R.E., Krupa, T.M., Law, M.C., Larivière, N. & Levasseur, M. (2015). Do-live-well": A Canadian framework for promoting occupation, health, and well-being. *Canadian Journal of Occupational Therapy / Revue Canadienne D'Ergothérapie*, 82(1), 9–23. https://doi.org/10.1177/0008417414545981.

Mori, A. B., Champagne, T., & May-Benson, T. A. (2017). *Occupational therapy using a sensory integration–based approach with adult populations. American occupational therapy association*. Available at: https://www.aota.org/~/media/Corporate/Files/AboutOT/Professionals/WhatIsOT/PA/Facts/SI-and-Adults-Fact-Sheet.pdf.

Mosey, A. C. (1989). The proper focus of scientific inquiry in occupational therapy: Frames of reference. *OTJR (Thorofare N J)*, 9(4), 195–201.

Moth, R., Thomas, P., McArdle, L., & Saundry, R. (2020). The business end": Neoliberal policy reforms and biomedical residualism in frontline community mental health practice in England. *Competition and Change*, 24(2), 133–153.

Nicholls, L., Cunningham, P. J., de Sena Gibertoni, C., & Daniel, M. (Eds.). (2013). *Psychoanalytic thinking in occupational therapy: Symbolic, relational and transformative*. Chichester: John Wiley and Sons Ltd.

O'Hagan, M. (2004). Guest Editorial. *Australian e-Journal for the Advancement of Mental Health*, 3(1), 5–7. https://doi.org/10.5172/jamh.3.1.5.

Occupational Therapy Association of South Africa (OTASA). (2015). OTASA Position statement on therapeutic group work in occupational therapy | Council | South African Journal of Occupational Therapy. *South African Journal of Occupational Therapy*, 44(3), 43–44. Available at: https://www.sajot.co.za/index.php/sajot/article/view/318/170.

Outdoorprescription. (2019). *Occupational therapy in mental health treatment*. Available at: https://outdoorprescription.wordpress.com/2019/07/11/occupational-therapy/.

Paxson, D., Tobey, T., Johnston, S., Winston, K. & Iwama, M. (2012). The Kawa model: Therapists' experiences in mental health practice. *Occupational Therapy in Mental Health*, 28(4), 340–355. https://doi.org/10.1080/0164212X.2012.708586.

Pentland, D., Kantartzis, S., Clausen, M. G., & Witemyre, K. (2018). *Occupational therapy and complexity: Defining and describing practice*. London: Royal College of Occupational Therapists.

Pettican, A., & Bryant, W. (2007). Sustaining a focus on occupation in community mental health practice. *British Journal of Occupational Therapy*, 70(4), 140–146.

Plastow, N. A., & Bester, J. (2020). Embedding graduate attributes during occupational therapy curriculum development: A scoping review and qualitative research synthesis. *Australian Occupational Therapy Journal*, 67(5), 498–511.

Plastow, N. A., Joubert, L., Chotoo, Y., et al. (2018). The immediate effect of African drumming on the mental well-being of adults with mood disorders: An uncontrolled pretest--posttest pilot study. *American Journal of Occupational Therapy*, 72(5), 1–6.

Rebeiro, K. L., & Polgar, J. M. (1999). Enabling occupational performance: Optimal experiences in therapy. *Canadian Journal of Occupational Therapy*, 66(1), 14–22. https://doi.org/10.1177/000841749906600102.

Rehm, J., & Shield, K. D. (2019). Global burden of disease and the impact of mental and addictive disorders. *Current Psychiatry Reports*, 21, 10. https://doi.org/10.1007/s11920-019-0997-0.

Rethink Mental Illness. (2011). *Detention under the mental health act factsheet. Rethink mental illness*. London. Available at: http://www.rethink.org.

Robinson, K., Kennedy, N., & Harmon, D. (2012). Happiness: A review of evidence relevant to occupational science. *Journal of Occupational Science*, 19(2), 150–164. https://doi.org/10.1080/14427591.2011.634780.

Rogers, A., & Pilgrim, D. (2014). *A sociology of mental health and illness*. Maidenhead, England: Open University Press.

Rose, D. (2017). Service user/survivor-led research in mental health: Epistemological possibilities. *Disability & Society*, 32(6), 773–789. https://doi.org/10.1080/09687599.2017.1320270.

Royal College of Psychiatrists. (2015). *See think act* (2nd ed.). Royal College of Psychiatrists Quality Network for Forensic Mental Health Services. Available at: https://www.rcpsych.ac.uk/docs/default-source/improving-care/ccqi/quality-networks/secure-forensic/forensic-see-think-act-qnfmhs/sta_hndbk_2nded_web.pdf?sfvrsn=90e1fc26_4.

Sarfo, F. S., Jenkins C., Singh A. (2017). Post-stroke depression in Ghana: Characteristics and correlates. *Journal of the Neurological Sciences*, 379, 261–265. https://doi.org/10.1016/j.jns.2017.06.032.

Slade, M., Amering, M., Farkas, M., et al. (2014). Uses and abuses of recovery: Implementing recovery-oriented practices in mental health systems. *World Psychiatry*, 13(1), 12–20.

Slade, M., Amering, M., & Oades, L. (2008). Recovery: An international perspective. *Epidemiologia e Psichiatria Sociale*, 17(2), 128–137.

Sumsion, T. (1999). A study to determine a British occupational therapy definition of client-centred practice. *British Journal of Occupational Therapy*, 62(2), 52–58.

Taylor, R. R. (Ed.). (2017). *Kielhofner's model of human occupation: Theory and application*. Wolters Kluwer.

Trimboli, C. (2017). Occupational justice for asylum seeker and refugee children: Issues, effects and action. In D. Sakellariou, & N. Pollard (Eds.), *Occupational therapies without borders* (2nd ed.) (pp. 460–467). London: Elsevier.

Trombly, C. A. (1995). *Occupation: Purposefulness and meaningfulness as therapeutic mechanisms 1995 eleanor clarke slagle lecture*. Available at: http://aota.org/terms.

Warren, A. (2002). An evaluation of the Canadian model of occupational performance and the Canadian occupational performance measure in mental health practice. *British Journal of Occupational Therapy*, 65(11), 515–521.

Wilcock, A. (2001). *Occupation for Health: A journey from self health to prescription* (Vol. 1). London: College of Occupational Therapists.

Wilson, L., Bryant, W., Lawson, J., & Reynolds, F. (2015). Therapeutic outcomes in a museum? "You don't get them by aiming for them". How a focus on arts participation promotes citizenship and wellbeing. *Arts & Health, 7*(3), 202–215.

de Witt, P. (2014). Creative ability: A model for individual and group occupational therapy for clients with psychosocial dysfunction. In R. Crouch, & V. Alers (Eds.), *Occupational therapy in psychiatry and mental health* (pp. 3–32). Oxford: John Wiley & Sons, Ltd. https://doi.org/10.1002/9781118913536.ch1.

World Federation of Occupational Therapists (WFOT). (2017). *Minimum standards for the education of occupational therapists.* Available at: https://www.wfot.org/resources/new-minimum-standards-for-the-education-of-occupational-therapists-2016-e-copy.

World Health Organization (WHO). (2004). *Promoting mental health: Concepts, emerging evidence, practice: Summary report from the World Health Organization.* Department of Mental Health and Substance Abuse in collaboration with the Victorian Health Promotion Foundation (VicHealth) and The University of Melbourne. Available at: www.who.int/mental_health/evidence/en/promoting_mhh.pdf.

World Health Organization (WHO), 2018. International classification of functioning, disability and health (ICF), WHO. World health organization. Available at: http://www.who.int/classifications/icf/en/ (Accessed: 9 November 2018).

Worth, E. (2018). A tale of female liberation? The long shadow of de-professionalization on the lives of post-war women. *Revue Française de civilisation Britannique.* https://doi.org/10.4000/rfcb.1778.

5

ASSESSMENT AND OUTCOME MEASUREMENT

MARY BIRKEN

CHAPTER OUTLINE

INTRODUCTION

Assessment is a crucial stage of the occupational therapy process because it involves systematically identifying issues before addressing them. Careful consideration, of what areas to assess and which assessment methods and tools to use, ensures that interventions can be targeted at a person's priority areas and accurate recommendations can be reported. The contribution of occupational therapy, to meeting the person's goals and the aims of a service, is demonstrated by measuring outcomes. The outcome data can be collected using standardized measures to meet expectations set by many healthcare services to monitor quality and effectiveness. Clearly communicating findings and outcomes facilitates person-centred

practice and teamwork, as well as informs commissioners of health services. Therefore assessment and outcome measurement need to be conducted accurately and ethically to benefit people engaging with occupational therapy.

In this chapter, assessment and outcome measurement in occupational therapy and mental health are defined and described, followed by a discussion of the ethical considerations and contemporary challenges. Several different methods of assessment are explored. The difference between outcome measures and assessments is explained, with information about what makes a measure standardized. There are barriers to formal assessments and routine outcome measurements in practice. These are explored with observations about the implications for professional practice. The chapter concludes with a section on the process of collaborating with researchers to develop a standardized tool. This might happen when a suitable one does not exist to measure an aspect which is important for the people receiving occupational therapy, occupational therapists and service managers.

Assessment Defined

Assessment Involves Several Stages

> *"collecting, analysing and interpreting information about people's functions and environments, using observation, testing and measurement, in order to make intervention decisions and to monitor changes."*
>
> *Creek 2010 p.25*

Occupational therapists start an assessment by gathering information from different sources and discussing, with the person being assessed, what the information gathered could mean. Assessment involves building a relationship with them to understand their perspective and how their mental health problems impact their daily lives. Professional reasoning will guide what is assessed and explored further (see chapter 3).

There may be specific consequences of having a mental health problem that need to be considered during assessment. For example, a person may self-stigmatize or anticipate discrimination, affecting how they see their problems and the possibility for change. Along with the instability caused by mental health problems and multiple admissions, they may have lost friends and other social identities and struggle to maintain routines and habits. Therefore the assessment may take place over several sessions, using screening tools, observations, structured interviews, testing and measurement (Creek 2010).

Outcome Measurement Defined

In healthcare settings, an outcome can be defined as the observed or measured consequence of an intervention (Laver Fawcett 2007). Therefore outcome measurement has been defined as:

> *"the process undertaken to establish the effects of an intervention on an individual."*
>
> *Laver Fawcett 2007 p.12*

Clearly, deciding on the specific effects of the intervention to measure and when is important. Laver Fawcett (2007) goes on to say:

> *"Outcome measurement is achieved by administering an outcome measure on at least two occasions to document change over time in one or more trait, attribute or characteristic to establish whether that trait/attribute/characteristic has been influenced by the intervention to the anticipated degree to achieve the desired outcome."*
>
> *Laver Fawcett 2007, p. 12*

This definition indicates that careful choice of outcome measure ensures that meaningful change is detected following an intervention. By using outcome measures, occupational therapists also demonstrate whether the outcomes of their interventions meet the aims of the service being delivered. Managers, funders and those monitoring the quality of services require accurate information about the services being delivered and the outcomes for people using these services. This information is used to decide what to invest in and where to withdraw funding from, if required.

CONSIDERATIONS FOR PRACTICE

A range of factors influences assessment and outcome measurement, which can be summarized into three aspects to consider:

- the person being assessed,
- the therapist conducting the assessment,
- the service where the assessment is taking place.

Regular reflection on practice and in practice, alone and with colleagues, enables these different aspects to be considered carefully (see chapter 3). The World Federation of Occupational Therapists (WFOT) states that participation is the outcome of occupational therapy (WFOT 2012). Whilst measures of participation are not routinely used, aspects of participation can be measured. For example, changes in how people use their time can show a change in variety and time spent in occupations.

Participation can also be observed through the person's occupational performance and how they describe it. Therefore it is critical that occupational therapists assess and provide interventions focused on participation and occupational performance. Engagement in an occupation is also considered a key focus of occupational therapy (Wilcock 1993) and therefore will be assessed and monitored as an outcome in conjunction with occupational performance and participation. Participation, occupational performance and engagement are discussed further in Chapter 2.

The Person Being Assessed

Choices of assessment areas and outcome measures need to take account of the person engaging with occupational therapy, considering their cultural beliefs and values, symptoms and capacity to consent. A person's current life situation, for example, being a parent or a student, influences assessment choice. Symptoms and impairments associated with ill-health may also influence the assessment and outcome measurement process. The occupational therapist determines the impact of symptoms and impairments, whether this impact is likely to change and, if so, how and when.

The person may be too unwell to assess at the time of the referral, raising an ethical issue of consent. Considering a person's capacity to consent involves ensuring that they understand the aim of the assessment and what is involved, before deciding to give informed consent to take part. If the person is unable to consent because of cognitive impairment, consent from a relative or a person who knows the person can be obtained. Therefore occupational therapists identify and follow local procedures in line with legislation regarding a person's ability to consent. In the United Kingdom the Mental Capacity Act (Department of Health 2005) requires consent to be regularly confirmed during contact with healthcare services. Chapter 9 offers more information about ethics, including consent.

The Occupational Therapist

Knowledge, skills and professional reasoning guide assessment and interpretation of findings (see Chapters 2–4). Occupational therapists draw on knowledge of occupational performance, participation, mental health and the properties of a measure relating to reliability, validity and use, which is discussed in a section later in this chapter. Effective assessment requires communication and observation skills, gaining and interpreting information from interaction with the person, connecting with their skills, interests, abilities, motivation and mental health.

Using knowledge and skills in this way forms part of an occupational therapist's professional reasoning. For example, routine practice might involve using a questionnaire that people are required to complete. In that case, the occupational therapist will consider the procedure of completing the questionnaire (procedural reasoning), what they know about approaching and working with the person the person (interactive reasoning) and whether the questionnaire is directly relevant to this situation (conditional reasoning). These different ways of reasoning are discussed in detail in Chapter 3.

Building rapport and a therapeutic relationship are necessary for carrying out assessments and outcome measures. The Intentional Relationship Model sets out to explain the therapeutic relationship within occupational therapy practice (Taylor 2008). The description of this model includes guidance for self-assessment, with tools to enable occupational therapists to identify and draw on their relevant interpersonal skills to facilitate person-centred assessment and outcome measurement.

Barrier

One barrier to routine assessment and outcome measurement is limited time to use assessment tools, which may result in the occupational therapist never gaining familiarity with the tool over time (Asaba et al. 2017). However, workplace culture can have the biggest impact on the use of assessment tools (Asaba et al. 2017). Assessments are not always carried out routinely, and outcome measurement is even less frequently assessed in occupational therapy practice in community mental health settings (Birken et al. 2017; Rouleau et al. 2015). Barriers to using assessment tools in practice have also been identified (Asaba et al. 2017). In Canada, Rouleau and colleagues (2015) found that 68% of occupational therapists working with people with mental health problems reported using a standardized assessment. However, the rate of repeating assessments during the intervention (0%–26%) was low, indicating that the occupational therapists did not rigorously monitor progress during interventions (Rouleau et al. 2015). A study conducted in the United Kingdom found the 41% of community mental health occupational therapists surveyed did not measure the outcome of occupational therapy interventions (Birken et al. 2017).

The Service

Assessment and outcome measurement are influenced by the aims of the service, time constraints and financial resources to buy tools. Practice models used across a large service can influence which areas are assessed and which outcomes are measured. One barrier to routine assessment and outcome measurement was limited time to use assessment tools, which may result in the occupational therapist never gaining familiarity with the tool over time (Asaba et al. 2017). However, workplace culture had the biggest impact on the use of assessment tools (Asaba et al. 2017). For example, for people engaging with occupational therapy over long periods, such as those with learning difficulties or using forensic or rehabilitation services, the frequency and consistency of assessment and outcome measures need to be considered. Using the same valid and reliable assessments and outcome measurements will enable information to be shared and compared between services. Therefore it is best to reach an agreement between occupational therapy teams regarding which tools to use. This will reduce the need to complete the process again if a team member moves to a different service or department. Outcomes can be more reliably captured if the same measures are used in different but related settings.

Confidentiality policies may affect who can be approached to gather information from and who the findings can be shared with. In their induction programme, a new occupational therapist or student finds out what local policies are in place, especially for sharing information between services. Increasingly, local policies may specify that service users have to receive a copy of all letters about them.

Services evolve over time because of political and social changes, so occupational therapists review and revise which assessments and outcome measures are used regularly to address current expectations. At a national level, agreeing on a core set of outcome measures across all similar services could enable the routine collection of outcomes to contribute to national data collection, such as the NHS benchmarking services in the United Kingdom (NHS Benchmarking Network 2016). This would ensure the outcomes of occupational therapy are recognized as contributing to the outputs of services.

ASSESSMENT

The occupational therapy process is often described as linear, with assessment coming before planning and intervention phases (see Chapter 4). However, in practice, the occupational therapist often assesses during the intervention phase, for example, observing the person participate in an activity which also offers opportunities for continued assessment. In this situation, once the initial assessment is completed and goals are set with the person, it may become apparent that further detailed assessment is required to understand the person's occupational performance more fully. An example of this is observing motor or processing difficulties whilst carrying out an activity and then carrying out an Assessment of Motor and Process Skills (AMPS) (Fisher and Bray 2014) with the person.

The purpose of the assessment is determined by the reason for referral, the aims of the service and the context of the person being assessed. In some areas of practice, such as an inpatient rehabilitation unit, the occupational therapist is expected to assess everyone in the unit, deciding how to assess and when.

Assessment can use a *bottom-up* or a *top-down* approach (Fig. 5.1), with different implications for each in practice (Kramer et al. 2003). A bottom-up approach examines a person's skills or occupational performance components separately, for example, their capacity to maintain eye contact with the occupational therapist appropriately. In contrast, a top-down approach takes an overall perspective and focuses on the person's participation in their living contexts to determine what is important and relevant to them.

Top-down occupational therapy assessment has been conceptualized as a hierarchy, with the most significant aspect of occupation being the highest so that people can be assessed as occupational beings (Hocking 2001) (see Fig. 5.1). The meanings of occupations are at the top, and, below that are the functions or purposes of occupations in the individual's life. Then there are the forms that those occupations take, and, lastly, the occupational performance components. Meanings in this context are constructed by the person as a unique individual so that meaningful occupations reflect their identity rather than a positive psychological focus on what makes them happy. Hocking (2001) also offered an ethical perspective on the type of assessments carried out, checking that the person is not being put through unnecessary assessments, as illustrated in Box 5.1.

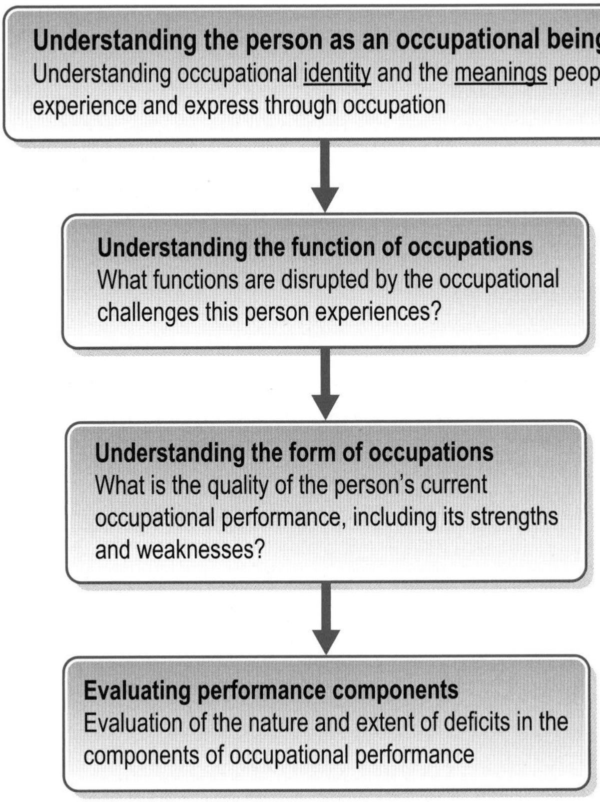

Understanding the person as an occupational being
Understanding occupational <u>identity</u> and the <u>meanings</u> people experience and express through occupation

↓

Understanding the function of occupations
What functions are disrupted by the occupational challenges this person experiences?

↓

Understanding the form of occupations
What is the quality of the person's current occupational performance, including its strengths and weaknesses?

↓

Evaluating performance components
Evaluation of the nature and extent of deficits in the components of occupational performance

Fig. 5.1 ■ Top-down occupational therapy assessment process conceptualized by Hocking (2001).

BOX 5.1
DAN COOKS A MEAL

Dan was preparing to move from an acute unit to a rehabilitation hostel whilst emerging from a serious episode of psychosis. During the initial assessment, he identified that cooking for himself was one of his strengths, and he was keen to reconnect with this strength to prepare for the transition. He proposed cooking a simple meal and identified the ingredients without prompting in the early stages of planning. The occupational therapist, Sam, knew from previous informal contact and the initial assessment that Dan's concentration was much improved, so assessment of occupational performance components such as concentration related to food preparation was not necessary. It would be unethical to delay Dan's move for an unnecessary assessment. Once Dan had eaten his meal, they discussed other aspects of the transition that might require further assessment.

Initial Assessment/Screening

The first stage is an initial assessment, which is sometimes called a screening assessment. This involves finding out if the person:

- is ready and willing to engage with occupational therapy,
- has occupational needs that can be addressed within the service,
- is in a situation where further assessment of occupational needs is feasible, necessary and appropriate.

This approach also ensures the best use of an occupational therapist's time so that, following an initial assessment, they can prioritize and decide which more detailed assessments are urgent and which cases do not require a more detailed assessment. A generic screening assessment may be undertaken by a duty worker in some settings, which provides a basis for the first contact between the occupational therapist and the person. The occupational therapist obtains general information about the person and their situation where this does not happen.

Before engaging in the initial assessment, the occupational therapist considers how to approach the person to ensure this part of the occupational therapy process is person-centred and therapeutic (see chapter 3 and 4). Thoughtfully and decisively drawing on interpersonal skills, such as those described by Taylor (2008) in the Intentional Relationship Model, will enable a therapeutic relationship to develop. This applies whether the occupational therapist first approaches in person or via a telephone call or video link.

In many inpatient and residential settings, the initial assessment may not occur when first meeting the person, as it can take time to build up the relationship and trust. The person may need to get to know the occupational therapist and gain an understanding of their role before discussing how occupational therapy could help them. An example is when the person is new to the service or is acutely unwell on a mental health inpatient unit. Whilst the occupational therapist can build rapport with the person, an initial assessment may be delayed until this can be jointly agreed upon. During this time, the occupational therapist will informally assess the person and their situation using their interpersonal and observational skills to gather information.

The form and structure of the initial assessment will vary between settings. If there is access to standardized assessment tools, the following examples could be used:

- The model of human occupation screening tool (MOHOST) (Parkinson et al. 2006)
- Occupational therapy circumstances assessment and rating scale (OCAIRS) (Forsythe et al. 2005)
- Occupational performance history interview II (OPHI-II (Kielhofner et al. 2004)
- Occupational Self-Assessment (Baron et al. 2006).

Assessment Methods

If the findings of the initial assessment indicate occupational needs that can be addressed, a more detailed assessment is used to gather information to inform goals and interventions, using a variety of assessment tools and methods. At this stage, specific outcome measures should also be identified as the selected assessments may not be suitable for measuring the outcome of the interventions. Assessments that do not provide a baseline score for occupational performance in specific areas will not have scope to capture later changes for comparison.

A range of methods are used by occupational therapists to complete a comprehensive assessment, as

---

BOX 5.2
HANNAH SEEKS A JOB

Hannah was a young woman supported by a community mental health team, who agreed with her occupational therapist, Kim, that the focus of the assessment was how Hannah performed the occupation of job seeking. This involved considering multiple aspects of her occupational performance, including exploring what jobs appealed most to her, identifying where to search for them, completing application forms, remembering to attend interviews and dressing appropriately. Hannah's participation in any of the activities relating to job seeking could be identified as outcomes and measured accordingly. Therefore the assessment might cover typical areas such as self-care, productivity and leisure, although Creek (2010) emphasizes that defining these areas varies between different theories and may be useful for the occupational therapist but not for the person being assessed.

BOX 5.3
ROSEMARY FINDS IT HARD TO LEAVE HOME

Rosemary was referred to occupational therapy following referral to a community mental health team by her GP. She had been diagnosed with late-onset schizophrenia and experienced paranoia, which had affected her occupational performance and participation in many valued aspects of life. She had become preoccupied with her thoughts and lost track of her usual routines and activities. The occupational therapist, Al, initially met Rosemary at the community mental health centre but agreed to meet her at her home next time, as Rosemary found it difficult to leave home because of her paranoid thoughts. At her home, the Occupational Therapy Circumstances Assessment and Rating Scale was used as a detailed assessment to identify areas of occupation that mattered to her that she had stopped doing. When walking together in her neighbourhood, Rosemary pointed out places she used to go and bus routes she used to take. This included a bus route to her church. This, along with observing religious items in her home, prompted Al to ask more. Rosemary identified that participating in religious activities was very important to her and could be a focus for intervention.

---

illustrated by the case stories in Boxes 5.2 and 5.3. Most often, the first method involves gathering information by discussing the need for occupational therapy with colleagues or those making the referral and reviewing clinical records. Following this, assessment methods such as interviewing the person and observing them in different situations are helpful in specific mental health settings. The occupational therapist could ask the person to complete a questionnaire, which is a self-report method to gather information in a structured way.

Standardized interview tools also offer a clear structure, such as the OCAIRS (Forsythe et al. 2005) or the OPHI-II, if they have not already been used in the initial assessment. A comprehensive assessment will give priority to hearing the person's perspective on their past, present and future occupational selves to help understand the impact of their mental health problems.

Observational tools such as AMPS (Fisher and Bray 2014) involve a detailed assessment of a person's performance of an everyday task. This is useful when a person is unaware of their difficulties or is struggling to articulate them. An assessment of a person's home environment gives the occupational therapist insight into the barriers to occupational performance. An example of such an observational assessment is the Residential Environment Impact Scale- Short Form (REIS-SF) (Parkinson et al. 2011).

Areas of Assessment

Mental health problems can impact multiple aspects of a person's life, so occupational therapists carefully consider what to assess and when. Using an occupational therapy theoretical framework can also clarify which areas of occupation to assess, such as performance and participation. The European Conceptual Framework for Occupational Therapy (Creek 2010) offers a comprehensive guide or map (see Fig. 5.2).

Performance

Performance is defined in the European Conceptual Framework as

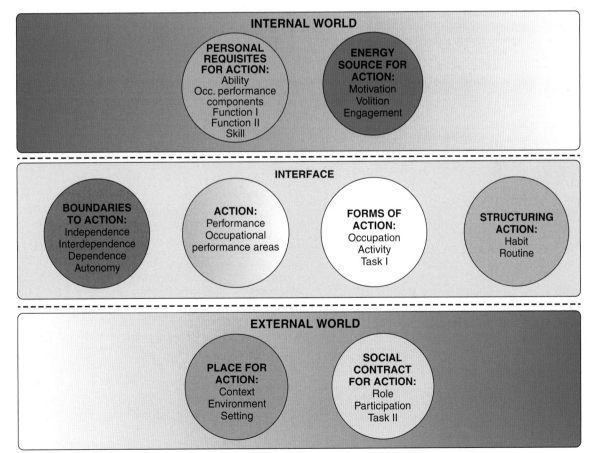

Fig. 5.2 ■ **The European Conceptual Framework for Occupational Therapy.**

"Choosing, organising, and carrying out occupations... in interaction with the environment" (Creek 2010, p. 25)

In this sense performance connects with occupations, activities and tasks, which are forms of action (see Fig. 5.2). Assessing action as an area of assessment links with a person's internal and external worlds. Multiple links can be tracked between performance and these other elements of the framework, providing an overview of connected areas to assess.

For example, in Box 5.3, Rosemary walked around the neighbourhood, an activity which is a form of action which her occupational therapist could assess as they did it together. The assessment findings suggested she was engaged with this activity (internal world/energy source for action). Seeing the bus (external world/environment) prompted her to share thoughts about her routine of catching a bus to church (interface/structuring action/routine). This insight might develop into a recommendation from the assessment on how to support her to develop this routine into a habit.

Participation

If participation is an anticipated outcome of occupational therapy, then assessment of it is required to measure change or indicate its qualities (WFOT 2012). The World Health Organisation (2001, p. 10) defines participation in the International Classification of Functioning as *"involvement in a life situation,"* indicating the commitment and context for what people do. Participation in the European Framework (Creek 2010, p. 180) is defined as *"involvement in life situations through activity within a social context,"* signalling that involvement or commitment to participate requires action, and that *life* situations are centred on the external world. Occupational performance is shaped by participation so that different people performing the same occupation will have different reasons for doing so. For example, Hannah in Box 5.2 could be an occupational therapist who has experienced post-natal psychosis and a long absence from work. Finding a new job will be shaped by her life situation. Rosemary (Box 5.3) could be an older woman who has only recently

TABLE 5.1	
Suggested Areas of Assessment	
Areas of Occupation	**Aspects of Occupation**
Spirituality	Meaning
Religious practice	Value
Rest and sleep	Beliefs
Leisure	Interests
Domestic activities of daily life: (Washing clothes, cleaning home, meal preparation, food and clothes shopping, money management)	Roles
	Habits
	Routine
Personal activities of daily life: Showering/bathing, hair and nail care, teeth care, skin care, dressing/undressing	Motivation
	Occupational balance
Productivity	Occupational engagement
Paid employment, voluntary work, education	Passive occupations (such as watching television)
	Active occupations (such as sudoku or cooking)
Performance Skills	**Environment**
Motor skills	Social
Process skills	Physical/built/terrain
Communication skills	Home
Sensory processing	Community
Participation	**Risks Relating to Occupations**
Time use	Historical risks
Social participation	Environmental risks
Balance between passive and active occupations, at home and in the community	Physical safety
	Personal risks

begun to experience serious difficulties with psychosis and has many established habits and routines to draw on in her recovery.

Further Considerations

Table 5.1 lists suggested areas that could be included in an assessment. These reflect the different ways occupation is understood and categorized (see Chapter 2). Specific models and approaches may help identify which areas to focus on (see Chapters 3 and 5). There may be areas of occupation that are less frequently assessed by occupational therapists but are very important to the person. For example, few assessment tools cover religious practice, but this may be an occupation the person would like to return to as a priority, as shown in Box 5.3. Reflecting on the areas in Table 5.1 offers insights into areas that tend to dominate assessments in practice and those that might get overlooked. Understanding why this is happening could point to continuing professional and service development opportunities.

Special consideration can be given to the assessment of skills with people who have become seriously unwell as children or young people, as the development of independent living skills can be disrupted. In addition, diagnoses such as schizophrenia are associated with cognitive deficits, and medication may affect concentration. An assessment of skills may also be particularly useful with children, new parents or those moving from a high support environment to lower support or community settings.

Interpreting and Sharing Findings

The information gathered from an assessment is described as findings, which are interpreted by thinking about them carefully and drawing conclusions. The context will strongly influence the interpretation: contrasting an assessment conducted in a person's home with one in a hospital setting reveals this influence. For example, often for pragmatic reasons, occupational therapists assess food and drink preparation in a therapy kitchen in a hospital or clinic setting rather than the person's kitchen at home. When interpreting the assessment findings from a session in a therapy kitchen, occupational therapists take into account that the person being assessed is likely to be unfamiliar with both the immediate environment and the assessment

process. Assessment of food preparation, with food supplied in a therapy kitchen in a hospital, might not reflect their usual occupational performance difficulties and therefore limits the conclusions that can be drawn from the assessment findings.

Like any investigation, the findings of an assessment will be of interest to the person, the occupational therapist and others involved in the person's care. Findings can be shared in different ways, including with the person who has been assessed, either immediately afterwards or in the next occupational therapy session. Sharing the findings enables goals and possible interventions to be identified, which are discussed in chapter 6. Deciding who to share the findings with involves the person in this may be when the person indicates with whom the report could be shared. Sharing the findings with others involved includes a discussion about progress and a formal report for the records. Asking "so what?" about assessment findings will clarify implications and recommendations.

When reporting findings, whether in person or in writing, it is very helpful to be easily understood. Clear conclusions regarding the outcome of the assessment and implications inform the next steps for the person who has been assessed and the multidisciplinary team. Profession-specific terms related to the assessment tools may be confusing and should be avoided, for example, the terms "effort" or "efficiency" as used in AMPS (Fisher et al. 2014). Often multidisciplinary

---

BOX 5.4
THE OUTCOMES OF RELAXATION TRAINING FOR CHRIS

Chris attended occupational therapy sessions in the community to learn how to address anxiety and agitation using relaxation techniques. These techniques had no impact on Chris's agitation. On observing this outcome, the occupational therapist switched approaches, as Chris was still keen to learn how to manage his agitation. Together they agreed to address his concerns about work. This was successful, with Chris obtaining a new role in security work that suited his persistent restlessness. Several years later, the occupational therapist heard from a colleague that Chris had Huntington's disease. The agitation had been an early sign. Carefully attending to the outcomes during the occupational therapy process had enabled success in the short term, even though the bigger problem had been unknown.

team members are too busy to read lengthy reports and may skip to the conclusion and recommendations. Therefore reports are concise and informative. Details can be discussed if required. Focusing on participation and occupational performance ensures there are clear suggestions and recommendations for the person's day-to-day life.

OUTCOME MEASUREMENT

In the intervention phase of the occupational therapy process, identifying and tracking outcomes guides people engaging with therapy and their therapists. Changes need to be considered in terms of their meanings to a person and significance in their everyday lives. Box 5.4 offers an example of this.

Using valid and reliable outcome measures (Box 5.5) assures the quality and effectiveness of occupational therapy and informs strategies for service improvements and developments. To secure ongoing funding of services, occupational therapy managers require evidence of outcomes. Where health funding is limited, this evidence is essential to fund service improvements and new areas of practice. Conversely, lack of evidence of outcomes could result in occupational therapy services being reduced or funding being stopped.

Carefully chosen outcome measures can produce accurate and consistent results, especially when used at the end of every intervention to detect and track significant change. They can also provide evidence about the effectiveness of an occupational therapy service by combining scores from all individuals receiving the service. When choosing an outcome measure, it will be apparent that some assessment tools may not detect a change and therefore cannot be used. For example, an interview assessment tool provides rich information as part of an assessment but may not include baseline scores, which can be repeated to detect a change in occupational performance, engagement or participation. Instead, a suitable outcome measure needs to be chosen after the person's goals have been agreed and before starting the occupational therapy intervention or interventions.

Important Features

Occupational therapists consider different features of outcome measures to ensure that their choice is most likely to detect a change in the areas of occupation that are the agreed focus for intervention. Three different features are briefly introduced here, with more detail in the following section on standardized assessments and outcome measures.

Sensitivity of Measure

Measuring outcomes involves detecting changes. Sensitive outcome measures detect subtle but important changes in a person's progress following intervention when measured over a specific period (Laver Fawcett 2007). Therefore sensitivity to defined changes is an essential quality of an outcome measure. For example, the outcome measure might have four levels through which a person can progress, or a detailed scoring system, for example, out of 100, which is more sensitive to change over time.

Floor and Ceiling Effects

A *floor effect* occurs when a person scores the minimum score, but this still does not measure the full extent of their difficulties (Laver Fawcett 2007). Positive changes achieved following an intervention may not be detected on the outcome measure because it is not sensitive enough. A *ceiling effect* occurs when a person scores the highest score the first time the outcome measure is used so that an improved score is not possible following occupational therapy interventions. In both cases, a different outcome measure will be required.

What to Measure

Anticipated changes in occupational performance following the intervention will direct the choice of outcome measure. For example, using Table 5.1, if the intervention aims to introduce alternative active occupations to passively watching television, measures that can capture changes in occupational engagement, motivation, volition and/or time use could be used. Other data, such as length of hospital stay or time to discharge back to primary care, are also often collected to measure changes indicating the effectiveness of interventions as outcomes of a service.

Examples of outcome measures that can be used by occupational therapists addressing mental health issues are:

- Canadian Occupational Performance Measure (Law et al. 2005). This measures performance and satisfaction in self-care, productivity and leisure from the person's perspective.

The Australian Therapy Outcome Measures-Occupational Therapy (Unsworth and Duncombe 2014). This measures functioning outcomes for people of all ages and all diagnoses. It also measures impairment, activity, participation and well-being outcomes (Unsworth and Duncombe 2014).

STANDARDIZED ASSESSMENT AND OUTCOME MEASURES

To use a standardized assessment, measure or test, three main components are required: a tool, a manual and a reference list (adapted from Cole et al. 1995, p. 22):

- A published tool, designed for a specific purpose in a given population
- A manual providing detailed instructions on:
  - when and how the tool can be used
  - how to score and interpret the results
- A reference list of published papers investigating the tool's reliability and validity.

The tool will usually consist of different items rated on a scale by the person assessed (self-report) or the assessor. An item is like a question in a survey, so each one is carefully designed to measure a different aspect of the domain covered by the tool or what is being assessed. The scores for each item are used to provide a baseline for future comparison and/or compared with each other to identify areas of strength and difficulty. Reliability and validity are useful and relevant concepts to understand and are described briefly in Box 5.5.

Tools are selected which provide precise, relevant, and reliable findings and outcomes, as investigating and recording vague, irrelevant and unreliable results is unethical and unprofessional, potentially harming the person receiving occupational therapy. Therefore standardizing tools is a valuable part of research and development within occupational therapy. For occupational therapists addressing mental health issues, using standardized tools for the purposes they were designed for ensures that the results of assessments and outcomes are reliable and valid. In-house and locally designed tools are unstandardized and can undermine confidence as the findings may be subjective, unreliable, irrelevant and not understood clearly by others. Standardized assessment and outcome measures are not suitable to be adapted, for example, by using only a subscale or leaving out questions, as this invalidates the tool, introducing the same issues as for unstandardized tools.

Choosing a Standardized Tool

Investigating an assessment or outcome measure before using it involves reading the manual to understand what it is designed to measure and how it was validated. The manual will also state the population the tool has been standardized for. Following up the references and more recent citations indicates its reliability and validity (see Box 5.5). Trying the tool out on a colleague may also reveal its usefulness. Health service policy determines what each service measures, depending on current frameworks used, such as recovery or social inclusion. However, the recommended tools may not be reliable or valid, being politically driven rather than evidenced as a robust tool. A second tool that is suitable for specifically measuring the outcomes of occupational therapy will need to be identified. Therefore choosing standardized assessments and outcome measures requires a team approach, piloting new tools in several settings before agreeing on which are suitable for the service being used.

Levels of Measurement

A standardized tool has a clearly defined structure, with specific items to be measured. The different ways in which items within a scale relate to each other are described as *levels of measurement*. For example, a thermometer marks off every degree at the same distance in contrast to a customer feedback survey, which might have a variety of rating scales and boxes. These levels of measurement form a foundation for using standardized assessment and outcome measures as intended. The level of measurement informs how the scores and results are to be interpreted and what statistical analysis can be used if any. A more detailed description can be found in specific textbooks covering this area, such as that by Laver Fawcett (2007).

There are four levels of measurement that can be found in standardized tools: nominal, ordinal, interval and ratio:

1. Nominal scales classify items by quality and can be used to describe the characteristics of a person's occupations, difficulties or abilities. The numbers in each classification can be counted, but the scores cannot be added together or used for other calculations.
2. Ordinal scales rank items in order, but the distance between the items does not have a

numerical value. The values of ordinal scales can be summarized by how frequently they occur. An ordinal scale is used in the MOHOST (Parkinson et al., 2006), which has four values for rating levels of occupational participation: facilitates, allows, inhibits and restricts.
3. Interval scales have an equal size or uniform intervals between the values that are a standard unit of measurement, for example, minutes as a measure of time. Arithmetic calculations can be performed to compare values, such as whether someone is getting quicker at completing a task.
4. Ratio scales have an absolute zero in addition to having a uniform interval between values. The absolute zero and the uniform interval between values makes it possible to state that one score is, for example, twice another score. Other statistical tests could be conducted, which is why ratio scales are seen as the best option for quantitative research.

Accessing and Developing Standardized Tools

Creating and standardizing assessment and outcome measures involves many validation stages, which can be expensive. Services may need to prioritize which ones to purchase or explore alternative funding options. Some free standardized assessment and outcome measures are available. Because there can be difficulty accessing appropriate tools, a solution might appear to be making an in-house tool specifically for the setting. Disadvantages of using in-house unstandardized assessment and outcome measures have been discussed. This practice carries risks of inaccurate and irrelevant results, which could adversely affect occupational therapy and is therefore potentially unethical. In addition, it can take several years and in-depth knowledge of scale development to make, test and validate a standardized assessment or outcome measure.

The best approach to addressing the problem of not being able to access a standardized assessment or outcome measure is to collaborate with occupational therapy or mental health researchers based in universities or research institutes who have skills and experience in developing a validated tool for use in practice. As part of the collaboration, the involvement of occupational therapists working in mental health services is often required, which can be a valuable way of developing a professional understanding of the validation process.

Stages of the Validation Process

To create and validate a new standardized assessment or outcome measure, there are three distinct stages:

1. Identify the need
2. Identify potential items for the scale
3. Standardization

These stages are documented in peer-reviewed published papers and books, for example, Streiner et al. (2014). Examples relevant to occupational therapy and mental health include the Pool Activity Level Checklist for use with older people with dementia (Wenborn et al. 2008) and MOHOST (Kielhofner et al. 2010). Both of these involved people using occupational therapy services in mental health settings and occupational therapists in the validation process.

Identify the Need

Having established research partnerships, the first step is to consider what needs to be measured, which is not already covered by existing standardized assessments and outcome measures. This will help identify relevant concepts. A literature review of these concepts will broaden understanding and enable the team to refine their ideas. The literature review can be extended to include existing measures to clarify if any are suitable. There may be one that could be revalidated for use with people encountered in a specific setting rather than developing a new measure from scratch.

Identifying Potential Items

A literature review provides a foundation for developing and refining items to include in the new scale. This helps to avoid bias from drawing only on personal experience. The concepts used for the literature review inform the list of potential items, which are then presented and discussed with a group of experts to establish the validity of the items. The group will consist of

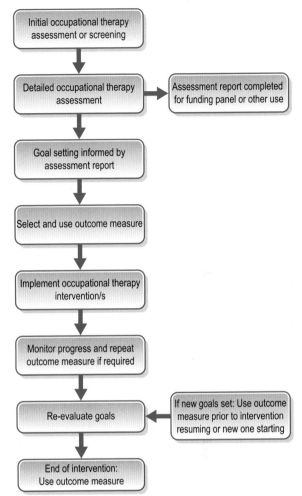

Fig. 5.3 ▪ Stages of assessment and outcome measurement process.

people who have used/are using occupational therapy services, their carers and occupational therapists. The aim is to explore their views on the list of items and reduce the number to those most relevant to the new tool. They could also advise on the format of the scale(s) for the items.

Then the draft tool can be tried out or piloted with the people for whom the assessment or outcome measure is being designed. This will help further refine the measure, ensuring it is feasible for use in practice and confirming it is acceptable and relevant. This stage ensures the manual accompanying the tool has clear and concise instructions.

Standardization

A new assessment or outcome measure is standardized when it has been thoroughly and systematically tested with a large group of the people it is designed for across different locations. This final stage of validation is to test reliability and validity.

The collaborative partnership which initiated the validation process continues throughout these stages, networking with others in research and practice at key points. Each stage is written up, reported and published to provide evidence for others who use the new standardized assessment or outcome measure and those who develop it in the future. When the validation process is collaborative, there are potential benefits for everyone involved, and it is more likely to be completed. A resource is jointly produced to develop occupational therapy and mental health professional practice in the long term.

APPLYING THIS CHAPTER TO PRACTICE

Fig. 5.3 summarizes the stages of assessment and outcome measurement, offering a structure for reflection and review. As societal and healthcare contexts change, reflections and reviews ensure that the most relevant and robust tools are used. It is helpful to analyse where a service fits in the journeys people take to address their mental health problems. What is the next step for the person? Is the service preparing the person for this next step or discharge to primary care (for example)? Do the targets or objectives of the service have to be met within a specific time scale?

Reflecting on the aims of the occupational therapy service could include any changes to the population the service is offered to. This will inform critical analysis of current assessment and outcome measures in use, checking that the most recent versions are being used. Journal clubs and communities of practice may help identify other assessment and outcome measures that could be useful in particular settings.

Outcome measures generate data that can be anonymized and collected routinely to evidence the value

and effectiveness of occupational therapy to commissioners and funders of services. Therefore regular team discussions identify the best outcome measures to use to match the aims of the service.

SUMMARY

Conducting assessments and outcome measurement is central to practice in occupational therapy. Assessment is a stage in the occupational therapy process, covering screening, detailed assessment, interpreting findings, measuring outcomes and reporting them. There are ethical considerations and practical challenges in identifying, accessing and using suitable tools for specific settings. A valid and reliable tool is most likely to provide relevant and consistent results when used for the population and purpose it is designed for. Standardized assessment and outcome measures are comprised of a tool, a manual and a reference list of a body of published peer-reviewed literature. The validation process to standardize them is systematic and best undertaken by collaborative partnerships. Assessment shapes the direction for planning and implementing interventions, the focus for the next chapter.

QUESTIONS FOR CONSIDERATION

1. List the stages of a typical occupational therapy process to show where assessment usually happens.
2. What makes an assessment tool appropriate for measuring occupational therapy outcomes?
3. What activities could Hannah participate in to help her meet her desired outcome (Box 5.2)?
4. Suggest a way in which an occupational therapist could measure the outcome of the intervention for Rosemary (Box 5.3).
5. Why is it important to measure outcomes?
6. What were the significant outcomes in Chris's story (Box 5.4)?
7. What are the four levels of measurement and the three stages of the validation process?
8. What is an example of a reliable tool? How would you define it?

SERVICE USER COMMENTARY

This chapter outlines a number of key considerations in assessments and advocates for building a standardized assessment. Based on my own experiences, I will reflect on the importance of the therapeutic relationship, evolving and flexible assessments, and the value of long term-follow up.

Firstly, I agree that building a relationship with patients is vital. In my experience, finding the occupational therapist to be a trusted ally and not noticing that I was being assessed was key. On a busy hospital ward, being left a questionnaire underneath my door or clearly seeing that notes were being taken during assessment felt demeaning. When a therapeutic relationship developed, I felt more able to share parts of my life.

Second, I agree that assessments should continue through the intervention phase, and goals may change over time. When first admitted to eating disorder wards because of poor physical health, I did not have the capacity for many occupational therapy activities and struggled to identify 'meaningful' activities. At that time, an amazing occupational therapist came and crocheted with me or did a crossword or watched television with me. She came alongside me. Later, as the occupational therapist got to know me better, she and I found that I did have some interests.

Third, it is important to measure effectively whether assessment goals are being achieved and not just through attendance. One of the best occupational therapy experiences I had was at a large hospital where amazingly broad hospital-wide occupational therapy activities included pottery, fruit picking, gardening, art, computers and textiles.

Simple attendance measures would not do justice to the value I, and many others, placed on these sessions. Assessments and outcome measures should include things like mood measures before and after the sessions or observing how engagement and enjoyment changed over time. Staff running sessions or escorting and the occupational therapists themselves could report on these.

Finally, repeated and long-term outcome measures are important. As an inpatient, I gained a great deal from a singing group. My engagement and enjoyment of the group were clear when I was discharged. Yet 6 months down the line, I was even more aware of the positive effects of the group on my confidence, sense of belonging, and love of music. Fortunately, the leader of the group contacted me for a follow up, but this was not part of a standardized outcome measure. It would be a shame if assessment and outcomes were so standardized that they cannot capture the ongoing impacts of interventions, especially when the person is returning to a community setting. After all, the aim of the intervention is not about making the ward environment bearable, it's about stimulating change within the person for their life going forward.

In conclusion, I agree that rapport and the therapeutic relationship are cornerstones of good assessments, and therefore interventions. If standardized measures are introduced, adaptability of goals over time and long-term follow up would help capture change from assessment to outcome.

Poppy Waskett

REFERENCES

Asaba, E., Nakamura, M., Asaba, A., & Kottorp, A. (2017). Integrating occupational therapy specific assessments in practice: Exploring practitioner experiences. *Occupational Therapy International*, 7602805, https://doi.org/10.1155/2017/7602805.

Baron, K., Kielhofner, G., Iyenger, A., Goldhammer, V., & Wolenski, J. (2006). *Occupational self-assessment (OSA) version 2.2. Model of human occupation clearinghouse*. Chicago, IL: University of Illinois at Chicago.

Birken, M., Couch, E., & Morley, M. (2017). Barriers and facilitators of participation in intervention research by mental health occupational therapists. *British Journal of Occupational Therapy*, 80(9), 568–572.

Cole, B., Finch, E., Gowland, C., & Mayo, N. (1995). *Physical rehabilitation outcome measures*. London: Williams and Wilkins.

Creek, J. (2010). *The core concepts of occupational therapy: A dynamic framework for practice*. London: Jessica Kingsley Publishers.

Department of Health. (2005). *Mental capacity act*. https://www.legislation.gov.uk/ukpga/2005/9/contents.

Fisher, A. G., & Bray Jones, K. (2014). Assessment of motor and process skills. In *User manual* (8th ed.) (Vol. 2)Fort Collins, CO: Three Star Press.

Forsyth, K., Deshpande, S., Kielhofner, G., Henriksson, C., Haglund, L., Olson, L., et al. (2005). *OCAIRS or occupational performance history interview II (OPHI-II)*. Chicago, IL: Model of Human Occupation Clearinghouse, University of Illinois at Chicago.

Hocking, C. (2001). The issue is...implementing occupation-based assessment. *American Journal of Occupational Therapy*, 55(4), 463–469.

Kielhofner, G., Fan, C.-W., Morley, M., Garnham, G., Heasman, D., Forsyth, K., et al. (2010). A psychometric study of the model of human occupation screening tool (MOHOST). Hong. Kong. *Journal of Occupational Therapy*, 20(2), 63–70.

Kielhofner, G., Mallinson, T., Crawford, C., Nowak, M., Rigby, M., Henry, A., et al. (2004). *Occupational performance history interview II (OPHI-II), version 2.1*. Chicago: MOHO Clearinghouse.

Kramer, P., Hinojosa, J., & Royeen, C. B. (2003). *Perspectives in human occupation: Participation in life*. Philadelphia, PA: Lippincott Williams and Wilkins.

Laver Fawcett, A. (2007). *Principles of assessment and outcome measurement for occupational therapists and physiotherapists: Theory, skills and application.* Chichester: Wiley.

Law, M., Baptiste, S., Carswell, A., McColl, M., Polatajko, H., & Pollock, N. (2005). *Canadian occupational performance measure* (4th ed.). Ottawa, ON: CAOT Publications ACE.

NHS Benchmarking Network. (2016). *United Kingdom, NHS benchmarking network.* Available at: www.nhsbenchmarking. nhs.uk/.

Parkinson, S., Fisher, G., & Fisher, J. (2011). *The residential environment impact survey-short form, version 2.2. Model of human occupation clearinghouse.* Chicago, IL: University of Illinois at Chicago.

Parkinson, S., Forsyth, K., & Kielhofner, G. (2006). *The model of human occupation screening tool (MOHOST), version 2.0.* Chicago: University of Illinois at Chicago.

Rouleau, S., Dion, K., & Korner-Bitensky, N. (2015). Assessment practices of Canadian occupational therapists working with adults with mental disorders. *Canadian Journal of Occupational Therapy, 82*(3), 181–193.

Streiner, D. L., Norman, G. R., & Cairney, J. (2014). *Health measurement scales: A practical guide to their development and use* (5th ed.). Oxford: Oxford University Press.

Taylor, R. R. (2008). *The intentional relationship. Occupational therapy and the use of self.* Philadelphia: FA Davis.

Unsworth, C. A., & Duncombe, D. (2014). *AusTOMs for occupational therapy* (3rd ed.). Melbourne, Victoria: La Trobe University.

Wenborn, J., Challis, D., Pool, J., Burgess, J., Elliott, N., & Orrell, M. (2008). Assessing the validity and reliability of the pool activity level (PAL) checklist for use with older people with dementia. *Aging and Mental Health, 12*(2), 202–211.

Wilcock, A. (1993). A theory of the human need for occupation. *Journal of Occupational Science, 1*(1), 17–24.

World Federation of Occupational Therapists. (2012). Position statement: Occupational therapy 2010. (Vol. 66. World Fed. *Occupational Therapy Bulletin,* 15.

World Health Organisation. (2001). *International classification of functioning, disability and health (ICF).* Geneva, Switzerland: World Health Organisation.

6

PLANNING AND IMPLEMENTING INTERVENTIONS

CLAIRE KEMBLE ■ NICOLA ANN PLASTOW

■ ■ ■ ■ ■ ■ ■ ■ ■ ■ ■ ■ ■ ■ ■ ■

CHAPTER OUTLINE

INTRODUCTION

After the initial assessment, the occupational therapist and service user discuss needs, skills and priorities relating to goals for functional recovery. Assessments also provide a baseline from which the outcome of an intervention will be measured. Following on from Chapter 5, the next stages of the occupational therapy process, that is planning and implementing an intervention, are explored in this chapter. First the occupational formulation is used to organize the assessment findings. Then the expected outcomes of occupational therapy are determined. The occupational therapy formulation and outcomes form goal setting, which is a collaborative process between the occupational therapist and service user. Then the therapist is ready

to plan, implement and evaluate interventions, which are the actions the occupational therapist and service user take to achieve the service user's goals. These actions are guided by the aims and objectives of the intervention.

'Functional recovery' is a term used in this chapter to describe how people's recovery is monitored by occupational therapists by observing and measuring improved function in its broadest sense. Pinar and Sabanciogullari (2020) indicate that functional recovery includes gaining insight and being able to engage successfully in daily living, work and social activities. Personal and functional recovery are distinct domains of recovery (Best et al. 2020). In contrast to focusing on a person's perceptions of their personal recovery (see Chapter 2), functional recovery can be indicated with standardized measurements of executive functioning (Bitter et al. 2020), as well as clinician ratings of overall functioning and quality of life (Santesteban-Echarri et al. 2017).

OCCUPATIONAL FORMULATION

Once relevant information has been gathered from the initial assessment, it is brought together into an occupational formulation to determine the next steps for the intervention. In many health professions, case formulations are structured statements about the factors that cause and maintain a person's symptoms and problems and the potential targets for treatment (Gates et al. 2021). They have been used in mental health practice to identify the individual needs of service users, rather than focusing exclusively on the diagnosis or a particular theoretical approach (Gazzillo et al. 2019). Writing an occupational formulation is a systematic way of explaining the difficulties that an individual is currently encountering and how these impact their occupational functioning.

Brooks and Parkinson (2018) suggest that creating an occupational formulation is a three-step process, following a narrative or story that describes:

- where the person is coming from (occupational influences);
- where the person is now (occupational presentation);
- and where the person wants to go from here (occupational focus).

This means that the therapist uses narrative reasoning, which pulls together all the threads of the story, when developing the formulation (see Chapter 3). Although it is the therapist who writes the formulation, the service user's experiences and difficulties are the central focus.

The terms used in a formulation may be grounded in a particular practice model, frame of reference or practice framework (see Chapter 4). Different practice models facilitate different ways of understanding occupational dysfunction, which then influence the terms used by the therapist to describe experiences and what the therapist focuses on during intervention. These influences are balanced with the service user's priorities in person-centred practice (see Chapter 4). Using different theories will also lead to different ways of interpreting the presenting

TABLE 6.1	
Occupational Formulation Using a Practice Model	
Occupational Formulation	**MOHO (Kielhofner 2009)**
Occupational Influences	The person's occupational identity, as revealed in their: ■ Participation in past and present roles, relationships and interests and turning points in their life; ■ Volitional context, including importance, satisfaction, personal causation and goals.
Occupational Presentation	The person's occupational competence, revealed by how well their occupational identity is matched with their current routines, skills (communication & interaction, process & motor skills) and performance and environmental supports.
Occupational Focus	The person's capacity for occupational adaptation, indicated by their skills, performance and participation.

MOHO, Model of human occupation.

issues. For example, using a cognitive behavioural frame of reference would guide the formulation to focus on antecedents to behaviours (e.g., situational triggers), what reinforces particular behaviours and how the person thinks about their situation (cognitions) (Mumma et al. 2018). In contrast, using the model of human occupation (MOHO) would guide the formulation to focus on occupational identity, occupational competence and occupational adaptation (Brooks and Parkinson 2018). Table 6.1 gives an example of how the occupational formulation structure is influenced by MOHO.

With more experience, formulations can be more person-centred, but novice-expert differences mean a therapist with less experience in a field might have to give more attention to their selected practice models to support and direct their reasoning. In contrast, with more experience, the service user's story is kept at the centre of a therapist's reasoning, while contextual, theoretical and practical aspects are considered in a more flexible way (see Chapter 3). The structure and terminology used in a formulation will offer insights to the service user and other team members about the occupational therapist's reasoning.

Case Study 6.1 provides an example of occupational formulation using Brooks and Parkinson's (2018) three-step process with an individual receiving support from an adult mental health service. The second person is used as a way of addressing the individual directly and making the formulation more personal to the individual.

OCCUPATIONAL THERAPY OUTCOMES

After creating the formulation and before goal-setting, the therapist considers the service user's expected response to occupational therapy as part of conditional reasoning (Mattingly and Fleming 1994, see Chapter

---

CASE STUDY 6.1

Writing an Occupational Formulation with Samantha

Samantha is a 32-year-old woman presenting to mental health services for the first time with a diagnosis of postnatal depression. Following initial assessment with the occupational therapist, Samantha's occupational formulation is expressed as a second-person narrative in the three sections proposed by Brooks and Parkinson (2018).

OCCUPATIONAL INFLUENCES

You participated in a range of occupations during your childhood, which were mainly determined by your family life and your own interests. You enjoyed your time at school and valued opportunities to participate in a wide variety of after-school activities, including gymnastics, netball, and choir. You left home at 18 years old and went on to university to study law. You successfully graduated 3 years later and earned yourself a training contract at a prestigious law firm. You then went on to forge a successful career as a commercial lawyer, building a busy social life around you. You were financially stable and met your future husband on a night out. You gave birth to your daughter, Sophie, 7 months ago: she is very much loved by you and your husband.

From the first day of starting your maternity leave, you missed your usual routine of going to work. You thought that you would be able to adjust to these changes once Sophie was born, however, the feelings of isolation worsened. You would like to feel okay with your new role as a mother and you recognize the importance of re-establishing a structured daily routine.

OCCUPATIONAL PRESENTATION

Following the birth of Sophie, you started to feel guilty about wanting to be at work. You avoided mixing with other new mums, feeling that you had nothing in common with them. You became less interested in going out and started to neglect domestic tasks. Your husband started to notice a change in your behaviour a couple of months ago and supported you to consult your GP.

You are currently struggling to find the energy to look after your personal care and household tasks; however, you have not lost the knowledge of how to do these things. Although your energy levels are low, you have no difficulties with your mobility or physical strength. You feel that currently you do not relate well to others; however, your husband thinks that you cope better in social situations than you give yourself credit for. You have responded positively to the structured support provided by perinatal peer support groups and you have expressed an interest in becoming more actively involved in local mother and baby groups.

OCCUPATIONAL FOCUS

You have identified four key areas that you want to focus on for intervention:

　　Feeling confident in your parenting skills;
　　Improving your relationship with your husband;
　　Developing new interests;
　　Preparing for the end of your maternity leave.

3). The term 'occupational therapy outcomes' refers to the results of the intervention (Royal College of Occupational Therapists (RCOT) 2015) and is estimated using professional expertise; research evidence; and individual, social and environmental factors affecting the person.

Individual factors influencing the outcomes of the intervention include:

- Personal characteristics (e.g., age, gender, ethnicity, religious beliefs);
- Medical/and or family history;
- How the mental health problems have presented in the past and are presenting now;
- Response and adherence to other treatments so far;
- The length of time that symptoms have been present;
- Whether or not there are other health issues present;
- The response to occupationally-focused interventions in the past.

Social and environmental factors are also known as social determinants (see Chapter 12) and influence the outcomes of occupational therapy:

- The quality of social networks and relationships: People recover better when they have social and emotional support networks. However, just because a service user lives with someone does not mean they are receiving that support.
- Experience of loneliness and isolation.
- Negative attitudes towards mental health issues or stigma delay access to intervention and reduce the level of social support available (see Chapters 11 and 12).
- Area of residence: People living in a well-resourced community are likely to have more positive outcomes than those living in social and economic deprivation.
- Access to mental health services: There are wide disparities in access to mental health services between high-income and low- to middle-income countries. Access may also be limited by people's ability to pay for the service and/or the transport costs to get there.
- Policy and legislation: Some countries like the United Kingdom have robust policy and legislation that supports the delivery of mental health services in the community. Other countries have outdated legislation based on institutional models of care (Zhou et al. 2018).

Considering the likely outcomes helps the therapist and the individual to set relevant and achievable goals.

GOAL SETTING

The occupational formulation and the expected outcomes enable the therapist and the individual to identify specific goals for the intervention. This part of the occupational therapy process is commonly referred to as goal-setting, and it is when the therapist and service user develop a shared understanding of what they hope to achieve. There are differences between setting goals (long term), aims (medium term) and objectives (short term), and the use of this terminology in this chapter is explained in Box 6.1.

A goal is a written or spoken statement of what the service user wants to achieve (Ponte-Allan and Giles 1999). The statement should be functional and recovery-oriented, so that it includes an intention to engage in a specific occupation, either at a previous or new level of performance, or an indication of how the service user would like to live their lives (see Recovery in Chapter 4). This is important because recovery from a mental health problem may include adopting a new lifestyle with new goals and aims (Kirsh et al. 2019).

Goal-setting enables the service user to move from ideas about what they wish to achieve to a concrete plan for how they are going to get there. The occupational therapist guides and supports the service user to set goals that present the right amount of challenge in the context of their current functional abilities. With skilled use of activity (see later section), goal-setting also involves considering how a goal can be realized with smaller, achievable steps or aims and objectives.

Collaborative goal-setting is led by the service user, when possible, in partnership with the therapist who carefully guides the process and focuses on attainable goals (Kessler et al. 2019). Some outcome measures include a facilitated process of goal-setting, including the Canadian Occupational Performance Measure (Law and Laver-Fawcett 2013) and Occupational Self Assessment (Kielhofner et al. 2009). Some service users are able to take full control of the goal-setting

BOX 6.1
GOALS, AIMS AND OBJECTIVES

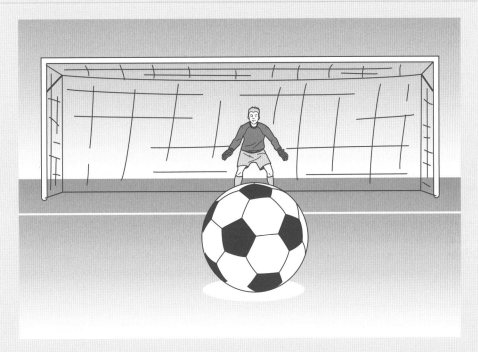

The words 'goal,' 'aim' and 'objectives' are used interchangeably by occupational therapists. In this chapter, as in football, a 'goal' is what the occupational therapist and service user are aiming for together. This means that 'aims' are the way they direct themselves towards the goal, and 'objectives' are set for each step. The outcome is whether a goal is scored or not, as a result of the actions taken during therapy.

Time is another way of thinking about the differences between goals, aims and objectives. Goals are what the service user wants to achieve in the long term. This may extend beyond the time that they are actively engaged in occupational therapy. Aims reflect what the occupational therapist and service user plan to achieve during occupational therapy, sometimes within one session. Objectives are the small steps that will be taken in the short term to achieve each aim.

process, which is likely to lead to better outcomes in terms of goal achievement. If service users are fully invested in the goals they have set, then their motivation to engage in therapy is greater.

Some people require more support from the therapist, depending on the trajectory of their illness. Goal-setting can be challenging for people who are acutely unwell and/or lack the insight to realistically appraise what they wish to work on. For example, a person who is experiencing a manic episode may overestimate their current abilities, leading to their expressed goals being unrealistic at the present time. In contrast, a person with high levels of anxiety may find thinking of goals as too overwhelming. In these instances, goal-setting

is often led by the therapist in conjunction with the rest of the multidisciplinary team and identified carers/family members, if applicable. Case Study 6.2 illustrates how goal setting can take place in partnership with a service user and spouse. The occupational therapist directs the decision on what is achievable and relevant in the hospital setting.

Setting SMART Goals

Occupational therapists often use the SMART formula to set goals that are specific, measurable, achievable, relevant and time-bound (Bowman et al. 2015). Writing clear, measurable goals, aims and objectives can be challenging, particularly for students and newly qualified

---

CASE STUDY 6.2

Setting SMART Goals, Aims and Objectives with Aanya

Aanya is a 43-year-old woman who has been admitted to the local acute mental health unit with a diagnosis of psychotic depression. Prior to her admission to hospital, Aanya's mental health had deteriorated to the level whereby she was not able to initiate her basic activities of daily living, including bathing and changing her clothes.

Aanya has been in hospital for 7 days now and continues to remain in bed for prolonged periods of the day. She is unable to initiate any of her personal care tasks but does respond to gentle, verbal prompting. The ward occupational therapist has met with Aanya and her husband together, and it is apparent that she is not yet able to formulate her own goals for therapy. Aanya's husband feels that her motivation to get out of bed and participate in the ward program me will improve if she is able to establish a morning routine to include waking up at the same time every day and having a shower. The occupational therapist works in collaboration with Aanya and her husband to set goals.

Goal: In 6 months, Aanya will have returned to work full-time from 8:00 to 17:00, Monday to Friday, and will be able to meet her job demands without accommodations.

Aim: In 4 weeks to discharge, Aanya will have increased her occupational engagement to the level that she is able to perform the following activities well, using the Occupational Self Assessment (Kielhofner et al. 2009): taking care of herself, managing her basic needs and getting along with others including her husband.

Objective: In 7 days, Aanya will get up and shower by 10:00 each day.

SPECIFIC	The objective is specific: we know exactly which part of Aanya's morning routine we are going to focus on first.
MEASURABLE	The objective is measurable: we can review if it has been met after 7 days.
ACHIEVABLE	It is the therapist's judgement that Aanya will be able to meet this objective. As you gain more experience in your clinical area, you will have a much better idea of what constitutes an achievable' goal, aim or objective.
RELEVANT	This objective is relevant to Aanya and her husband, as they have both discussed this as area of need with the occupational therapist during the information-gathering stage.
TIME-BOUND	The time-line for achieving Aanya's first objective has been set at 7 days.

---

occupational therapists. Using the SMART formula, the therapist starts by naming the *specific* occupation, performance component or aspect of the environment that will be addressed. The goal is made *measurable* by being clear about the extent to which limitations will improve or be maintained, so in Case Study 6.2 Aanya can look ahead to working full time without accommodations. Based on the formulation, the occupational therapist ensures the agreed goals, aims and objectives are *achievable* and *relevant*. The occupational therapist should also decide on the *time* needed to achieve the

goals, aims and objectives. This may be a review date, when the occupational therapist and the person decide if the goal has indeed been met or may extend beyond the expected end of occupational therapy.

In Case Study 6.2 the aims are focused on what will be achieved by the time Aanya is discharged. Goals should be written in a way that represents the service user voice rather than in the technical language sometimes used by healthcare professionals. In Case Study 6.2 an example SMART objective is getting up and showering every day.

Goals: What We Aim For in Occupational Therapy

Goals express what the service user wants to achieve in the long term. They are usually driven by the individual's future aspirations, personal life goals, and hoped-for possible self (Christiansen 1999). People may wish to work towards valued goals that relate to their previous occupations before becoming unwell and that support their ongoing personal recovery. The realistic timeframe for a goal to be achievable may extend beyond the time available for occupational therapy. The role of the therapist is to support and encourage the service user to work towards achieving their goals, providing opportunities for personal growth, maintaining hope and generating positive expectations for the future. In Case Study 6.2, as well as returning to work, Aanya's long-term goals could be restarting a previously loved leisure interest. Setting goals too early may cause anxiety if the service user is not able to visualize achieving them at all. In this case, it is still important for the therapist and service user to know the direction they want to take, even if this is not expressed as a SMART goal. For example, a person may aspire to find a sexual partner but be reluctant to state that as a goal. Nonetheless, this aspiration could provide some of the motivation for setting and working towards aims and objectives, such as managing personal hygiene and learning how to initiate a conversation.

Aims of Intervention: The Direction We Are Heading Towards

Aims are agreed statements that reflect what the occupational therapist and the service user plan to achieve in the medium term, for example, by the end of occupational therapy. By setting aims, the therapist and service users identify intermediate steps to help them achieve the goals for the future.

Aanya's overall ability to manage her activities of daily living independently was impaired prior to her admission to the hospital (see Case Study 6.2). An agreed aim was, therefore, to build her occupational engagement throughout the week so that her sense of occupational competence improved. As well as the objective to establish a morning routine, the aim could include attending various therapeutic groups within the hospital or accompanying her husband to a local café. All these activities would contribute to her ongoing functional recovery and, in the longer-term, lead to her goal of being able to return to work.

Objectives: Steps to Achieve the Aim

Objectives are the steps needed to achieve the aim of intervention and primarily address the here and now issues. Objectives are often designed to focus on specific components of task performance and are graduated so that the easiest steps are made first. For example, Aanya's first aim included re-establishing a morning routine, and the first objective was to address her self-care (see Case Study 6.2). By supporting Aanya to attain this first objective, the occupational therapist enables her to move onto her next objective, which could be regularly attending breakfast on the ward.

Depending on the setting, objectives tend to have a completion timeframe of days and weeks as opposed to months. They are reviewed regularly and, if necessary, modified depending on the functional recovery of the service user. For example, if the individual relapses, affecting their functional abilities. Then objectives are reviewed and re-graduated to be relevant and achievable. Similarly, if the individual is making quick progress in achieving their objectives in a measurable way, the occupational demands of the aims can be reviewed and new objectives set. If Aanya established a new morning routine of getting up and showering after four days rather than seven, then a new objective could be set sooner. This might be to get ready to go out for a walk every day in the morning after breakfast, reflecting her aim of meeting her husband at a café.

INTERVENTION PLAN

The intervention plan is a programme of activities designed with a graduated approach to achieving successive aims and their objectives. After goal-setting, the service user and occupational therapist work together to develop an intervention plan, discussing how to achieve the goals, aims and objectives. For the occupational therapist, this discussion will refer to the focus of therapy or approach to intervention (see Chapter 4) and the types of intervention available (see later in this chapter). In mental healthcare settings, an intervention plan usually includes a mixture of individual and group work and may involve collaboration with carers or other healthcare professionals.

As well as what they will be doing, the service user is likely to require information about who will implement the plan and how often they will see the occupational therapist, technician or assistant. The plan also indicates how long occupational therapy is likely to last (Boop et al. 2020). Developing an intervention plan is a shared responsibility. As with goal-setting, the therapist could take the lead in some discussions or in the generation of ideas, for example, if the service user is struggling to think of feasible and appropriate activities or tasks for the setting. Planning an intervention requires occupational therapists to reason about several aspects together, including how to match action and motivation and choosing a frame of reference.

Matching Action and Motivation

Collaboratively creating an intervention plan may be challenging when energy is low, limiting a service user's motivation and therefore capacity for action. By creating just the right level of challenge for service users to be interested and develop their skills, occupational therapists facilitate them to identify appropriate activities (Rebeiro and Polgar 1999). For example, after initially meeting in a ward day room or clinic room, discussing the plan in a setting that offers different activity options such as an activity room, occupational therapy department, or arts or leisure centre could energize and inspire service users.

Various theories offer slightly different explanations of how to support someone to identify activities that are at the right level for them and engage in those activities to promote growth and development. For example, the Vona du Toit model of creative ability defines creative ability as a person's ability to bring about change in themselves and reach their potential. There are two components of creative ability: a person's motivation or drive towards action and the externalization or expression of that motivation which is observable in action (Van der Reyden et al. 2019). Thus the level of motivation or drive that someone presents with determines the level of action at which they are able to function. This model suggests priorities for intervention at each level of action and how to structure activities for just the right level of challenge. In selecting activities, the therapist will also think about what skill components are required for occupational performance, such as fine motor skills or cognitive skills, and how the activity can be graded to continue meeting just the right level of challenge as the person's performance changes. The process of identifying the skills required for the performance of an activity is referred to as activity and task analysis, discussed later in this chapter.

Choosing a Frame of Reference

In Chapter 4 a neighbourhood analogy was introduced to understand how theories inform occupational therapy practice. Using that analogy, an occupational therapist organizes the occupational therapy process within a practice model (Ikiugu et al. 2019) in the same way that our daily lives are organized within a building. Similar to being in different rooms in a house, an occupational therapist can draw on different frames of reference to complement their organizing model of practice (Ikiugu et al. 2019). In a systematic review of mental health practice, Ikiugu et al. (2017) found that interventions drawing on the cognitive behavioural, psychodynamic, client-centred and occupational adaptation frames of reference may improve occupational performance and well-being when complemented by MOHO and the Canadian Model of Occupational Performance and Engagement (Ikiugu et al. 2017).

By being clear about the chosen frame of reference in an intervention plan, the occupational therapist can explain the design and adaptations to activities to service users and colleagues. For example, African drumming may lead to a significant reduction in tension, depression, fatigue, anger and confusion and experiences of enjoyment among adults with acute depression (Plastow et al. 2018). Different frames of reference will offer details for an intervention plan.

- When drumming is done at the correct intensity and duration, it can be a moderate form of exercise (Smith et al. 2014). Specifying a sensory-motor frame of reference could indicate the plan is to use drumming as a physical means of releasing anger and tension.

- When applying a psychodynamic frame of reference, the occupational therapist might use drumming as an expressive activity that enables group members to become aware of the significance of their emotions and thoughts, expressing and exploring them non-verbally.
- Using a cognitive behavioural frame of reference, African drumming could be an alternative to other relaxation strategies. The occupational therapist would facilitate group discussions before and after the drumming to compare how the participants' thoughts and actions changed, associated with feeling tense and then relaxed.

For all of these frames of reference, new insights and learning could lead to other activities to benefit mental health, which could be explored outside of an occupational therapy session.

IMPLEMENTING THE INTERVENTION

Having agreed on an intervention plan, the occupational therapist then implements it. In this section, interventions are defined, then we explore the use of activities in occupation-centred practice. Consideration is given to choosing activities and how they are used as therapy in mental health settings. Finally, social prescribing and telehealth are discussed as emerging trends, which present new issues for implementing interventions.

Defining Interventions

Interventions are the actions taken by the occupational therapist and service user(s) to achieve the goals identified in the plan. In this context, service users could be individuals, groups of people, or whole communities. Interventions can be provided directly, when the occupational therapist works with an individual, a family or a group with similar goals. Alternatively, interventions can be provided indirectly, such as when occupational therapists work:

- in partnership with a community of interest that comes together to address a particular issue (Lauckner et al. 2019);
- in a consultative capacity, for example, in services for people with intellectual and developmental disabilities (Umeda et al. 2017);

- or at a systems or policy-level in which the focus is on the structures and systems that support or hinder mental well-being (Lauckner et al. 2019).

Occupation-Centred Interventions

Enabling health and well-being by engaging in occupations and activities is a cornerstone of occupational therapy (Boop et al. 2020). Occupation is defined as a set of activities that have personal and socio-cultural meaning and support participation (Brea et al. 2012). A person interacts with the world by doing activities. Changes in function and performance can be achieved by using activities as therapy because activities are flexible and adaptable and can be used with all people to achieve a multitude of different outcomes.

There is strong evidence that occupation-based interventions improve participation in activities of daily living and instrumental activities of daily living and moderate evidence for leisure participation for adults with severe mental health problems (D'Amico et al. 2018). Interventions are particularly effective when they directly address service users' goals. There is further discussion and guidance for the use of a wide range of occupations as therapy in the other chapters of this book, including physical activity (Chapter 13), learning occupations (Chapter 14), creative activities (Chapter 16), play (Chapter 17), self-care (Chapter 18), nature-based practice (Chapter 19) and work (Chapter 20).

Using Activities for Therapeutic Purposes

Ideally, occupational therapy always involves activity in part or all of a session. For example, an occupational therapist designs and facilitates a creative writing session on an acute mental health ward, where the activity is continued for the duration of the session. In contrast, an occupational therapist working in a community mental health setting adopts a psychoeducational approach, first discussing options for how to adapt an occupation for therapeutic purposes and then trying out one of the options. Maintaining a focus on occupation is supported by approaches such as Recovery Through Activity (Parkinson 2017), which enables service users to recognize the long-term benefits of occupational participation by exploring a range of activities.

When implementing an intervention, the occupational therapist considers many factors to ensure that an activity is therapeutic. The way the therapist thinks about these factors will be informed by theories of occupation (see Chapter 2) and structures for practice (see Chapter 4). For example, theories, models and frameworks, which emphasize the relationships between the person, their occupations and the environment, might lead the therapist to think about the environment for the intervention. The factors considered might include any unforeseen risks that need to be managed immediately or how best to facilitate occupational engagement in a busy room. Reflection-in-action (see Chapter 3) guides adjustments and adaptations during the flow of the activity to increase or reduce its difficulty based on how well the person is able to engage in the activity. As occupational therapists develop professional artistry, they become more skilled and fluent in reflection-in-action and using activities as therapy (see Chapter 3).

There are no hard and fast rules as to what activities should or should not be implemented in a mental health setting. The occupational therapist reasons through the options (see Chapter 3), framing thoughts with relevant key principles such as those associated with person-centred practice (see Chapter 4). To implement the intervention, all aspects of a session are considered, from preparation to evaluation (see Chapter 4).

Person-Centred Practice

Enabling service users to choose activities that will help them achieve their goals embraces the principles of person-centred practice. Selecting activities that people find interesting, pleasurable and appropriate will also help to sustain their motivation and engagement, thus increasing the likelihood of successful recovery. There are occasions where a service user may not be able to easily identify activities that they would like to engage in. Reasons for this difficulty include:

- The person is acutely mentally unwell and therefore unable to identify or articulate their preferences easily;
- The person has a cognitive deficit that impacts on their ability to understand or articulate their preferences easily;
- The person has been deprived of valued occupation for a prolonged period of time (for example, due to environmental constraints or chronic depression) and does not know what they would enjoy.

In the event that an individual is struggling to identify activities of interest, talking with family members or others who know the person well could generate ideas for starting the intervention. The occupational therapist could also use prompts, such as an interest checklist that is suitable for the local context (Klyczek et al. 1997; Nakamura-Thomas et al. 2014) to stimulate ideas. Choosing activities in resource-constrained settings can also be challenging, especially when working with people who live in poverty or experience deprivation. In these settings it is important to:

- use recycled or sustainable materials;
- avoid using foods that will be thrown away (e.g., making a picture using pieces of dried pasta);
- ensure costs per participant are as low as possible (affordable);
- use items that are accessible within the home or community;
- and produce a usable end-product as far as possible.

The therapist may not always have skills for or experience of a particular activity chosen by the individual. To ensure the activity is successful, the therapist may need to carry out further exploration or learning to identify the skills and steps involved in the activity.

Effective Facilitation

To get started, there are recognized dos and don't in relation to how a session should be facilitated. This is applicable to both one-on-one and group interventions. Table 6.2 provides some practical tips for effective facilitation of therapy sessions.

Strategies

When implementing interventions, occupational therapists use strategies to achieve the best fit between people, the environment, and the occupations or activities. These strategies include activity analysis, activity synthesis, activity adaptation, activity grading, activity sequencing and task analysis. Each of these strategies is introduced briefly in this chapter, illustrated by the case story of James returning to work in Box 6.2.

Activity analysis is the process of 'breaking up an activity into the components that influence how it is chosen, organized and carried out in interaction with

TABLE 6.2	
Practical Tips for Effective Facilitation of Therapy Sessions	
DO	**DON'T**
Allow freedom of thought and discussion. Actively listen and ensure that your body language reflects this.	Dominate the session with your own thoughts or opinions.
Be prepared to cut the session short or modify the content if the individual/s is/are struggling to engage or finding it difficult to sustain focus.	Carry the activity on unnecessarily. If engagement has clearly ceased, then so should the intervention.
Encourage people in a group session to identify ground rules to ensure a safe space for therapy.	Ignore the ground rules if a group member is consistently breaching what was agreed. Instead, be confident in asking the member to modify their behaviour or to step outside the session to take a breather.
Inform individuals that the therapy session is a confidential space; however, highlight that if anything is disclosed that could suggest a serious risk to themselves or others, then this will be shared with other members of the healthcare team.	Do for people, aim to *do with*. The therapist's role is to facilitate participation in the session, not to take over doing the activity.
Arrive on time and inform people in good time if the session will be starting later than planned.	Be too reliant on the session plan. This flexibility will become easier as the therapist gains experience; however, it is important to learn not to try to fit the individual into the intervention if it becomes apparent that this type of intervention is not suited to their needs.
Be sensitive to the non-verbal cues that session participants are giving. Are they yawning more often than usual? Do they seem distracted? Are they distressed? Be prepared to modify the plan or stop if need be.	Forget to document your observations soon after the session has ended. This includes collating any feedback received and completing pre-/post-outcome measures.

the environment' (Creek, 2010. p. 25). A component of activity could be any aspect such as the time it takes or a performance skill required, as suggested in Table 5.1 in Chapter 5 and in practice frameworks (Boop et al. 2020). When analysing the components of an activity, the occupational therapist evaluates the therapeutic potential and keeps in mind the specific interests of the individual and their motivation to participate. In Box 6.2 the occupational therapist, Marek, analysed the activities involved in James' work as a police officer and going to an outdoor gym. Being physically fit and alert were components that were common to both activities.

Activity synthesis is used in situations in which activity components can be combined to create new activities, guided by aims and objectives. Marek could have offered general encouragement to James to use the outdoor gym, but, instead, he and James considered how the temporal, physical and social components of the activity offered scope to synthesize it into forms which were similar to the demands of James' job.

Activity adaptation is adjusting or modifying an activity to suit the individual's needs, skills, values and interests. As well as getting more physically fit, James wanted to become more alert, make decisions under pressure and negotiate with other people. Adapting the time he visited the outdoor gym enabled him to practice this.

Activity grading is a way of adapting the activity so that it becomes progressively more difficult as the individual's skills improve or easier as their function deteriorates. The proximity of the second outdoor gym to James' work made him agitated and was initially too challenging, so Marek graded the activity of travelling to the work location and made it easier by meeting him at a café nearby.

Activity sequencing means finding or designing a sequence of different but related activities that will incrementally increase or decrease the demands. Occupational therapists sequence activities as people's performance improves or deteriorates to ensure the level of challenge is appropriate. It is used as an adjunct or alternative to activity grading. By suggesting meeting at a café rather than the gym, Marek added a new activity into the sequence, which could then be graded

James was on sick leave from his job as a police officer, because he had become anxious and agitated, unable to think clearly and make decisions at work. With his community occupational therapist, Marek, he identified his goal to return to work. They planned how he was going to achieve this, starting with an **activity analysis** of the demands of his job which included being alert, physically fit and able to use negotiation skills. Marek suggested they meet at an outdoor gym in the local park, which appealed to James as he thought getting fit was a relevant and appropriate first aim. However, by analysing the outdoor gym as an activity with many **components**, Marek could see how it offered scope to address the other demands of James' job. He **synthesized the activity** so the objective in the early sessions was to arrive at the gym at 10 am and stay for 30 minutes, requiring James to be alert to time and place. Then Marek suggested **adapting the activity**, so James arrived earlier at 8 am when it was busy and he had to negotiate use of the equipment. Then James suggested using another outdoor gym near to where he worked on the other side of town. Marek recognized this would **grade the activity**, increasing the demands such as the time taken and James' exposure to anxieties associated with his work.

However, James became agitated so Marek thought about what was needed to change about the activity. Together, they developed a new **activity sequence,** so initially James met Marek in a café near to work, then he met a supportive colleague there, and then he established the habit of going to the outdoor gym 4 days a week. Marek used the strategy of **task analysis** to identify that going to the gym reduced James' anxiety by becoming more alert, getting physically fit and negotiating equipment use. However, the prospect of making the journey to work raised new issues. James' agitation related to an assault he had experienced at work. Task analysis enabled Marek and James to identify how to synthesize new activities which felt achievable and relevant. These included servicing his bike so it felt safe to use, downloading and listening to music that helped him relax at home, and his supportive colleague accompanying him to an informal meeting at work. The process of preparing people to return to work is discussed in detail in Chapter 20.

into a meeting with a colleague outside of occupational therapy.

Task analysis is used to identify all of the steps or tasks a person needs to complete to do an activity. An occupational therapist may do a task analysis to identify specific steps which a person may find difficult to complete so that this step can be adapted or

eliminated. Task analysis is also useful for activity adaptation so that the objective of the session is met or to decide the best way of teaching an activity to a person (Mccullough 2014). James found his journey to work challenging because of having to negotiate with other people on public transport and worrying about what would happen when he got there. Marek's task analysis of these challenging steps in James' journey to work led to an activity synthesis, suggesting bicycle maintenance to make the journey feel safer and organizing relaxing music before and after work. The challenge of the destination was adapted by setting an informal meeting at work. The strategies used by Marek to ensure the activities were therapeutic for James also required consideration of the environment where they were taking place.

Adapting the Environment

In Chapter 2 the ways in which different dimensions of the environment shape participation is explained. Occupational therapists carefully analyse the environment where the person engages in occupation to identify factors that facilitate or inhibit occupational engagement. The choice of theory, model or framework will influence the way in which the environment is analysed. Case Study 6.3 illustrates different questions about the environment an occupational therapist, Jess, could ask when planning a cooking intervention, depending on which theory, model or framework is used.

Implementing an intervention includes adapting the environment as well as working directly or indirectly with people. For example, for a person with dementia, home adaptations may enable them to live in their own home for longer (Soilemezi et al. 2019) or improve the delivery of person-centred care in a care home (Sjögren et al. 2017). There is a strong link between mental health recovery and social inclusion (Saavedra et al. 2018). Whatever the setting, the therapist considers the importance of place to the recovery of the service user (Doroud et al. 2018) and tries to maintain the service user's close link with community settings as much as possible. If it is not possible for the intervention to be delivered in a community setting, then the therapist works to create an environment that affords opportunities for the service user to feel socially connected and valued. Chapter 29 presents a case study on how opportunities for engagement can

CASE STUDY 6.3

Planning a Cooking Session in a Forensic Setting

Charlie, a service user on a forensic mental health ward, identifies that they would like to engage in some cooking sessions to increase their independent living skills. The occupational therapist, Jess, needs to plan how this will be possible in the constraints of a secure environment. The way in which Jess analyses the environment will be influenced by her understanding of particular theories, models or frameworks. The table below illustrates some questions Jess could ask.

OCCUPATIONAL INJUSTICE (THEORY)	MODEL OF HUMAN OCCUPATION	INTERNATIONAL CLASSIFICATION OF FUNCTIONING, DISABILITY AND HEALTH (FRAMEWORK)
How do service users use their time on the ward?	What space is available that is suitable for a cooking session?	What are the rules and regulations of the institution that affect the type of activity Charlie may participate in?
Is cooking restricted in the ward environment?	Are the tools and equipment needed for cooking Charlie's choice of meal available and safe to use?	Are the tools and equipment needed for cooking Charlie's choice of meal available and safe to use?
How do the restrictions in access, time and resources for cooking affect Charlie's participation?	Who is available to escort Charlie to the session?	Do the attitudes of other staff facilitate engagement in cooking during occupational therapy?
What institutional supports are available for cooking as a therapeutic activity and how can they be activated?	How are Charlie's cooking skills likely to be impacted by the lack of expectation that they prepare any meals on the ward?	

be created for homeless people, leading to improved occupational performance and social inclusion.

Interventions to Support Mental Health

While any activity can be used to address occupational dysfunction related to mental health issues, some categories of interventions are used more commonly than others, such as peer support and group work. In mental health settings, many interventions are also used by other mental health professionals, sometimes working as a cotherapist. Some of these interventions are techniques that require specific skills and abilities. When using these interventions, the occupational therapist may become more aware of the boundaries between generic and specialist practice (see Chapter 4). For occupational therapists, the focus of the intervention is to promote occupational performance. For example, Jan has difficulty going to the shops due to his social phobia, which he discusses with his psychologist. Breathing exercises are known to increase relaxation and reduce anxiety symptoms. Jan's

occupational therapist teaches him a range of breathing exercises that he can do when he is out shopping. Then they visit a local building supplies store together so that Jan can practice his new breathing skills in context. Synthesizing the breathing exercises with shopping, as a new activity, grades Jan's occupational therapy and focuses on his occupational performance.

Common categories of interventions in mental health settings are:

Cognitive approaches: A range of time-limited and collaborative interventions in which people develop new ways of thinking about themselves and the world, changing their behaviour. The focus is on the present, collaborating with service users to agree priorities for change, duration and evaluation date of therapy (Lee and West 2014).

Cognitive stimulation: A range of enjoyable activities that provides general stimulation of cognitive skills, usually in a social setting like a small group. Cognitive stimulation has been used extensively with people with dementia across a range of cultures and settings (Aloyce 2017; Chen et al. 2019; Gibbor et al. 2021; Stoner et al. 2021) (see Chapter 23).

Group work: A method of implementing an intervention plan which is selected when there are other service users with similar occupational needs and goals or when available resources are shared to address the goals of as many service users as possible (Engelbrecht et al. 2018). Therapeutic activities are at the core of an occupational therapy group, with aims and objectives clearly communicated to the participants (Occupational Therapy Association of South Africa (OTASA) 2015). The occupational therapist engages with each participant to explore how group participation will enable them to achieve their goals. When occupational therapists facilitate group interventions, they use their knowledge of social interaction, leadership and group dynamics to facilitate learning and skill development (Boop et al. 2020). Theoretical and practice considerations for client-centred groups are presented in detail in Chapter 15.

Motivational interviewing: A person-centred, semi-directed intervention that uses empathy and increasing self-awareness to enhance intrinsic motivation for change (Smedslund et al. 2009). Motivational interviewing is particularly useful for people who need to change their behaviours to achieve better mental health and well-being, for example, people in recovery from substance dependence (Smedslund et al. 2009; Park et al. 2019) (see Chapter 27).

Multisensory stimulation: A method of implementing an intervention plan which focuses on self-regulation using activities or environments that stimulate the senses in a way that is calming or arousing. Ayers sensory integration©, African drumming and reminiscence groups are a few examples of interventions that use multisensory stimulation to achieve service users' goals (Carr et al. 2013; Bodison and Parham 2018; Plastow et al. 2018; Park et al. 2019) (see Chapters 16, 19, 23 and 25, which all touch on a variety of sensory approaches).

Peer support: An approach which involves people who have direct or lived experience of mental health problems and services offering support to others in the same situation. Many people who have recovered or are recovering successfully can offer useful support, encouragement and hope to their peers (Walker and Bryant 2013). Peer support may offer service users greater levels of self-efficacy, empowerment and engagement and so it is recognized as a core component of the multidisciplinary team in a wide variety of mental health settings (Farkas and Boevink 2018). Peer support can work effectively in partnership with occupational therapy or as a stand-alone intervention, such as an internet café in an occupational therapy department led by peer support workers (Birken and Bryant 2019). When peer support workers cofacilitate sessions with an occupational therapist, they provide a beneficial, added emphasis on sustaining recovery and well-being (see Chapter 21).

Psychoeducation: An approach which focuses on educating people and their family/carers about the symptoms, management and prognosis of mental health disorders (Xia et al. 2013). Occupational therapists use psychoeducation alone or in combination with other approaches (Engelbrecht et al. 2018; Kirsh et al. 2019) (see Chapter 14).

Relaxation techniques: A range of strategies to achieve a calm state of mind and low level of physiological arousal that includes those focused on the body (e.g., progressive muscle relaxation), the mind (e.g., visualization) or a combination of both (e.g., brief relaxation techniques).

Social skills training: A range of strategies to target the underlying performance skills that are needed for social interaction (Wauchope et al. 2016; Storebø et al. 2019) (see Chapters 14 and 18 on Learning Occupations and Self Care).

Emerging Trends

The effectiveness of an intervention emerges as knowledge about it advances (see Chapter 2), and it is widely evaluated as part of evidence-based practice (see Chapter 4). Telehealth describes the innovative approaches emerging with technological advances. Social prescribing is an organizational response to increased awareness of how to promote mental health using social and occupational approaches.

Telehealth

Telehealth is the use of information and communication technologies (ICT) to implement any part of the occupational therapy process when the occupational therapist and service user are in different locations (World Federation of Occupational Therapists (WFOT) 2014). The terms 'telerehabilitation,' 'telecare' and 'teletherapy are also used. Emerging evidence suggests therapy provided through ICT is at least as effective as face-to-face interventions (Gigantesco and

Giuliani 2015; Hung and Fong 2019; Dahl-Popolizio et al. 2020). Telehealth has the potential to improve access to mental health services, for example, for those living in rural areas and gives service users the option to receive therapy in their own home (Hung and Fong 2019). Nevertheless, there are a number of practical and ethical considerations when using this approach (WFOT 2014), which means that occupational therapists should develop their telehealth competencies before using this approach with service users.

Social Prescribing

Social prescribing connects service users in primary care with non-medical community services to improve their health and well-being (Wakefield et al. 2020; Aggar et al. 2021; Vidovic et al. 2021). With an awareness of the social determinants of health, primary care health professionals, including occupational therapists, assess a person's social needs and refer them to a care coordinator or link worker (Wildman et al. 2019). Social needs might arise from unemployment, debt, poor housing, loneliness, sedentary living or poor diet (see Chapter 12). From a social prescribing perspective, these needs can be addressed by engagement with non-medical community services such as art projects, nature-based activities, physical exercise groups, volunteering, befriending and sources of benefits, tenancy and legal advice.

As well as being referrers, occupational therapists provide community activities, grounding their practice in different theories such as:

- Addressing occupational injustices associated with deprivation and health inequalities (Thew et al. 2017);
- Using occupation as a means (Trombly 1995) to tackle specific needs and support people's progress from statutory services to the mainstream community;
- Conducting activity analysis and adaptation to maximize engagement by people of all levels of ability (see earlier in this chapter).

Practical challenges in social prescribing arise when service users need more support. Signposting by link workers may be insufficient to ensure connections with community activities actually happen. More involvement may be required because of stigma, with people preferring to have a supportive and flexible travel *companion*, rather than a travel *agent* (who signposts

referrals) (Deitchman 1980; Fieldhouse 2012). A further challenge is the constraints on the funds available linked with how the effectiveness of social prescribing is evaluated. Narrow health economics and performance indicators could overshadow the holistic practice the pioneers had hoped for (Kimberlee 2018).

Role-emerging placements indicate new areas for social prescribing (Thew et al. 2017), such as the Skills, Learning and Educational Activities for Kids (SLEAK) Project that uses leisure activities to develop the prevocational skills of children aged 10 to 13 in a Cape Town suburb with high levels of gangsterism and substance use (Bester and Kloppers 2016). These placements offer great flexibly for de-constructing a professional philosophy and knowledge-base and re-casting it according to new frameworks (Dancza et al. 2019).

Keeping the Intervention Safe

Before beginning an intervention, the therapist carefully identifies any potential risks that need to be addressed. These could be risks related to the individual, the environment or the therapist themselves. It is important that occupational therapists are risk-aware rather than risk-averse, because therapeutic or positive risk taking is important for mental health recovery (Nugent et al. 2017, see also Chapter 22 about community). The risk assessment and management process does not stop once the activity has started: it is a dynamic process that can change quickly during the intervention. The therapist needs to respond quickly and adapt the session accordingly. In Chapter 7 on Professional Accountability, positive risk taking is discussed with a risk assessment matrix that can be used to analyse the potential risks of an intervention.

EVALUATING THE INTERVENTION

To evaluate something is to judge its quality (Collins English Dictionary 2021). Evaluating an intervention is a fluid and continual process of judging how well individual goals are being addressed and whether modifications are required. Evaluation could involve considering the relevance, acceptability, effectiveness and efficiency of occupational therapy. Occupational therapists use qualitative feedback and outcome measurement to evaluate interventions.

Relevance is considered in SMART goal setting but also has ongoing importance. People may experience occupational therapy as irrelevant if they do not think that engaging in activity will improve their mental health. In Chapter 2 beliefs and values are discussed to indicate how understandings differ between people and their therapists about mental health problems and what improves occupational performance. Interactive reasoning (Chapter 3) and therapeutic use of self (Chapter 4) guide the therapist's choice of method for evaluating relevance: if a person seems to want to share how their understanding of their mental health has changed through engaging in occupation, it is very important to encourage this even if it might seem obvious to the therapist.

Acceptability is related to relevance, considering whether service users accept and find occupational therapy appropriate. Evaluation could include whether service users attend their occupational therapy appointments; their thoughts about and feelings towards their intervention; and their perceptions of whether the intervention helped them achieve their goals or not (Sekhon et al. 2017).

Effectiveness of an intervention is evaluated by judging how well the service user's goals and the aims and objectives for occupational therapy have been achieved (Burches and Burches 2020). When interventions are not as effective as expected, the occupational therapist may need to modify the intervention plan or the interventions used, using the strategies explained previously to ensure the activity is therapeutic. Ongoing evaluation could suggest the intervention might take longer than planned to meet the aims, because there are more steps to functional recovery than anticipated. This reflects the complex interactions between people, environments and their occupations. It is not a failure of conditional reasoning (see Chapter 3) or the intervention. Evaluation of effectiveness will inform the therapist's decision about repeating any part of the intervention cycle: this might mean reviewing the formulation; adjusting goals, aims and objectives; redesigning the plan; and reconsidering how to implement an existing plan. This cycle could be repeated multiple times when an occupational therapist is working with people intensively or over many months and years.

Efficiency indicates if occupational therapy *input* (e.g., number of contacts and therapy hours) maximizes *outputs*, which could be use of health services

(e.g., number of healthcare visits, number of admissions, days in hospital) or mental health outcomes (e.g., improved occupational performance) (Engelbrecht et al. 2019; Burches and Burches 2020).

Evidence-based practice can inform decisions about how to balance efficiency with effectiveness, for instance, when evaluating whether sufficient input has taken place for an improvement in occupational performance to be sustained (see Chapter 4). New issues are often addressed by other services, requiring the occupational therapist to make a referral. For example, the person may be returning home after an in-patient stay, so community mental health occupational therapy can continue the intervention plan.

Gathering Qualitative Feedback

After each session and at the end of therapy, feedback is discussed with service users to evaluate the intervention. Professional reasoning and therapeutic use of self will guide choices about the method(s) for eliciting useful feedback. Organizations may have established procedures and tools for evaluation (see Chapter 3), but occupational therapists usually gather additional feedback to include occupational performance and engagement. Feedback about the quality of the intervention is sought directly from the service user and relevant family members/carers about their view of the person's progress. Gaining qualitative feedback is crucial in understanding of views of personal recovery. Sharing qualitative feedback enables people, and the people who care about them, to take an active role in the evaluation process. Informal discussion about the details of the person's experience can inform evaluation beyond what is captured in an outcome measure (see Chapter 5).

Measuring Outcomes

Evaluation of interventions also involves measuring outcomes to capture significant changes in a person's occupational performance or participation. Chapter 5 provides detailed guidance on selecting and using assessments and outcome measures. Measuring a change requires a baseline to be recorded as well as the outcome and so the same outcome measurement tool is used at assessment and evaluation. Sharing the results of outcome measurement with the service user and discussing the significance of any changes will facilitate decisions about the next stage of achieving goals.

SUMMARY

In this chapter, stages of planning and implementing interventions are detailed with particular reference to mental health. Following on from the initial assessment, the occupational therapist collaborates with the service user to create an occupational formulation and agree d-upon goals for functional recovery. Interventions can be provided in a range of different media, including on an individual basis, in a group or as a combination of both. Occupational therapists deliver their interventions in a wide variety of settings, including hospitals, secure environments, schools and communities. When possible, service users are supported to engage with their local communities to enable them to feel socially connected, giving them a greater hope of achieving and sustaining recovery.

Careful consideration is given at all times during interventions to assessing and managing risk, taking into account the environment and the tools that are being used in the activity. The occupational therapist uses their skills in task and activity analysis, synthesis, adaptation and grading to ensure that activities are therapeutic and related to the person's goals. Evaluating the intervention, both during and at the end of the process, allows the therapist and service user to ascertain what progress has been made and whether further therapy is required. This evaluation paves the way for identifying the next steps to take. As an intervention, occupational therapy enables recovery and hope for a better future through engagement in activities which are planned and implemented to develop or regain valued occupations.

QUESTIONS FOR CONSIDERATION

1. How would you describe occupational formulation in your own words?
2. Using the SMART model in Table 6.2, identify at least two personal or professional goals for yourself.
3. Are there other goals, aims and objectives you might encourage Aanya and her husband to consider See Case Study 6.2?
4. Is there a difference between using occupations and activities during intervention?
5. Choose one activity that may improve your health and well-being. How can you apply the strategies in this chapter to modify the activity so that it is the best fit for you?
6. Give reasons behind the Do and Don't outlined in Table 6.2.
7. What does peer support offer which occupational therapists cannot? Is this approach universally beneficial to service users?
8. How might you attain quantitative feedback in your service?

Acknowledgements

We would like to acknowledge Jon Fieldhouse for his contribution on social prescribing and Jennifer Creek for her assistance with editing earlier versions of this chapter.

REFERENCES

Aggar, C., Thomas, T., Gordon, C., Bloomfield, J., Baker, J. (2021). Social prescribing for individuals living with mental illness in an Australian community setting: A pilot study. *Community Mental Health Journal, 57*(1), 189–195. https://doi.org/10.1007/s10597-020-00631-6.

Aloyce, K. (2017). Cognitive stimulation therapy as a sustainable intervention for dementia in sub-Saharan Africa: Feasibility and clinical efficacy using a stepped-wedge design. *International Psychogeriatrics, 29*(6), 979–989. https://doi.org/10.1017/S1041610217000163.

Bester, J., & Kloppers, M. (2016). Evaluation of outcomes associated with a leisure-time activity program for disadvantaged youth. *The Open Journal of Occupational Therapy, 4*(1). https://doi.org/10.15453/2168-6408.1171.

Best, M. W., Law, H., Pyle, M., Morrison, A. P. (2020). Relationships between psychiatric symptoms, functioning and personal recovery in psychosis. *Schizophrenia Research, 223*, 112–118. https://doi.org/10.1016/j.schres.2020.06.026.

Birken, M., & Bryant, W. (2019). A photovoice study of user experiences of an occupational therapy department within an acute inpatient mental health setting. *British Journal of Occupational Therapy, 82*(9), 532–543. https://doi.org/10.1177/0308022619836954.

Bitter, N., Roeg, D., van Nieuwenhuizen, C., van Weeghel, 2020. Recovery in supported accommodations: a scoping review and synthesis of interventions for people with severe mental illness. Community Ment. Health J. 56, 1053–1076. doi: 10.1007/s10597-020-00561-3.

Bodison, S. C., & Parham, L. D. (2018). Specific sensory techniques and sensory environmental modifications for children and youth with sensory integration difficulties: A systematic review. *American Journal of Occupational Therapy*, *72*(1). https://doi.org/10.5014/ajot.2018.029413.

Boop, C., et al. (2020). Occupational therapy practice framework: Domain and process fourth edition. *American Journal of Occupational Therapy*, 1–87. https://doi.org/10.5014/ajot.2020.74S2001.

Bowman, J., Mogensen, L., Marsland, E., Lannin, N. (2015). *The development, content validity and inter-rater reliability of the SMART-goal evaluation method: A standardised method for evaluating clinical goals*. https://doi.org/10.1111/1440-1630.12218.

Brea, M., Creek, J., Meyer, S., Stadler-Grillmaier, J., Pitteljon, H., & Faias, J. (2012). Understanding the European conceptual framework for occupational therapy: For what it is worth. *World Federation of Occupational Therapists Bulletin*, *65*(1), 12–19. https://doi.org/10.1179/otb.2012.65.1.004.

Brooks, R., & Parkinson, S. (2018). Occupational formulation: A three-part structure. *British Journal of Occupational Therapy*, *81*(3), 177–179. https://doi.org/10.1177/0308022617745015.

Burches, E., & Burches, M. (2020). Efficacy, effectiveness and efficiency in the health care: The need for an agreement to clarify its meaning. *International Archives of Public Health and Community Medicine*, *4*(1), 3–5. https://doi.org/10.23937/2643-4512/1710035.

Carr, C., Odell-Miller, H., & Priebe, S. (2013). A systematic review of music therapy practice and outcomes with acute adult psychiatric in-patients. *PLoS One*, *8*(8). https://doi.org/10.1371/journal.pone.0070252.

Chen, J., Duan, Y., Li, H., Lu, L., Liu, J., & Tang, C. (2019). *Different durations of cognitive stimulation therapy for Alzheimer's disease: A systematic review and meta-analysis*. https://doi.org/10.2147/CIA.S210062.

Christiansen, C. H. (1999). Defining lives: Occupation as identity: An essay on competence, coherence, and the creation of meaning. *American Journal of Occupational Therapy*, *53*(6), 547–558. https://doi.org/10.5014/ajot.53.6.547.

Creek, J. (2010) *The core concepts of occupational therapy: A dynamic framework for practice*. London and Philadelphia: Jessica Kingsley Publishers.

Dahl-Popolizio, S., Carpenter, H., Coronado, M., Popolizio, N. J., & Swanson, C. (2020). Telehealth for the provision of occupational therapy: Reflections on experiences during the COVID-19 pandemic. *International Journal of Telerehabilitation*, *12*(2), 77–92. https://doi.org/10.5195/ijt.2020.6328.

D'Amico, M. L., Jaffe, L. E., & Gardner, J. A. (2018). Evidence for interventions to improve and maintain occupational performance and participation for people with serious mental illness: A systematic review. *American Journal of Occupational Therapy*, *72*(5). https://doi.org/10.5014/ajot.2018.033332.

Doroud, N., Fossey, E., & Fortune, T. (2018). Place for being, doing, becoming and belonging: A meta-synthesis exploring the role of place in mental health recovery. *Health & Place*, 110–120. https://doi.org/10.1016/j.healthplace.2018.05.008.

Engelbrecht, R., Plastow, N., Botha, U., Niehaus, D., & Koen, L. (2018). The effect of an occupational therapy mental health day treatment centre on the use of inpatient services in the Western Cape, South Africa. *Disability & Rehabilitation*. https://doi.org/10.1080/09638288.2018.1453873.

Farkas, M., & Boevink, W. (2018). Peer delivered services in mental health care in 2018: Infancy or adolescence? *World Psychiatry*, *17*(2), 222–224. https://doi.org/10.1002/wps.20529.

Gates, V., Hsiao, M., Zieve, G. G., Courry, R., & Persons, J. B. (2021). Relationship to CBT outcome and dropout of decision support tools of the written case formulation, list of treatment goals and plot of symptom scores. *Behaviour Research and Therapy*, *142*, 103874. https://doi.org/10.1016/j.brat.2021.103874.

Gazzillo, F., Dimaggio, G., & Curtis, J. T. (2019). Case formulation and treatment planning: How to take care of relationship and symptoms together. *Journal of Psychotherapy Integration*, 1–13. https://doi.org/10.1037/int0000185.

Gibbor, L., Yates, L., Volkmer, A., & Spector, A. (2021). Cognitive stimulation therapy (CST) for dementia: A systematic review of qualitative research. *Aging & Mental Health*, *25*(6), 980–990. https://doi.org/10.1080/13607863.2020.1746741.

Gigantesco, A., & Giuliani, M. (2015). A quality assessment of systematic reviews on telerehabilitation: What does the evidence tell us? *Annali dell'Istituto Superiore di Sanita*, *51*(1), 11–18. https://doi.org/10.4415/ANN_15_01_04.

Hung, G. K., & Fong, K. N. (2019). Effects of telerehabilitation in occupational therapy practice: A systematic review. *Hong Kong Journal of Occupational Therapy*, *32*(1), 3–21. https://doi.org/10.1177/1569186119849119.

Ikiugu, M. N., Nissen, R. M., Bellar, C., Maassen, A., & Van Peursem, K. (2017). Clinical effectiveness of occupational therapy in mental health: A meta-analysis. *American Journal of Occupational Therapy*, *71*(5), 1–10. https://doi.org/10.5014/ajot.2017.024588.

Ikiugu, M. N., Plastow, N. A., & van Niekerk, L. (2019). Eclectic application of theoretical models in occupational therapy: Impact on therapeutic reasoning. *Occupational Therapy in Health Care*, *0*(0), 1–20. https://doi.org/10.1080/07380577.2019.1630884.

Kessler, D., Walker, I., Sauvé-Schenk, K., & Egan, M. (2019). Goal setting dynamics that facilitate or impede a client-centered approach. *Scandinavian Journal of Occupational Therapy*, *26*(5), 315–324. https://doi.org/10.1080/11038128.2018.1465119.

Kielhofner, G. (2009). *Conceptual Foundations of Occupational therapy Practice* (4th ed.). Philadelphia: F.A. Davis Company.

Kielhofner, G., Forsyth, K., Kramer, J., & Iyenger, A. (2009). Developing the occupational Self assessment: The use of Rasch analysis to assure internal validity, sensitivity and reliability. *British Journal of Occupational Therapy*, *72*(3), 94–104. https://doi.org/10.1177/030802260907200302.

Kirsh, B., Martin, L., Hultqvist, J., & Eklund, M. (2019). Occupational therapy interventions in mental health: A literature review in search of evidence. *Occupational Therapy in*

Mental Health, 35(2), 109–156. https://doi.org/10.1080/016421 2X.2019.1588832.

Klyczek, J. P., Bauer-yox, N., & Fiedler, C. (1997). The interest checklist: A factor analysis. *American Journal of Occupational Therapy, 51*(10), 816–823. https://doi.org/10.5014/ajot.51.10.815.

Lauckner, H., Leclair, L., & Yamamoto, C. (2019). Moving beyond the individual: Occupational therapists' multi-layered work with communities. *British Journal of Occupational Therapy, 82*(2), 101–111. https://doi.org/10.1177/0308022618797249.

Law, M., & Laver-Fawcett, A. (2013). Canadian model of occupational performance: 30 years of impact!. *British Journal of Occupational Therapy, 76*(2), 519–519. https://doi.org/10.4276/0 30802213X13861576675123.

Lee, S., & West, R. (2014). Cognitive approaches to intervention. In W. Bryant, J. Fieldhouse, & K. Bannigan (Eds.) *Creek's Occupational Therapy and Mental Health* (5th ed.) (pp. 224–238). Edinburgh: Elsevier

Mattingly, C., & Fleming, M. H. (1994). *Clinical Reasoning: Forms of Inquiry in a Therapeutic Practice.* Philadelphia: F.A. Davis Company.

Mccullough, S. (2014). Planning and implementing interventions. In W. Bryant, J. Fieldhouse, & K. Bannigan (Eds.), *Creek's Occupational Therapy and Mental Health* (5th ed.) (pp. 86–102). Edinburgh: Elsevier.

Mumma, G. H., Marshall, A. J., Mauer, C., & Gregory Mumma, C. H. (2018). *Person-specific validation and testing of functional relations in cognitive-behavioural case formulation: Guidelines and options.* https://doi.org/10.1002/cpp.2298.

Nakamura-Thomas, H., Kyougoku, M., & Forsyth, K. (2014). Relationships between interest, current, and future participation in activities: Japanese interest checklist for the Elderly. *British Journal of Occupational Therapy, 77*(2), 103–110. https://doi.org/ 10.4276/030802214X13916969447317.

Nugent, A., Hancock, N., & Honey, A. (2017). Developing and sustaining recovery-orientation in mental health practice: Experiences of occupational therapists. *Occupational Therapy International.* https://doi.org/10.1155/2017/5190901. 5190901.

Park, J., Gross, D. P., Rayani, F., et. al. (2019). Model of Human Occupation as a framework for implementation of motivational interviewing in occupational rehabilitation. *Work, 62*(4), 629–641. https://doi.org/10.3233/WOR-192895.

Park, K., Lee, S., Yang, J., Song, T., & Son Hong, G.-R. (2019). *A systematic review and meta-analysis on the effect of reminiscence therapy for people with dementia.* https://doi.org/10.1017/ S1041610218002168.

Plastow, N. A., Joubert, L., Chotoo, Y., et. al. (2018). The immediate effect of African drumming on the mental well-being of adults with mood disorders: An uncontrolled pretest-posttest pilot study. *American Journal of Occupational Therapy, 72*(5), 1–7. https://doi.org/10.5014/ajot.2018.021055.

Ponte-Allan, M., & Giles, G. M. (1999). Goal setting and functional outcomes in rehabilitation. *American Journal of Occupational Therapy, 53*(6), 646–649. https://doi.org/10.5014/ajot.53.6.646.

Rebeiro, K. L., & Polgar, J. M. (1999). Enabling occupational performance: Optimal experiences in therapy. *Canadian*

Journal of Occupational Therapy, 66(1), 14–22. https://doi. org/10.1177/000841749906600102.

Royal College of Occupational Therapists (RCOT). (2015). *Research Briefing: Measuring Outcomes.* Available at: https://www. rcot.co.uk/sites/default/files/Research-Briefing-Measuring-Outcomes-Nov2015.pdf.

Saavedra, J., Pérez, E., Crawford, P., & Arias, S. (2018). Recovery and creative practices in people with severe mental illness: Evaluating well-being and social inclusion. *Disability & Rehabilitation, 40*(8), 905–911. https://doi.org/10.1080/0963828 8.2017.1278797.

Santesteban-Echarri, O., Paino, M., Rice, S., (2017). Predictors of functional recovery in first-episode psychosis: A systematic review and meta-analysis of longitudinal studies. *Clinical Psychology Review,* 59–75. https://doi.org/10.1016/j. cpr.2017.09.007.

Sekhon, M., Cartwright, M., & Francis, J. J. (2017). Acceptability of healthcare interventions: An overview of reviews and development of a theoretical framework. *BioMed Central Health Services Research, 17*(1), 1–13. https://doi.org/10.1186/s12913-017-2031-8.

Sjögren, K., Lindkvist, M., Sandman, P.O., et al. (2017). Organisational and environmental characteristics of residential aged care units providing highly person-centred care: A cross sectional study. *BioMed Central Nursing, 16*(44), 1–9. https://doi. org/10.1186/s12912-017-0240-4.

Smedslund, G., Lindkvist, M., Sandman, P.O., (2009). Motivational interviewing for substance abuse. *Cochrane Database of Systematic Reviews* (4). https://doi.org/10.1002/14651858. CD008063.

Smith, C., Viljoen, J. T., & McGeachie, L. (2014). African drumming: A holistic approach to reducing stress and improving health? *Journal of Cardiovascular Medicine, 15*(6), 441–446. https://doi.org/10.2459/JCM.0000000000000046.

Soilemezi, D., Drahota, A., Crossland, J., & Stores, R. (2019). The role of the home environment in dementia care and support: Systematic review of qualitative research. *Dementia, 18*(4), 1237–1272. https://doi.org/10.1177/1471301217692130.

Stoner, C. R., Lakshminarayanan, M., Durgante, H., & Spector, A. (2021). Psychosocial interventions for dementia in low-and middle-income countries (LMICs): A systematic review of effectiveness and implementation readiness. *Aging & Mental Health, 25*(3), 408–419. https://doi.org/10.1080/13607863.2019 .1695742.

Storebø, O. J., Andersen, M. E., Skoog, M., et al. (2019). Social skills training for attention deficit hyperactivity disorder (ADHD) in children aged 5 to 18 years. *Cochrane Database of Systematic Reviews, 2019*(6). https://doi.org/10.1002/14651858.CD008223. pub3.

Trombly, C. A. (1995). *Occupation: Purposefulness and Meaningfulness as Therapeutic Mechanisms 1995 Eleanor Clarke Slagle Lecture.* Available at http://aota.org/terms.

Umeda, C. J., Fogelberg, D. J., Jirikowic, T., et al. (2017). Expanding the implementation of the Americans with disabilities act for populations with intellectual and developmental disabilities: The role of organization-level occupational therapy consultation. *American Journal of Occupational Therapy*, 7104090010p1–7104090010p6. https://doi.org/10.5014/ajot.2017.714001.

Vidovic, D., Reinhardt, G. Y., & Hammerton, C. (2021). Can social prescribing foster individual and community well-being? A systematic review of the evidence. *International Journal of Environmental Research and Public Health.* https://doi.org/10.3390/ijerph18105276.

Van der Reyden, D, Casteleijn, D., Sherwood, W., & De Witt, P. (2019) *The Vona du Toit Model of Creative Ability: Origins, constructs, principles and application in occupational therapy.* Pretoria: Vona and Marie du Toit Foundation.

Wakefield, J. R. H., Kellezi, B., Stevenson, C. (2020). Social prescribing as "social cure": A longitudinal study of the health benefits of social connectedness within a social prescribing pathway. *Journal of Health Psychology.* https://doi.org/10.1177/1359105320944991.

Walker, G., & Bryant, W. (2013). Peer support in adult mental health services: A metasynthesis of qualitative findings. *Psychiatric Rehabilitation Journal*, 36(1), 28–34. https://doi.org/10.1037/h0094744.

Wauchope, B., Terlich, A., & Lee, S. (2016). Rel8: Demonstrating the feasibility of delivering an 8-week social skills program in a public mental health setting. *Australasian Psychiatry*, 24(3), 285–288. https://doi.org/10.1177/1039856215612992.

Wildman, J. M., Moffatt, S., Penn, L., O'Brien, N., Steer, M., & Hill, C. (2019). Link workers' perspectives on factors enabling and preventing client engagement with social prescribing. *Health and Social Care in the Community*, 27(4), 991–998. https://doi.org/10.1111/hsc.12716.

World Federation of Occupational Therapists (WFOT). (2014). World Federation of occupational therapists' position statement on telehealth. *International Journal of Telerehabilitation*, 65195(110), 37–40.

Xia, J., Zhao, S., & Jayaram, M. B. (2013). Psychoeducation (brief) for people with serious mental illness. *Cochrane Database of Systematic Reviews*, 2013(11). https://doi.org/10.1002/14651858.CD010823.

Community Mental Health Journal (2020) 56:1053–1076. https://doi.org/10.1007/s10597-020-00561-3 ORIGINAL PAPER Recovery in Supported Accommodations: A Scoping Review and Synthesis of Interventions for People with Severe Mental Illness Neis Bitter1 · Diana Roeg1 · Chijs van Nieuwenhuizen1,2 · Jaap van Weeghel1,3,4

Section 3

THE CONTEXT OF OCCUPATIONAL THERAPY

SECTION OUTLINE

7 MANAGEMENT AND LEADERSHIP

GABRIELLE RICHARDS

INTRODUCTION

Many occupational therapists start their careers as practitioners and move into management roles over a period of time. They do not always have specific training in these roles and many develop 'on-the-job' experience. Occupational therapists often make very good managers, but we have to start recognizing ourselves as leaders as well. According to Orman (2018) it is crucial we recognize our expertise and clearly articulate how we can apply it within service delivery. However, it is also important to have an underpinning knowledge of management principles and theory to be a good manager in practice. An understanding of the organization worked in is invaluable as a manager. Getting to grips with its purpose, vision and direction of travel can help managers define the unique contribution occupational therapy makes to realizing an organization's aims. As Braveman (2016 p.33) reflected, 'we can get aggressively involved in our organizations. Volunteer or assertively ask to be a member of committees and initiatives to streamline care, broaden your

intervention... we can become the "go-to" person on the team.' Knowing both the internal and external factors that can influence the environment occupational therapists work in reinforces their ability to look ahead and manage with confidence.

Alongside management, the importance of leadership in healthcare has grown in significance in recent years. Rodgers (2012) proposed that occupational therapists identify themselves as leaders wherever they are, position themselves within organizations or in their professional lives and take on leadership roles no matter how big or small. This means that occupational therapists should identify and sieze opportunities to lead. Occupational therapists are able to recognise the potential for change in the people, communities, institutions and societies in which they work, and have the leadership skills needed to be agents of change.

From the day occupational therapists commence practice they are faced with many challenges associated with applying the theory of what they have learnt as undergraduates and transitioning to the rigors of practice. This includes applying management and leadership theory. New graduates have to manage high workloads with diverse populations in very complicated service delivery systems. McCombie and Antanavage (2017) proposed that having a mentor, high job satisfaction and a good clinical fit helped new graduates as in many instances they are also working in new and emerging practice settings.

Most commentators would agree management skills needed for new graduates should not only include, for example, time management and planning, but they should also include skills related to leadership such as resolving conflict and difficult staff relations. It is crucial that not just senior occupational therapists but also newly qualified ones understand the importance of leadership and, where possible, take on a leadership role for the profession. Having leadership skills, particularly clinical ones, can enhance new practitioners' ability to successfully function within their teams. Learning different skills, styles and behaviours associated with leadership will only add to an individual's effectiveness. Managers, be they occupational therapists or health managers in general, look for practitioners who can meet the challenges and have competencies to cope in rapidly changing work environments (Morley 2009; Spyby 2012). This raises the question of whether the leadership and management skills sets learnt for traditional healthcare practice are adequate for the super-complex environments in which occupational therapists work. Hendricks and Toth-Cohen's (2018) study of leadership development among Black occupational therapy students in South Africa suggests that authentic leadership is complex and includes the self, others and the systems in which occupational therapists work. Future practice to develop authentic leadership could include promotion of storytelling as a means of reflection on authentic leadership skills and knowledge.

This chapter explores the concepts of management and leadership, particularly the differences between the two, before examining what this means for occupational therapists working in mental health settings that exist in modern, ever-changing health and social care systems across the world. One of the big changes for occupational therapists is the growing emphasis of the allied health professions' (AHP) agenda. Anecdotally, mental health occupational therapy managers

BOX 7.1
A SUMMARY OF THE REASONS WHY ORGANIZATIONS NEED MANAGERS

Drucker (1955)

1. Set objectives – set goals for the group and determine how to best meet those
2. Organize – divide work into manageable activities and assign these to relevant team members
3. Motivate and communicate – communicate decisions clearly and create a team ethos amongst staff
4. Measure – establish appropriate yardsticks and targets, and analyse and interpret performance
5. Develop people – develop staff as company assets

and leaders are taking increasing responsibility for line managing or professionally supporting other allied health professionals and, in many cases, changing the title of 'occupational therapy head' to 'allied health professional head.' This is interesting in itself and will be reflected on later in the chapter. Another significant advance in mental healthcare is the concept of coproduction of service development and sometimes delivery with people and their carers who use mental health services. This will be discussed under the Power section. Most of the occupational therapy examples are from the United Kingdom—a model of leadership competence from a leading mental health trust is presented to illustrate the discussion. The chapter presents these concepts as a useful toolkit for occupational therapists to use for management and leadership success. At the same time, occupational therapists need to think about the specific cultural issues that may shape management and leadership practices differently, such as in the South African example referred to earlier.

MANAGEMENT

Many commentators have posed the question, 'Why do organizations need managers?' Peter Drucker, widely known as the person who first started writing about management in organizations, provided some reasons which are still pertinent to organizations today (Box 7.1). Many people refer to 'management' as the individuals charged with running the organization and, as such, management presumes a business-oriented focus. A commonly quoted view from Drucker (1955) refers to getting things done through others, but there are different ways of viewing management. Some assert that the aim of management is to support their employees' efforts to be fully productive members of their organizations and citizens of the community in which they operate (Mirvis and Googins 2018). Definitions generally refer, in some way, to the process of directing and leading a programme of work in an organization. Managers are the people charged with the responsibility for this process and use many different types of management to achieve this (Box 7.2).

In health and social care systems, management is seen as accomplishing a series of tasks, often through the effort of others. That is, it is not oriented around a production line; it is about people conducting the business as well as managing the resources. Managers can accomplish so much more through others by building resilience, providing good supervision and performance managing. This means there needs to be more understanding of what managers actually do in practice to be effective. This includes the organizational processes of strategic planning, setting objectives, managing resources, and deploying the human and financial resources needed to achieve organizational objectives. Traditionally, the term 'management' refers to the activities (and often the group of people) involved in the four general functions: planning, organizing resources, leading and controlling and coordinating. All of these four functions occur at all levels in organizations and are highly integrated throughout. Management tasks also involve recording of information, setting performance targets and measuring results. It also assumes that there is a cycle in which management activities are planned, executed and measured through a series of ongoing processes.

Planning

Occupational therapists are used to planning their work for the people for whom they provide services. They carry out assessments, then provide interventions based on those assessments in collaboration with the service user. There is an expectation that the work they do has goals that are specific, measurable (outcome-oriented), achievable, relevant and time-based, often referred to as *s*pecific, *m*easurable, *a*chievable, *r*elevant, *t*ime-based (SMART). As Kate Miller described, 'When I think about what it is that we do

as occupational therapists in everyday clinical practice ... we apply very certain and definite kind of steps and approaches to our work, it includes listening, gaining an understanding or taking another perspective of the person we are trying to gain an understanding about. We don't make judgements about others and don't force our beliefs on others, we try to engage people in activities and motivate them to improve or regain function. We think outside the box on an everyday basis because we need to make situations and environments work for people so they can continually engage as they want to' (Rodger 2012, p. 176).

This same discipline can be applied to the planning and development of occupational therapy services. For example, most organizations carry out an annual business planning process to determine the budget to provide services, set targets and judge performance against the agreed plan. This is different from a strategic plan which might be more long term and visionary. For example, occupational therapy services usually have an annual working business plan based on the organization's goals and the budgets set for the provision of services. However, they may also have a strategy which includes a high-level mission statement and a plan that incorporates the aims and objectives as to how the overall mission will be achieved. A good example is the UK's Royal College of Occupational Therapists' (RCOT, 2006) strategy, 'Recovering ordinary lives – a vision for the next ten years,' which clearly describes key messages for the profession and others to work towards improving mental health services. As the document states, 'the aims of this strategy are twofold: to reassert the importance of occupation to health and well-being, and to develop a vision and principles that will guide occupational therapy practice within rapidly changing social and political environments' (RCOT 2006, p. ix). Several mental health occupational therapy services in the United Kingdom have based their strategic plans on the RCOT's (2006) strategy document as a way of framing their own strategy development.

Other types of planning also feed into both annual and strategic plans. The most common are workforce and project planning.

- 'Workforce planning' refers to how an organization estimates its future workforce requirements and calculates the numbers, nature and

BOX 7.2
A SUMMARY OF THE DIFFERENT TYPES OF MANAGEMENT

- **Change management** is a structured approach for ensuring that changes are thoroughly and smoothly implemented and that the lasting benefits of change are achieved (MindTools). It could involve service reconfiguration and redesign, staff changes or disinvestment (budget cuts), for example.

- **Information management** includes the use of both physical and electronic information. Managers need to manage all sources and formats of information, for example, paper, electronic, video and audio. Importantly, it is not only about how knowledge and information are gathered, but also how they process them, digest them and use them to best effect.

- **Knowledge management** is a series of tools and activities to capture the range of information available to an organization. It can be used to enhance efficiency, increase productivity, audit and research and effect change. Knowledge management is the systematic management of information and learning. It turns personal information and experience into collective knowledge that can be widely shared throughout an organization and a profession (Association of Project Management 2019).

- **Operational management** refers to the responsibility of day-to-day organizing and coordinating of services and resources, liaising with practice staff and other professionals, dealing with the public, managing complaints and anticipating and resolving service delivery issues (see NHS operational management). In the health service this role has often been carried out by general managers, but people with a professional background, like occupational therapists, also carry out this role.

- **People management** is one of the manager's most important tasks. Managing people often involves planning individuals' work tasks, setting workloads and carrying out supervision and appraisal processes.

- **Performance management** relates to assessing a person's ability to perform to the best of their ability (Armstrong 2005). If a person, team or organization is unable to perform adequately, processes should be put in place to monitor and support improvement.

- **Personal management** is about how an individual manages their own work life, goals, time management and career development. Access to opportunities for mentoring, coaching, shadowing and further training will help develop the competencies to be an effective manager.

- **Personnel management** is not to be confused with people management. Personnel management is traditionally performed by the human resources department and includes activities such as recruitment processes, screening and interviewing applicants and developing and overseeing employment policies.

- **Professional management** refers to the process of setting the standards expected for the profession in the organization, providing supervision, assessing competence and defining quality.

- **Project management** is the application of knowledge, skills, and techniques to execute projects effectively and efficiently (Project Management Institute 2012). It is usually a time-limited activity with an identified beginning, middle and end with an agreed remit, budget and time allocation and an intended agreed outcome.

sources of potential employees who might meet that demand. In other words, it is about getting the right number of people with the right skills in the right place and at the right time. Occupational therapy managers are asked to predict the numbers of staff and what grades they need to meet the work priorities and demands from their business and strategic planning processes. This may also extend to influencing the number of undergraduate places that are commissioned for occupational therapy training to meet future workforce demands.

- 'Project planning' is the application of the techniques of planning, implementing and managing the resources available in relation to a specific project. It is usually a time-limited activity with an identified beginning, middle and end with an agreed budget and time allocation and an agreed outcome. Examples of these may be setting up a new service or indeed closing a service. It might also include carrying out a feasibility study or marketing and launching a new product or intervention.

Organizing Resources

Managing resources is about being responsible for a whole range of available resources, that is, people, finances and physical resources such as buildings and materials. Understanding these resources helps the manager maintain control of the budget allocated for their services. A budget is the sum of money allocated for a particular purpose. Budgets are usually set out on a yearly basis as described in the planning section (above) and serve both a planning and controlling function. Budgets can include a complex mix of information related to the resources required, so appropriate training in budgetary management is advised if occupational therapy managers are to successfully utilize and maintain budgetary control.

In recent years budgets in mental health services, particularly in the United Kingdom, have been held in general management or operational systems, not by individual professional groups. General management was intended to offer active, strategic direction and to devolve responsibility through a clear structure of line management and devolved budgets. As a result, occupational therapy managers over the years have had less direct control of staffing budgets, as these may be held in the

integrated services. Therefore the role of the occupational therapy manager is one involving much more influence in relation to making the best use of resources rather than direct responsibility for them. Workforce development is a good example of how occupational therapy expertise is essential in recommending the appropriate grades of occupational therapists to provide activity within services and how those occupational therapy resources are deployed. As an example of organizing resources, in the United Kingdom the occupational therapy mental health indicative care packages for mental health 'Payment by results' set out potential occupational therapy assessment, interventions and outcomes for service users as well as recommended staffing levels for carrying out the activity (Department of Health (DH) 2011; Morley et al. 2011). A more recent initiative is the development of the Model Hospital, a digital information service designed to help NHS providers improve their productivity and efficiency. This is where comparisons can be made of the AHP workforce deployment across different organizations, bench mark and prompt some challenge in the way resources are made available to maximize the patient and clinical outcome.

Leading

Leading is about 'setting the direction of travel' for the organization and realizing its vision through leading teams and individuals and influencing them to follow that direction. As stated previously, this is an important area of development for all grades of occupational therapists. Examples of leadership activity include establishing strategic direction (vision, values, mission and/or goals) and championing methods of organizational performance management to pursue that direction. This is discussed further in the section on Leadership (below).

Controlling and Coordinating

Controlling and coordinating is about the processes and systems designed to manage an organization's structures and data as effectively and efficiently as possible to reach its goals and objectives. The analysis of data in a modern healthcare organization can be particularly complex and detailed. It involves the ongoing collection of feedback, monitoring and adjustment of systems, processes and structures to meet demands. Data that exist can be financial; they can be the findings from research or audit. Data can be used in producing policies and procedures, performance management processes and measures to avoid risks. The key point is to control and coordinate these data to support the delivery of services. Using SMART goals could be one way of providing a framework with which to control and coordinate systems and processes as they can provide a purpose and clarity for evaluating whether a service is meeting its identified standards. Identifying these SMART goals with a range of stakeholders from superiors, peer subordinates and service users can ensure clarity and purpose and hold people accountable for the delivery of services. Smyth (2017) reported on a project in which occupational therapists working as Health and Work champions were training staff to 'ask the work question' as part of everyday consultations. In doing so, 60 occupational therapists have trained in excess of 500 NHS staff to improve clinicians' knowledge and confidence to talk about employment. The strap line for the project was 'occupational therapists can help the whole NHS turn a million patient contacts every 36 hours into a million opportunities to talk about work'. Occupational therapy managers and practitioners on the ground need to be astute in utilizing information like this to their advantage.

LEADERSHIP

There has been a growing interest in recent years about the importance of leadership and management skills in the delivery of health and social care. This has led to a proliferation of literature about the significance of leadership. In 2015 a review of leadership in the NHS (Kings Fund 2015) concluded that there is clear evidence of the link between leadership and a range of outcome within health services, including patient satisfaction, organizational financial performance, staff well-being, engagement, and overall quality of care. Braveman (2016) emphasized it is important to distinguish between the act or process of leading, that is, leadership, and the individuals who are in the position of guiding others, that is, the leaders. He also proposed the following definition of leadership: "Leadership is the process of creating structural change wherein the values, vision and ethics of individuals are integrated into the culture of a community as a means of achieving sustainable change" (p. 6).

Leaders are the inspiration and directors of the action; they are the people who possess the combination of

TABLE 7.1

A Summary of Different Characteristics of Management and Leadership

Management	Leadership
Processes	People
Facts	Feelings
Intellectual	Emotional
Head	Heart
Position power	Persuasive powers
Control	Commitment
Problem-solving	Possibility thinking
Reactive	Proactive
Doing things right	Doing the right things
Rules	Values
Goals	Vision
Lights fire under people	Stokes the fire within people
Written communications	Verbal communications
Standardization	Innovation

personality and skills that makes others want to follow their direction.

The Differences Between Leadership and Management

Leadership and management are distinct but complementary concepts (Table 7.1). The terms have been used interchangeably, but recently there has been growing recognition of the differences between the two and the need to be a good leader and an effective manager. For example, in 2014 the American Occupational Therapy Association (AOTA) implemented leadership development programmes for academics, middle managers and emerging leaders focusing on leadership styles and outcomes. Current thinking tends to separate them and recognizes that having clarity about how they differ will help individuals to maximize their performance. Management is generally seen to involve overseeing day-to-day operations, accomplishing goals and achieving tasks, while leadership spans a wider remit that includes influencing and inspiring others, generating ideas and defining a strategy and vision. Managers are not confined to management, and leaders are not restricted to leadership. The critical issue is to find the right balance for your job.

It is important to note that one set of characteristics is not better than the other. Both are needed for success, and many people will use them interchangeably to be effective in their roles.

Leadership Styles

Within leadership there are different leadership styles. In the 1930s Kurt Lewin proposed three leadership styles which are still relevant to understanding different approaches to leadership today:

1. 'Autocratic leaders' make decisions without consulting their teams. This is considered appropriate when decisions genuinely need to be taken quickly, when there's no need for input, and when team agreement is not necessary for a successful outcome.
2. 'Democratic leaders' allow the team to provide input before making a decision, although the degree of input can vary from leader to leader. This type of style is important when team agreement matters, but it can be quite difficult to manage when there are lots of different perspectives and ideas.
3. 'Laissez-faire leaders' do not interfere; they allow people within the team to make many of the decisions. This works well when the team is highly capable and motivated and when it does not need close monitoring or supervision. However, this style can arise because the leader is lazy or distracted, and, here, this approach can fail.

An effective leader should be aware of the different styles and know when to use them for different outcomes required. For example, a leader might find an open democratic style on a day-to-day basis is preferable and effective most of the time, whereas during times of sudden increase in workload or deadlines a more directive or autocratic style might be required. Leadership style can depend on the situation; there are other factors which can also influence which style is most effective and which one to use. This includes the manager's personality, values and work experience. It can also be influenced by the employees' individual preferences of how they like and respond to various leadership styles. Lastly, the values, philosophy and ethos of an organization can also influence leadership styles. Some are based on a spirit of partnership in decision-making, while others operate in a more directive fashion. Box 7.3 provides a summary of some of the key competencies needed for effective leadership.

Power

Another important aspect in considering the concept of leadership is power. As Clark (2010, p. 265), the internationally renowned occupational therapy researcher

---

BOX 7.3

A SUMMARY OF THE COMPETENCY DEFINITIONS RELATED TO LEADERSHIP

- **Analytical reasoning:** Analyses data to reach sound decisions, thinks creatively and innovates
- **Communicating and influencing:** Communicates effectively both in person and in writing, gains buy-in from others, fosters open communication
- **Leading people:** Coaches and develops others, empowers teams and leads on change
- **Overseeing and supporting the business:** Drives for results, pursues business opportunities, manages financials, delivers on plans and manages time and priorities
- **Cultivating relationships:** Builds effective relationships with others, adopts a collaborative approach, manages conflict and values everyone's contribution
- **Managing self:** Is motivated and self-confident, copes under pressure, acts with integrity and models the organization's values
- **Partnership and engagement:** Understands partners, works with internal and external stakeholders and manages high-stakes interactions
- **Strategic focus:** Develops a compelling vision for the organization, understands its strategic position and designs and implements strategies

---

and past president of the AOTA, stated, 'many of our practitioners are uncomfortable with the word "powerful."' She proposed that this unease exists because it could be seen as the opposite of caring, it has masculine attributes (in a predominantly female profession) and it is associated with domination. She observed that power is neither good nor bad, but how an individual uses or misuses power ultimately colours the perception of power in the views of others. Davidson (2012) questioned, for a predominantly female professional group such as occupational therapy, whether we are sufficiently aware of the impact of gender leadership and the use of power to ameliorate negative impact and actively promote female advantage. She proposed that the challenge for occupational therapists is to achieve their potential while balancing the development of leadership skills and use power in a way that strengthens and promotes female leadership skills and behaviours.

The combination of leadership, power and influence within management in an organization is constantly developing. There are five different powers that affect leadership style. These are expert power, referent power, legitimate power, reward power and coercive power. Some are more effective than others. For example, coercive power is generally not thought to be very efficient as workers can feel threatened or punished, whereas reward power is where the leader has the ability to reward workers in some way (UK Essays 2019).

The personal power of a leader comes from being an expert where skills, experience and knowledge are valued leadership traits; referent power comes from being trusted and respected as a leader. All of these aspects of power are influenced by the:

- personal characteristics of the leader;
- attitude, needs and other personal attributes of the employees;
- nature of the organization the leader operates in, such as its purpose, structure and the tasks to be performed; and
- the wider social, economic and political environment.

The concept of sharing power with the people who use services is not new in healthcare. Kemp (2010) wrote service users' involvement has now established itself as a significant feature in the landscape of mental health provision. The term 'nothing about us without us' is commonly used in relation to service users and carer involvement to communicate the idea that no policy or service development should be done without the participation of the people who use those services. The 'Expert Patient Programme also acknowledges that patients take the power by running and providing self-management education for people with chronic conditions based on their own experiences.

In essence, it is important to understand the concept of power and how it affects and influences the development of the occupational therapy profession to manage and lead successfully. It is also important to consider the involvement and influence of the people we provide services to. Coproduction, where professionals, people who use services and those who care for them share power to plan and deliver services or projects together,

undoubtedly impacts on the power dynamic that a leader has to consider. For occupational therapists to have a successful experience of coproduction, they have to make a shift in their thinking and working relationships, which may mean giving up power to have a successful shared outcome for both the professionals and the people who use the services. Powerful leaders appreciate their personal attributes, understand the organizations they work in and grasp the bigger picture of the environment around them. The Kings Fund (2012) report on leadership and engagement referred the need to move from a hierarchy-driven system where power comes from authority to one in which managers need to exert influence, or soft power, across a matrix of organizations. To do this, leaders need to deploy a range of leadership styles and behaviours to support the creation of a strong culture of engagement in which power and responsibility are shared within service users, carers within teams, organizations and the wider healthcare system.

Leadership Success

Occupational therapy needs strong leaders to support the profession to flourish (Hankinson 2012). Bradd's et al. (2017) research found that there was less knowledge about allied health leadership than other clinical professions. However, although leadership success is a complex set of interactions between many variables, it can be reflected on from other industries. The main message is that there is no right style of leadership, but it is worth understanding that a range of leadership skills and attributes are as important as management capability. According to Kumar and Khiljee (2016) effective leadership is vital in modern healthcare settings and needs leaders to adopt a style that is inclusive and meets the needs of the healthcare professionals they work with, that is, a more collective leadership style. Goleman (1995) popularized the idea of emotional intelligence to help with the understanding of what makes leadership success. He said there are five main elements of emotional intelligence:

1. Self-awareness: If you are self-aware, you always know how you feel. Being self-aware in a leadership role means you know your strengths and weaknesses.
2. Self-regulation: This is about staying in control and not making rushed or emotional decisions.
3. Motivation: Self-motivated leaders work towards their goals.

4. Empathy: Leaders with empathy have the ability to put themselves in someone else's situation to help develop others, listen, challenge and give constructive feedback.

5. Social skills: Leaders with emotional intelligence are good communicators and experts at getting their team to support them and be excited about a new mission or project.

Leaders must have a solid understanding of their emotions and how their actions affect the people around them. The concept of 'authentic leadership' is important here. Davis (2017) proposed that authentic leadership is more about being true to your word and demonstrating by example than it is about getting people to follow you and telling others what to do. The better a leader relates to and works with others, the more successful he or she will be. 'Others' should now explicitly include the people we provide a service to.

MANAGEMENT AND LEADERSHIP IN OCCUPATIONAL THERAPY

Having considered management and leadership in general terms, this section considers management and leadership in occupational therapy from an historical perspective, management and leadership today and leadership for the future; all illustrated using management and leadership in the United Kingdom (note the comment above about the importance of culture in shaping management and leadership). To bring theory and practice together, this section ends with a case study that presents a day in the diary of an occupational therapy leader in mental health.

The Historical Perspective

Occupational therapists have always held management roles. For example, in the United Kingdom the chief occupational therapist in 1955 was responsible to the medical superintendent for the development and progress of the whole occupational therapy department. 'While delegating immediate responsibility for the working details to her respective occupational therapists she will act in a supervisory capacity under the direct authority of the medical superintendent and collaborate with the various medical officers in the sections allocated to them' (O'Sullivan 1955, p. 52). In one of their first textbooks Willard and Spackman (1963) recommended that management

responsibility should be established: 'effective administration is a means of getting things done through people and of making the institution a good place in which to work' (p. 17).

Over the years occupational therapy management roles have changed. In the 1970s district occupational therapists had an advisory role, only moving to holding managerial responsibility later in the decade. In the early 1980s a wider interpretation of management was introduced with the inception of the general manager role in health organizations. This person was someone who did not necessarily have a health professional qualification. As a result, a wide variety of individually determined management structures proliferated. It is the same today, with general management integral in organizations. However, there is also a greater number of professional staff, including occupational therapists, carrying out these managerial and operational roles.

In the past it was more common for occupational therapy managers to have had direct responsibility for holding budgets for services. They were given a predetermined amount to run an occupational therapy service within an organization based on the annual planning process. This role included being responsible for 'pay costs,' that is, costs incurred by the employment and payment of staff, and 'non-pay costs', that is, expenses incurred from running the service, for example, stationery, equipment, training and travel costs. It could also have included generating income from any activity, for example, external training provided and sale of goods.

Management and Leadership Today

In the ever-evolving healthcare system occupational therapy managers find themselves having to differentiate and understand a variety of management and leadership activity they have to undertake in their roles. In the United Kingdom many occupational therapy manager roles have less direct operational management responsibilities and have to use leadership skills, such as influencing to promote and profile the profession. This is particularly the case in mental health as occupational therapy managers, as stated earlier, increasingly take on AHP management and leadership roles. Collectively, AHPs 'are the third largest workforce in the NHS and their 'Allied health professionals into action: using allied health professionals to transform healthcare and wellbeing' (NHS 2017) outlines the transformative potential and power of a collective voice. At a similar time, in 2018 the RCOT launched their strategic intentions document, which focused on the importance of leadership. However, Rodger (2012) reiterated now, more than ever, whatever their professional role or stages of career development, occupational therapists need to embrace leadership opportunities, no matter how small.

One way to do this is to maintain the unique perspective of the occupational therapist at any level of occupational therapy or AHP leadership by focusing on 'our strength in being experts in both understanding occupation and its impact on health and how to use occupation to improve or maintain health and sharing our expertise with others will mark us out as truly a mature profession' (Molineux 2011, p. 95). This could be said of a student or a new therapist learning to find their professional voice as a lone worker in a team of specialists who bring a distinct skillset to their posts and of occupational therapy consultants leading the way forward in education, clinical expertise and research. To paraphrase Rodger (2012, p. 178), if we can provide an occupational perspective to address issues of importance to individuals whose performance and participation are limited, as well as to healthcare organizations and society more generally, occupational therapy will be more recognized and leadership will be celebrated as part of the profession's territory.

Leadership for the Future

Finally, there has also been great stock put on the value of marketing occupational therapy services and knowing about political influencing (Galheigo 2011; Morley and Rennison 2011). Generally speaking, marketing is seen to be about advertising and selling goods and services. It is also associated with identifying the particular wants and needs of a target market of customers; in health terms, a whole range of stakeholders from service users and their carers to commissioners. Marketing goes on to analyse customers' needs and makes strategic decisions about product design, pricing, promotion and distribution. Some of that marketing strategy for occupational therapy could be, for example, the professional bodies lobbying political parties through to an individual occupational therapist, creating new and inventive interventions to support changes in practice and to trigger a policy development at a local level. An example of this is the RCOT's series of documents 'Occupational Therapy: Improving lives, Saving Money' (2018). The documents provide overarching recommendations to improve health and well-being outcomes for people whilst demonstrating a strong return on investment. They have been very successful in highlighting how occupational therapy services can save money and improve health outcomes in mental health, and prisons, reducing pressures on hospitals and care for older people. Professional bodies producing guidance created by the profession is a very powerful tool in setting the direction of travel for the future leadership of the profession.

So, what is the future of occupational therapy management and leadership? Modern healthcare sits with a range of providers, not just government-funded organizations. Great stock is placed in the need for the occupational therapy profession to be more entrepreneurial (Lachter and Szymanska 2016). Many occupational therapists now work outside traditional healthcare settings in corporate and non-governmental charitable organizations. In the United Kingdom, for example, there has been the rising development of social enterprises and the potential of occupational therapists leading and managing them. A social enterprise is a business whose objectives are primarily social and whose profits are reinvested back into its services or the community (DH 2012). For example, students working as volunteers in third-sector social enterprise initiatives (Raine et al. 2010) are profiling the role of occupational therapists in that setting. Stickley (2017) studied occupational therapists who were working in social enterprises and concluded they were able to practice according to their professional philosophy and experience job satisfaction and professional autonomy. A second growth area refers to occupational therapists increasingly working in private practice, for example, paediatrics, acquired brain injuries and medicolegal work. This is seen by occupational therapists as a viable career choice with greater autonomy and financial flexibility. It does pose a question: Are there different skills sets required for occupational therapists as leaders and managers in this practice setting?

The AOTA developed a list of emerging practice areas in which occupational therapists may play a role. Those in mental health included depression, recovery and peer support model; sensory approaches and veterans and wounded warriors. It follows that with the increase of role emergent placements across the world comes the creation of role-emergent posts and occupational therapists that are equipped with confidence, autonomy and independence in service development (Ullah and Klaentschi 2011; Kearsley 2012).

SUMMARY

Far from being straightforward and simple, good management and leadership skills also require a great degree of intuition, influencing, pragmatism, and political awareness. Today's occupational therapists, from newly qualified practitioners to occupational therapy managers, are constantly challenged to provide the best evidence-based services possible. As outlined in the introduction to this chapter, it is essential for all practitioners to understand the concepts of management and leadership to provide that quality service. This chapter has reviewed the foundations of occupational therapy management, the growing importance of leadership skills and the changing nature of a widening brief of allied health professional management and leadership

alongside coproduction of services with service users and their carers within the modern healthcare system. Understanding the different types and styles of management and leadership will enhance occupational therapists' ability to perform the various tasks and activities required of them in their job role. Being an excellent professional and moving into management is not enough. Occupational therapists need to know what the essential components of management are to maximize their effectiveness. While known to be important and growing in significance, leadership does not always come naturally. Having a toolkit of techniques available to an aspiring professional or manager can enhance their performance as a leader. The model presented in this chapter brings together the competencies needed for both those management and leadership roles.

CASE STUDY 7.1

A Day in the Diary of an Occupational Therapy Leader Working in a Mental Health Service

Every day in the life of an occupational therapy manager and leader is different. Here are some examples of the tasks and activities a typical day might look like (the leadership qualities and skills and types of management that may be deployed in that day are in brackets).

- Plan and prepare for the day ahead (personal management, self-awareness, self-regulation)
- Read and respond to emails (personal management, motivation, information management, operational management)
- Convene and co-chair (with a service user) an organization-wide service user committee. The function of the meeting is to discuss service user involvement in the Trust's operational services and report back where service users are involved in the development of new services, quality initiatives and evaluating services (knowledge management, change and project management, influencing, personal and connection power)
- One-to-one professional supervision meeting (professional and people management, performance management, coaching, empathy, social skills, personal power)

- Spend time carrying out tasks (operational, project and information management, self-regulation)
- Chair an organization-wide project: functions include developing a community care plan on the organization's electronic system, gathering and coordinating contributions from a variety of stakeholders, staff, service users and their families (change, project and performance management, influencing, personal and connection power)
- Meet with the deputy medical director who is leading on a seclusion policy and wants occupational therapists to be involved in the implementation plan (change, professional and personnel management, influence and personal power)
- Meet with the AHP leads to begin developing a new strategy (knowledge, project and professional management)
- Read and respond to emails (personal management, information management, operational management, motivation)

QUESTIONS FOR CONSIDERATION

1. What management skills may help the transition from undergraduate to occupational practice?
2. What is your answer to the question, 'Why do organizations need managers?'
3. What might a manager consider and prioritize when practicing *Workforce* or *Project* planning?
4. Analyse your own attributes for each of the three key leadership styles, and suggest your own approach.
5. Based on Case Study 8.1, do you think your own leadership skillset would suit this role? If not, what might be an area that you need to develop?
6. Looking at each of the five main elements of emotional intelligence, determine your strength in each area and what that means for your leadership ability.

REFERENCES

Armstrong, M., & Baron, A. (2005). *Managing performance*. London: Chartered Institute of Personnel and Development.

Association of Project Management. (2019). Available at: https://www.apm.org.uk.governance. Accessed 24/3/19.

Bradd, P., Travaglia, J., & Hayen. (2017). A leadership in allied health: A review of the literature. *The Asia Pacific Journal of Health Management, 12*(1), 17–24.

Braveman, B. (2016). *Leading and managing occupational therapy services, an evidence-based approach* (2nd ed.). Philadelphia: F.A Davis Company.

Braveman, B. (2016). *You have a seat at the table, now what? Indiana occupational therapy Association conference, Nov 5*th. (presentations) www.Brentbraveeman.com.

Clark, F. (2010). Power and confidence in professions: Lessons for occupational therapy. *Canadian Journal of Occupational Therapy, 77*(5), 264–269.

Clouston, T. J., & Whitcombe, S. W. (2008). The professionalization of occupational therapy. *British Journal of Occupational Therapy, 71*(8), 314–320.

College of Occupational Therapists (COT). (2006). *Recovering ordinary lives. The strategy for occupational therapy in mental health services 2007–2017*. London: College of Occupational Therapists.

Davidson, H. (2012). A leadership challenge for occupational therapy. *British Journal of Occupational Therapy, 78*(8), 390–392.

Davis, J. (2017). *The power of authentic leadership*. eBookIt.com.

Department of Health (DH). (2011). *Payment by results. Mental health factsheet No. 15, Gateway reference 15828*. London: Department of Health.

Department of Health (DH). (2012). *Top tips for establishing a healthcare social enterprise*. Available at: http://webarchive.nationalarchives.gov.uk/+/www.dh.gov.uk/en/Managingyourorganisation/Socialenterprise/index.htm.

Drucker, P. (1955). *The practice of management*. Oxford: Elsevier.

Fund, K. (2015). *Leadership and leadership development in health care*. Available at: https//www.kingsfund.org.uk/publications/leadership-and-leadership-development-health-care.

Galheigo, S. M. (2011). What needs to be done? Occupational therapy responsibilities and challenges regarding human rights. *Australian Journal of Occupational Therapy, 58*(2), 60–66.

Goleman, D. (1995). *Emotional intelligence: Why it can matter more than IQ*. London: Bantam Books.

Hankinson, N. (2012). Editorial words from Naomi Hankinson – chair of BAOT council. E-newsletter. *The College of Occupational Therapists specialist section – mental health, 1*(2), 2–3.

Hendricks, F., & Toth-Cohen, S. (2018). Perceptions about authentic leadership development: South African occupational therapy students' camp experience. *Occupational Therapy International*.

Kemp, P. (2010). The creative involvement of service users in the classroom. In J. Weistein, & J. Kingsley (Eds.), *Mental health, service user involvement and recovery* (pp. 171–185). London: Jessica Kingsley Publishers.

Kumar, R. D. C., & Khiljee, N. (2016). Leadership in healthcare. *Anaesthesia and Intensive Care Medicine, 17*(1), 63–65.

Local Government Improvement and Development. (2012). Available at: http://webarchive.nationalarchives.gov.uk/20120202153716/http://idea.gov.uk/idk/core/page.do?pageid=1.

McCombie, R. P., & Antanavage, M. E. (2017). Transitioning for occupational therapy students to practicing occupational therapy students: First year of employment. *Occupational Therapy in Health Care, 31*(2), 126–142.

McGregor, D. (1987). *The human side of enterprise*. London: Penguin.

Mirvis, P., & Googins, B. (2018). Engaging employees as social innovators. *California Management Review, 60*(4), 25–50.

Molineux, M. (2011). Standing firm on shifting sands. *New Zealand Journal of Occupational Therapy, 58*(1), 21–28.

Morley, M. (2009). An evaluation of a preceptorship programme for newly qualified occupational therapists. *British Journal of Occupational Therapy, 72*(9), 384–392.

Morley, M., Garnham, M., Forsyth, K., et al. (2011). Developing occupational therapy indicative care packages in preparation for mental health payment by results. *Occupational Therapy in Mental Health, 16*(1), 15–19.

Morley, M., & Rennison, J. (2011). Marketing occupational therapy: everybody's business. *British Journal of Occupational Therapy, 74*(8), 406–408.

NHS operational management. Available at: http://www.nhscareers.nhs.uk/explore-by-career/management/careers-in-management/operational-management/.

NHS England. (2017). *Allied health professions into action*. Available at: https://www.england.nhs.uk/publications.ahps-into-action/.

Orman, K. (2018). *Why is leadership such a hot topic for occupational therapists right?* Available at: www.rcot.co.uk.

O'Sullivan, E. N. M. (1955). *Textbook of occupational therapy.* London: HK Lewis.

Project Management Institute. (2012). Available at: http://www.pmi.org/uk-landing.aspx.

Raine, R., Eyres, P., Luscombe, A., et al. (2010). *Developing social enterprise. Volunteering opportunities of occupational therapy students.* Available at: http://uplace.org.uk:8080/dspace/handle/10293/784?show=full.

Rodger, S. (2012). Leadership through an occupational lens: Celebrating our territory. *Australian Occupational Therapy Journal, 59*(3), 172–179.

Royal College of Occupational Therapists. (2018). *Improving lives, saving money.* Available at: www.rcot.co.uk.

Smyth, G. (2017). *Occupational therapy promoting employment.* Available at: www.rcot.co.uk.

Spyby, M. (2012). Let the sparks fly! The College of occupational therapists specialist section – ment. *Health, 1*(2), 5–6.

Stickley, A. J., & Hall, K. J. (2017). *Social enterprise: A model of recovery and social inclusion for occupational therapy practice in the UK.* Mental Health and Social Inclusion, 21(2), pp. 91–101. https://doi.org/10.1108/MHSI-01-2017-0002.

The Kings Fund. (2012). *Leadership and engagement for improvement.* London: The Kings Fund.

UK Essays. (2018). *Use of power in Organisations.* Available at: https://www.ukessays.com/essays/management/the-use-of-power-in-organizations—management-essay.php?vref=1.

Ullah, M. M., & Klaentschi, C. (2011). 'Role emerging' placements – a global phenomenon? *Occupational Therapy News, 19*(4), 36.

Willard, H. S., & Spackman, C. S. (1963). *Occupational therapy* (3rd ed.). Philadelphia, PA: Lippincott.

8 PROFESSIONAL ACCOUNTABILITY

BOB COLLINS

CHAPTER OUTLINE

INTRODUCTION

Over the last century occupational therapy has developed into an autonomous healthcare profession (World Federation of Occupational Therapists (WFOT) 2007; Loh et al. 2017). However, with professional autonomy comes accountability, and therefore practitioners are personally responsible for what they do (Royal College of Occupational Therapists (RCOT) 2017), are answerable to others for their actions and must be able to justify their decisions (Health & Care Professions Council (HCPC) 2013). Set in the context of trust, this chapter explores professional accountability and how it affects the working lives of occupational therapists in mental health. It also explores how accountability might be accomplished whilst maintaining the core values of the profession.

What is Professional Accountability?

Simply deconstructed, the term 'accountability' refers to the ability to give account; to describe or document an action or event. Associated dictionary definitions include the term to 'bring to account'; to give reasons for or justify what has been done. In their article about professionalism, Nortje and De Jongh identify that the word 'profession' derives from the Latin, meaning 'public declaration' and a professional's 'main aim is to profess on how best to organize and deliver health care' (2017, p. 43). Professional accountability is therefore understood to be not only about providing best care but doing that openly and under the scrutiny of others.

A Crisis of Trust?

Traditionally, the public rarely questioned the care they received from healthcare providers, holding the fundamental belief that a professional would provide a good service. Opinion shows that the public are able put their trust in health professionals with an expectation that they will do their job well, for the benefit of others, or at the very least they will do no harm, take advantage of, deceive or exploit others (Smith 2017). Nobody suspected UK doctor Harold Shipman or nurses Beverly Allitt, Lucy Letby and numerous other cases worldwide (Medical Error Action Group 2019) because they were 'trusted' professionals. However, harm at the hands of a malicious minority has prompted stringent legislation for professional registration and staff regulation, and subsequently systems have been implemented to protect the public (Department of Health (DH) 2019). Unfortunately, these systems have often failed, and the public remains at risk, resulting in a well-documented 'crisis of trust' (Hutchinson 2018; Gille, Smith and Mays 2015).

Shortfalls in healthcare continue to be reported on a global scale, with headlines suggesting that death and suffering are linked to low quality healthcare in low- and middle-income countries; medical staff are the third largest cause of death in America; and unavoidable deaths in hospitals are the 'biggest scandal in global healthcare.' Alongside nationally renowned failings such as the Esidimeni scandal in South Africa (143 deaths) (Makgoba 2017), the Winterbourne View (physical and psychological abuse suffered by people with learning disabilities) (Flynn 2012) and Mid-Staffordshire Trust (patients routinely neglected) (Francis 2013) enquiries in the United Kingdom, there is a perception that trust in health services is at a critically low level and that professionals may no longer be deemed to be trustworthy (Huang et al. 2018).

Failing public trust has brought about the urge to make services more transparent for professionals to share and cascade facts and figures and make information widely accessible to the public through media and technology (Roberts 2017). However, where there is greater transparency there is a greater risk of a breach or abuse of confidentiality, or misinformation and deception. 'Health professionals are regulated in order to ensure that they have the skills, competence, health and attitudes that command public trust and patient confidence' (DH 2019, p. 9).

Also, in the ongoing economic downturn and climate of austerity there is growing pressure to show effectiveness, to provide indicators of performance, and to reach payment by result targets (Wanna, Lee and Yates 2015).

The consequence of accumulating public mistrust has led to further sanctions that make governments, institutions and professionals ever more accountable. Increasingly there is an expectation on professionals to provide evidence of their actions and monitor interventions. The increase in stringent measures to regulate, scrutinize and control has created a culture of bureaucracy which inhibits the performance of the professional and hinders their ability to do the job itself (O'Neill 2002). Systems of accountability implemented to limit the crisis of trust are actually having the opposite effect. Accountability tasks that 'tick the boxes' are distracting people from doing their job, with a midwife account saying, 'It takes longer to do the paperwork than deliver the baby' (O'Neil 2013, p. online). For occupational therapists, rising expectations to fulfil accountability processes jeopardizes therapeutic time and threatens the fundamental philosophy of person-centred work, which underpins their practice.

Any frameworks implemented to improve practice do, in principle, raise standards. There are now UK policies, such as Whistle Blowing and Freedom to Speak Up, that encourage staff to report on any practice that falls below expected standards. Yet there is a conflict between expectations to undertake accountability processes, which are driven by management, and an approach in keeping with occupational therapy values and beliefs. Accountability processes undertaken at a clinical level may detract from person-centred working because more time has to be spent in training and governance obligations (Royal College of Nurses (RCN) 2017). These processes seem to only meet the 'paymasters'' needs for continued commissioning or attempts to regain the trust of a litigious society. O'Neill (2013) challenges whether we do in fact need to trust more and rebuild trust. Instead, she encourages the public to trust more intelligently and place trust in the trustworthy, asking professionals to provide simple and adequate evidence that they can be trusted by being competent, honest and reliable.

WHO ARE OCCUPATIONAL THERAPISTS ACCOUNTABLE TO?

The issue of who occupational therapists are accountable to is complex and multifaceted. Ultimately, and most importantly, occupational therapists are accountable to the people they serve, but there are also demands from employers and governing bodies for performance quality and governance requirements. As a healthcare professional your behaviour and decision-making should align with the standards expected by yourself, your profession and the public. Both the WFOT (2016) and the Council of Occupational Therapists for the European Countries (COTEC) (2009) document these three levels of quality and obligation as Level one—to self, Level two—to a second person and Level three—to groups and society.

Level One—Self

In her inaugural presidential address to the American Occupational Therapy Association, Lamb (2016) asks her audience to reflect on their career as occupational therapists and how their personal values led to that choice of profession. She asserts that by being authentic to our values in our everyday working lives we are able to drive the profession to meet the needs of the public. 'Values and ethical responsibilities (one's sense of what is important, of what is right and wrong) inform and direct professional behaviours, which, in turn, affect one's level of professionalism' (Hordichuk, Robinson and Sullivan 2015, p. 153). Professional accountability starts with integrity and authenticity of the self.

Level Two—A Second Person

The Recipient of Occupational Therapy

A core value of the occupational therapy profession is person-centred practice, which upholds collaboration and shared decision-making. Occupational therapists have always upheld the person at the centre and worked 'with' people rather than 'for' people (Creek 2003). Although the therapeutic relationship should be as equal as possible, ultimately the responsibility lies with the therapist to ensure that the nature of the relationship always remains professional. There is a difference between providing social interventions in a person-centred, friendly way and becoming

friends with people. It may be acceptable to attend a social function as a therapeutic intervention as long as boundaries and professional integrity are discussed (HCPC 2016), see Case Study 8.1 for clinical contexts).

Occupational therapists need to be able to effectively communicate personal boundaries in the context of their professional standards. If any problems remain, they should use supervision to discuss and explore any issues to establish a resolution and manage any blurring of professional boundaries.

Employers

Occupational therapists are accountable to their employers and must work within the terms and conditions of their employment and job description. They may face disciplinary action or dismissal if they

---

CASE STUDY 8.1
Personal and Professional Boundaries

An occupational therapist invites an individual to attend a social function and questions whether it is acceptable to drink a small quantity of alcohol to normalize the social situation. Practitioners should refer to professional standards to know what is acceptable. The UK Code of Ethics and Professional Conduct states, 'You must not undertake any professional activities when under the influence of alcohol, drugs or other intoxicating substances' (Royal College of Occupational Therapists (RCOT) 2015, p. 25). Therefore even a small amount of alcohol would not be acceptable.

If an occupational therapist is going to have lunch with someone, it is not usually appropriate for the therapist to eat as it may be seen as financial abuse or exploitation (RCOT 2015) if the person always buys and cooks lunch for the occupational therapist. As the person may find this difficult to understand and be offended by the decision, it is important for the occupational therapist to explain the circumstances in relation to their professional responsibilities. Also, if the individual misinterprets the invitation as anything other than professional, they may be vulnerable to emotional rejection if the situation was not clarified in advance.

do not. All employees are expected to demonstrate certain standards in communication, development, safety, improvement, quality and diversity. Professionals employed in posts with higher profiles are expected to take on higher levels of proficiency and responsibility, handle diverse data and work with complex information, collaborate and develop working relationships, work safely and successfully assess and manage risk (HCPC 2013). Employers expect occupational therapists to critically evaluate outcomes, be able to reflect and review practice and solve problems, have excellent interpersonal skills to relate sensitively to others and have an aptitude to learn and undertake self-improvement (Skills for Health 2008). Employers also expect employees to keep up to date with mandatory training requirements such as:

- fire training
- moving and handling
- infection control
- data protection

And depending on the job role, other competency requirements may include:

- basic life support
- managing aggression and violence, conflict resolution and breakaway
- safeguarding adults
- child protection
- food hygiene
- carer awareness

Employers develop local policies to ensure that employees work within the frameworks of policy and legislation, and staff training is just one standard by which NHS services are governed to ensure high standards (Box 8.1). To maintain the core values of their profession, occupational therapists should engage in training to maximize the quality and safety of service provision.

Level Three—Groups and Society

The Profession

Occupational therapists are accountable to their profession and have a responsibility to define their role, provide an explanation of occupational therapy and uphold what makes the profession unique. 'Underpinning your practice is the belief that occupation

---

BOX 8.1
CLINICAL GOVERNANCE

In the United Kingdom the NHS has developed a regulatory structure called Clinical Governance defined as 'the system through which NHS organizations are accountable for continuously improving the quality of their services and safeguarding high standards of care by creating an environment in which clinical excellence will flourish (Scally and Donaldson, 1998, p.61).' It is an umbrella term that includes working in partnership with service users, carers and the public to develop and deliver services, manage risks, audit services and ensure that they are effective and based on the best available evidence and ensure that staff are recruited and managed effectively. Healthcare institutions in the United Kingdom are now regulated by the Care Quality Commission, which reports to the public about the quality of services delivered. There are five things that are asked of services: are they safe, caring, responsive, effective and well led (Care Quality Commission 2018)? As well as being responsible for the quality and safety of services, many organizations now have to be financially accountable through the status of Foundation Trusts. Although these systems are developed to regulate the NHS, many providers in the United Kingdom use them to monitor the quality of their services under the banner of Clinical Governance.

---

and activity are fundamental to a person's health and wellbeing' (RCOT 2015). In 2018 the RCOT published their new report for occupational therapy in mental health. Part of the *Improving Lives Saving Money* series, 'Getting my Life Back' aims to consolidate the profession's place in delivering mental health and well-being through occupation (RCOT 2018). Accountability to the profession necessitates knowing and using occupation to deliver on health and social care outcomes. In early 2019, NHS England published The NHS Long Term Plan (NHS England 2019). The RCOT response to this document expresses reassurance that the key themes promoted in the document around prevention, care closer to home and integrated services reflect the values recommended by the College, which 'places the profession in a key role to help deliver the plan's vision for the NHS' (Scott 2019, p. online). It seems that the profession is now at the forefront of change necessitated by challenges facing modern health services (RCOT 2018) (Care Quality Commission, Public

Health England, NHS 2015). Occupational therapists and other health professions have seized the opportunity to inspire and transform health and social care systems (Chief Allied Heath Professions Officer's Team 2017).

National Standards

In the United Kingdom occupational therapists are regulated by the HCPC. A few examples of the regulatory bodies for other English-speaking countries are:

- National Board for Certification in Occupational Therapy (United States)
- Allied Health Practitioners Registration Authority (Australia)
- Occupational Therapy Board of New Zealand (New Zealand)
- Health Professions Council of South Africa (South Africa)
- Council of Occupational Therapists for European Countries (Europe)
- Association of Canadian Occupational Therapy Regulatory Organizations (Canada)

The title 'occupational therapist' is protected by law in many countries, and it can only be used by those registered with their relevant bodies such as the HCPC (2018), who keep a register of health professionals that meet a set of standards for health, training, professional skills and behaviour. To be able to register, an accredited course must be completed and standards maintained for continued registration. Occupational therapists are also accountable to wider society via the criminal justice system. If a criminal offence is committed, they are subject to criminal justice proceedings and could be tried in a criminal court (RCOT 2017). Indemnity insurance is used to protect occupational therapists from the personal financial cost of this, but they may be struck off the HCPC register.

Wherever in the world occupational therapists work and whether that is in health, social care or non-traditional, role-emerging/diverse practice or independent settings, they will be subjected to fluctuating and evolving working environments (Wimpenny and Lewis 2015). Despite the changes they have to withstand they are expected to continuously provide excellent and effective services. To enable them to reach these high expectations of care many are able to perform their duties based on a set of guidelines published by the occupational therapy professional council of their country of practice.

The UK Code of Ethics and Professional Conduct (RCOT 2015), though not legally binding, provides occupational therapists with an accountability framework upon which to base professional standards and behaviours whilst remaining person-centred and retaining integrity. It can be used as evidence in any civil or criminal proceedings as a measure of reasonable and acceptable practice. It would be difficult to put up a defence against allegations of negligence if these standards had not been followed. Equally, it would be difficult to substantiate a claim of unfair dismissal before an employment tribunal if an employer could establish a persistent failure to meet these standards.

International Standards

The WFOT places responsibility for competent, ethical and professional behaviour on each of its associate country's lead professional organizations. Any authority that has not developed standards for practice in occupational therapy is expected to follow those of WFOT (2016). Membership countries of the COTEC are all expected to have a Code of Ethics and Professional Conduct to ensure excellent, safe and equitable services are provided with the best interests of the public they serve at heart. 'An overall mission of Code of Ethics is to promote high professional standards and quality in occupational therapy practice based on client-centred or user-oriented principles and social responsibilities' (COTEC 2009, p. 4).

Professional accountability will be illustrated in this chapter by focussing on the systems used to regulate occupational therapists working in the United Kingdom. The Code of Ethics and Professional Conduct published by the UK College of Occupational Therapists (RCOT 2015) is used extensively in this chapter to highlight the professional standards occupational therapists are expected to abide by in the United Kingdom. This code is similar to the codes of conduct published in other countries (if expressed slightly differently), and readers are encouraged to access their local codes of conduct and consult any related pieces of legislation (e.g., mental health act). If you do not work in the United Kingdom, the reality of this practice may not be directly relevant to you, but the underlying principles will be. Hence this chapter is suitable to students and occupational therapists both working in the United Kingdom and across the globe. The code is divided into the following sections:

- Service provision including risk management and record keeping;
- Service user welfare and autonomy including consent and confidentiality;
- Professionalism including personal and professional integrity;
- Professional competence and lifelong learning;
- Developing and using the profession's evidence base.

These headings have been used to structure the discussion over the rest of this chapter.

SERVICE PROVISION

The service provided by occupational therapists will always be structured around the therapy process, from referral and assessment to planning, implementation, review and discharge. Creek (2003) identifies a more detailed version of what a complex intervention is, but the idea of an on-going cycle of reflection on the situation and negotiation with people remains constant. Occupational therapists have a responsibility to ensure that they provide a fair and equitable service in accordance with the law in their country and the Human Rights Act (Her Majesty's Stationary Office 1998). Many services use referral criteria to assess the need for occupational therapy and prioritize the workload to maximize resources. The reality is that occupational therapists work within finite resources, and there are often times when service demand exceeds the capacity to meet it. For example, one week lots of people meet the referral criteria but not everyone can be seen, maybe due to staff shortage because of annual leave or sickness absence. Another week, with staff at full capacity, there might be more people who meet the high priority criteria and so those lower down the priority list may not be seen. Either way, those with lower

priority needs may have to wait longer for therapeutic intervention, so it is important that decisions are as fair as possible and can be justified against specific criteria. One such document is the Community Health Occupational Therapy Priority Tool—Adult (Victoria State Government 2018), which is used to screen referrals and can be made publicly available for people to make sense of any decisions that affect access to care. This is a good example of transparent decision making. Consideration may need to be given to how transparency is achieved as care records will only document decisions about individual interventions and not service management decisions. A poster displayed in accessible areas may be an appropriate way of publicizing how referrals are prioritized. However, efforts to provide transparent information can be counterproductive as it can breed suspicion and mistrust (O'Neill 2002). Rather than providing open access information to the public, it may be better to justify decisions discretely to individuals as needed.

A common dilemma for occupational therapists working in mental health, particularly those who are employed as case managers or care coordinators, is that priority is given to referrals or cases which present with high risk. It may become a challenge to work beyond minimizing risk and to find capacity to work with people's occupational needs that affect quality of life. The following section suggests possibilities to optimize occupational participation and effectively manage risk.

Risk Management

Risk management involves identifying potential hazards or negative incidents and providing adaptive strategies to reduce the likelihood of these occurring or minimizing the harm caused if they do (NHS Improvement 2018). Occupational therapists are accountable to the systems designed to ensure that any risks are identified and reduced wherever possible to maintain duty of care to the people they serve and the general public. For example, they have a duty to safeguard children and vulnerable adults with whom they come into contact and need to ensure that abuse is recognized and dealt with effectively. Another important system for those working in mental health in the United Kingdom is the Mental Health Act (Her Majesty's Stationary

Office 2007), which is a law designed to assess and treat people in the interest of their own or others health and safety. Inevitably, despite attempts to manage risk, incidents do occur, and both public and staff will at times be exposed to risk. Therefore many organizations have systems for recording incidents and near misses.

The National Patient Safety Agency (2008) published a version of a widely recognized risk management tool for use in the NHS. The five-by-five matrix requires risk to be defined and the seriousness of the outcome ranked on a five-point scale including negligible, minor, moderate, major or catastrophic. A negligible consequence would have minimal impact, for example, an incident resulting in a graze or bruise requiring no or minimal intervention. A catastrophic outcome would be, for example, a major incident leading to multiple, permanent injuries or death or an incident involving large numbers of patients. The probability of the incident occurring is then established using a five-point scale including rare, unlikely, possible, likely, probable and almost certain. Rare incidents would probably never recur and 'almost certain' incidents would undoubtedly recur, possibly frequently (Fig. 8.1).

A risk score is calculated by multiplying the consequence by the likelihood. Consequence (C) × Likelihood (L) = Risk (R). A green incident between 1 and 3 = low risk, yellow between 4 and 6 = moderate risk, orange between 8 and 12 = high risk, and a red incident between 15 and 25 = extreme risk (The National Patient Safety Agency 2008). Every incident or near miss can be scored in this way and should be recorded for review and escalated to the senior clinician, management and risk management team as required. Staff should be clear about what to report and when to effectively manage risk, identify what can be done to prevent any further incidents and consider whether any risks are acceptable. Once a risk score (1 to 25 and green to red) has been identified, clinicians should refer to published criteria and local risk management policy to identify what action should be taken if an incident occurs. An incident identified as low risk (green) may only require review by a local team manager, resolved only by minimal action and only require ongoing monitoring for any repetition. Any repetition of incident or near miss may escalate the likelihood of the incident to a moderate or high risk and require further action (Case Study 8.2).

If the consequence is very serious and/or it is very likely that the incident will happen again, giving a high risk score, it needs to be given high priority in terms of resources. Any high or extreme risk should trigger further investigation either by an internal incident investigator or by external sources. For example, a suicide by ligature on an in-patient ward would score as red or as an extreme risk incident. A serious incident investigation would be undertaken, and a coroner's inquest may require reports from all parties involved in that person's care. Immediate action would be taken to assess risk to individuals and update all risk assessments, increase observations where necessary, assess the environment and ligature points and minimize access to any ligatures. Any internal or external review should identify any failing in current systems or

Likelihood by consequence risk matrix (the national patient safety agency 2008)				
	Likelihood			
Consequence	1	2	3	4	5
	Rare	Unlikely	Possible	Likely	Almost certain
5 Catastrophic	5	10	15	20	25
4 Major	4	8	12	16	20
3 Moderate	3	6	9	12	15
2 Minor	2	4	6	8	10
1 Negligible	1	2	3	4	5

Fig. 8.1 ▪ Likelihood by consequence risk matrix. (The National Patient Safety Agency 2008.)

protocols, and a thorough review of practice may identify need for change of working practice, staff training or extra funding to improve environments.

This risk management tool is used across many industries, professions and diverse settings. It can be used to manage clinical risk such as self-harm, health and safety such as the spillage of a hazardous substance and financial risks such as lack of funding for safe

---

CASE STUDY 8.2
Monitoring Adverse Events to Reduce Risk

A group of occupational therapists working in mental health services for older people participated in the organization's incident reporting system since its inception. Whenever a low-risk incident or near miss occurred, they filled in a report and submitted it to the risk manager. Once a month they received information that summarized the incidents that had taken place. This was reviewed in the monthly occupational therapy meeting so that consideration could be given to how risks could be reduced, both for a one-off incident and for those with emerging trends. Between February and April there was an increase in the number of incidents reported in the occupational therapy garden. There were four reports of near misses, describing how service users had stumbled on the way out to the greenhouse, and one report of an incident in which a service user had fallen, with minimal harm, in the same place. Examination of previous reports revealed that the reason for the falls was a patio slab that had become raised during the hard frost of the winter to create an uneven piece of ground, thus escalating the likelihood of the risk to 'likely' and overall risk score to 'high.' As a result of this analysis, a requisition was put into the works department and the slab was re-laid to make the ground even again. Consequently, there were fewer incident and near miss reports submitted in May, and no service users were reported to have stumbled or fallen on the patio. To ensure that this risk did not occur in other parts of the organization, the Risk Management Department circulated a memorandum highlighting the risk and asking managers to check patio areas.

---

staffing levels. It is used to standardize risk management processes, identify trends and disseminate information so that practice can be changed to improve safety.

Positive and Defensive Risk Management

In mental health settings in which there are potentially high levels of risk, professionals might be inclined to spend a disproportionate amount of time completing risk assessments to ensure that they are not accountable if a risk incident occurs. Worse still is when all possible risk situations are avoided, leading to a negative cycle of defensive practice. Following any major untoward incident, media attention and management scrutiny on practice can provoke fear amongst staff and public, which may lead to reduced confidence and the practice becoming even more risk averse (Felton & Stickley 2018). It is important to find a balance between ensuring safety and providing opportunities for people to engage in activities that promote health and well-being. A cycle of defensive risk management (Department of Health & Social Care 2009) that leads to occupational deprivation (see Chapter 3) may increase risk levels and should be avoided. A risk management approach which engages the person in a collaborative process provides a more positive experience and reduces risk because strategies for risk management are sought and implemented. This then leads to further collaboration and reduced risk.

Positive Risk Taking

There are comprehensive clinical risk management tools available for use in specific situations, such as A Pocket Guide to Risk Assessment and Management in Mental Health (Hart 2014), which is used across services including acute wards, crisis intervention and longer term community mental health teams. The guide encourages a positive approach by undertaking an assessment of risk, identifying a formulation and developing a risk management plan. It promotes risk management as a dynamic process and taking risks to produce positive outcomes. Weighing up potential risk with potential benefits and deciding what is acceptable risk is as important as minimizing harmful consequences of risk (Fig. 8.2).

This alternative matrix proposed by the author of this chapter emphasizes to the reader that risk taking

Likelihood by consequence benefit matrix (authors interpretation of diagram 1)					
	Likelihood				
Consequence	1	2	3	4	5
	Rare	Unlikely	Possible	Likely	Almost certain
5 Astronomic	5	10	15	20	25
4 Major	4	8	12	16	20
3 Moderate	3	6	9	12	15
2 Minor	2	4	6	8	10
1 Negligible	1	2	3	4	5

Fig. 8.2 ■ Likelihood by consequence benefit matrix. (Author's interpretation of Fig. 8.1.)

can lead to potential benefits and not just harm. It uses the same principal but this time considers the outcome as benefit rather than harm. Consequence (C) × Likelihood (L) = Benefit (B) score. A red score is between 1 and 3 = low benefit, orange between 4 and 6 = moderate benefit, yellow between 8 and 12 = high benefit, and a green between 15 and 25 = extreme benefit. This benefit matrix can be used by occupational therapists and other professionals to evidence the benefit of engagement in activity, in planning and evaluating groupwork and in providing a therapeutic environment. A red or low benefit score could mean that not many people benefit from a certain intervention, perhaps offering a group activity that only appeals to a few people or that an activity is not a good fit for someone and so they have no motivation to engage. An orange or moderate benefit may be an activity that involves several people but only significantly benefits one person. An example of a high benefit or yellow score might be to allow a person to use sharp knives in the kitchen to prepare a meal. The session provides opportunity for mastering a skill and succeeding, which improves confidence and motivates more achievements. Another example of high benefit might be the fitting of mirrors to inpatients' en-suite bathrooms. Once effectively risk managed, this provides an opportunity for all people in that environment to engage with activities of daily living effectively, to undertake self-care tasks and to improve self-esteem, self-worth and positive identity and thus move further along on their journey of recovery. Finally, a green score, or extreme benefit, could be described as something that involves wider groups and populations such as a stakeholder event with arts and music or a football tournament involving people with lived experience of mental health from other parts of the country where there are multiple benefits to both physical and mental well-being.

These are only a few examples of the potential benefits derived from meaningful occupation, therapeutic environments and opportunity for self-care and social or leisure activity. When considering an intervention, if the probability of a risk or harm incident occurring is reduced by positive risk management and the likelihood of there being major therapeutic benefits to the person, then the intervention can be justified. This focus on benefit rather than risk fits with a wider, modern context of mental health recovery, which looks at the positives and identifies strengths rather than deficits and encourages more of what works to aid self-efficacy, reconnection and recovery. As an occupational therapist in mental health it may be that you are the only person to put your trust in a person and brave enough to take risks, but when managed effectively you can have amazing outcomes with positive risk taking (Case Study 8.3).

Record Keeping

In whatever setting, reports enhance the collaborative process to produce efficient and effective services (Buchanan, Jelsma and Siegfried 2016). Record keeping is fundamental to the profession as it ultimately improves care. 'Records primarily support and enable the provision of care to the service user, but they also demonstrate that you have carried out your

CASE STUDY 8.3

Positive Risk Taking

A man on a section in a mental health ward had assaulted another patient and was subsequently denied leave. The following week his risk behaviour escalated, and there were several other incidents of physical abuse to staff and patients on the ward. Staff began to become fearful of him and avoid any contact with him, and he continued to be denied leave for fear of unpredictable behaviour in the community. His lack of opportunity to engage in any meaningful activity on and off the ward contributed to a further deterioration of his mental health, and the cycle of risk, fear and occupational deprivation continued. During the initial assessment on the ward the occupational therapist had ascertained that the young man had been a keen rock climber. The occupational therapist discussed this with him and they agreed this would be something to work towards. During the multidisciplinary team meeting the occupational therapist suggested that she could take him to a local climbing wall. The team thought that this would be unsuitable due to his mental state and unpredictability, but the team agreed with him this would be a good goal to work towards. A plan was agreed to engage him in other activities on the ward and take a graded approach to building up escorted leave. Over the next few weeks the young man's behaviour was less destructive, and his escorted leave went well. The occupational therapist undertook the necessary risk assessments and took the decision that the benefits of a focused physical activity in a controlled environment outweighed the potential risk involved, and he was granted leave to go with the occupational therapist to the climbing wall. The activity was a success and the sessions continued on a weekly basis until the man was well enough to go home where the activity continued with the community team.

responsibilities in line with legal, professional and local requirements' (RCOT 2018, p. 1). Care records can include any media that holds information collected as part of an individual's care provision. Materials can be handwritten, electronic, auditory or visual and would include computer or digital data, images, auditory or visual recordings, letters, notes, emails, text messages and duplicate copies (RCOT 2018). All occupational therapists must follow local and national legislation with regard to record keeping. For example, in the United Kingdom the Care Programme Approach provides a framework to assess need, plan care and undertake reviews to ensure needs are being met.

Reports should provide a full, precise and justifiable account of what interventions are planned and delivered and should adhere to any national guidelines. Written notes should be accurate, legible, updated after each contact and contemporaneous, that is, written as soon after the event as possible (RCOT 2017). Some local policies maintain that best practice should be within 24 hours. Notes should clearly identify the person's name, date of birth, any identifying reference if used (this is the NHS number in the United Kingdom) and are chronological with a clear date and time. It is also good practice for records to be written with the person and written in terms they can understand without any overcomplicated terminology or confusing abbreviations (RCOT 2018). For example, in electronic communication 'lol' has been used and confused as meaning 'laugh out loud,' 'lots of love' and more offensively, 'little old lady'. Thus most occupational therapy services avoid abbreviations altogether, although some will allow them in accordance with local policy that has a list of accepted abbreviations included within the notes.

Records should also provide an account of the assessment, the intervention planned and provided and the arrangements for continuing contact. It is often useful to link interventions to the care plan so it is clearly seen how interventions are meeting the person's needs. Best practice also suggests that people's care records demonstrate that care is based on evidence; this is a particular requirement in insurance-funded health systems. Also, the person's views and any action taken responding to their needs, including any information provided, explanations given or warnings delivered, should be recorded. It is useful to base care records on a clear structure. For example, 'SOAP' notes use the headings Subjective, Objective, Analysis and Plan to ensure all elements of good record keeping are included (Gately and Borcherding 2016).

In the United Kingdom, although there are no laws specifically addressing record keeping, there are several pieces of related legislation:

- The Data Protection Act (2018) relates to how records are kept and information is shared.
- The Freedom of Information Act (2000) refers to people accessing their medical records (unless they include third party information or disclosure information which is harmful to the person).
- The Access to Health Records Act (1990) applies to relatives of deceased patients.
- The Human Rights Act (1998) relates to people's right to complain about how they are treated, and records may be cross referenced as evidence.

Therefore record keeping is one of the most important elements of professional accountability, not only to the person but also to the legal framework, particularly if records are called upon for legal proceedings; 'if it's not written down, it didn't happen' (Andrews and St. Aubyn 2015). 'An adequate medical record can be defined as one that enables you to reconstruct consultation without reference to memory. It doesn't mean that you need to write every detail, but when you come back to look at the record, you should be able to identify exactly what you would have done and said at the time' (Hegan 2004, p. 44). Both formal records and informal notes, for example, those taken during a home visit, in a case discussion or made in a diary, contain information that should be held safely under conditions of information governance.

Keeping records is an expected part of working practice but staff complain that the amount of record keeping is often unnecessary and a bureaucratic exercise (Moss 2017). It can seem as if the majority of time is spent undertaking accountability processes for the benefit of the management, but, ultimately, they are in place to benefit and protect the public. Occupational therapists need to keep their person-centred philosophy in mind and make all records relevant and pertinent to individual needs.

SERVICE USER WELFARE AND AUTONOMY

Capacity and Consent

Once a therapeutic relationship between a member of the public and a professional has been established, the professional takes on responsibility to ensure the well-being of that person. Firstly, someone's ability to make decisions, in other words their mental capacity, should be assessed. The Mental Capacity Act (2005) states that capacity should be assumed unless proved otherwise and is considered for each individual situation. If a person is deemed as lacking capacity, action should be taken in the person's best interest and in the least restrictive way (see Chapter 9 on Ethics for a wider discussion on mental capacity). When someone is referred to the occupational therapy service, it is then important to obtain informed consent for assessment and for further interventions. Gaining consent is not a one-off event but an on-going process, and individuals should be aware that they can refuse intervention at any time (RCOT 2015). It is not about signing a piece of paper or giving verbal consent once, but, as in deciding capacity, gaining consent is considered for each situation.

As far as possible, individuals should be able to make informed decisions about the therapeutic activities with which they wish to engage. Occupational therapists working in mental health may find times when people lack motivation to do an activity because they perceive they will not get any satisfaction from it.

CASE STUDY 8.4

Informed Choice

An occupational therapist works within a long-stay rehabilitation environment. The people she works with have been living in an institution for many years and may have attended Industrial Therapy units. They have never been able to explore what it is they enjoy and make informed choices about the activities they do and do not want to participate in (Fjellfeldt et al. 2016). The occupational therapist needs to offer a wide variety of activities and use her skills to encourage people to sample these so that they are able to make informed choices in the future. A refusal to participate may not be because they do not wish to engage in the activity but because they are not feeling mentally well enough to participate on that day. The occupational therapist needs to be patient and persistent without being coercive and keep offering opportunities to engage in meaningful activity.

Confidentiality

When members of the public pass personal information to professionals, they can expect to do so with the confidence that it will be looked after correctly and trust it will not be disclosed to other parties without permission. Occupational therapists have a responsibility to keep information safe and maintain confidentiality. The basic principle that they need to be aware of is that information should not be disclosed without the consent of the individual concerned. Where consent is given, this should be documented in the person's records, providing details of what information can be shared and with whom. However, there are exceptions to the rules around consent for disclosure, and the issue can be complex (DH 2003) (see Chapter 9 on Ethics for a more detailed discussion about confidentiality). Explaining circumstances of how, when and with whom information is shared is vital to ensure the rights of the individual are met and the correct procedures

related to risk are followed. Occupational therapists should be clear about what their responsibilities are around when and how information is shared with other members of the team, third parties and friends and family.

PROFESSIONALISM

Personal and Professional Integrity

It is hard to separate personal and professional integrity because your core values inform the decisions you make about a chosen profession. It would be inconsistent if someone with no hesitation about harming others were to choose a profession which requires the promotion and protection of others' well-being (Stemwedel 2007). There are times when it is necessary or useful to differentiate the boundaries between the personal and the professional, but these are not easy to define and can be ambiguous (Occupational Therapy Board of New Zealand 2016). Sometimes professional duties may take priority over personal values (e.g., putting aside personal feelings when providing a service for people with history of serious offences in a forensic setting or working in acute mental health settings where the maintenance of professional boundaries are required to maintain safety).

In clinical settings a uniform not only functions as appropriate work wear for health and safety reasons (DH 2010), but also it allows the wearer to distinguish between the personal and work role, to feel more professional and to be identified as an occupational therapist (HCPC 2011). Appearance plays an important role for the professional image of occupational therapy. What someone wears provides clues to others regarding their social standing and expected behaviour. Therefore professional conduct whilst wearing a uniform is important because the public expects continuity between behaviour and appearance behaviour (HCPC 2011).

In mental health practice the development of therapeutic relationships can be difficult. Nevertheless, Kannenberg et al. (2016) recognize the use of self as a core skill of the occupational therapist. Therapists need to 'adopt an approach which centres on the service user and establish appropriate professional relationships in order to motivate and involve the service user in meaningful occupation' (HCPC 2013, p. online). In a community mental health situation, wearing jeans and

---

CASE STUDY 8.5

Confidentiality

A young man has been admitted to a mental health unit on a police section after being arrested for breach of the peace. He does not want his parents to know the circumstances and does not consent to the ward sharing any information with his family. His family is informed by the police that he has been taken to hospital and is enquiring after his well-being. When the family arrives at the hospital the occupational therapist is asked to deal with the situation. She informs the young man that his parents are in the building and asks if he is willing to see them, and if not what information he will give. He is adamant he does not want to see them or want them to know what happened. The occupational therapist informs the parents that the young man is in good hands on the ward, but he is not willing to let them know what happened at this time. The occupational therapist apologizes and explains that until their son gives his consent, due to confidentiality policies, they cannot divulge any other information. The occupational therapist suggests that they contact the ward later in the week to see if the situation has changed and the family is directed to contact the police regarding the situation around the arrest.

a t-shirt and a hooded top or sportswear and adopting a more relaxed manner may at first sight seem unprofessional, but this approach may help the engagement process. In this case professionalism is more about considering what impact the therapist's presentation has on the person in their own social context. When working closely with people in the community and their own homes, occupational therapists also need to consider their conduct for optimizing meaningful occupation.

PROFESSIONAL COMPETENCE AND LIFELONG LEARNING

Lifelong learning spans all levels of personnel from support workers, those in education, to new graduates and specialist workers, up to those undertaking post-graduate and research scholarships. The range of learning activities through which professionals develop throughout their career is defined as 'continuing professional development (CPD).' CPD and lifelong learning are necessary for the development of everyone who works in health and social care and for the experience of service users. CPD and lifelong learning support a workforce that is capable of designing, delivering, evaluating and improving high-quality care and services' (Broughton and Harris, 2019, p. 5). Individuals are responsible for their own learning and development and are required to engage in a cyclical process of reflection and action which ensure they maintain their capacity to practice safely and legally (RCOT 2017). Evidence of CPD can come from a wide variety of learning activities and can be in whatever format suits the learning needs of the individual. Examples of CPD activities are shown in Table 8.1.

It is not simply the participation in a wide range of activities that contributes to good CPD; it is equally important to engage in the process of reflection and learning from those experiences. The RCOT has launched a series of resources to encourage CPD activity which includes a reflective log to help professionals consider what they have learned and how it can be put into practice.

In the United Kingdom the HCPC requires registrants to meet five standards of CPD which includes: i) keeping a record of CPD activity, ii) demonstrating that CPD activity is relevant to practice, iii) that it improves quality and iv) is of benefit to people using the service, and, if requested, v) submitting a

TABLE 8.1	
Continuing Professional Development Activities	
Categories	Examples
Work-based learning	■ Learning by doing ■ Case studies ■ Reflective practice ■ Audit of service users ■ Coaching from others ■ Discussions with colleagues ■ Peer review ■ Work shadowing ■ Secondments ■ Job rotation ■ Journal club ■ In-service training ■ Supervising staff or students ■ Expanding your role ■ Significant analysis of events ■ Project work ■ Filling in self-assessment questionnaires ■ Gaining and learning from experience ■ Involvement in the wider, profession-related work of your employer (for example, being a representative on a committee)
Professional activity	■ Lecturing or teaching ■ Mentoring ■ Being an examiner ■ Being a tutor ■ Involvement in a professional body, specialist-interest group, or other groups ■ Maintaining or developing specialist skills (for example, musical skills) ■ Giving presentations at conferences ■ Organizing journal clubs or other specialist groups ■ Organizing accredited courses ■ Being an expert witness ■ Supervising research or students ■ Being a national assessor
Formal and educational	■ Courses ■ Further education ■ Research ■ Attending conferences ■ Writing articles or papers ■ Going to seminars ■ Distance or online learning ■ Planning or running a course ■ Going on courses accredited by a professional body
Self-directed	■ Reading journals or articles ■ Reviewing books or articles ■ Keeping a file of your progress ■ Updating your knowledge through the internet or TV
Other	■ Relevant public service or voluntary work

Adapted from Health & Care Professions Council (2018).

written portfolio of CPD activity for quality assessment (HCPC 2018). To ensure professionals are engaged in meaningful, good quality CPD activity, the HCPC audits a sample of registered occupational therapists every two years. If selected, the registrant must present their professional profile with a summary report of current practice and statement about how CPD standards have been met along with relevant supporting evidence (HCPC 2017). A CPD portfolio should include a career history, a current job profile description, a personal development plan, the most current performance appraisal, reflective logs and a sample of achievements of learning (e.g., research papers, improved outcomes for the individual in practice and design of new rehabilitation programmes. Portfolios may also include course certificates and testimonials from colleagues, individuals and their families. Keeping a CPD portfolio is good practice, whether it is expected by a registration body or not, because reflecting on practice and learning experience improves professional competence. This ultimately leads to improvement in the quality of service experienced by people using them.

Professional competence also relates to occupational therapists only providing services that they are educated and qualified for. Any activity over and above their level of competence should be undertaken with planning and guidance. Occupational therapists have the right to refuse a request to undertake a task beyond their capabilities. Likewise, tasks should not be delegated to other team members without ensuring that they are capable and supervised (RCOT 2015). Competence also requires professional knowledge and skills to be maintained by an awareness and adherence to current evidence, legislation and guidance.

DEVELOPING AND USING THE EVIDENCE BASE

Occupational therapists must ensure compliance with national and international evidence-based recommendations and implement those that are relevant to the service they deliver. However, national guidance does not cover every intervention. This means that occupational therapists have a professional responsibility to ensure that their work is based on the best available evidence (RCOT 2015). Research and development in the field of occupational therapy and mental health is growing worldwide. Occupational therapists need to keep up to date to ensure that they can provide interventions based on available practice evidence. Some occupational therapists will want to contribute to the evidence base by carrying out research, but all occupational therapists need to be able to search for the evidence, critically appraise it and use it to inform their practice (HCPC 2013). One of the ways that occupational therapists can show that their practice reflects the evidence base is through clinical audit.

Clinical Audit

Clinical audit is sometimes confused with research (see Chapter 9); 'research is finding out what we ought to do, while audit is finding out if we are doing what we ought to do.' (Paton, Ranmal and Dudley 2015). For example, an occupational therapist may want to:

- survey colleagues to see which risk management tools are currently in use (research),
- complete a research project to establish which risk management tool is most appropriate for use within their setting (research), or
- complete an audit to see whether the risk management tool is being used in accordance with specified standards (audit).

It is important to be clear that the aim of auditing is to measure whether written standards or guidelines have been achieved. Standards for clinical practice may be audited against standards produced nationally or against internal audit criteria. Examples of audit could be how a service compares with:

- national standards and published guidelines
- other care providers delivering similar services
- standards set by the organization
- local standards relating to specific therapeutic interventions

The National Institute for Health and Care Excellence (NICE) regularly publishes sets of guidance and quality standards relating to various different conditions across the health and social care sector. Staff can use the guidance to ensure they are providing the best, most up-to-date and cost-effective care in their setting. One such example is the NICE guidelines published for psychosis and schizophrenia, which include information about early detection and management of psychosis and the standards to be followed for access to early intervention psychosis teams and the core interventions they should provide, including anti-psychotic medication, cognitive behavioural therapy for psychosis, family interventions, carer support, physical health checks, physical interventions and employment interventions (NICE 2016). Occupational therapists can form part of a wider multidisciplinary team to deliver on these guidelines to reduce the impact of the illness on the person to achieve successful recovery.

Although clinical audit is well established within health and social care services and the use of national guidelines are critical to maintaining best practice, local audit and scrutiny of services should be undertaken with caution. Local audits do not always lead to changes in service delivery, and there is little empirical evidence to suggest they improve care (Boyle and Keep 2018). Problems with audit include:

■ Lack of clarity about the issue being audited
■ Setting the standards without rigorous research
■ Poor feedback about results
■ Little time to implement any changes in practice

If occupational therapists do undertake an audit exercise, it is important to clarify what is being audited, measure against good quality data, identify what change needs to take place, actually implement some change and then monitor the effects of change. Occupational therapists have a responsibility to ensure that they share the lessons learned from their audit activity so that practice can be improved. In modern mental health services in the United Kingdom there is much less emphasis on local audit processes with increased focus on national programmes overseen by independent organization, Healthcare Quality Improvement Partnership, which aims to improve quality of services measured against standard NICE guidelines.

SUMMARY

This chapter has explored professional accountability using the Code of Ethics and Professional Conduct published by the UK RCOT (2015). Many European and worldwide organizations have a similar code of ethics and professional conduct so the principles are likely to be widely applicable. Although some of the processes associated with professional accountability can sometimes seem to exist for the benefit of the organizations, the practitioners work within there is an ultimate professional responsibility to ensure that people using services receive the best possible care. This means ensuring that professional accountability is more than a set of merely bureaucratic processes designed to reassure the public. It is also a framework for maintaining practitioners' focus on the person-centred values of occupational therapy.

QUESTIONS FOR CONSIDERATION

1. Describe what each of the three levels of quality and obligation might mean for you in your current role or in a prospective role.
2. Name the regulatory body for occupational therapy in your country and one publication that defines the professional standards and behaviours in your context.
3. Using Fig. 8.2, suggest examples of risks that would likely fit each level of the matrix in your practice setting.
4. What records are occupational therapists expected to keep?
5. Following an audit, what could be done as good practice for implementing changes?

REFERENCES

Andrews, A., & St Aubyn, B. (2015). 'If it's not written down; it didn't happen. *Journal of Community Nursing, 29*(5), 20–22.

Boyle, A., & Keep, J. (2018). Clinical audit does not work, is quality improvement any better? *British Journal of Hospital Medicine, 79*(9), 508–510.

Broughton, W., Harris, G., & on behalf of the Interprofessional CPD and Lifelong Learning Group (2019). *Principles for continuing professional development and lifelong learning in health and social care.* Bridgewater: College of Paramedics.

Buchanan, H., Jelsma, J., & Siegfried, N. (2016). Practice-based evidence: Evaluating the quality of occupational therapy patient records as evidence for practice. *South African Journal of Occupational Therapy, 46*(1), 65–73.

Care Quality Commission, Public Health England, National Health Service. (2015). *Five year forward view.* London: NHS England.

Chief Allied Health Professions Officer's Team. (2017). *nAHPs into action. Using allied health professions to transform health, care and wellbeing*. London: NHS England.

Council of Occupational Therapists for the European Countries (COTEC). (2009). *Developing codes of ethics: COTEC policy and guidelines*. Athens: COTEC.

Creek, J. (2003). *Occupational therapy defined as a complex intervention*. London: College of Occupational Therapists Ltd.

Department of Health (DH). (2003). *Confidentiality: NHS code of practice*. London: Her Majesty's Stationary Office.

Department of Health (DH). (2010). *Uniforms and workwear: Guidance on uniform and workwear policies for NHS employers*. Available at http://www.dh.gov.uk/prod_consum_dh/groups/dh_digitalassets/@dh/@en/@ps/documents/digitalasset/dh_114754.pdf.

Department of Health (DH). (2019). *Promoting professionalism, reforming regulation*. Leeds, UK: Crown Copyright. Available at https://assets.publishing.service.gov.uk/government/uploads/system/uploads/attachment_data/file/655794/Regulatory_Reform_Consultation_Document.pdf.

Department of Health & Social Care. (2009). *Assessing and managing risk in mental health services*. London: DHSC.

Felton, A., & Stickley, T. (2018). Rethinking risk: A narrative approach. *J. Ment. Health Train. Educ. Pract., 13*(1), 54–62.

Fjellfeldt, M., Eklund, M., Sandlund, M., & Markström, U. (2016). Implementation of choice from participants' perspectives: A study of community mental healthcare reform in Sweden. *Journal of Social Work in Disability & Rehabilitation, 15*(2), 116–133.

Gately, C., & Borcherding, S. (2016). *Documentation manual for occupational therapy writing SOAP notes* (4th ed.). Thorofare, NJ: Slack Incorporated.

Gille, F., Smith, S., & Mays, N. (2015). Why public trust in health care systems matters and deserves greater research attention. *Journal of Health Services Research and Policy, 20*(1), 62–64.

Hart, C. (2014). *A pocket guide to risk assessment and management in mental health*. London: Taylor and Francis.

Health & Care Professions Council (HCPC). (2011). *Professionalism in healthcare professionals*. London: HCPC.

Health & Care Professions Council (HCPC). (2013). *Standards of proficiency: Occupational therapists*. Available at https://www.hcpc-uk.org/standards/standards-of-proficiency/occupational-therapists/.

Health & Care Professions Council (HCPC). (2016). *Standards of conduct, performance and ethics*. London: HCPC.

Health & Care Professions Council (HCPC). (2017). *Continuing professional development and your registration*. Available at https://www.hcpc-uk.org/globalassets/resources/guidance/continuing-professional-development-and-your-registration.pdf.

Health & Care Professions Council (HCPC). (2018a). *Professions and protected titles*. London: HCPC.

Health & Care Professions Council (HCPC). (2018b). *Standards of continuing professional development*. Available at https://www.hcpc-uk.org/standards/standards-of-continuing-professional-development/.

Hegan, T. J. (2004). A smile a day keeps the lawyers away! the importance of effective communication in preventing litigation. *Malta Medical Journal, 16*(02), 42–45.

Her Majesty's Stationery Office. (1990). *Access to health Record Act*. London: HMSO.

Her Majesty's Stationery Office. (1998). *Human Rights Act*. Available at http://www.legislation.gov.uk/ukpga/1998/42/contents.

Her Majesty's Stationery Office. (2000). *Freedom of Information Act*. Available at http://www.legislation.gov.uk/ukpga/2000/36/contents.

Her Majesty's Stationery Office. (2005). *Mental Capacity Act*. London: Her Majesty's Stationery Office.

Her Majesty's Stationery Office. (2007). *Mental health Act*. London: HMSO.

Her Majesty's Stationery Office. (2018). *Data Protection Act*. Norwich: The Stationary Office.

Hordichuk, C. J., Robinson, A. J., & Sullivan, T. M. (2015). Conceptualising professionalism in occupational therapy. *Australian Occupational Therapy Journal, 62*, 150–159.

Huang, E. C. -H., Pu, C., Chou, Y.-J., & Huang, N. (2018). Public trust in physicians—health care commodification as a possible deteriorating factor: Cross-sectional analysis of 23 countries. *Inquiry, 55*, 1–11.

Hutchinson, M. (2018). The crisis of public trust in governance and institutions: Implications for nursing leadership. *Journal of Nursing Management, 26*(2), 83–85.

Kannenberg, K., Amini, D., & Hartmann, K. (2016). Occupational therapy in the promotion of health and well-being. *American Journal of Occupational Therapy, 70*, 1–15.

Lamb, A. J. (2016). The power of authenticity (inaugural presidential address). *American Journal of Occupational Therapy, 70*(6).

Medical Error Action Group. (2019). *Cask*. Available at https://www.medicalerroraustralia.com/spotlight/cask/.

Moss, B. (2017). *Communication skills for health and social care*. London: Sage Publications.

NHS England. (2019). *Mental health and the NHS long term plan*. Available at https://www.longtermplan.nhs.uk/areas-of-work/mental-health/.

NHS Improvement. (2018). *Issue and risk management*. London: NHS Improvement.

Nortje, N., & De Jongh, J. (2017). Professionalism-a case for medical education to honour the societal contract. *South African Journal of Occupational Therapy, 47*(2), 41–44.

O'Neil, O. (2013). *What we don't understand about trust*. Available at https://www.ted.com/talks/onora_o_neill_what_we_don_t_understand_about_trust/transcript#t-68937.

O'Neill, O. (2002). *Reith lectures 2002: A question of trust- lecture 3 'called to account'*. Available at http://www.bbc.co.uk/radio4/reith2002/lecture1.shtml.

Occupational Therapy Board of New Zealand (OTBNZ). (2016). *Professional boundaries: An occupational therapist's guide to the importance of appropriate professional boundaries*. Wellington: OTBNZ.

Paton, J., Ranmal, R., & Dudley, J. (2015). Clinical audit: Still an important tool for improving healthcare. *Archives of Disease in Childhood Education and Practice, 100*, 83–88.

Roberts, L. W. (2017). Is a doctor like a toaster? Earning trust in the profession of medicine. *Academic Psychiatry*, *41*, 305–308.

Royal College of Occupational Therapists (RCOT). (2015). *Code of ethics and professional conduct*. London: College of Occupational Therapists.

Royal College of Occupational Therapists (RCOT). (2017a). *Career development framework: Guiding principles for occupational therapy*. London: RCOT.

Royal College of Occupational Therapists (RCOT). (2017b). *Professional standards for occupational therapy practice*. London: RCOT.

Royal College of Occupational Therapists (RCOT). (2018a). *Getting my life back: Occupational therapy promoting mental health and wellbeing in England*. London: RCOT.

Royal College of Occupational Therapists (RCOT). (2018b). *Keeping records - guidance for occupational therapists*. London: RCOT.

Royal College of Occupational Therapists (RCOT). (2018c). *Our strategic intentions*. London: RCOT.

Scally G. and Donaldson L.J. (1998). Clinical governance and the drive for quality improvement in the new NHS in England. *British Medical Journal*, *317*(7150), 61–65.

Scott, J. (2019). *Royal College of occupational therapists response to the NHS long term plan*. Available at https://www.rcot.co.uk/news/royal-college-occupational-therapists-response-nhs-long-term-plan.

Skills for Health. (2008). *Employability skills matrix for the health sector*. Bristol: Skills for health.

Smith, C. P. (2017). First, do no harm: Institutional betrayal and trust in healthcare professions. *Journal of Multidisciplinary Healthcare*, *10*, 133–144.

Stemwedel, J. D. (2007). *Personal integrity and professional integrity*. Available at https://scienceblogs.com/ethicsandscience/2007/02/28/personal-integrity-and-profess.

The National Patient Safety Agency. (2008). *A risk matrix for risk managers*. London: The National Patient Safety Agency.

Victoria State Government. (2018). *Community health occupational therapy priority tool – adult*. Available at https://www2.health.vic.gov.au/primary-and-community-health/community-health/community-health-program/ch-demand-management/occupational-therapy-priority-tool-adult.

Wanna, J., Lee, H.-A., & Yates, S. (2015). *Managing under austerity, delivering under pressure: Performance and productivity in public services*. Acton: Australian National University Press.

Wimpenny, K., & Lewis, L. (2015). Preparation for an uncertain world: Professional agency and durability in the practice preparation of mental health in occupational therapy. *South African Journal of Occupational Therapy*, *2*(45), 22–28.

World Federation of Occupational Therapists (WFOT). (2007). *Occupational therapy: Professional autonomy*. Available at http://www.wfot.org/ResourceCentre.aspx.

World Federation of Occupational Therapists. (WFOT). (2016). *Code of ethics - ethical core of occupational therapy*. Columbia: WFOT.

9

ETHICS IN PRACTICE AND RESEARCH

LANA VAN NIEKERK ▪ MATUMO RAMAFIKENG

CHAPTER OUTLINE

INTRODUCTION

This chapter introduces ethics in occupational therapy mental health practice and research. The chapter starts by differentiating between three closely related concepts: professionalism, morality and ethics. A brief overview of theories of ethics that underpin the ethical principles used to guide ethical reasoning is provided. Case Studies are used to highlight some of the ethical dilemmas that occupational therapists face when applying ethical principles in day-to-day practice and research.

Ethics is 'a branch of philosophy which, through formal and systematic analysis, attempts to critically examine human conduct focusing on the rightness and wrongness … of actions (Grodin 1995, p. 7). Ethics is used to guide moral behaviour; hence it has been described as 'the critical study of morality' (Campbell 2013, p. 14) and 'the science of morals' (Duncan et al. 2017, p. 300).

In occupational therapy practice and research, ethical principles are used to guide ethical reasoning when therapists have to make decisions about what is the right thing to do to 'do good' (Beauchamp and Childress 2013) and to minimize harm. Ethical reasoning refers to applying ethical principles to guide decision-making, reasoning, and actions when ethical issues emerge. These issues refer to situations when circumstances arise that require the application of ethical principles to resolve them and there is a clear solution.

ETHICS, MORALITY AND PROFESSIONALISM

Ethics, morality and professionalism are so closely related that sometimes people assume they mean the same thing. Being clear about the differences between these terms helps with understanding the theories behind ethical, moral and/or professional reasoning in practice.

Morality 'refers to a set of values that are widely shared and relatively stable within a community' (Horner 2003, p. 263). In societies such as South Africa, communities are diverse, therefore there are likely to be competing sets of values upheld by different communities. Similarly, occupational therapists are members of the occupational therapy community, regardless of any differences in terms of geographical location, ethnicity, place of work and economic background. The profession has a set of agreed core values and principles that guide behaviour and actions. Morality 'encompasses many standards of conduct, including moral principles, rules, ideals, rights and virtues' (Beauchamp and Childress 2013, p. 3). In comparison to ethics, morality is not principles-based but focuses on upholding or enacting values. These values guide moral reasoning and actions which aim to foster the greater good of everyone in the community (Horner 2003). Case Study 9.1 illustrates an example in which a therapist's moral values with regard to smoking inform her actions in refusing to buy cigarettes for a service user.

Professionalism is not easy to define. It is a subjective, complex, multifaceted concept (Aguilar et al. 2012) that is socially constructed and open to interpretation. Hence there is no consensus on its definition within occupational therapy (Hordichuk et al. 2015). The difference between professionalism and ethics is that professionalism 'extends beyond ethics' (Nortje and De Jongh 2017, p. 41). Therefore professionalism encompasses ethics.

Twelve attributes of professionalism often cited in occupational therapy literature are 'clinical competence, cultural competence, altruism, leadership, accountability, interpersonal skills, respect, continuous professional development, ethical behaviour, legal compliance, appearance, and education' (Nortje and De Jongh 2017, p. 42). Professionalism forms the basis for good practice. Sound professional reasoning ensures provision of quality health services. This is because professionalism requires 'specific knowledge, attitudes, and values–all manifested by professional behaviours' (Kasar and Muscari 2000, p. 43) (see also Chapter 8 on Professional accountability). Professionalism is often regulated by professional bodies that set standards and guidelines for professional practice. These standards are informed by ethical principles, legislation, and agreed guidelines for conduct that also highlight professional responsibilities.

Professional reasoning refers to 'the cognitive and meta-cognitive processes that guide action and decision-making in occupational therapy practice' (Ramafikeng 2017, p. 209) regardless of the setting. Professional reasoning is dynamic in nature and influenced by context. It also evolves with expertise and requires collaborative decision-making (Turpin and Higgs 2010). Professional reasoning includes scientific, hypothetico-deductive, diagnostic and ethical reasoning (Schell and Schell 2008), as well as various forms of clinical reasoning: procedural, interactive, conditional (Mattingly and Fleming 1994), pragmatic and narrative (Neistadt 1998) (see Chapter 3).

CASE STUDY 9.1

Refusing a Request

Cheryl (an occupational therapist) is on her way to Ann's home. Ann is a woman with serious mental health problems that make it impossible for her to leave her house. Cheryl receives a message from Ann asking her to pick up cigarettes on the way. Cheryl refuses because of her personal anti-smoking beliefs, despite awareness that this decision might cause significant distress to Ann.

CASE STUDY 9.2

Professional Misconduct

Participants in a research study on students' perceptions of professionalism in occupational therapy practice shared experiences of witnessing unprofessional behaviour among other members of a multidisciplinary team. One participant recounted an incident where carers at an institution for people with intellectual disabilities were behaving unprofessionally. The participant was engaged in an intervention session with a person diagnosed with intellectual disability, and, during the session, the caregivers would tease the person, deliberately provoking anger outbursts. This made the person quite agitated and impacted on the intervention process (Fodo et al. 2018).

Case Study 9.2 illustrates how unprofessional conduct can lead to the violation of ethical principles. The occupational therapy students could first try to contain the feelings of the service users by applying handling principles. Then, in collaboration with the supervisor, the student could consider how to facilitate continued professional development sessions covering professionalism and ethical principles. The supervisor should inform the contacts in the setting (if known). The ultimate aim would be to make it clear that taunting people constitutes unprofessional conduct.

Theories About Ethics

There are many theories about ethics to draw on when discussing ethical issues. When practitioners do not agree, being able to recognize ethical theories can shed some light on points of disagreement. Sharing these theories could focus the discussion and inform the outcome. When ethics theories that inform reasoning are made explicit, practitioners might better understand why members of a health or research team can hold different opinions, despite them sharing the same professional background. For these reasons occupational therapists can benefit from having some knowledge of the main ethical theories. Some of the key ethical theories commonly informing occupational therapy are briefly highlighted and illustrated by Case Studies 9.1 and 9.3.

CASE STUDY 9.3

Exaggerating Symptoms to Facilitate Admission

Mpho is a 23-year-old young woman diagnosed with schizophrenia. She has been relatively stable for six months. Mpho's family brings her to a psychiatric hospital for re-admission. They provide false information about her symptoms, stating that Mpho is irritable and sometimes fights with family members, talks to herself as if she is hearing voices and roams around aimlessly. However, in reality Mpho is relatively stable. The family is exaggerating her symptoms to facilitate her admission so as to exclude her from her sister's wedding ceremony. The family does this to ensure her safety during the celebration and to protect her and the family's dignity. Mpho, who is very unhappy with her family's actions, has thus become agitated and is refusing to be admitted voluntarily. Legislation makes provision for involuntary admission. The occupational therapist is part of the team that decides on the admission.

Utilitarian ethics considers ethics on the basis of positive and negative consequences. Emphasis is placed on achieving the greater good, which means achieving the best outcome for the largest number of people in a particular situation. The consequences of possible outcomes guide decisions for the best course of action.

In Case Study 9.3 Mpho's family is exaggerating her symptoms to secure admission to a hospital while the family is away attending a wedding. Securing admission to a hospital, in their minds, will protect Mpho from being ridiculed (which might be the case if she attends the wedding) and prevent her from roaming the streets (which is what she tends to do if left alone). If the occupational therapist goes along with what the family wants and supports Mpho's admission, one might argue that this will achieve the best outcome for the largest number of people.

Virtue ethics focus on the character of the person; being a good person with associated positive character traits, such as compassion, honesty and courage. The core assumption is that people of good moral character conduct themselves in a virtuous manner and do good (Cotterill 2014). 'Emphasis is placed on the whole moral life, rather than incidents of moral choice or dilemma' (Campbell 2013, p. 35). Ethical reasoning underpinned by virtue ethics emphasizes being honest and having compassion. In Case Study 9.3 the occupational therapist could be courageous and confront the family, counsel them to recognize the negative consequences of exaggerating Mpho's symptoms and then attempt to assist with finding a solution for the problems identified by the family.

Deontological ethics strongly emphasizes accepted codes of behaviour and doing one's duty. Rules or principles that guide ethical behaviour are often found in guidelines or codes produced by professional organizations or ethics committees to guide action. Workplace norms, practice standards and even job descriptions usually contain principles that guide ethical reasoning. Strict adherence to rules and guidelines regardless of a situation is the core of deontological ethics. Referring to Case Study 9.3 once more, an occupational therapist who relies strongly on deontological ethics will follow the rules for admission to the hospital and thus not admit Mpho if admission is not warranted.

Relational ethics is primarily informed by respect and consideration for the people that the practitioner works with and seeks to understand. It refers to 'the appreciation of the responsibility of health professionals that extends beyond fidelity to duty and obligation of respect for the person or to submission to general rules, but also to the development of a relational commitment between the caregiver and one for whom he or she is responsible' (Barbosa 2012, p. 227). Respect for autonomy is therefore the primary consideration in ethical reasoning underpinned by relational ethics. Using Case Study 9.1 as an example, if Cheryl's ethical reasoning was primarily informed by relational ethics, she might have bought the cigarettes Ann asked for because of the value placed on self-determination and autonomy.

Ecological ethics emphasizes the interdependent nature of relationships and thus strives to consider decisions within their broadest possible context. Consequences of actions are judged in accordance with the broader impact on the context or community. Consideration for doing the greater good extends beyond just the people involved and includes the broader context. Returning to Case Study 9.1, if Cheryl's reasoning was informed by ecological ethics, she would not buy the cigarettes Ann requested because of the long-term negative health consequences. She would also generalize the situation to other people and other therapists and recognize the pitfalls of similar requests in other forms and situations. Her decision to not buy the cigarettes would be informed by the broader potential implications.

Ethical Principles

Ethical principles that guide ethical reasoning are derived from the theories outlined above. The principles of respect for autonomy, beneficence, nonmaleficence, veracity, fidelity and justice are discussed here and illustrated by Case Studies 9.1 to 9.5.

Autonomy

Respect for autonomy refers to considering a person's right to have opinions, make choices and act on choices based on their values and beliefs (Beauchamp and Childress 2013). Occupational therapists empower people and create conditions that enable them to make autonomous choices and participate in decision-making processes. This can be challenging in mental health service settings, especially when engaging with service users whose mental health is fluctuating. Case Studies 9.1 and 9.3 illustrate examples where Ann and Mpho's autonomy is not respected.

Respect for autonomy is not simply about having a tolerant attitude towards others' choices; it also includes deliberate action to ensure that the capacity to make choices is enabled, protected, and enhanced (Beauchamp and Childress 2013). Among the conditions created to enable decision-making is the provision of information so that a person can make an informed choice. Health professionals are obliged to provide accessible information, ensure understanding, and ensure that the process of decision-making is indeed voluntary. Discussing information will help understanding and provide a sense of autonomy (Beauchamp and Childress 2013). Hence the process of negotiating informed consent in research is a strategy for adhering to the principle of respect for autonomy. Adherence to this principle entails ensuring and enabling others to freely make and act on their choices according to their beliefs and values, provided this does not cause harm to other people and themselves as illustrated in Case Study 9.4.

In Case Study 9.4 Donovan is exercising his right to make a choice about not disclosing his diagnosis to the employer. However, this might not be an informed

---

CASE STUDY 9.4
Advocating for Fair Opportunities

Donovan, a 35-year-old man diagnosed with uncontrolled epilepsy, has recently been discharged from a psychiatric hospital in South Africa where he underwent vocational rehabilitation. Due to numerous admissions Donovan has struggled to secure permanent employment and has been unemployed for four years. During a follow-up appointment Donovan informs the occupational therapist that he has found work as an assistant on a construction site. Some of his duties include climbing ladders and scaffolding frames to collect materials and clear rubble. Donovan has not disclosed his diagnosis to the employer and informs the therapist that he does not wish to disclose for fear of losing the job.

decision if he is putting himself and others at risk by failing to disclose. The occupational therapist could discuss this with Donovan, exploring relevant information to enable him to make a more informed decision.

Beneficence

The principle of beneficence requires practitioners to have an 'attitude of goodwill towards others' (Campbell 2013, p. 45), to help others and to act for their benefit (Beauchamp and Childress 2013). In essence this principle is about a commitment to do good. For example, ensuring that interventions are therapeutic is one way in which occupational therapists adhere to the principle of beneficence.

In practicing beneficence, we try to prevent harm, to remove that which is harmful, to counterbalance any harm with benefit and actively promote the well-being of others (Campbell 2013, p. 45). For example, countering the side effects of psychopharmacological drugs for mental health service users through active engagement in occupations would be of benefit to them. In Case Study 9.1 the occupational therapist attempts to prevent Ann from experiencing the harmful effects of smoking by refusing to buy her cigarettes.

However, this principle bears the risk of promoting paternalism, especially in practice. A form of paternalism would be imposing treatment on people despite their choice not to receive such treatment thereby breaching the principle of autonomy (Campbell 2013). Case Study 9.3 shows a complex example of how adherence to the principle of beneficence potentially breaches the principle of autonomy through imposing admission on the service user despite her objection to it, even though it might be to her own good. The risk of paternalism is particularly significant in mental health service delivery as service users are sometimes unable to make their own decisions; therefore others make decisions on their behalf. Paternalism refers to restricting a person's autonomy for their own good. This is often done by caregivers or others in authority such as was the case in Case Studies 9.1 and 9.4. Paternalism is different from abuse as the intent in an abusive act is to cause harm, such as is the case in Case Study 9.2. Teasing a service user constitutes harm and is therefore abusive.

Non-Maleficence

This principle refers to the obligation to intentionally avoid actions that cause harm to others (Beauchamp and Childress 2013). For example, adhering to precautions, implementing safety measures and refraining from physical or psychological harm during interactions with mental health service users would be adhering to the principle of non-maleficence. On the one hand Case Study 9.2 illustrates how this principle can be breached by professionals causing psychological harm through their actions towards the service users. On the other hand Case Study 9.1 illustrates the therapist's adherence to the principle of non-maleficence by refusing to buy cigarettes for the service user.

Veracity

Veracity refers to the quality of information: its accuracy, whether it is given in a timely fashion and comprehensively and how the professional ensures understanding of the information provided (Beauchamp and Childress 2013). Use of language that the service user understands is particularly important in ensuring adherence to this principle. Case Study 9.5 contains the observations of a participant, an occupational therapy student who recognized that language was key to accurate assessment and treatment of mental health service users.

CASE STUDY 9.5

The Impact of Language and Translation on Practice

Unathi, a participant in a research study, shared her concerns about the impact of language on service delivery for mental health service users with active symptoms affecting attention and concentration. She considered them doubly disadvantaged when treatment is not in a language that they are proficient in. She said, 'If you're speaking a language that they don't understand, it's even harder to get their attention.' Later in the interview she commented, 'People seemed less psychotic when you speak a language they understand, coz when they speak to other people and they like form sentences in English … people just think oh my gosh this guy is so crazy and then when you speak to them in Xhosa, you're like he is not that crazy he just doesn't understand what you're trying to say to him.' This excerpt indicates Unathi's awareness of the importance of language in enabling accurate assessment of service users (both acute and chronic) in mental health practice (Ramafikeng 2017).

The principle of veracity is closely related to the principle of respect for autonomy. However, veracity extends beyond respect for choice to respect for the person as a human being. Veracity is founded on obligations to respect the person and the promise to provide information truthfully and to develop and maintain trust in the relationship between the professional and the service user or research participant (Beauchamp and Childress 2013). Falsifying information as in the case illustrated in Case Study 9.3 breaches the principle of veracity. However, it is important to bear in mind that adherence to this principle can be challenging for occupational therapists and other professionals as, at times, when mentally unwell, people can provide inaccurate information, which can cause harm to others, such as false accusations of abuse.

Fidelity

Fidelity refers to promise-keeping and honouring agreements, both explicitly or implicitly, given the nature of the relationship between the health professional and the service user (Beauchamp and Childress 2013). Fidelity is based on the virtues of trustworthiness and loyalty. Case Study 9.2 illustrates a case in which professionals who are contractually in an agreement with service users fail to honour that agreement.

Justice

Justice refers to commitment 'to equal share and fairness' (Orb et al. 2001, p. 95). A basic feature of this principle is the fair distribution of costs and benefits and not simply calculating the potential cost and benefits as this can undermine the principles of beneficence and non-maleficence (Campbell 2013). Applying this principle prevents the abuse and exploitation of people, as illustrated in Case Study 9.6.

Case Study 9.6 illustrates students' need for awareness of distribution of resources and how this can influence health and access to quality health services. They could take affirmative action as advocates based on their awareness of the principle of justice. In other words, they could counteract the negative consequences of discrimination by creating opportunities or providing support specifically to individuals known to have been marginalized. Affirmative action is a form of

> ### CASE STUDY 9.6
> #### Students Confronted by Reality in Practice
>
> During an ethics lecture with final-year occupational therapy students, the lecturer picks up that students are struggling to reconcile the reality of providing services with ideal scenarios taught in the classroom. High demand for services within resource-constrained environments meant that opportunities to offer intervention were restricted, unavailable or not affordable for people to access. The students tended to internalize the negative consequences of not being able to offer the best intervention to people. This was taking a toll emotionally, adding a layer of anxiety which students found difficult to manage.

redress and can be considered to be positive discrimination (De Asís Roig 2016).

Ethical Dilemmas

Making ethical principles explicit will not necessarily resolve ethical dilemmas; however, it will help prioritize considerations during ethical reasoning. When ethics are referred to in practice, it is often with reference to ethical reasoning to resolve ethical dilemmas, but ethical reasoning is not only applied when there is a dilemma. An ethical dilemma occurs when several approaches are possible but none are ideal because all will involve breaching one or more ethical principles. Practitioners thus face the predicament that none of the solutions are deemed fully satisfactory (Wells 2007). An example of an ethical dilemma is presented in Case Study 9.4. Arguably the best option for the occupational therapist will be to counsel Donovan to inform his employer that he has uncontrolled epilepsy to ensure his own and coworkers' safety in accordance with the principle of non-maleficence. However, this will probably lead to Donovan losing the job, thus bringing harm to him and his family. Therefore neither option available would constitute non-maleficence. When faced with an ethical dilemma it is important to work in close collaboration with the service user and other professionals to arrive at a decision. In addition, caution should be taken to not break confidentiality.

Factors that Complicate Ethical Reasoning in Mental Health Practice

A number of factors can complicate ethical reasoning in the field of mental health. Some pertain to personal factors while others originate from the context.

Fluctuation in Mental Health Status

The nature of mental health problems is such that symptoms experienced during acute phases are likely to have a significant impact on the decision-making of service users. However, when not experiencing active symptoms, service users are capable of making decisions for themselves. Practitioners thus need to remain vigilant in balancing the principles of autonomy and non-maleficence. In addition, caregivers often take on the responsibility of making decisions for service users but do not relinquish this responsibility once the person is well. In such cases occupational therapists have a responsibility to educate caregivers about mental health and recovery while advocating for the rights of service users to maintain autonomy for their own decisions. Also, occupational therapy–specific knowledge about grading decisions within activities is particularly useful in reducing a polarized approach.

Health professionals or committee structures who are responsible for making decisions on behalf of persons with mental health problems have a tendency to question the autonomy of service users and often exaggerate their vulnerability. In such cases the tendency will be to err on the side of being paternalistic. When such professionals or committees are not adequately informed about the capacity of mental health service users to give consent and make decisions, an advocacy role should be taken by occupational therapists. It is important to involve service users in practice-related decisions as much as possible. Furthermore, they should be included in planning research because this is a mechanism to show what mental health service users are capable of (refer to Faulkner (2005) for guidelines).

Scarcity of Resources Affecting Access to What Service Users Need for Recovery

Limitations in human and material resources lead to ongoing ethical tension associated with not being able to offer occupational therapy to the many people requiring it. Furthermore, mental health services are often not prioritized, thereby exacerbating the relative neglect of persons with mental health problems. The scarcity of resources is a global theme that impacts delivery of occupational therapy services (Bushby et al. 2015; Durocher et al. 2016). As highlighted in Case Study 9.6, scarcity of resources impacts practice, and therefore occupational therapists are required to advocate for access to resources to provide quality services.

Disjuncture Between Policy Frameworks and Resource Availability

Policy frameworks can create challenges or barriers to optimum service delivery for mental health service users. Often what is proposed in the frameworks does not align with current resource availability, thereby creating a mental health treatment gap that stems from policy implementation. For example, the National Mental Health Policy of South Africa advocates for deinstitutionalisation and continuation of care within communities. However, there is a lack of both material and qualified human resources to provide mental healthcare services in the community (Thornicroft et al. 2016).

The principle of justice will be the most important when challenged by macro-environmental factors to ensure distribution of scarce resources. In addition, creative strategies to optimize intervention would be called for, and advocacy should be a consistent and explicit component of occupational therapy practice.

CONCLUSION

Ethical reasoning is required on a day-to-day basis to achieve the best possible outcomes in practice and research. An ethical practitioner considers potential approaches critically, with an explicit focus on ethical principles that could be applied in each situation. Ethical theories underpin ethical reasoning and can explain why particular ethical principles should be prioritized. Ethical reasoning remains a personal responsibility of occupational therapy practitioners and should be applied consistently.

QUESTIONS FOR CONSIDERATION

1. List six ethical principles and identify how each one might guide an occupational therapist's ethical reasoning in a mental health setting.
2. Consider how occupational therapists might differ in their ethical reasoning from their team colleagues, particularly in relation to the autonomy and vulnerability of service users.
3. Identify the key factors of ethics, morality and professionalism that would help you separate them.
4. Which theory of ethics do you feel most relates to you in your day-to-day life? How strictly to you adhere to those principles, and how do you respond to your beliefs being challenged?
5. Consider a potential situation such as the one in Case Study 9.1 in which a service user requests something you feel unable to grant. What are the different ethical perspectives on it?
6. If you were involved in a scenario like the one from Case Study 9.3, who would you discuss your thoughts with? When and why?
7. What is an ethical dilemma, and what is important to consider in justifying a decision?
8. In Case Study 9.4, is there Is there legislation that could protect Donovan (in any country) from being refused employment, despite his fears and experiences?

SERVICE USER COMMENTARY

Ethics, morality, professionalism–technical and specific words for attributes that are 'within' us. Yet they are not fixed and are influenced by many things. Where we live, how we were raised as children, maybe a faith, the systems that we live and work in affect our thinking and reasoning about people. These attributes reside within each of us, and become noticeable whenever we work with others, be they colleagues or patients.

As a patient with bipolar disorder, I have had a lifetime of involvement with medical and support services, including occupational therapists. I have never asked any professional about their ethics, morality, or professionalism. This may be because there are many more important things to focus on. However, I have certainly been able to tell the difference between a confident yet reflective professional and one who is just 'going through the motions'. The professional who has become jaded and cynical, has lost the hope that patients can recover and improve and shows their frustrations and unhappiness in their work.

Like many professions that involve working with others, there will have been an initial reason why you have chosen occupational therapy as your career. Sometimes, with the stresses and strains of the job, many of which are beyond your control, it is easy to lose sight of that initial desire that led to this choice. This can be like a slow wearing away, like a stone where there is dripping water, the water is a persistent drip, that over the months and years can wear a hole in the stone. The limitations of the profession, the organization you work for, the larger health system that you work in can all be like the water dripping onto the stone. Then you realize that there is a hole within you. These things have nothing to do with the patient you are working with and they will be more powerless than you may feel.

So how to prevent this from happening? Be aware that it is a possibility, be aware that your patients and colleagues will notice this within your practice, maybe before you. Ensure that you spend time with colleagues discussing professional development and exploring how your profession changes you as a person. Training will be an important part of this process. Take as many opportunities that are on offer to continually improve your practice. Do not be threatened by situations or knowledge that is new or different to your own, see these as a way of testing and even challenging your beliefs. Read about your profession, what new approaches there are, examples of good practice, and patient feedback. All these things will take your time, and it might be that you are not working in an environment that values these things, where the workload can be overwhelming, where it is more important to be seen 'doing' occupational therapy. Remember that it is not just your knowledge of occupational therapy that you are applying, it is the whole of your being, of who you are, of the ethics, morality and professionalism that are within you.

Fiona Naylor

REFERENCES

Aguilar, A., & Stupans, I. (2012). Exploring professionalism: The professional values of Australian occupational therapists. *Australian Occupational Therapy Journal*, 59(3), 209–217. https://doi.org/10.1111/j.1440-1630.2012.00996.x.

Barbosa, A. (2012). *Relational ethics and psychosomatic assessment.* Karger Publishers.

Bushby, K., Chan, J., Druif, S., Ho, K., & Kinsella, E. A. (2015). Ethical tensions in occupational therapy practice: A scoping review. *British Journal of Occupational Therapy*, 78(4), 212–221. https://doi.org/10.1177/0308022614564770.

De Asís Roig, R. (2016). Reasonableness in the concept of reasonable accommodation. *Age of Human Rights Journal*, 6(6), 42. https://doi.org/10.17561/tahrj.v0i6.2929.

Duncan, E. M., Ramachandran, & Dsouza, S. A. (2017). Ethics and professionalism in occupational therapy Ppactice. In S. A. Dsouza, R. Galvaan, & E. L. Ramugondo (Eds.), *Concepts in occupational therapy: Understanding Southern Perspectives* (pp. 298–315).

Durocher, E., Kinsella, E. A., McCorquodale, L., & Phelan, S. (2016). Ethical tensions related to systemic constraints: Occupational alienation in occupational therapy practice. *Occupational Therapy Journal of Research (Thorofare N J)*, 36(4), 216–226. https://doi.org/10.1177/1539449216665117.

Faulkner, A., & Joseph Rowntree Foundation (2004). *The ethics of survivor research: Guidelines for the ethical conduct of research carried out by mental health service users and survivors.* Policy Press.

Hordichuk, C. J., Robinson, A. J., & Sullivan, T. M. (2015). Conceptualising professionalism in occupational therapy through a Western lens. *Australian Occupational Therapy Journal*, 62(3), 150–159. https://doi.org/10.1111/1440-1630.12204.

Kasar, J., Muscari, M.E., (n.d.). A conceptual model for the development of professional behaviours in occupational therapists KEY WORDS Career planning and development Professional development Professional-student relations.

Mattingly, C. (1994). In M. H. Fleming (Ed.), *Clinical reasoning: Forms of inquiry in a therapeutic practice* Davis.

Nortje, N., & De Jongh, J.-C. (2016). Client confidentiality: Perspectives of students in a healthcare training programme. *The South African Journal of Bioethics and Law*, 9(1), 31. https://doi.org/10.7196/SAJBL.2016.v9i1.460.

Orb, A., Eisenhauer, L., & Wynaden, D. (2001). Ethics in qualitative research. *The Journal of Nursing Scholarsh*, 33(1), 93–96. https://doi.org/10.1111/j.1547-5069.2001.00093.x.

Ramafikeng, M. (2017). Professional reasoning. In S. A. Dsouza, R. Galvaan, & E. L. Ramugondo (Eds.), *Concepts in occupational therapy: Understanding Southern Perspectives* (pp. 205–215). Manipal University Press.

Schell, B. A., & Schell, J. W. (2008). Political reasoning as a basis for practice. In *Clinical and professional reasoning in occupational therapy*. Lippincott Williams & Wilkins.

Thornicroft, G., Deb, T., & Henderson, C. (2016). *Community mental health care worldwide: Current status and further developments.* (n.d.).

Turpin, M., & Higgs, J. (2010). Clinical reasoning and evidence-based practice. In T. Hoffmann, S. Bennett, & C. M. Mar (Eds.), *Evidence-based practice across Health Professions* (pp. 300–317). Elsevier Australia.

Wells, J. K. (2007). Ethical dilemma and resolution: A case scenario. *Indian Journal of Medical Ethics*, IV(1). https://doi.org/10.20529/IJME.2007.010. 2006–2008.

10 PERSPECTIVES ON USING SERVICES

ANNE-LAURE DONSKOY ■ ROSEMARIE STEVENS

INTRODUCTION

Both authors are service users who have used occupational therapy in the context of mental health services in the United Kingdom. The chapter aims to draw on experiential knowledge (the authors' and that of other service users) of using services to help occupational therapists develop their practice.

The social and political environment within which people access mental health services has evolved greatly in many countries since the last edition of this book. The 'recovery agenda' has become central and drives the discussion in this chapter. User involvement and access to occupational therapy are also explored as well as peer-led services.

RECOVERY

"Recovery is often a complex, time-consuming process. Recovery is what people with disabilities do. Treatment, case management, and rehabilitation are what helpers do to facilitate recovery."

Anthony 1995, p. 7

The idea that people 'recover' from psychosocial distress should not be contentious. Indeed, recovery has been a primary influence on mental health service development in the 21st century. However, due to erosion and colonization by proponents of the medical model, recovery is now often little more than the expectation that people with mental health

159

problems will 'get better' by returning to a former state of health; the recovery concept now seemingly owned by policymakers (Beresford 2015). Consequently, many service users are now extremely wary of recovery (Pilgrim and McCranie 2013; Beresford 2015), leading to many polarized debates.

Recovery is frequently understood very differently by service users and survivors of psychiatry compared with mental health service providers (Pilgrim and McCranie 2013). For service users recovery is a personal, complex, individual and self-defined process concerned with regaining hope and independence (Chamberlin 1978; Deegan 2001; Turner-Crowson and Wallcraft 2002; Beresford 2015) and 'what works for one person may not work for another' (Ásmundsdóttir 2009, p. 116). When listening to service users discuss their recovery, common themes include 'recovering hope, developing a perspective on the past to move on, taking control of one's own life, repairing or developing new, valued relationships and social roles, developing new meaning and purpose in life and persevering in spite of reverses and ongoing problems' (Wallcraft 2005, p. 203).

Anthony's definition of recovery 'as a way of living a satisfying, hopeful and contributing life even with limitations caused by the illness' (1995, p. 7) is well known. However, it is often truncated in the literature to fit a narrow, service-orientated view of mental healthcare (Boniface et al. 2015). The part frequently left out is presented on the previous page. Arguably, it is omitted because it challenges psychiatric orthodoxy, placing treatment, case management and rehabilitation (services, in other words) in a subsidiary role to service users' own momentum.

Significantly, Diksy et al. (2015) and Rossi et al. (2018) have shown that self-reported recovery and clinical recovery can be very different things, and many service users/survivors think that the concept of recovery has been taken over and abused by mental health professionals (Burstow 2015), reflecting the colonization of recovery (Mills 2014a; Burstow 2015).

The Colonization of Recovery

Who would not want to recover? One author (RS) was recently asked by an occupational therapist, 'you do want to get better, don't you?' This was felt to be a loaded question, allowing for only a restricted response; one that effectively bypassed RS' experiential knowledge of her of own mental health and, arguably, reflected the 'hijacking' of a self-determined recovery process by a service-led one:

> *Researchers and activists have highlighted the complex ways in which recovery discourse is entangled and imbricated with wider policy imperatives, such as reducing welfare spending, curtailing commitment to long term social care and promoting 'back to work' agendas.*
>
> *Woods et al. 2019, p. 6*

O'Donnell and Shaw (2016) argue that there has been an 'ideological colonization of the recovery model' (p. 12) by service providers which has diluted it. This is evidenced by the renaming of community mental health teams as 'recovery teams,' for example, and recovery itself has been reconfigured to become increasingly aligned with welfare-to-work policies (Deacon and Patrick 2011; Friedli and Stern 2015). This places pressure on the individual to move into paid employment wherever possible (and sometimes when it is not) to be deemed a responsible (productive) citizen.

One author (A-L D) experienced this shift in occupational therapy services herself; from occupation being offered as a means of promoting her recovery (that is, promoting a sense of self, building her confidence and developing life skills, for example) to focusing primarily on moving from welfare benefits into paid work, seemingly obeying the 'work is good for you' mantra. However, this was not what she felt she needed.

This shift has sometimes been discreet and gradual, but at other times, startling. Regardless of how protected from this shift occupational therapists think their seemingly person-centred professional reasoning may be, their practice will inevitably be shaped and constrained by any dilution of recovery principles.

This is, arguably, an expression of neoliberalism, as implemented within mental health services. The neoliberal agenda influences social and economic ideas globally, promoting a shift away from state provision and placing the onus of responsibility onto individual citizens for their socio-economic well-being and welfare (Farnsworth and Irving 2018). In the United Kingdom, especially since New Labour (mid-1990s until 2010), there has been a move away from a 'welfare society' (which, its critics alleged, created dependency) to an 'active society' which promotes responsible individual agency. This has led to the introduction of gradually more severe and/or punitive welfare policies, including sanctions and conditionality for many people. It reflects a *responsibilization* agenda (see later), whereby individuals are held responsible for things which would have previously been the concern of the state (Watts et al. 2014; Watts 2018). One can argue this runs counter to a social model of disability and to fundamental occupational therapy ideas about the interactive roles that person, environment and occupation all play in a holistic view of a person's life.

This apparent redefinition of recovery has sometimes resulted in the misuse of outcome measures such as the Recovery Star or the Wellness Recovery Action Plan. Of course, outcome measures are merely tools, and it is how they are implemented that is the decisive factor in how they are experienced by end-point service users. Whilst they may provide a useful focus for support when used appropriately, they can also be mishandled and applied in a prescriptive, reductionist and atomizing manner, becoming disconnected from the wider context in which the person lives. For example, they can ignore the impact of societal stigma, social exclusion, poor housing, an increasingly punitive welfare system and limited life choice options, in fact, any external life stressors that may influence recovery. This can be experienced as patronizing, humiliating and pressuring for service users who may feel 'tested' rather than supported. Life and recovery can go in many different directions and this requires a flexible, intuitive and properly paced approach. The different domains highlighted on the Recovery Star and the UnRecovery Start (see later) illustrate this tension very well.

> Seen from this 'colonization' perspective, 'recovery,' like the 'happiness and well-being' or the 'resilience' discourses, arguably have a common underpinning: a reductionist positive psychology approach which negates the multiple, dialectical, complex aspects of human emotion.
>
> *Ferrier and McGregor 2016*

> *Positive psychology (a growth area within psychology since the late 1990s) emphasizes the individual's commitment to creating 'the good life' for themselves through using personal strengths (Seligman 1990). Nevertheless, it arguably misses out both the societal pressures (which operate beyond the 'person') and the importance to some individuals of opposition and activism in relation to mental health service provision; 'I have the right to be angry and to express that anger, to hold it as my motivation to fight, just as I have the right to love and to express my love for the world, to hold it as my motivation to fight.'*
>
> *Freire 2008, p. 58*

Colonization and Peer Support

Peer services can 'provide hope, role modelling and simple, safe strategies for recovery' (Mead 2006, p. 8). Peer support workers have direct personal experience of mental health challenges and of working towards their own recovery. This expertise can be invaluable, for instance, providing practical and emotional support to other service users and exchanging information about aspects of services. For some individuals this advice can help them overcome the barriers to engagement in services.

However, there are potential tensions for peer support workers, particularly if expectations are placed on them to undertake tasks associated with other staff roles. Darby Penney is a long-time activist and researcher in the human rights movement in the United States for people with psychosocial disabilities. She has defined two categories of peer support: peer-developed peer support and the peer staff model (Penney 2018). The former refers to the development, in the 1970s, of forms of peer support which offer 'an interpersonal process with the goal of promoting healing and growth' (Penney 2018). The aim is to support the integration of a person's relational experiences (such as friendship, romance), how they feel about themselves and their familial experiences (such as tensions, ruptures, support) and develop a greater awareness of how these domains interact and impact the person's life. The original idea behind peer support is to take a radical view of the social structures that impose definitions of mental illness on individuals and to create a new model that accepts difference (Mead 2001).

Peer support workers are employees with a history of mental health problems who work in paraprofessional roles in traditional mental health programmes and similar positions in mental health programmes (Penney 2018); they may be called 'peer mentors,' 'peer support specialists,' 'recovery support specialists' or 'recovery coaches.' However, reflecting a cost-cutting agenda, they may additionally be asked to take on clinical duties normally performed by a nurse, for example, such as encouraging/checking that a service user takes their medication (Penney 2018). This may mean they become involved in coercing service users to comply with treatments (Mead and MacNeil 2006) and ultimately be subsumed into the dominant medicalized culture, thus compromising their 'survivor' identity. This act of appropriation by a controlling culture is what is referred to by the term 'colonization.'

Although peer programmes would like to think they are uniquely different to other providers, this role blurring around medication supervision or quandaries around 'managing' challenging behaviour can result in colonization of peer support. Peer support workers' work environment and the training they receive will be decisive factors in this process. Thus the cultural context in which peer programmes are created is important, as the following international examples illustrate.

France

In France peer programme initiatives were initially strongly opposed by health trade unions who viewed the introduction of peer support workers within clinical teams as a threat to their members' employment. In addition, some well-known psychiatrists were also contemptuous of service users as 'pair-aidants' (peer support workers) (Baillon 2011).

Some French survivor activists warned against the medicalization of the peer support worker role, especially when they were expected to 'educate' service users about being compliant with treatment, including medication (CRPA 2013).

Significantly, the training and accreditation of peer support workers is now under the management of the educational arm of the World Health Organization in Lille. In this model, they are fully integrated into the clinical team, either as volunteers or remunerated workers, and are expected to follow and support the medical model. The job descriptions and language used arguably reflect the intrusion of the neoliberal agenda, equating service user empowerment with responsibilization.

Netherlands

Sometimes, as Penney (2018) notices, peer support projects have been taken over by mainstream mental health services, as this observation of Dutch recovery colleges by a Dutch service user shows:

At first they [psychiatrists] took over educational programmes, followed by the competency framework and redefined what constitutes a peer support worker and what this position comprises. Gradually, peer support workers who had been trained in the social model of disability had to integrate the psychiatric model too. The consequence is that a lot of peer support workers no longer apply the core values and principles of peer support as defined and advocated by the service user movement. Can they still be called peer-support workers or regular mental health workers?

Anonymous 2019a

United Kingdom

Open Dialogue (OD) is a model of involving service users in their care that originated in family therapy in Finland and uses peer support workers. In the United Kingdom it is mainly referred to by the modified title of Peer-Supported Open Dialogue (POD). Conversations that the authors have had with trainees (Anonymous 2019b) highlight concerns that the original model may have become diluted through the influence of a psychiatric or medicalized paradigm – as noted elsewhere by Razzaque and Stockmann (2016) – and by a lack of consistency in the types of training offered. For instance, POD now has a reduced training time (from three years to one year) and there is a concern that recovery will lose its multifaceted narratives. Similarly, an advertisement by a UK mental health service provider recruiting an OD Peer Support Worker appears to emphasize the lived experience of peer support workers:

"If you have lived experience and are trained or being trained in Peer Support Open Dialogue this role may well be for you...' (Devon Partnership Trust 2019)."

However, subsequent references in the advertisement to providing 'formalized peer support,' adopting the broad principles of 'the Recovery Approach' (note the capitals) and the requirement of being accredited to the Association of Peer Support Open Dialogue or in training suggests that recovery has become a systematically formalized – as distinct from a personalized – process.

Recovery Colleges, found in the United Kingdom and other English-speaking countries, see people as students in their own recovery (Health Foundation 2019) who can develop the skills needed for life and work. While these colleges are gaining popularity across mental health services, with a strong focus on 'hope' and 'agency,' they can be criticized for changing the nature of recovery by introducing a more 'medical model' (cooptation) version. All this is far removed from the original intention behind peer support, as described by Shery Mead, founder of *Intentional Peer Support*, which had more of an activist, political focus:

> As peer support in mental health proliferates, we must be mindful of our intention: social change. It is not about developing more effective services, but rather about creating dialogues that have influence on all of our understandings, conversations, and relationships.
> *Intentional Peer Support website – see Useful Resources*

A further outcome of cooptation may be the sequestering of the peer voice into a position in which it will pose no threat to the dominant medical model. This is described by one of the foremost proponents of Critical Discourse Analysis, Norman Fairclough, as 'the capacity to "naturalize" ideologies (i.e., to win acceptance for them as non-ideological "common sense")' (Fairclough 2010, p. 27). In practice this had led to pressure on service users to discuss positive narratives of recovery, rather than any negative experiences they had (Recovery in the Bin (RitB) 2019a). For example, author RS was involved as a service user volunteer in a programme of risk training for mental health workers, with her personal experiences being used as an example for training. However, over time, it was suggested that she and other service user volunteers pick

positive examples of good practice and avoid negative experiences. The stated reason for this was that people learn better from positive stories. Whilst this may be true in principle, it resulted in the service user's voice becoming distorted and a misrepresentation of their reality.

This cooptation trend has been reported by survivors in many countries, including the United States, France, Sweden and Germany and across many domains of service user activities, including research (Pascal and Sagan 2018). It illustrates the tensions that still exist between experiential knowledge and evidence-based practice and the difficulties of interweaving both approaches (Noorani et al. 2019).

Such shifts are also an expression of the influence of psychiatry 'producing colonizing standards' (Burstow 2015, p. 155) whereby peer support workers not only become instrumental to the continued dominance of the medical model, but also the service user/survivor voice gets contained (Mills 2014a).

The Responsibilization Agenda

The responsibilization discourse takes a 'moral' perspective, drawing on notions of self-governance, autonomy, positive risk-taking and reduced dependency on the welfare system and the state (Lidenberg et al. 2013; Andersson et al. 2016; Roy and Buchanan 2016; Pyysiäinen 2017). This reliance on moral values firmly places the onus for well-being, personal agency and (good) citizenship on the individual (Peeters 2017), thus creating moral obligations for service users. Safety nets such as the welfare state either disappear or become difficult to access (Liedenberg et al. 2013). This agenda (individualization) contrasts strongly with a social model of disability, which sees 'society' itself as a having a crucial disabling or enabling role in people's lives.

A Moral Obligation to Be Active

There is a paradox in conceding to the moral obligation to be 'active.' On the one hand it may indeed be beneficial, but on the other hand it may only be an outward sign of compliance with staff, unconnected with any therapeutic purpose (Mills 2014b). For instance, two participants in a study in a forensic setting in which good behaviour determined release said that attending occupational therapy was primarily about appearance:

> 'You go to the right groups ... for two years ... You've got to do all that before they let you go ... you've got to appear to be keen ... because you'll never get out of this place, you know you've got to get motivated and all that' (Craik et al. 2010, p. 342).

Becoming more active is widely regarded as a sign of 'recovery,' and developing new interests a sign of 'growth.' However, someone may have very good cultural, ethical or practical reasons for not wanting to engage in occupations (Friedman 2012). Additionally, some service users might be reluctant to be seen as active for fear of being considered to have 'recovered' and, consequently, being discharged from services before they are ready.

In the United Kingdom the Department of Work and Pensions requires individuals to report any change in circumstances that can affect their benefit entitlement; therefore premature discharge is a real fear amongst service users. The sense of being scrutinized may be pervasive, particularly when - as Watts (2018) noted - welfare agencies have gained access to people's social media accounts (for example, gym membership records) or CCTV footage from public places such as supermarkets, to check the legitimacy of people's claims about their disability.

Similarly, the emphasis on 'being active' can feel paternalistic to service users, reflecting a moral belief in the benefits of activity for its own sake (Friedman 2012). It echoes the moral treatment movement of the 19th century, which can be linked back to the work of William Tuke and Phillipe Pinel (Bing 1981). This movement not only stressed the corrective benefits of 'activity' (Peloquin 1989), but it also significantly relied on constant surveillance of patients and created moral chains of obligation to the doctor and the asylum (Foucault 1965).

A Moral Obligation to Be Productive

A key feature of the responsibilization agenda is workfare. In the United Kingdom, for example, this refers to government welfare policy which requires individuals to undertake work in return for benefit payments or risk losing them. This is controversial because, whilst some people claim it supports people to move into jobs, others see it as government coercion into a kind of indentured labour, motivated by a desire to reduce welfare payments.

Workfare Coercion

Policies aimed at influencing people to 'regulate their own behaviour to ensure this is consonant with the interests of the state' (Pierson 2004, p. 75) are not new (Dwyer 2004). The corrective aspect of workfare coercion can be seen in the use of behavioural and positive psychology techniques aimed at those deemed inactive and non-productive.

For instance, the Behavioural Insights Team (UK Government 2019) set up by the UK Government in 2010 earned the nickname the 'Nudge Unit' after the work of American economists and behavioural psychologists Thaler and Sustein (2009) who applied behavioural techniques to the implementation of policy on benefit sanctions and conditionality for people with disabilities. The Nudge Unit developed techniques to nudge, or push, people into action by implying that they were personally responsible for change. In addition, it used negative reinforcement on people's job-searching habits–such as by calling them into job centres for 'a chat' about their job search, sending them for medical assessments (which have been heavily criticized for their poor quality and heavy handedness), sending motivational text messages about job searching several times a week (Friedli and Stern 2015) or demanding firm commitments from an individual about what they will do to find work. Furthermore, not being able to find work has been considered as a sign of mental ill-health that needs to be addressed and corrected (Friedli and Stern 2015). In 2015 this led the United Kingdom to introduce behaviour therapists within job centres to target the long-term unemployed and those with health issues to change the way they think about their situation (Jones 2015). This is achieved by obligating people to join back-to-work schemes as a condition of benefit payments. Welfare benefit sanctions are then applied with grave outcomes for those who are considered non-compliant, including poverty, homelessness, removal of support and sometimes death (Butler 2018; Watts et al. 2018; Dwyer 2019). For the authors, this kind of pressurizing has been acutely felt. For example, RS was recently told to 'do her bit' to help reduce the state deficit caused by the 2008 financial crisis.

Jones (2015) describes this linking of welfare payments with therapy or positive psychology intervention as a form of 'gaslighting'; a 'form of psychological manipulation in which a person seeks to sow seeds of doubt ... making them question their own memory, perception, and sanity' (Wikipedia 2019). These techniques have been described as forms of psychocompulsion and psychopolitics, or points where human psychology and politics interact (Friedli and Stern 2015; Thomas 2016). They reflect Foucault's concepts of biopower and biopolitics whereby political technology is used to regulate or manage people in large groups (Adams 2017). Such policies create a moral discourse about work which 'continually places paid employment at the pinnacle' (Cole 2009, p. 40). Coming off benefits and becoming a productive citizen (that is, one who does not rely on the state for their income) becomes a moral imperative. In this model the argument that 'work is good for you' (Prior et al. 2013, p. 658) seemingly becomes the answer to everything, whilst ignoring:

> those dissenting voices which argue that without strong provisos (taking into account the complexity of individual circumstances, choice, timeliness, appropriateness as much as the quality of support and work on offer) the argument is both unhelpful and counterproductive, and can have devastating consequences for those concerned.
>
> *Donskoy 2016*

Of course, paid employment pays a major part in most people's lives. This is reflected in the views of service users in a study evaluating vocational services:

> Work provided a sense of purpose and structure to their lives, which in turn had positive impacts on their lived experiences of mental illness. Other perceived beneficial aspects of work extended to a sense of achievement, valued opportunities for enjoyment in other occupations, and access to financial and other resources to engage in their own recovery.
>
> *Hitch et al. 2107, p. 722*

However, the 'wrong' type of work for the individual can be a 'source of stress and pressure, which may in turn be detrimental to mental well-being and recovering' (Hitch et al. 2017, p. 722; see also Apostolopoulos et al. 2016). Kamerãde et al. (2019) showed that whilst having a small amount of work (1–8 h/wk) can improve mental health, it is far less clear if working longer hours has the same effect or can, in fact, be detrimental.

Individual Placement and Support

Individual Placement and Support (IPS) schemes operate in several European countries (Fioritti et al. 2014); for instance, the United Kingdom, Italy, Netherlands, Spain, Portugal, and Germany (see Useful Resources). Where they are properly funded they offer a flexible, imaginative and tailored way for people to engage with a work role, allowing plenty of time and fully accommodating a person's vocational needs and wishes. In Portugal, for example, the IPS scheme supports people to try out different types of employment and training or to explore the option of higher education if this is what the person chooses to do. Such schemes are gaining ground in the United Kingdom, too (NHS England 2019b), although their future may be in doubt due to the severe financial pressures the NHS has been under (Hutchinson et al. 2018). The practicalities of the IPS model are explored fully in Chapter 20.

To truly tackle long-term unemployment for people with psychosocial disabilities, 'a separate strategy that actually reflects the barriers they face and promotes their human rights' (Mental Health Europe 2016) is required. Occupational therapists have a vital role to play, having more specific rehabilitative expertise compared with staff in mainstream employment services (Machingura 2017). Strategies must also fully implement the United Nations (UN) Convention on the Rights of Persons with Disabilities (UN 2006).

Decolonization of Recovery

Many user activists have taken a critical perspective on how recovery has been colonized, using the analogy of imperial colonialism to explain how the psychiatric model infiltrates and gradually transforms such grassroot approaches to fit its ideology (Mills 2014a; Mills 2015):

I am not alone in taking a step or two backwards when exposed to excessive enthusiasm, a rallying battle cry or a drive to push from the dark into the light. As George Bernard Shaw said, 'The fact that a believer is happier than a sceptic is no more to the point than the fact that a drunken man is happier than a sober one.' I heard Anne Milton during her brief stint as health minister [UK govt. 2010-2012] talk about commissioning miracles . . . The recovery agenda has right on its side: 'You don't want the recovery we offer? Then I am not sure you deserve our help.' . . . A nice little shaming prod.

Boyt 2013

Recovery in the Bin

RitB is the main UK survivor voice critic of the colonization of recovery, offering critical and theoretical reflection on the process. RitB's membership includes not only service users and carers, but also mental health professionals and academics. The group has gained recognition for its important work in the United Kingdom and on social media (see Useful Resources).

RitB focuses on 'the idea that recovery was a radical idea which has been coopted by mainstream policy-makers to pursue a neoliberal agenda' (Woods et al. 2019). It has developed its own concept of 'UnRecovery' as illustrated in its *20 Principles of Recovery* (RitB 2019b) and in the 'The UnRecovery Star' (see https://recoveryinthebin.org/unrecovery-star-2/) which includes domains reflecting societal issues (not just personal ones) that are frequently excluded from conversations about recovery, such as unstable housing, sexism, loss of the welfare state, loss of rights, economic inequality, homophobia/transphobia, racism, discrimination, trauma/iatrogenic trauma, and poverty.

The concept of 'UnRecovery' does not mean that people want to remain 'unwell' or 'ill' but that they want greater acknowledgement of the impact of societal pressures on their mental health. Specifically, RitB promotes the idea of rights, solidarity, social justice and collective action. It is intended as a counterbalance to the responsibilization agenda which places the onus of responsibility for self-management solely on the individual, who is expected to strive to become a 'worthy citizen'.

Mad Studies

Mad Studies, developed by survivors of psychiatry in the early 2000s in Canada (LeFrançois et al. 2013), is another voice offering critical reflection on colonization. Mad Studies is not about substituting one dominant discourse (such as psychiatry's 'medical model') with another (the survivor discourse) but, instead, about reclaiming narratives of madness through intellectual enquiry and activism in research.

SERVICE USERS' INVOLVEMENT IN THEIR OWN CARE

In many Western countries, for the past 30 years, policies have morphed the patient into a consumer (Abelson et al. 2010; Andersson et al. 2011; Beresford 2013, 2019). In the United Kingdom patient and public involvement in healthcare has been one of the central tenets since New Labour's health modernization agenda (Pascal and Sagan 2018). However, service users want to be treated as more than mere 'consumers' of services; they want to have a genuine say in how they are designed and delivered on a personal level and collectively. They have experienced 'client-centred practice' as a quasi-mantra, more often than not devoid of genuine meaning or intent and defined without reference to clients' perspectives (Hammell 2013).

Being properly involved means being given all the relevant information in a timely manner and in a format that suits the needs of the person so that they can make informed choices about interventions and occupations. According to NHS England, the regulatory body for England's public health, involving people in their care and treatment means:

supporting people to manage their own health and wellbeing on a daily basis. It means supporting them to become involved, as much as they want or are able to, in decisions about their care and giving them choice and control over the NHS services they receive. It means focusing on what matters to the individual within the context of their lives, not simply addressing a list of conditions or symptoms to be treated.

NHS England 2017a

However, when 'involvement' in one's care is redefined as 'self-management', its purpose shifts dramatically so that the individual is deemed to be solely responsible for his or her well-being and choices rather than doing so in collaboration with a therapist. This is especially complex in mental health in which, overall, the power remains mostly in the hands of professionals, especially in cases in which the person may be the subject of a legal order which can severely restrict or annul their agency.

Care Planning

Involving someone in their care may be a formal or informal process. In the United Kingdom the formal Care Programme Approach (CPA) dominates. It implements national standards as defined in the United Kingdom by a national body, the Care Coordination Association (formerly the CPA Association) (see Useful Resources). Involving someone in their care plan, or similar schemes, should be more than a bureaucratic exercise. The CPA is intended to be an 'equitable partnership between service users, carers and providers of services' (DoH 2008).

Good practice would see service users, with appropriate support if needed, ask for a CPA meeting, decide who attends and lead it if that is what they want. However, the reality is that the process is still largely owned by professionals. Care plan meetings are usually organized around the professionals' own needs – time of day, length and location of the meeting, agenda, etc. (Donskoy and UFM 2009) – and 'there is substantial evidence that many users and carers are marginalized and removed from the care planning process' (National Institute for Health and Care Excellence 2012), denying them their human rights under the UN United Convention on the Rights of Persons with Disabilities (UN 2006).

These shortcomings are widely evident. The care plan itself, which is a formal record of what has been decided, should create opportunities for genuine engagement from all parties, sense-checking by all and empowerment, while acknowledging that a patient's journey is often non-linear but comprises twists and turns (like life itself). Instead, partly due to the formality of the process, it is often an objectifying and largely administrative exercise. A care plan will usually only provide a summary of the meeting. Consequently, it can become disconnected and distorted from the original intention, especially when read by someone not involved in the original discussions. Nuance and complexity are often lost.

Experience indicates that, despite good intentions, care plans often remain highly bureaucratic, prescriptive and one-sided affairs. This rigidity prevents the creation of the sort of space needed, especially in complex cases, to fully support the person to express their stories, needs and wishes and for everyone's voice to be heard. Clearly, the idea of an 'equitable partnership' (DoH 2008) often remains but a laudable intention. Having outlined frequent failings of the CPA process, it is also important to acknowledge that some people may not wish to be involved in decisions about their care

Open Dialogue and Care Planning

Open Dialogue (OD) (see earlier) enjoys the input of genuine peer support and involves a firm commitment to person-centredness. This is because power dynamics in OD are much more evenly distributed between health professionals and service users, who are given a greater voice (Aaltonen et al. 2011; Seikkula et al. 2011). Meetings become dialogical spaces in which multiple viewpoints are elicited in an embodied (openly expressed) way, including narratives which are sometimes difficult, angry or conflictual or express uncertainty (Olson et al. 2014), qualities which may be harder to accept within traditional mental health services' more bureaucratized CPA processes.

ACCESSING OCCUPATIONAL THERAPY

The geographical location and the nature of the local service provider contract will greatly influence what is on offer for people who may need or want occupational therapy. Additionally, a range of barriers exist for many people such as insufficient information about services, service-orientated organizational culture, geographical inaccessibility, cost of transport and prohibitive referral/acceptance criteria.

Sharing Information

To access occupational therapy a person first needs to know that it exists, of course. Up-to-date information about services (their location, purpose, the occupation/media used and the referral process for gaining access) should be available in different formats. It is also important to bear in mind that occupational therapy may not be familiar to all service users, especially if they are new to mental health services.

Significantly, in many cases, it will not be an occupational therapist but a mental health nurse or a psychiatrist who first mentions or suggests occupational therapy to a service user. The danger is that if occupational therapists are not clear in their communications with interprofessional colleagues about what occupational therapy can offer, this relaying of information by a third party may create a misleading (perhaps 'medicalized') picture of occupational therapy from the outset. Service users may then feel under pressure to fit themselves into a somewhat distorted picture of occupational therapy, especially if these introductory conversations are initiated by their psychiatrist. This coercive influence is illustrated by a situation that arose when the authors were conducting a research interview with a service user in a forensic unit. The service user said he had felt under pressure to agree to participate in the research because it had been suggested by his psychiatrist, and he felt he needed to be seen to be cooperative or it may harm his chance of being discharged. It is therefore important for therapists to publicize what they do (in ward environments, for example) and to ensure they have preparatory conversations with service users directly, face-to-face when possible.

Organizational Barriers to Accessing Services

Access to occupational therapy is often limited to working hours and weekdays with little or no service provision at weekends and evenings (Notley et al. 2012). For service users on hospital wards, access to other hospital resources at those times (such as kitchens or art rooms) may also be denied, limiting the opportunities for service users to progress with their occupations and start to translate the skills acquired in therapy to more real-world settings (Townsend 1996). Le Granse et al. (2006) found the following example from a study of occupational therapy in the Netherlands, Belgium and Germany:

> 'The occupational therapist encourages the client to make his own cup of coffee. On the ward, however ... he is not allowed to do that himself. The client wants

> to go to the cinema, but he can't because the night nurse locks the doors around 22.00 hours' (Le Granse et al. 2006, p. 151).

Location

The way occupational therapy services are accessed has changed considerably over the past decade in the United Kingdom, with the gradual disappearance of day hospitals in favour of community mental health teams (DoH 1999). These have a largely brokering or bridge-building role, assisting people to engage with mainstream supports wherever possible (Carpenter and Raj 2012), and frequently, such teams offer very limited in-house service provision themselves. This can be positive and facilitate social inclusion, provided the person is fully informed and supported to explore community-based activities and the settings in which they take place. However, accessing community resources can be challenging. While disability access issues are often considered in terms of challenges presented by the physical environment, analysis of the psychosocial elements of the mainstream community can be just as important. The social model of disability, for example, highlights societal attitudes (including stigma and prejudice) as a primary barrier and cause of disability (Tew 2005; French and Swain 2008; Oliver and Barnes 2012), referring in part to the *discrimination* featured in the UnRecovery Star (see earlier).

A major development in the United Kingdom's mental health services has been the Improving Access to Psychological Therapies (IAPT) project. Many people in the United Kingdom who visit their general practitioner regarding their mental health (especially regarding anxiety or depression) are now likely to be referred to outsourced primary IAPT services, which use psychotherapy and cognitive therapies and are often located away from traditional mental health services (see Useful Resources). In IAPT services, occupational therapists are not usually employed in a profession-specific, occupation-focused role as the emphasis is on 'talking therapies,' as distinct from 'doing' or occupation-focused intervention. Due to this separation of service provision there may be a loss of holism in the way IAPT services approach an individual's care.

Related to the location, the availability and cost of transport to potentially dispersed community-based resources are also important factors to consider.

Referral Criteria

Service users may be denied access to community and hospital services due to prohibitive referral acceptance criteria and risk assessment policies over which individual service users have no control. Organizations set the referral criteria for their services so that resources can be targeted efficiently and effectively. This can impact on occupational therapists' choices about provision and hence the choice offered to service users and can exclude people who are deemed to be more challenging to engage. Commitment to the occupational therapy process cannot begin to take place when the service user's agency is effectively thwarted from the start.

One service user, in a study of occupational therapy in an acute admissions unit, felt excluded when they were told occupational therapy was targeted exclusively to skill acquisition rather than meaningful occupation:

> They said it was for people who need to learn and they said … I didn't need to be here, there, doing it, which I thought was a bit unfair.'
>
> **Bryant et al. 2011, p.164**

The assessment of risk is an everyday practice in mental health services, including the risk individuals pose to themselves and to other people. It may be linked to the service users' legal status under legislation such as the United Kingdom's Mental Health Act 1983/2007, but it is generally becoming standard practice. The capacity of organizations to manage reasonable risk is a crucial factor in service users' recovery (Langan 2010). Unfortunately, such risk assessments are often undertaken without the knowledge or involvement of the service user themselves. This lack of sharing, combined with services often being risk averse, may result in people being denied access to opportunities to acquire new skills and take control of their own recovery. The negative effect of such denial of services is compounded if the service user is unaware of the real reason (such as covert risk management decisions) for the denial of a learning opportunity (Langan 2008). This issue is still an ongoing problem as indicated by Simpson et al. (2016) who comment that 'risk was a significant concern for workers, but this appeared to be rarely discussed with service users, who were often unaware of the content of risk assessments' (p. vi).

Positive risk-taking is not only an important enabler of learning but is also underpinned by a social perspective of mental health (Ramon 2005) and an awareness of human rights (Dimond 2010) that emphasize that people should be treated equally and fairly as a member of society (UN 2006).

NEGOTIATING MEANING

An occupational therapy assessment may have profound unanticipated consequences for service users' sense of identity. The individual may interpret the assessment as a judgement; a perception of failings, perhaps, which may start them wondering, 'What is the occupational therapist seeing that leads them to think I need occupational therapy?' How first encounters are handled is vitally important.

Author RS's experience of being introduced to the activities in a day service's therapeutic programme shows how opportunities for engagement can be missed if a therapist presumes to be able to bestow meaning on an activity from their own perspective. Meaning must be negotiated and confirmed by the service user and therapist collaboratively.

> This member of staff showed me around and I saw this guy doing mosaic on glass. I love working with colours and that grabbed my attention. I asked if I could do that too but the member of staff said 'no' I could not do it because this other person was already doing it and so I was shown to a table where these women were doing some sewing. Now I hate sewing, it just isn't me but she was adamant it would be a good activity for me. That was the end of my interest in OT.

As recovery is such a personal and unique journey, it requires the therapist to have a whole-person approach to engage with the service user's narrative and to understand the different reasons why a person might want to engage in a particular occupation. This includes the meanings that a person has already ascribed to an occupation (based on past experience, for example) and which they bring with them to the 'doing' and the meanings that arise for them through participation in occupation in the moment of 'doing' (Tew 2005; Wilcock 2006). It may be that the therapist is able to unlock a dormant interest or pique a person's curiosity by simply suggesting an activity they may not have considered before.

Survival: The Art of Staying Alive

Wilcock's (2006) doing-being-becoming-belonging synthesis highlights the significance of occupation not just in terms of doing but also in terms of being; a necessary stage before becoming or 'change' can be anticipated or perhaps even imagined.

For many service users, survival is a hard struggle that dominates their everyday life. This simple fact may be so obvious as to be overlooked in professional literature and therapists' training. The notion of meeting basic needs is also about recognizing the need to simply 'be'. To facilitate this the therapist must keep an open mind, avoid making assumptions about what represents a step forward for the service user and keep their sense of humanity and respect for personal identity alive.

Consequently, it is important not to underestimate the value of an individual's occupational engagement at what might first appear to be a basic level. Watching television, smoking and sleeping may be regarded by staff as time wasted, despite the fact that many people in their everyday lives engage in these occupations unquestioned. For service users in the early stages of recovery or living with long-term psychosocial distress, filling time in these ways can be helpful.

> 'We wanted them to provide distraction from the feelings that we experience' (College of Occupational Therapists 2006, p. 8).

Boredom can be a distressing experience if a person feels trapped by it. At the same time, apparent boredom may indicate to an occupational therapist that an individual may be open to exploring what they might want to do. However, in some hospital settings, there is no choice of activity on offer outside of working hours (Bejerholm 2010), and this can undermine someone's recovery, as noted earlier.

It is acknowledged that presenting occupational therapy as a way to 'structure time, relax and relieve boredom' (Lim et al. 2007, p. 27) may be problematic for therapists who do not want their therapeutic role to be devalued as something purely diversionary. However, 'filling time' is not merely about providing entertainment. Giving a person a reason to get up in the morning and engage in something stimulating is a motivator for occupation; a possible step forward from 'being' to 'doing'. It was better to be doing something rather than nothing, according to a service user in a forensic setting;

> 'You feel good with yourself knowing that you've done something for the day, instead of just doing nothing ... even if you don't like the lesson. But you're doing it ... not because you have to, it's because you want to' (Craik et al. 2010, p. 342).

Creative Activities

Creativity can improve someone's sense of worth and reduce anxiety (Pöllänen 2015). In addition, it is a trait highly valued in society. Creative activities are widely used in occupational therapy (see Chapter 16). Someone with a bipolar diagnosis commented that being creative 'makes you feel like you're you,' as 'ultimately, those ideas are your own' (Taylor 2015, p. 661).

However, the frequent association between mental health problems and creativity may imply there is a direct correlation, so careful critical reflection on this cliché is necessary. Drawing on Weisberg's (1994) quasi-experimental test of the hypothesis that manic-depression increases creativity, Murray and Johnson (2010) note that, although the sheer volume of output may be higher during manic periods than depressive ones, the work done when someone is 'high' may be of poorer quality because creativity requires attention to detail and critical reflection as well as spontaneous generation of new ideas. They also note that 'it may be helpful to share with clients evidence that creativity is not specifically related to manic periods, that people with a history of hypomania are more likely to have creative accomplishments than those with mania' (p. 11). These considerations should be kept in mind by occupational therapists choosing creative activities that focus primarily on self-expression and process (using a psychodynamic approach, perhaps) versus those selected mainly with an end-product (an artwork) in mind.

Of course, creative activities are not just activities done within an occupational therapy context. For example, author RS had a talented artistic friend who, but for his mental health difficulties, might have pursued a career as an artist. Some of his work was displayed as an art show in the corridors of the psychiatric hospital without his consent and, seemingly, as a showcase for the hospital rather than for his talent (Lancashire Evening Post 2011). This raises a number of issues, such as the extent to which service users 'own' their own artwork (particularly if the individual is an artist who would normally sell their work) and the importance of confidentiality. Indeed, output from creative activities, which may be offered as therapy and have a strong projective element, should be treated as confidential material. Accordingly, occupational therapists should always make it clear in advance what service users' creative output may be used for to set therapeutic boundaries, reduce inadvertently inappropriate disclosure, and maximize service users' safety.

OCCUPATION-FOCUSED, USER-LED SERVICES

User-led initiatives with an interest or focus on occupation are to be found primarily in the voluntary or non-statutory sector. They might be specifically commissioned, or a user-led project may already be part of an organization's activities. For example, Clubhouse International (see Useful Links) offers an innovative model for providing occupation-focused activities as therapy, community participation and inclusion in the community.

The Swedish Club House model, for instance, has a strong recovery orientation with a specific focus on agency and self-determination, on learning through doing and through listening to people's stories (see Useful Resources). At the Fontänhuset (Fountain House) Club House in Stockholm there are programmes with 'real life' outcomes, such as learning to cook in a professional kitchen attached to a café or learning information technology and communication skills in a professionally set up newsroom, leading to the production of a successful magazine. Users are referred by health and social care services, or they can self-refer.

CONCLUSION

This chapter has critically reflected on recovery as a key international policy driver shaping mental health services. Whilst bringing real, tangible hope to people is important, the way recovery is implemented can be contentious in which it is felt to be an enactment of a responsibilization agenda which fails to account for the wide range of social and societal factors that create and maintain disability.

For occupational therapists this means taking into account the wider socio-economic and political context of people's lives beyond 'the person' and rebooting their notion of 'person-centredness' or 'client-centred practice' accordingly. This would create spaces in which occupation becomes a genuine means of sharing experiences and exploring new possibilities that enable people not only to survive and recover but also to flourish as human beings.

USEFUL RESOURCES

- **Behavioural Insights Team:** https://www.gov.uk/government/organisations/behavioural-insights-team
- **Care Coordination Association**: http://www.cpaa.org.uk/welcome-to-the-cca.html
- **Club Houses:** http://www.iccd.org/mission.html
- **Clubhouse International**: https://clubhouse-intl.org/
- **Foucault, Michel:** see for instance: http://criticallegalthinking.com/2017/05/10/michel-foucault-biopolitics-biopower/
- **Fountain House, Sweden:** http://www.fountain-house.org/category/tags/training
- **IAPT:** https://www.england.nhs.uk/mental-health/adults/iapt/
- **Individual Placement and Support:** https://www.centreformentalhealth.org.uk/what-ips
- **Intentional Peer Support:** https://www.intentionalpeersupport.org/what-is-ips/?v=79cba1185463
- **Peer Workers France:** https://www.solidarites-usagerspsy.fr/s-engager/les-pairs-aidants/
- **Recovery Colleges:** https://www.mentalhealth-today.co.uk/recovery-colleges-bridging-the-gap-in-mental-health-service-provisionhttps://www.health.org.uk/article/increasing-the-emphasis-on-recovery-in-mental-health-services
- **Recovery in the Bin:** http://www.recoveryinthe-bin.org

QUESTIONS FOR CONSIDERATION

1. Why is supporting recovery so important in occupational therapy?
2. If the service user is the expert on 'the life being lived,' then where does the expertise of the occupational therapist lie in recovery-orientated practice?
3. Are there any aspects of your own occupational therapy practice or of the institutional context in which you work that might be experienced as stigmatizing by service users?
4. Why do you think paid work is considered as a sign of recovery in society? Do you think this is justified?
5. Are there any other domains you would suggest adding to the UnRecovery Star?
6. Can you think of ways of ensuring that a 'care plan' is meaningful to the service user?
7. What might have been a good method for the occupational therapist to communicate the purpose of the sewing activity to 'author RS' that would have encouraged engagement?
8. Do you see any tensions between a 'top down' recovery as policy agenda and the service user's understanding of their own recovery needs?

SERVICE USER COMMENTARY

My name is Jerome Sewell. I am a former service user at the Bethlem Royal Hospital, London, UK, and have worked there as a group facilitator, peer trainer and expert by experience.

When we are told in this chapter about Anthony's (1995) idea that recovery-orientated services have 'a subsidiary role to service users' own momentum' we should realize, from an occupational therapy standpoint, that therapy only works if it is interwoven with service users' own convictions and passions in life. For example, it was my desire to attain certain career goals and make progress in my life that led me to engage with occupational therapy. It allowed me to express my personal abilities and encouraged my desire to deliver services also.

To ensure the process of therapy and service users' goals are interwoven it would be beneficial for occupational therapists to analyse the occupational, vocational, spiritual and philosophical life of a person. Occupational therapists should do a comprehensive assessment of what the person's goals are, what is important to the person, what has shaped their life so far and what are the prosocial elements of their life. From that point of initial assessment the aim should be to deliver services which address that holistic range of needs. In short, the main thing is to establish what someone wants in their life and help them achieve it. This will lead to more sustainable outcomes, potentially having a life-changing effect.

Regarding patient involvement in mental healthcare, I would go one step further than advocating more holistic assessment by saying that the service user has a right to identify their own needs and what they want from the services they use. In addition, there is a need for service users to design services themselves. There is not enough emphasis on service users becoming 'practitioners', to assist in delivering services whereby they can help themselves and each other instead of being the passive recipients of care.

I have also learnt that occupational therapists who serve inpatients do not always do enough to enhance the work habits and vocational skills of service users with theoretical knowledge such as specific, measurable, achievable, relevant, time-based goal-setting or using continuing professional development.

In terms of how this relates to the meaning of occupational therapy, my journey highlighted to me that the occupational therapist's greatest asset was in being a skills-based, vocational and occupational professional. In other words, occupational therapists should be interested in what you do and skilled in facilitating what you *can* do. It worked for me because I made a point of combining my own interests in the mainstream community with work that I could get on with in hospital. This included editing a short film I had made before admission with the aim of having it released after discharge and script-writing for another film I am now making.

To conclude, I was fascinated by the chapter's seemingly quite radical argument that neoliberal ideology has had an effect on mental health services and the idea that the delivery of recovery-orientated services is being controlled by this. For example, I agreed with the observations about the CPA and wish I had more scope to write more about other issues I picked up on.

Jerome Sewell

REFERENCES

Aaltonen, J., Seikkula, J., & Lehtinen, K. (2011). The comprehensive open-dialogue approach in Western Lapland: I. The incidence of non-affective psychosis and prodromal states. *Psychosis, 3*(3), 179–191.

Abelson, J., Montesanti, S., & Li, K. (2010). *Effective Strategies for Interactive Public Engagement in the Development of Healthcare Policies and Programs.* Ottawa: Canadian Health Services Research Foundation. Available at https://www.cfhi-fcass.ca/Libraries/Commissioned_Research_Reports/Abelson_EN_FINAL.sflb.ashx.

Adams, R. (2017). *Michel Foucault: Biopolitics and Biopower. Critical Legal Thinking: Law and the Political.* Available at http://criticallegalthinking.com/2017/05/10/michel-foucault-biopolitics-biopower/.

Anderson, L., Spanjol, J., Jeffries, J. G., et al. (2016). Responsibility and well-being: Resource integration under responsibilization in expert services. *Journal of Public Policy & Marketing, 35*(2), 262–279.

Andersson, E., Fennell, E., & Shahroth, T. (2011). *Making the Case for Public Engagement: How to Demonstrate the Value of Consumer Input.* Eastleigh: INVOLVE. Available at https://www.involve.org.uk/resources/publications/practical-guidance/making-case-public-engagement.

Anonymous. (2019a). *Private Communication with Service User.* The Netherlands, 20 June.

Anonymous. (2019b). *Private Communication with Open Dialogue Trainee.* United Kingdom, 8 August.

Anthony, W. (1995). *Toward a Vision of recovery.* Available at: http://mentalhealth.ohio.gov/assets/recovery/toward-a-vision-of-recovery.pdf.

Apostolopoulos, Y., Sönmez, S., Hege, A., & Lemka, M. (2016). Work strain, social isolation and mental health of long-haul truckers. *Occupational Therapy in Mental Health, 32*(1), 50–69.

Ásmundsdóttir, E. E. (2009). Creation of new services: Collaboration between mental health consumers and occupational therapists. *Occupational Therapy in Mental Health, 25*(2), 115–126.

Baillon, G. (2011). *Les pairs-aidants, pseudo générosité et dérives sur la psychiatrie, en réponse à Pluriels.* Available at https://blogs.mediapart.fr/edition/contes-de-la-folie-ordinaire/article/060211/les-pairs-aidants-pseudo-generosite-et-deri.

Bejerholm, U. (2010). Relationships between occupational engagement and status of and satisfaction with sociodemographic factors in a group of people with schizophrenia. *Scandinavian Journal of Occupational Therapy, 17*(3), 244–254.

Beresford, P. (2013). *Introductory comments at recovery and social justice: Transforming mental health at individual, service and societal levels* (Unpublished) (9 October). Preston, England.

Beresford, P. (2015). Distress and disability: Not you, not me, but us? In H. Spandler, J. Anderson, & B. Sapey (Eds.), *Madness, Distress and the Politics of Disablement* (pp. 245–259). Bristol: Policy Press.

Beresford, P. (2019). Public participation in health and social care: Exploring the co-production of knowledge. *Front. Soc., 3*(41), 1–12.

Bing, R. K. (1981). Occupational therapy revisited: A paraphrastic journey. *American Journal of Occupational Therapy, 35*, 499–518. https://doi.org/10.5014/ajot.35.8.499.

Boniface, G., Humpage, S., Awatar, S., & Reagon, C. (2015). Developing an occupation- and recovery-based outcome measure for people with mental health conditions: An action research study. *British Journal of Occupational Therapy, 78*(4), 222–231.

Boyt, A. (2013). *The R Word. Blog post.* November. Available at: https://drinkanddrugsnews.com/the-r-word/.

Bryant, W., McKay, E., Beresford, P., et al. (2011). An occupational perspective on mental health service user involvement in research. In F. Kronenberg, N. Pollard, & D. Sakellariou (Eds.), *Occupational Therapies without Borders.* Amsterdam: Elsevier.

Burstow, B. (2015). *Psychiatry and the Business of Madness.* New York: Palgrace MacMillan.

Butler, P. (2018). *Benefit Sanctions Found to be Ineffective and Damaging.* Available at https://www.theguardian.com/society/2018/may/22/benefit-sanctions-found-to-be-ineffective-and-damaging.

Care Coordination Association. (2014). *The Care Standards Handbook.* Available at: http://www.cpaa.org.uk/care-standards-handbook.html.

Carpenter, M., & Raj, T. (2012). Editorial introduction: Towards a paradigm shift from community care to community development work. *Community Development Journal, 47*(4), 457–472.

Cercle de Réflexion et de Proposition d'Actions sur la psychiatrie - CRPA. (2013). *Submission to the rapporteur on mental health.* November https://psychiatrie.crpa.asso.fr/IMG/pdf/2013-11-21-audition-par-la-mismap-texte-word-positions-crpa.pdf.

Chamberlin, J. (1978). *On Our own: Patient-Controlled Alternatives to the mental health System.* New York: Hawthorn Books.

Cole, M. (2008). Sociology contra government? The contest for the meaning of unemployment in UK policy debates. *Work Empl. Soc., 22*(1), 27–43.

College of Occupational Therapists (COT). (2006). *Recovering Ordinary Lives: The Strategy for Occupational Therapy in mental health services 2007–2017, results from service User and Carer Focus Groups.* London: College of Occupational Therapists.

Craik, C., Bryant, W., Ryan, A., et al. (2010). A qualitative study of service user experiences of occupation in forensic mental health. *Australian Occupational Therapy Journal, 57*(5), 339–344.

Deacon, A., & Patrick, R. (2011). A new welfare settlement? The coalition government and welfare to work. In H. Bochel (Ed.), *The Conservative Party and Social Policy.* Bristol: Policy Press.

Deegan, P. (2001). Recovery as a self-directed process of healing and transformation. *Occupational Therapy in Mental Health, 17*(3/4), 5–21.

Department of Health. (2008). *Refocusing the Care Programme Approach: Policy and Positive Practice Guidance.* Available at https://webarchive.nationalarchives.gov.uk/20130124042407/http://www.dh.gov.uk/prod_consum_dh/groups/dh_digitalassets/@dh/@en/documents/digitalasset/dh_083649.pdf.

Devon Partnership NHS Trust. (2017). *It's Occupational Therapy Week - Jezz talks about how his OT role benefits patients, 6*

November. Available at https://www.dpt.nhs.uk/news/it-s-occupational-therapy-week-jezz-talks-about-how-his-ot-role-benefits-patients.

Devon Partnership NHS Trust. (2019). *Open Dialogue Peer Support Worker Job Advert*. https://www.jobs.nhs.uk/xi/vacancy/?vac_ref=915602369.

Diksy, J., Ramachandra, Lalitha, K., Desai, G., & Nagarajaiah (2015). Consumer perspectives on the concept of recovery in schizophrenia: A systematic review. *Asian J. Psych*, 14, 13–18.

Dimond, B. (2010). *Legal Aspects of Occupational Therapy* (3rd ed.). Oxford: Wiley Blackwell.

Donskoy, A.-L., & UFM Team. (2009). *The Experiences of the Care Programme Approach in Bristol: How Socially Inclusive is it?* Bristol: Bristol Mind.

Donskoy, A.-L. (2016). *Workfare Coercion in the UK: An Assault on Persons with Disabilities and Their Human Rights*. Available at: https://politicsandinsights.org/2016/04/27/workfare-coercion-in-the-uk-an-assault-on-persons-with-disabilities-and-their-human-rights-anne-laure-donskoy/.

Dwyer, P. J. (2004). *Creeping Conditionality in the UK: From Welfare Rights to Conditional Entitlements?* Available at http://usir.salford.ac.uk/id/eprint/12778/2/CREEPING_CONDTIONALITY.pdf.

Dwyer, P. J. (2019). *Dealing with Welfare Conditionality: Implementation and Effects*. Policy Press. https://policy.bristoluniversitypress.co.uk/dealing-with-welfare-conditionality.

Fairclough, N. (2010). *Critical Discourse Analysis* (2nd ed.). London: Routledge.

Farnsworth, K., & Irving, Z. (2018). Austerity: Neoliberal dreams come true? *Critical Social Policy*, 38(3), 461–481.

Ferrier, C., & McGregor, C. (2016). Who are we smiling for? Three contradictions of the happiness and wellbeing agenda in community practice. *Concept*, 7(3). Available at http://concept.lib.ed.ac.uk/article/view/2481.

Fioritti, A., Burns, T., Hilarion, P., et al. (2014). Individual placement and support in Europe. *Psychiatric Rehabilitation Journal*, 37(2), 123–128.

Freire, P. (2008). *Pedagogy of Indignation*. Boulder, Colorado: Paradigm Publishers.

French, S., & Swain, J. (2008). *Understanding Disability. A Guide for health Professionals*. Edinburgh: Churchill Livingstone/Elsevier.

Friedli, L., & Stern, R. (2015). Positive affect as coercive strategy: Conditionality, activation and the role of psychology in UK government workfare programmes. *Medical Humanities*, 41, 40–47.

Friedman, J. R. (2012). Thoughts on inactivity and an ethnography of 'nothing': Comparing meanings of 'inactivity' in Romanian and American mental health care. *North American Dialogue*, 15, 1–9.

Hammell, K. R. (2013). Client-centred practice in occupational therapy: Critical reflections. *Scandinavian Journal of Occupational Therapy*, 20(3). https://doi.org/10.3109/11038128.2012.752031.

Health Foundation (The). Increasing the emphasis on recovery in mental health services. An interview with Jane Melton. Available at https://www.health.org.uk/article/increasing-the-emphasis-on-recovery-in-mental-health-services.

Hitch, D., Robertson, J., Ochoteco, H., et al. (2017). An evaluation of a vocational group for people with mental health problems based on the WORKS framework. *British Journal of Occupational Therapy*, 80(12), 717–725.

Hutchinson, J., Gilbert, D., Papworth, R., & Boardman, J. (2018). Implementing supported employment. Lessons from the making IPS work project. *International Journal of Environmental Research and Public Health*. Available at https://www.ncbi.nlm.nih.gov/pmc/articles/PMC6069163/pdf/ijerph-15-01545.pdf.

Jones, K. S. (2015). The power of positive thinking is really political gaslighting. Blog post. 22 March. *Politics and Insight*. Available at https://politicsandinsights.org/2015/03/22/the-power-of-positive-thinking-is-really-political-gaslighting/.

Kamerāde, D., Wang, S., Burchell, B., Balderson, S. U., & Coutts, A. (2019). A shorter working week for everyone: How much paid work is needed for mental health and well-being? *Social Science & Medicine*. https://doi.org/10.1016/j.socscimed.2019.06.006. Available at:.

Lancashire Evening Post. (2011). Art show by patients. *Lancashire Evening Post* 4/11/2011.

Langan, J. (2008). Involving mental health service users considered to pose a risk to other people in risk assessment. *Journal of Mental Health*, 17(5), 471–481.

Langan, J. (2010). Challenging assumptions about risk factors and the role of screening for violence risk in the field of mental health. *Health, Risk & Society*, 12(2), 85–100.

Le Granse, M., Kinébanian, A., & Josephsson, S. (2006). Promoting autonomy of the client with persistent mental illness: A challenge for occupational therapists from The Netherlands, Germany and Belgium. *Occupational Therapy International*, 13(3), 142–159.

LeFrançois, B., Menzies, R., & Reaume, G. (2013). *Mad Matters: A Critical Reader in Mad Studies*. Toronto: Canadian Scholars' Press Inc.

Liedengerg, L., Unga, M., & Ikeda, J. (2013). Neo-liberalism and responsibilisation in the discourse of social service workers. *British Journal of Social Work*, 45(3), 1006–1021.

Lim, K. H., Morris, J., & Craik, C. (2007). Inpatients perspectives of occupational therapy in acute mental health. *Australian Occupational Therapy Journal*, 54(1), 22–32.

Machingura, T., & Lloyd, C. (2017). Mental health occupational therapy and supported employment. *Irish Journal of Occupational Therapy*, 45(1), 52–57.

Mead, S., Hilton, D., & Curtis, L. (2001). Peer support: A theoretical perspective. *Psychiatric Rehabilitation Journal*, 25(2), 134–141.

Mead, S., & MacNeil, C. (2006). Peer support: What makes it unique? *International Journal of Psychosocial Rehabilitation*, 10(2), 29–37.

Mental Health Europe. (2016). *Statement on the long-term unemployment recommendation*. Available at https://www.mhe-sme.org/mental-health-europes-statement-on-the-long-term-unemployment-recommendation/.

Mills, C. (2014a). *Decolonizing Global mental health. The Psychiatrization of the Majority World*. Hove: Routledge.

Mills, C. (2014b). Sly normality: Between quiescence and revolt. In B. Burstow, LeFrançois, & S. Diamond (Eds.), *Psychiatry Disrupted* (pp. 28–224). Montreal: McGill-Queen's University Press.

Mills, C. (2015). The global politics of disablement: Assuming impairment and erasing complexity. In H. Spandler, J. Anderson, & B. Sapey (Eds.), *Madness, Distress and the Politics of Disablement* (pp. 199–213). Bristol: Policy Press.

Murray, G., & Johnson, S. L. (2010). The clinical significance of creativity in bipolar disorder. *Clinical Psychology Review, 30,* 721–732.

National Institute for Health and Care Excellence. (2012). *Enhancing the Quality of service User Involved Care Planning in mental health services (EQUIP). Study report.* Available at https://www.nice.org.uk/sharedlearning/enhancing-the-quality-of-service-user-involved-care-planning-in-mental-health-services-equip.

NHS England a. (2017). *Involving People in Their own health and Care: Statutory Guidance for Clinical Commissioning Groups and NHS England.* Available at https://www.basw.co.uk/system/files/resources/basw_65419-2_0.pdf.

NHS England b. (2019). *Individual Placement and Support Offers Route to Employment for People with Severe mental health Conditions.* Available at https://www.england.nhs.uk/mental-health/case-studies/individual-placement-and-support-offers-route-to-employment-for-people-with-severe-mental-health-conditions/.

Noorani, T., Karlsson, M., & Borkman, T. (2019). Deep experiential knowledge: Reflections from mutual aid groups for evidence-based practice. *Evidence Pol, 15*(2), 217–234.

Notley, J., Pell, H., Bryant, W., et al. (2012). 'I know how to look after myself a lot better now': Service user perspectives on mental health in-patient rehabilitation. *International Journal of Therapy and Rehabilitation, 19*(5), 288–298.

O'Donnell, A., & Shaw, M. (2016). Resilience and resistance on the road to recovery in mental health. *Concept, 7*(3). Available at http://concept.lib.ed.ac.uk/article/view/2483.

Oliver, M., & Barnes, C. (2012). *The New Politics of Disablement.* Basingstoke: Palgrave Macmillan.

Olson, M., Seikkula, J., & Ziedonis, D. (2014). *The Key Elements of Dialogic Practice in Open Dialogue: Fidelity Criteria.* Available at https://www.umassmed.edu/globalassets/psychiatry/open-dialogue/keyelementsv1.109022014.pdf.

Pascal, J., & Sagan, O. (2018). Cocreation or collusion: The dark side of consumer narrative in qualitative health research. *Illness Crisis Loss, 26*(4), 251–269.

Peeters, R. (2019). Manufacturing responsibility: The governmentality of behavioural power in social policies. *Social Policy and Society, 18*(1), 51–65. https://doi.org/10.1017/S147474641700046X.

Peloquin, S. (1989). Moral treatment: Contexts considered. *American Journal of Occupational Therapy, 43*(8), 537–544.

Penney, D. (2018). *Who Gets to Define "Peer Support?".* Mad in America: Science, Psychiatry, and social justice. 10/02/2018. Available at https://www.madinamerica.com/2018/02/who-gets-to-define-peer-support/.

Pierson, C. (2004). *The Modern State.* London: Routledge.

Pilgrim, D., & McCranie, A. (2013). *Recovery and mental health: A Critical Sociological Account.* Basingstoke: Palgrave Macmillan.

Pöllänen, S. H. (2015). Crafts as Leisure-based Coping: Craft Makers' Descriptions of Their Stress-Reducing Activity. *Occupational Therapy in Mental Health, 31,* 83–100.

Prior, S., Maciver, D., Forsyth, K., Walsh, M., Meiklejohn, A., & Irvine, L. (2013). Readiness for employment: Perceptions of mental health service users. *Community Mental Health Journal, 49,* 658–667.

Pyysiäinen, J., Halpin, D., & Guilfoyle, A. (2017). Neoliberal governance and 'responsibilization' of agents: Reassessing the mechanisms of responsibility-shift in neoliberal discursive environments. *Distinktion, 18*(2), 215–235. https://doi.org/10.1080/1600910X.2017.1331858.

Ramon, S. (2005). Approaches to risk in mental health: A multidisciplinary discourse. In J. Tew (Ed.), *Social Perspectives in Mental Health. Developing Social Models to Understand and Work with Mental Distress.* London: Jessica Kingsley.

Razzaque, R., & Stockmann, T. (2016). An introduction to peer-supported open dialogue in mental healthcare. *BJPsych Advances, 22,* 348–356. https://doi.org/10.1192/apt.bp.115.015230.

Recovery in the Bin (RitB). (2019a). *Positivity, Terrorism, & Neorecovery.* Available at https://recoveryinthebin.org/2019/08/08/positivity-terrorism-neorecovery/.

Recovery in the Bin (RitB). (2019b). *20 Key Principles of recovery.* Available at https://web.archive.org/web/20170612062252/https://recoveryinthebin.org/recovery-in-the-bin-19-principless/.

Rossi, A., Amore, M., Galderisi, S., et al. (2018). The complex relationship between self-reported 'personal recovery' and clinical recovery in schizophrenia. *Schizophrenia Research, 192,* 108–112.

Royal College of Occupational Therapists (RCOT). Occupational Therapy and Primary Care. Removing the Barriers to Participation. Available at https://www.rcot.co.uk/sites/default/files/OT%20and%20Primary%20Care_A5%20ENG.pdf.

Roy, A., & Buchanan, J. (2016). The paradoxes of recovery policy: Exploring the impact of austerity and responsibilisation for the citizenship claims of people with drug problems. *Social Policy & Administration, 50*(3), 398–413.

Seikkula, J., Aaltonen, J., Alakare, B., Haarakangas, K., Keränen, J., & Lehtinen, K. (2006). Five-year experience of first-episode nonaffective psychosis in open-dialogue approach: Treatment principles, follow-up outcomes, and two case studies. *Psychotherapy Research, 16*(2), 214–228.

Seikkula, J., Birgitta Alakare, B., & Aaltonen, J. (2011). The comprehensive open-dialogue approach in Western Lapland: II. Long-term stability of acute psychosis outcomes in advanced community care. *Psychosis, 3*(3), 192–204.

Seligman, M. (1990). *Learned Optimism: How to Change Your Mind and Your Life.* New York: Free Press.

Simpson, A., Hannigan, B., Coffey, M., Jones, A., et al. (2016). Cross-national comparative mixed-methods case study of recovery-focused mental health care planning and co-ordination: Collaborative care planning project (COCAPP). *Health and Social Care Delivery Research, 4*(5). https://doi.org/10.3310/hsdr04050.

Taylor, K., Fletcher, I., & Lobban, F. (2015). Exploring the links between the phenomenology of creativity and bipolar disorder. *Journal of Affective Disorders, 174,* 658–664.

Tew, J. (2005). Core themes of social perspectives. In J. Tew (Ed.), *Social Perspectives in Mental Health. Developing Social Models to Understand and Work with Mental Distress*. London: Jessica Kingsley.

Thaler, R., & Susstein, C. (2009). *Nudge: Improving Decisions about health, Wealth and Happiness*. Caravan Books.

Thomas, P. (2016). Psycho politics, neoliberal governmentality and austerity. *Self Soc, 44*(4), 382–393.

Townsend, E. (1996). Enabling empowerment: Using simulations versus real occupations. *Canadian Journal of Occupational Therapy, 63*(2), 114–128.

Turner-Crowson, J., & Wallcraft, J. (2002). The recovery vision for mental health services and research: A British perspective. *Psychiatric Rehabilitation Journal, 25*(3), 245–254.

UK Government, 2019. Available at: https://www.gov.uk/government/organisations/behavioural-insights-team

United Nations (UN). (2006). *United Convention on the Rights of Persons with Disabilities and its Optional Protocol*. New York: United Nations.

Wallcraft, J. (2005). Recovery from mental breakdown. In J. Tew (Ed.), *Social Perspectives in Mental Health*. London: Jessica Kingsley Publishers pp. 200–2015.

Watts, J. (2018). *No Wonder People on benefits live in Fear. Supermarkets Spy on Them Now*. Available at https://www.theguardian.com/commentisfree/2018/may/31/benefits-claimants-fear-supermarkets-spy-poor-disabled.

Watts, B., Fitzpatrick, S., Bramley, S., & Watkins, D. (2014). *Welfare Conditionality: Sanctions, Support and Behaviour Change*. Available at https://www.jrf.org.uk/sites/default/files/jrf/migrated/files/Welfare-conditionality-UK-Summary.pdf.

Weisberg, R. W. (1994). Genius and madness? A quasi-experimental test of the hypothesis that manic-depression increases creativity. *Psychological Science, 5*(6), 361–367.

Wilcock, A. (2006). *An Occupational Perspective of health*. NJ: Thorofare: Slack Inc.

Woods, A., Hart, A., & Spandler, H. (2019). The recovery narrative: Politics and possibilities of a genre. *Culture Medicine and Psychiatry*. Available at: https://link.springer.com/content/pdf/10.1007%2Fs11013-019-09623-y.pdf.

11 TEACHING AND LEARNING

REBECCA LICORISH ■ WENDY BRYANT ■ JESSICA LING ■ ESTE LOUW

INTRODUCTION

Students prepare to become occupational therapists in multiple ways, with professional and educational requirements and standards shaping their experience. These requirements and standards evolve in response to changing priorities in higher education and practice. Most education programmes take place in universities, the term used in this chapter to describe where programmes are based. To use the protected title of occupational therapist, graduates need to register with a regulatory body, so pre-registration programmes are the focus of this chapter. Pre-registration programmes last two, three, or four years, integrating 1000 hours of placement education including a mental health setting (Rowan and Alsop 2016). The people who design and deliver pre-registration programmes are described as educators, with a distinction, where required, between placement educators and academics.

Teaching and learning are distinct experiences. The former involves facilitating the engagement of others with new knowledge, understanding and skills; the latter involves being transformed by this knowledge, understanding and skills (DeIuliis 2017). Often students learn and educators teach, but effective education is based on educators being open to learning from students (Barnett 2007). Students meanwhile are required to give voice to their learning like a teacher, writing, preparing and giving presentations and providing feedback to each other (Wellard and Edwards 1999; Barnett 2007).

Education is distinct from therapy. While both involve facilitating and enabling people to meet their occupational goals, in education, the goal of becoming a health professional is not negotiable unlike in therapy in which goals are negotiated (see Chapter 6). Educators and students analyse barriers to achieving the goal, identifying possible solutions which are enacted independently by the student or with support from other staff teams. Becoming a practice educator or an academic involves learning about university resources and requirements: the culture, structures and processes can be alien to a new educator despite their expertise as a practitioner. Change is a theme at every stage: including changes in understanding through learning, changing lives through occupational therapy and contextual changes in teams, services, and organizations.

This chapter is written for students, practice educators, and academics, so the context is explored initially before theories about teaching and learning are introduced. An overview of how effectiveness is appraised and measured is followed by specific considerations of how to prepare to be a mental health professional. Relevant future issues are discussed at the end of the chapter.

CONTEXT FOR TEACHING AND LEARNING

From changing identities to the intricate challenges of curriculum design, the context influences and is influenced by students and stakeholders.

Student Identities

Being a student is a socially constructed identity that involves particular expectations of behaviour such as working hard and staying out late to go to parties. The demands of an occupational therapy programme are not always congruent with this sense of being a student, especially during practice placements. This means that different student identities are noticeable at different times and places, known as 'identity salience' (Brenner et al. 2014). For example, Higgs and Hunt (1999) suggested that students could be identified as apprentices, professionals, problem-solvers, or technicians. Five contemporary identities are suggested below.

Consumers

Many students commit to tuition fees and formal assessment of their performance and so are identified as consumers or units in educational bureaucracy (Adie et al. 2018; Bentley 2019).

Agents

Students can be active agents in their own learning (Adie et al. 2018; Walsh and Pollard 2020).

Diverse Individuals

When education is seen as a human right, inclusion is addressed in terms of 'access, participation and achievement' (Hoffman et al. 2018, p. 2). Improving access and supporting participation enable students to achieve their goals. Sometimes students have to emphasize one identity over another because of lack of awareness about intersectionality, for example, seeking support for dyslexia rather than issues with depression (Miller 2018; see Chapter 12). However, students on health professional courses are often motivated by direct experience of health issues and also more likely to disclose this (Bentley 2019; McKenzie et al. 2020).

Activists and advocates:

Students can be instrumental in changing services, reflecting the different ways occupational therapists act as activists and advocates (Doel and Shardlow 2016; Bryant et al. 2019). A desire to improve people's lives can often be a motivation for starting a career as a mental health professional (McKenzie et al. 2020), developed by studying political competence (Walsh and Pollard 2020).

Emerging mental health professionals:

Gaining professional knowledge, skills and understanding of occupation and mental health develops professional identity as an occupational therapist (see

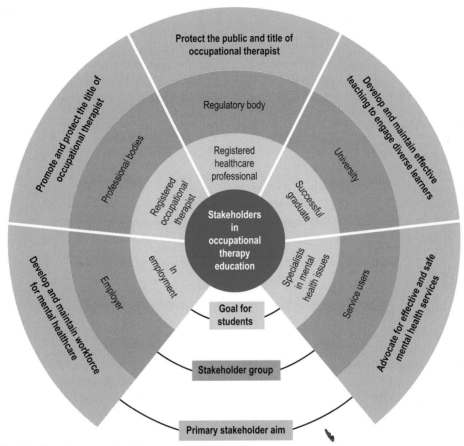

Fig. 11.1 ■ Stakeholders in occupational therapy education.

Chapter 3). One particular challenge is interprofessional education as students are initially focused on developing understanding of their own profession and find it difficult to appreciate the nuances of being a team member (Kent et al. 2020).

These and other identities influence preparations for practice. While the complex nature of working with people and their mental health problems is not always appreciated at the start, students anticipate the challenge and are keen to learn strategies to avoid burnout (McCombie and Antanavage 2017; Tétreault et al. 2020). However, students' priorities may not always align with those of stakeholders.

Stakeholders

The purpose of stakeholders is to monitor pre-registration programmes, ensuring that they adhere

to agreed standards and priorities (Shardlow and Doel 2016). Between them, they cover practice, research, and education (Craik 1995). In the United Kingdom the power and influence of different stakeholders varies. Elsewhere, there may be differences in how the stakeholders are grouped, their goals for students and their aims.

The stakeholder groups are identified in Fig. 11.1, working outwards in three layers:

- goal, what the stakeholders want for students,
- stakeholder group,
- primary stakeholder aim (how their work is directed so students achieve the goal).

The stakeholders with responsibilities for monitoring pre-registration programmes are the professional bodies, regulatory body, and university. They are influenced by the two other groups, employers and service users. Leaders of occupational therapy pre-registration programmes therefore work in multiple partnerships to address the aims of the stakeholders, which do not always align completely. The role that each stakeholder plays is explained below, starting with the employers' goal for students to become employees.

Employee in Workforce

Employers influence the structure and content of pre-registration programmes because they aim to develop and maintain the workforce for their service. They have a particular role to play in providing placement education. Practice educators represent their employers as stakeholders, an important role that has to be balanced with the demands of their job. Hosting a placement requires the careful organization of resources including time and space, which are usually shared and limited in multidisciplinary settings (Rowan and Alsop 2016). In England pre-registration education is currently expanding to include apprenticeships in which students are employed throughout their degree, so these employers are more formally linked with universities than others (Royal College of Occupational Therapists (RCOT) 2019b).

Registered Occupational Therapist

Professional bodies promote occupational therapy and protect the interests of members, providing resources to support practice and research. The World Federation of Occupational Therapists (WFOT) provides minimum standards for occupational therapy education (WFOT 2016), forming the basis for national guidelines (Occupational Therapy Council of Australia 2018; Health Professions Council of South Africa 2019; RCOT 2019a).

Registered Health Professional

A regulatory body, such as the Health and Care Professions Council (HCPC) in the United Kingdom, registers students as occupational therapists on graduation (HCPC 2018a). The HCPC protects the public by monitoring whether people claiming to be occupational therapists have the correct qualifications and are engaged in continuing professional development. It has the disciplinary power to remove registration for malpractice (see Chapter 7).

Successful Graduate

Leaders of occupational therapy programmes maintain and develop their courses aligning with university initiatives to recruit, retain, and successfully support students to employment. In the United Kingdom there is a national group of university leaders of health professional programmes, the Council of Deans, which influences national policy and funding decisions (Council of Deans 2021). All occupational therapy academic educators are required to obtain a postgraduate teaching qualification, which, in the United Kingdom, is accredited by an independent national body, Advance HE (Advance HE 2020). Placement educators are also required to complete local courses (Rowan and Alsop 2016). Awareness of effective teaching approaches is also part of widening participation.

Specialist in Mental Health Issues

The effectiveness and safety of mental health services is dependent on mental health professionals. Service users are valued as stakeholders because of their direct experience of services and shared understanding. In the United Kingdom pre-registration programmes have arrangements such as service user advisory panels to meet the requirements of the HCPC, the regulatory body (HCPC 2018b).

There are advantages and disadvantages of seeing students, educators and stakeholders as different systems involved in pre-registration education. One disadvantage is that in trying to define and solve a problem, pinpointing one of the systems could exclude others. For example, valuing students as agents in their own learning might fall short if their understanding of mental health work is focused on diagnosis and treatment. Mapping relevant resources and influences of different stakeholders is central to curriculum design.

Curriculum Design

The details of a programme are brought together in a curriculum covering 'the learning outcomes, educational methods and assessments for each component' (RCOT 2019a, p. 10). Often a curriculum is designed and reviewed by the team delivering it, although in places where occupational therapy is not established, a national curriculum may be used (Opoku et al. 2021). Fig. 11.2 shows a basic design structure.

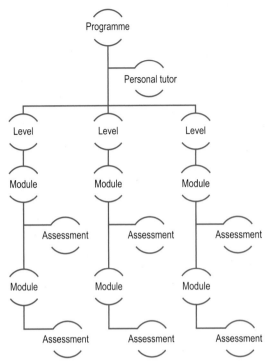

Fig. 11.2 ▥ Curriculum structure.

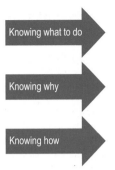

Fig. 11.3 ▥ Bringing knowledge and practice together.

When pre-registration programmes are designed locally the terminology for each component of Fig. 11.2 is different. For example, a module might be called a course or a study block. Levels may be seen as years or cohorts. However, all programmes will have a hierarchy of components and defined developmental stages or levels. Progress through the levels is sometimes described as spiral or scaffolded learning (Dadswell et al. 2021).

Designing, delivering, monitoring and reviewing a programme therefore involves many different components. In the review process questions are often raised about specific areas of practice. Sometimes there is anxiety that students do not know techniques for a setting. These concerns are often about knowing what to do and how to do it. However, pre-registration education is also concerned with knowing why something needs to be done, as shown in Fig. 11.3.

Occupational therapy education brings knowledge and practice together, learning by simultaneously advancing knowledge (what), deepening understanding (why) and acquiring professional approaches and skills (how) in what is sometimes known as a spiral curriculum (Dadswell et al. 2021). This is in contrast to programmes in which professional skills are not required such as an undergraduate psychology degree.

Table 11.1 brings Figs. 11.2 and 11.3 together to show how the different components of a curriculum might be designed to enable an occupational therapy student, Gloria, to learn about group work, mental health and occupational therapy. In Table 11.1 the curriculum structure forms a matrix with knowing what, why and how.

Learning Outcomes

A curriculum design has learning outcomes for programmes, modules and sessions. In self-directed learning, students create their own learning outcomes, mirroring goal-setting in practice (Rowan and Alsop 2016; see Chapter 4). Writing learning outcomes involves analytical thinking and creativity, allowing some ambiguity so that learning can take place. Highly detailed learning outcomes can limit scope for development of individuals and the curriculum itself (Barnett 2007).

While many students may be concerned with how well they achieve learning outcomes, educators are often concerned with enabling all students to meet the required standard to pass, where their work will be judged against the learning outcomes. Judgement occurs in peer groups as much as anywhere else, so as part of understanding how to achieve learning outcomes, it can be helpful to explore students' awareness of their 'mutual obligations' (Barnett 2007, p. 81) in terms of what they contribute and how they respond to others.

The Curriculum Review Cycle

There are continuous cycles of review in pre-registration education to enable development, reflection and

		TABLE 11.1	
	Gloria Learns about Group Work, Mental Health and Occupational Therapy		
	Knowing What	Knowing Why	Knowing How
Programme	Gloria learns throughout the programme that occupational therapy takes place with families, groups and communities who face issues with their mental health.	She understands that because social occupations are key to mental health, survival and well-being, groups can therefore be a valuable therapeutic modality (see Chapters 2 and 6).	She knows how to use the occupational therapy process to structure her practice in a wide range of settings (see Chapter 4).
Personal tutoring	At the end of a tiring term Gloria learns that challenging experiences with her peer student groups are partly due to ongoing group dynamics (see Chapter 15).	She understands that group dynamics can be addressed to facilitate participation when motivation is low and conflicts are occurring (see Chapter 15).	She knows how to share her reflections with her personal tutor, acknowledging her feelings and using the tutorial as a form of practice supervision (see Chapter 7).
Level	Midway, Gloria learns that therapeutic groups can be designed to address performance components such as making choices (Creek 2010).	She understands that groups become therapeutic with professional reasoning, analysing what happens and why some responses are more effective than others (see Chapters 3 and 15).	She knows how to write a group protocol and understands how to put the protocol into practice with therapeutic use of self (see Chapters 3 and 15).
Module	In Gloria's penultimate practice placement with people recovering from severe mental health problems, she learns that groups require effective leadership to function.	She understands why leadership is critical for protecting a group's boundaries, to keep it focused on the therapeutic aims (see Chapter 15).	She learns how to colead a short term closed group, experiencing increasing professional artistry as her placement progresses (see Chapter 3).
Assessment	In her final assessment, which includes a literature review, Gloria learns that there is limited evidence for the benefits of mindfulness as a group intervention in community mental health occupational therapy.	She understands why evidence might be limited for specific contexts even when systematic searching skills are used to find and analyse published research (see Chapter 4).	She knows how to conduct and write up a literature review of the evidence for an occupational therapy group intervention.

planning. Fig. 11.4 indicates the main points of the curriculum review cycle. Each point involves formal processes, including gathering feedback and other data, written reports and routine meetings with formal agenda.

Approval events involve a series of formal meetings that take place before a new programme is launched or when a curriculum is significantly changed. The new curriculum and the resources for teaching/learning are reviewed in a rigorous process (Schaber and Candler 2020):

- The regulatory body approves a programme if it is designed to educate occupational therapists who will adhere to professional standards and practice safely and effectively.

- The professional body accredits a programme if it meets the minimum standards set by the WFOT (2016).
- The host education institution validates the programme if it is designed according to institutional requirements, with appropriate use of institutional resources.

Other stakeholders and students give feedback on the new curriculum as required. However, minor curriculum developments are often prompted by informal and formal module reviews.

Module reviews involve students who complete formal evaluations. Informal feedback to academics is helpful, for example, for adjusting content during a

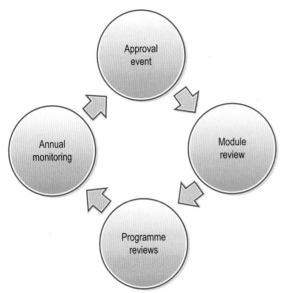

Fig. 11.4 ■ Curriculum review cycle.

Progress	• Through levels, teaching process • Bloom
Act	• To learn through experience • Dewey
Respect	• Students as people with many parts • Maslow, rogers
Reflect	• In cycles of learning • Kolb
Together	• Collaborating with peers • Vygotsky

Fig. 11.5 ■ Theorists influencing occupational therapy pedagogy.

module, signposting students to other resources and informing annual module reports, which then inform programme reviews.

Programme reviews and *annual monitoring* occur regularly with set agenda items, ensuring that there is continuous monitoring of the standards set at the approval event. The programme is also reviewed in examination boards, meetings with stakeholders, student evaluations on graduation, student-staff liaison meetings and teaching team meetings.

TEACHING AND LEARNING

Occupational therapy teaching and learning is informed by pedagogical knowledge (Mitcham 2014). Pedagogy is defined by DeIuliis (2017, p. 111) as the 'art, science and craft of teaching.' The pedagogy for occupational therapy has been influenced by various theorists, shown in Fig. 11.5, which draws on DeIuliis (2017).

These influences suggest how some types of knowledge are privileged over other ways of knowing about the world (see Chapter 2). For example, if a student believes that learning is mainly about gaining knowledge and memorizing facts, they will not recognize the value of reflection or collaboration, thus delaying

their professional development (Bonsaksen 2018). With awareness of other ways of knowing, students are socialised into the cultures of occupational therapy and higher education. These cultures recognize diverse knowledge about people, health and well-being, which might be historic and drawn from other disciplines. For example, Carper (1978) proposed that there are four different types of knowledge in nursing:

- empiric knowledge: of the scientific method, the facts and figures;
- ethical knowledge: of professional and legal obligations;
- personal knowledge: from a person's own narrative, their lived experience and culture;
- aesthetic knowledge: using tacit knowledge or intuition.

Chinn and Kramer (2008) added emancipatory knowledge of social and political understandings of health and well-being (see Chapters 2, 4 and 12). These types of knowledge influence design and reviews, pedagogical approaches, and discussions to orientate stakeholders and students. In this section three main components of teaching and learning are discussed: signature pedagogies, occupation as a threshold concept and transformation.

Signature Pedagogies

To understand how a profession teaches its future practitioners the concept of signature pedagogies has been developed by Shulman (2005), an educational psychologist. This concept has been taken up by professions including law (Bryant and Milstein 2007), medicine (Sullivan et al. 2007), social work (Wayne et al. 2010), and nursing (Crookes et al. 2019). A signature pedagogy guides the student on how to think, perform, and feel like a professional (Schaber and Candler 2020).

Schaber et al. (2012) reviewed past and current approaches to teaching occupational therapy and proposed a signature pedagogy framework. This brings together three established approaches: relational learning, affective learning and active contextualized learning.

Relational learning occurs through interacting with others. The student learns from observing their peers, placement educators, other team members and academics, attending to their interactions, values, attitudes and reasoning (DeIuliis 2017). In the COVID-19 pandemic, rapid adaptation ensured opportunities for relational learning were accessible, despite some limitations of e-learning (Gomez 2020).

Affective learning relates to the transformation of the student's personal and professional identities. Students are immersed into the culture of the educational programme and, through this, develop their professional values, attitudes and beliefs.

Active contextualized learning is a combination of 'learning-by doing' and place-based learning (Schaber et al. 2012, p. 188). The focus is on developing a professional for the broad contexts in which they might practice.

These aspects of the signature pedagogy align well with the occupational therapy ethos which is focused on occupation. Active contextualized learning has been used long before the formalization of occupational therapy education (Alsop 2006).

In Box 11.1 teaching strategies and signature pedagogies are linked together with examples. Some teaching strategies extend across the three categories. Problem-based, or enquiry-based, learning is widely used and follows a structure in which a group of students are given a topic to investigate, presenting their findings together (Alsop 2006; Abdullah et al. 2019).

> ### BOX 11.1
> ### TEACHING STRATEGIES FOR SIGNATURE PEDAGOGIES
>
> *Relational learning focused on interactions with others through:*
>
> - student/educator relationships mirroring the person/therapist relationship in lectures, seminars, personal tutoring, supervision of research/project/placement (Rowan and Alsop 2016);
> - narratives involving practitioners and people with direct experience of occupational therapy in their recovery and treatment;
> - interprofessional learning (Shardlow and Doel 2016).
>
> *Affective learning, developing professional values, attitudes and beliefs through:*
>
> - formal assessment of students' work, including direct feedback on performance and echoing the occupational therapy process;
> - interprofessional learning to compare values and attitudes with other health professionals, shaping identities (Rowan and Alsop 2016; Shardlow and Doel 2016);
> - guest speakers engaging students in emotional aspects of healthcare with detailed current accounts of practice both as therapists providing services and as people receiving them.
>
> *Active contextualized learning, through learning by doing and place-based learning in:*
>
> - workshops and group work, including simulation and problem-based, or enquiry-based, learning (Abdullah et al. 2019);
> - practice placements and real-world projects;
> - varied modes of delivery – online, hybrid, blended, web platforms, synchronous and asynchronous (Deluliis 2017).

They learn how to work together (relational learning), manage their feelings about the highs and lows of self-directed learning (affective learning) and address a problem or topic which is directly relevant to practising occupational therapy (active contextualized learning). All these elements of the signature pedagogy reflect occupational therapy in practice (Jensen et al. 2013; Krishnagiri et al. 2019).

Abrupt increases in student numbers and other changes can adversely impact on student access to appropriate learning opportunities, especially relational and active-contextualized learning (O'Brien et al. 2019). For example, a reduction in human connection could threaten the development of compassion and empathy (Jensen et al. 2013). Therefore stakeholders such as professional bodies carefully monitor student:staff ratios in annual monitoring. A signature pedagogy ensures a programme has relevant approaches to teaching and learning. The threshold concept ensures the programme content is relevant.

Occupation as a Threshold Concept

A threshold is a doorway or opening into a space and, as a metaphor, is a significant place to cross (Collins English Dictionary 2021). All academic disciplines engage in redefining and reviewing their threshold concepts. Occupation is considered the main threshold concept for occupational therapists, although Berg et al. (2019) suggest social determinants of health could be one, too. Students learn a threshold concept as a basis for understanding subsequent programme content (Sadlo 2016). For example, Mitcham (2014) suggests that learning about occupation is about 'seeing through an occupational lens,' then 'listening through occupational ears' and finally 'reasoning through our occupational mind' (Mitcham 2014, p. 642).

An occupation-centred curriculum tends to emphasize the links between occupation, health and wellbeing, rather than defining occupation as a concept or construct (see Chapter 2). This emphasis reflects the interests of occupational therapists as practitioners, scholars and researchers, rather than students studying it for the first time (Howarth et al. 2018). Hooper et al. (2020) suggest three aspects to teaching occupation: subconcepts of occupation, reasoning and professional identity. These aspects filter throughout a programme:

- experiencing occupation-based workshops followed by reflection;
- seminar discussions on theoretical publications;
- using practice frameworks applied to cases in problem-based, or enquiry-based, learning;
- observing someone's occupation on placement; and
- conducting interviews about occupation with other students.

However, occupation may not be always explicitly mentioned, leaving the student to make the connection for example, in understanding the link between housing as an essential space for occupational performance, case management and community mental health (Krishnagiri et al. 2019).

Occupation as a threshold concept can be introduced to the student in a staged way (Price et al. 2017):

1. occupation as a way of seeing the self,
2. occupation as a way of seeing others,
3. occupation as a way of seeing the profession.

These stages could form the basis of learning not just for practice, but also for life (Howarth et al. 2018). After exploring the self as an occupational being (Wilcock 1993; Clark 1997), students learn about the difference between occupation in theory and therapeutic occupation (Hinojosa 2017). Table 11.2 illustrates this using the different ways of thinking about theory introduced in Chapter 2 and referring to other chapters in which these perspectives are explored in more depth.

Transformation

The occupational therapists and students in Table 11.2 changed their practice based on how they thought about occupation. These changes are characteristic of the ongoing transformation associated with continuing professional development. A student commits to being transformed into a mental health professional, knowing there might be challenges and setbacks (Barnett 2007). Transformative learning describes the 'changes in attitudes, beliefs and values' (DeIuliis 2017, p. 117) of educators and students. Box 11.2 offers an example of transformation being considered in curriculum design.

A common experience in transformative and affective learning is having strong feelings, because changes can occur when engaging with uncomfortable areas of learning. For example, when expectations are challenged by real world realities or unexpected barriers arise in service learning or role-emerging placements (Clarke et al. 2015; Naidoo et al. 2019). Grenier et al. (2020) link transformative learning with a constructivist pedagogy in which students and educators shift their worldviews together by constructing new critical understandings of knowledge.

TABLE 11.2		
Perspectives on Occupation and Becoming an Occupational Therapist		
Worldview	This way of seeing the world is focused on occupation and its impact on well-being, health and survival.	See Chapters 2–4
Sam had studied psychology as an undergraduate, which influenced her worldview. She focused on cognitive and emotional aspects of her life and the people she encountered. In her second practice placement, which was with an assertive outreach team, she realized the significance of occupation as her new worldview. She wanted to learn more about how occupation-centred encounters with service users could be understood. She reflected on herself as an occupational being to understand more.		See Chapters 2, 3 and 22
Frames of reference	For understanding aspects of occupation, for example, sensory processing.	See Chapters 2 and 4
When Rob started working with a community team for people diagnosed with personality disorders, he learned about trauma-informed care. This was an important frame of reference for the team, but he found himself wondering about a frame of reference on citizenship to refocus occupational therapy on social inclusion. As a placement educator he supported a student to develop an in-service project exploring this perspective in practice.		See Chapters 4 and 12
Constructs	Categorizing and organizing structures to understand occupation and focus therapy, for example, Chapter 3 Being a therapist, Chapter 4 Structuring practice, Chapter 5 Assessment and outcome measurement and Chapters 13–20 covering specific occupations.	See Chapters 2–5 and 13–20
For an assignment, Toni reflected on their first placement with a horticultural therapy organization. They realized how therapeutic occupation could be distinguished from a passive appreciation of nature by analysing and adapting the forms, functions and meanings of horticultural occupations. It became clearer how to explain occupational therapy in this context.		See Chapters 2, 3 and 19
Concepts	Defining occupation as the grounds for practice and distinguishing it from other associated concepts such as behaviour, activity, task and skill.	See Chapters 2 and 3
Sophie had much experience leading people in activities: from youth groups and school. She was really good at enthusing people with her passion for arts and crafts. However, when she started covering a post with a community intellectual disabilities team, she had to rethink how she defined occupation and what it could mean for the people she was working with.		See Chapter 25

Formal assessment of their performance can provoke strong feelings in students, especially when learning to develop and communicate critical perspectives. Barnett (2007) suggested that critical pedagogy was much more than thinking, describing how educator and student are open and prepared to 'venture forward into unknown and probably discomforting frames' (p. 158). Occupational therapy is exciting to explore at the start of a programme. However, a student might feel overwhelmed when new ideas and perspectives have to be judged against standards (Barnett 2007). Understanding that self-doubt is part of being transformed into an occupational therapist can be supported by developing reflective practice.

Reflective Practice

Reflective practice is a professional expectation (see Chapter 3), and reflection is a stage in Kolb's cycle of learning (DeIuliis 2017). Students engage with their experiences and different ways of knowing by reflecting in varied ways, often by using one of many reflective models. For example, Johns' model which signposts Carper's types of knowledge previously discussed (Carper 1978; Johns 2017). Models offer structure

BOX 11.2
TRANSFORMATION AND CURRICULUM DESIGN

Placement modules were redesigned and given new titles in an overhaul of MSc and BSc pre-registration programmes. These titles were designed to convey expectations about what students do on placement at each stage of their transformation into occupational therapists:

Explore: learning-by-doing and enquiry-based learning;

Initiate: considering and justifying when, where, how and with whom to act;

Lead: acting independently in various aspects of practice;

Manage: strengthening professional identity through self-management.

but do not necessarily indicate what to reflect on or what makes a good reflection, provoking uncertainty in students when asked to present their reflections for assessment. Uncertainty can be addressed with clarity about the context and what the reflection is on or for. For example, reflections can be shared for assessment of understanding, to review placement experiences or to gather thoughts to underpin professional reasoning (see Chapter 3). The authenticity of a reflection can be hard to gauge if the context and purpose is not understood.

Authenticity

Authenticity in teaching and learning is about genuine, reliable and accurate experiences (Collins English Dictionary 2021). Hooper et al. (2020, p. 121) suggest that authentic learning experiences are evident in these situations:

- clearly meant to be a learning situation,
- students apply 'content and the thinking process they learned in one situation to apply to novel situations,'
- students take multiple perspectives,
- students reflect during and after on how they used core knowledge.

These aspects are particularly relevant to placement education. Students value being able to observe professionals at work, discussing their career aspirations, doing authentic routine and interesting tasks,

working autonomously, being able to practise, and get feedback and engaging in supervision to overcome doubts (Jackson 2019). Barnett (2007), a philosopher, suggested that students are transformed into authentic versions of what they want to be. In the process, educators and students voice their ideas in different ways. Those listening judge the authenticity of what they are saying: does it reflect their understanding or are they voicing what they have heard from others? Authenticity is also a useful quality in considering whether the expectations of both students and educators are met effectively.

EFFECTIVENESS

Effective occupational therapy programmes enable the majority of students to progress with minimal delay, register as occupational therapists and gain employment on graduation. Therefore effectiveness is indicated by the outcomes. Fig.11.6 suggests ways of considering effectiveness using an example of what influences graduates to choose a mental health setting for their first post. This choice is framed as a question to focus the evaluation (second level of Fig. 11.6), which could have been raised by local employers in a programme committee meeting. Two approaches to evaluating effectives are suggested: appraising and measuring. In Fig. 11.6 the lowest level suggests some sources of data or information for answering the question.

Appraising effectiveness takes a broad approach, considering the context and quality of student experience. In Fig. 11.6 information from programme committee meetings and placement education might reveal that a local mental health service is very involved in different aspects of the programme.

Measuring effectiveness involves collecting data on performance to evaluate how often targets are successfully met. Nationally, data from different education institutions are compared and published in league tables to inform student choice about which course to apply for. In Fig. 11.6 the evaluation might be prompted by the results of a local final year student survey about future employment plans.

There are many ways of considering effectiveness in education, so five main areas are considered here: assessment, expectations, placements, employability and advancing knowledge.

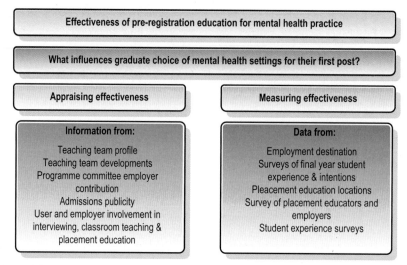

Fig. 11.6 ■ Appraising and measuring effectiveness.

Assessment

Assessment of students is an ongoing process of testing whether standards are being met, which are generally stated as learning outcomes. Educators may provide guidance to students preparing for their assessment by giving feedback on a formative assignment. This assignment is usually a draft form and is like a rehearsal for the summative assessment, which determines how well the student has met the required learning outcomes.

Echoing the varied ways of demonstrating effectiveness in practice, scholarship and research, methods and forms of assessment are used such as:

- group protocols;
- oral presentations;
- essays;
- designing and implementing the occupational therapy process on placement; and
- proposals for funding a new service, service improvement or research investigation of effectiveness, including a review of the relevant evidence.

Examinations in which a student has to give evidence of their learning under time pressure are not used exclusively. Producing evidence under pressure is part of professional practice but can be tested in other more accessible, relevant and inclusive ways.

Expectations

The effectiveness of teaching and learning is indicated by meeting expectations, defined by Golos and Tekuzener (2019, p. 2) 'as a person's beliefs that a certain behaviour or outcome will occur as a result of a specific event.' Students, educators and stakeholders have expectations, for example, that in a teaching team there will be educators with practice experience in mental health settings, evidenced in approval documents and staff profiles. It is helpful to question how realistic expectations are and explore the barriers to achieving them (Patterson et al. 2017; Golos and Tekuzener 2019). Effective ongoing review processes will facilitate dialogue and reflection on mismatched expectations, including results from surveys of student satisfaction.

Formal documents have details of the standards for the core 'values, beliefs, professional attributes, knowledge and skills,' which students are required to meet (RCOT 2019a, p. 4). At the beginning of their programme, students are introduced to codes of ethics and professional practice, which will apply throughout their career (RCOT 2021). Where national associations and regulatory boards have produced them, the terminology used and the order of the content varies, reflecting how the settings and priorities for occupational therapy differ (Singapore Association of Occupational Therapists 2012; Occupational Therapy Board

Australia 2014; American Occupational Therapy Association 2020). For example, working effectively with indigenous people is an expectation in Australia and New Zealand. While recognizing the need for local variations, the WFOT (2016) sets out expectations for what occupational therapist do (tasks) and who they are responsible to (responsibilities).

Placement Education

The effectiveness of placement education can be dependent on the quality of the relationship between universities and providers, so preparations, monitoring and debriefs for students and placement educators are carefully planned (Naidoo et al. 2019; O'Brien et al. 2019). Collaboration between academics and practice educators facilitates student learning about applying theory to practice and developing professional communication skills (Karp 2020). Echoing the requirements for academics, placement educators must have post-graduate practice experience and commit to post-graduate training in placement education (Rowan and Alsop 2016).

One challenge for the effectiveness of placement education is that mental health services are constantly changing, so it can be difficult to keep track and allocate students appropriately. Whereas change is a reality, it is helpful to question whether particular situations are too challenging for a student, distracting from their learning or restricting access to service users who are able to consent to be part of a student's education (Rowan and Alsop 2016). These challenges can be mitigated with skilled supervision (O'Brien et al. 2019).

Employability

Gaining and keeping a job in the first year after graduation is a significant indicator that a university programme is effective, signalling the university's contribution to the economy (Parutis and Howson 2020). Employability is defined as 'a multi-dimensional concept involving a set of skills for preparing graduates for employment' (Williamson et al. 2020, p. 8). The assumption that successful graduates simply have the skills required by employers ignores:

- skills valued by employers depend on the setting and may be generic and/or basic, more easily

> **BOX 11.3**
> **CAPITAL AND EMPLOYABILITY**
>
> Tomlinson's conceptual model (2017) offers different categories of capital, defined as 'key resources that confer benefits and advantages' (p. 339). There are three aspects to capital in education: recognizing different forms, knowing how to gain different forms of capital and how to develop it.
> **Human: 'knowledge, skills and future performance'** (p. 341) – qualifying to register to practice and articulating how general knowledge can be applied in a particular setting.
> **Social: 'networks and human relationships'** (p. 342) – using bridging ties beyond close social networks to find jobs by realizing the potential value of placements, external lecturers and career fairs.
> **Cultural: 'employability and cultural synergy and alignment'** (p. 343) – enabling all students to have insight into what they could do as occupational therapists and what is valued.
> **Identity: 'self-concept and personal narratives'** (p. 345) – reflecting on broader opportunities in the university and community beyond the profession expressed in portfolios.
> **Psychological: 'resilience and career adaptability'** (p. 347) – preparing for inevitable setbacks and disappointments with career, learning from newly qualified therapists as well as more experienced staff.

learned in the work environment (Tomlinson 2017; Hora et al. 2018);
- developing a professional identity involves more than skill acquisition (Jackson 2019);
- students with less direct experience of professional behaviours, for example, because of their age or social class may be disadvantaged in communicating their professional identity (Naidoo et al. 2019; Parutis and Howson 2020).

Tomlinson (2017) suggests that capital might be a better focus than skills for designing opportunities to increase employability (Box 11.3).

Experiences throughout a programme will influence job choice; therefore involvement of employers can encourage students to choose to work with people with mental health issues. Positive experiences in practice placements have a strong influence on influencing work preference (Jackson 2019). There

BOX 11.4
ADVANCING KNOWLEDGE ABOUT
TEACHING DIVERSITY

Grenier et al. (2020) conducted a scoping review of pedagogical approaches and paradigms to teaching diversity
to understand the implications of predominant practices.
They found that:

- few authors stated their position in terms of
  diversity;
- teaching cultural competency risked objectifying
  diverse people as other, alien and neutral;
- teaching social justice risked ignoring structural
  discrimination while focusing on student attitudes;
- addressing the hidden curriculum (policies,
  processes, resources) is a largely unacknowledged
  aspect of teaching diversity.

The review indicated that transformative learning extends beyond acquiring skills such as feeling more competent about diversity, to questioning and changing practices which reveal discriminatory beliefs, thoughts, feelings
and values.

BOX 11.5
TIME TO REFLECT...

During one of the first multidisciplinary team meetings
in an acute psychiatric ward where I started working, a
team member mentioned that the new admission was a
'revolving door client.' Immediately I sighed internally and
thought, 'Oh well, another one of those without hope.' I
caught my thoughts in that moment and realized how I
had already made up my mind regarding how the client
would be treated. Was I really going to give up on him
even before trying just because he had the label 'revolving
door client' attached to him? How would my attitude affect my students' interpretation of this label and the con-
sequent treatment they give to such clients?

are also indications that students who have previous
experience of mental health services are more inclined
to enter mental health practice areas on qualification
(Graessle 1997).

Advancing Knowledge

Pedagogical scholarship and research indicate effectiveness and advance knowledge, which can be shared
widely in publications such as the example in Box 11.4.
A broader perspective on advancing knowledge is in
Chapter 2. A simple example to distinguish between
scholarship and research is that students write scholarly assignments or essays before conducting research
projects. Anyone who studies can be considered a
scholar (Collins English Dictionary 2021). Scholarship
involves a process of investigating and writing about
an idea and exploring and critiquing different perspectives on its application. In contrast, in pre-registration
education, research is a process of generating evidence
for practice, with most students preparing a literature
review, proposal and investigation into a practice issue.
However, scholarly assignments involve many research
skills such as searching for, appraising and synthesizing relevant literature.

Roberts et al. (2020) observed that many published
studies were focused on the student experience despite

the need for more understanding about how to teach
and learn about core concepts such as occupation.
Box 11.4 offers an example of pedagogical scholar-
ship/research which critically questions the students'
experience.

MENTAL HEALTH DISCOURSES

People with mental health problems will be encountered in every practice setting, so in this section mental health is seen as a construct rather than an area of
practice. As a construct, mental health is understood
with many assumptions based on varied and sometimes competing discourses (Rose 2019). A discourse
uses informal and formal aspects of language to guide
understanding of the world and our experiences. For
example, psychiatry has a discourse that guides thinking and speaking about mental health and ill-health
using medical terminology (Rose 2019). Foucault
(1974) suggests that reality is constructed through
discourse; so distinct understandings of mental health
and its context are developed and expressed with specific language (Box 11.5).

When distinct understandings or discourses are
shared, interactions and working relationships are
influenced. The reflection in Box 11.5 considers how
the discourse would influence students' future practice. Dominant discourses are powerful, giving power
to some processes and people and marginalizing others. Students, educators and service users are exposed
to changing and conflicting discourses about mental
health, which have implications for education, practice

and everyday occupation (Rose 2019). Discourses about mental health conflict and inform each other:

- mind-body split vs. holism (Rose 2019);
- biomedicine vs. social determinants (see Chapter 12; Chapman et al. 2020);
- occupation as determinant for health and well-being vs. mental and physical health services (Hooper et al. 2020).

Recovery offers another example of conflicting discourses because there are differences between clinical, functional and personal recovery (Higgins and McGowan 2014; see Chapters 2 and 10). In a recovery service, service users may anticipate relief from symptoms (clinical recovery) whereas staff may be aiming for recovery of social and occupational functioning in a person's life (functional and personal recovery) (Keogh et al. 2014).

While some discourses may be more valued than others in practice by occupational therapists, exploring a range of discourses in pre-registration education will enable students to develop their professional reasoning and identity. For example, when coming in contact with a psychologist offering behavioural activation as a therapy, a student could reflect on their knowledge about frames of reference, therapeutic occupation and mental health to understand what makes occupational therapy different (see Chapter 3-4).

In pre-registration programmes mental health is more likely to be addressed as a theme throughout rather than in designated modules, apart from placements in mental health services (Keady and Thompson 2016; Egan and Cahill 2017; Tyminski et al. 2019). Many people, including students and educators, are aware of how to promote mental health and have experiences of mental health problems. These experiences influence how they engage with the theme of mental health and apply related topics in practice. One of these topics is stigma, which is discussed further in this section because of its significance in discourses about mental health problems.

Stigma

Mental ill-health is stigmatized in most communities (Thornicroft 2006; Pescosolido et al. 2010) and stereotypes can differ vastly between cultures (Bracke et al. 2019). With the stigma of mental ill-health being a dominant discourse, people can experience discrimination in work, family, social, civil and healthcare spheres. This discrimination can create self-stigma and poor outcomes (Thornicroft 2006; Stull et al. 2013). Stigma can come from external (society, culture, institutions) or internal (internalized public stigma) factors. Grappone (2018) identified seven types of stigma experienced by people with mental health problems. Public stigma occurs with discrimination, which often arises from prejudice or negative stereotypes about madness and distress. When people have internalised public stigma, they experience self-stigma. Staff and service users could experience perceived stigma, when they believe that others will be negative about mental health. When people avoid seeking help from services, label avoidance could be occurring. This form of stigma signals how diagnoses and places such as mental health units can be associated with prejudice and stereotypes, negatively labelling the people associated with them. Carers, families and others connected to people with mental health difficulties may experience stigma by association. This can occur in interactions with services especially, because of structural stigma indicated by discriminatory policies or other social practices. Grappone's (2018) seventh form of stigma is associated with health practitioners, who may lack awareness of their discriminatory attitudes to madness and distress. Unless they develop their knowledge and understanding of mental health difficulties and social determinants, they could perpetuate all forms of stigma (see chapter 12).

Implications for Teaching and Learning

Despite increasing awareness, stereotypical representations of mental health and ill-health continue to be prevalent in society, the media and the hidden curriculum (Corrigan 2004; Atanasova et al. 2019; Grenier et al. 2020). When mental ill-health is consistently considered and discussed (Krupa 2008), subtle differences in discourses can be explored. For example, considering the hidden curriculum might reveal the difference between working *with* mental health rather than working *in* mental health or in working with patients, clients or with people with mental health difficulties (see Chapter 2). There could be self-stigma by occupational therapists themselves

(Schulze 2007; Halter 2008) if their knowledge of mental health and ill-health is not viewed as authentic or valuable in some settings. In a pre-registration programme, sustained development of understanding and technical knowledge can enable stigma to be challenged (Waqas et al. 2020).

User Involvement

Stigma can be also addressed by involving people with direct experience of using mental health services in teaching and learning. The opportunities and challenges of user involvement in education reflect the broader context in which collaborative approaches such as coproduction have influenced many initiatives. There is tension between tokenism and authentic participation, as in the United Kingdom user involvement in pre-registration education is required, but approaches and methods are not prescribed (HCPC 2018b; Burke and Newman 2021) (see Chapters 2 and 12). Taking an occupational perspective on user involvement in education and research, Bryant (2021) focused on how to design occupational forms of involvement in a creative and respectful approach, navigating and acknowledging service users' capacities and identities. When considering how to involve users discourses about mental ill-health, risk and vulnerability have to be balanced with discourses about living with mental health problems and what students expect to learn as they develop their professional identity (Arblaster et al. 2015, 2018). As well as sharing their lived experiences and engaging with students in the classroom, service users are interested in shaping curricula (Arblaster et al. 2018).

NAVIGATING IDENTITIES

As well as working out how to involve users in pre-registration education, it is necessary for students and educators to navigate their own identities. At the beginning of this chapter student identities were briefly introduced. Navigating these and other identities is central to being a therapist (see Chapter 3) and a mental health professional. Three aspects are discussed here: disclosure, how identities are navigated and the tension between educator-therapist identities.

Disclosure

Nicola-Richmond et al. (2017) investigated reasons for students failing, which included non-disclosure because of self-stigma. When students choose to disclose direct experiences of mental ill-health or other personal details, their communication will be shaped by discourses about mental health as a construct. Their disclosure may be overshadowed by shame (see Chapter 3). Switching between different identities of professional and service user can be influenced by the power imbalance between these identities (Richards et al. 2016). There is also a danger of self-stigma being targeted for specialist intervention, missing critical discourses about structural social determinants (see Chapter 12). Yet disclosure can also have benefits, such as accessing reasonable adjustments for disabled students (Disability Rights 2021). The Coming Out Proud programme and others provide guidance on how to disclose (Corrigan et al. 2004). Public disclosure can help reduce the perception of stigma as a stressor (Modelli et al. 2021).

Strategies for Navigation

Reflection, different forms of reasoning and therapeutic use of self can guide strategies for navigating different identities and acknowledging self-stigma and other negative impacts of stigma. For example, in responding to the reflection in Box 11.5 in which there are negative attitudes from colleagues, there will be policies about anti-discriminatory practice (procedural reasoning), but considering and discussing the future impact on the person being described as 'revolving door' may be a more powerful discourse (conditional reasoning) (see Chapter 3). If the person reflecting had a close family member who had also been given this label, there would be another dimension to reflection and another identity to navigate. The person's thoughts and actions in this situation might be best guided by therapeutic use of self, working out ways of keeping therapeutic aims at the centre of interactions (see Chapter 3).

Navigating Therapist and Educator Identities

Being a therapist involves setting boundaries on occupational therapy, especially when addressing mental health issues (see Chapter 3). In navigating therapist and educator identities, an educator considers the boundary between therapy and education, especially in response to student distress. Signposting is essential to uphold the boundary as there is a thin line between aiming for the goal of becoming an occupational therapist and strategies to overcome barriers to achieving that. Where the strategies involve psychosocial or other therapeutic techniques, it is better facilitated by someone other than the educator, whether practice educator or personal tutor.

However, some studies report examples of using practice knowledge and skills with students, for example, applying the Goal Attainment Scaling measure to placement evaluations (Chapleau and Harrison 2015), applying an occupational adaptation frame of reference to understand placement failure (Krusen 2015), applying the concept of locus of control to understand student experience (Keptner 2019) and the significance of the relationship between practice educator and student (Rodger et al. 2014).

Emotional Labour

When a student has new experiences, such as hearing a presentation from a service user, thoughts and feelings can make them feel uncomfortable in different ways (Barnett 2007). For some students apprehension about working with people with mental health problems arises because of fears about being exposed to upsetting situations. These situations could be encountering self-harm, suicide, or people who evoke feelings about past losses and traumas. Person-centred practice is an ideal which might have to be compromised when having to restrict choices in the best interest of the person, which also conflicts with discourses about occupation, health and well-being (see Chapter 4). These conflicts and upsets provoke emotional reactions.

Emotional labour takes place when emotions are expressed in a way that is professionally desirable (Oxford Reference 2021), placing responsibility on the students to learn to manage their emotions whilst learning how to recognize and work with the emotions of others (see Chapter 3). A related concept is emotional intelligence, defined by Gribble et al. (2017, p. 9) as the 'need to recognize, understand, and convey emotions' and used in their study to understand the emotional reactions of students who were underperforming.

Working with people with mental health problems can stir difficult feelings, so it is helpful to learn strategies such as self-validation (Dialectical Behaviour Therapy 2021). Including stress management, strategies in teaching and learning can not only help students to manage academic stress (Gura 2010), but they also can be a way to develop the student's capacity for empathy (Kinsella et al. 2016). The necessary anxiety and stress of being a student is distinguished from incapacitating anxiety. This distinction mirrors that in psychiatry between mental distress and mental disorders (Rose 2019).

Professional Practice

Positioning occupation as a threshold concept (see earlier) creates challenges and opportunities for exploring how it relates to mental health and professional practice (Mitcham 2014). If a student appears unprepared for practice, being mindful of discourses about mental health and pedagogical approaches could broaden understanding. It could be that the student or new graduate has not yet had the opportunity to explore what particular practice situations could mean. It might not be obvious to them which professional skills are most relevant.

Professional reasoning can be undermined if skills are separated from the context into generic categories like report writing. Hora et al. (2019) analysed skills for engineers and nurses, observing the tendency to simplify skills into decontextualized competencies such

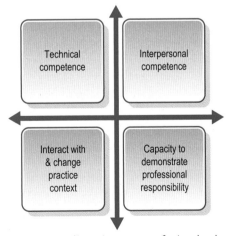

Fig. 11.7 ■ Four dimensions to professional education. (Higgs and Hunt 1999.)

as 'critical thinking, teamwork and communication' (p. 2222). Simplifying communication skills undermines the work done to understand and respond to situations in professional practice. Isolated skills also tend to be associated with 'normal' (Hora et al. 2019, p. 2257), which is especially problematic in mental health discourses, potentially reinforcing stigma and discrimination.

Higgs and Hunt (1999) suggested four dimensions to professional education, as shown in Fig. 11.7. The student becomes grounded in occupation and competent in the occupational therapy process and refined and specialized for mental health practice (see Chapters 2 and 4–6). They develop their interpersonal skills to be able to respond effectively to the particular challenges of working with people experiencing mental distress or disorders (see Chapter 3). With their professional reasoning they can interact and act on their practice setting so that occupational therapy can be beneficial (see Chapters 3 and 6). This is distinguished from other informal uses of occupation in a mental health setting when they demonstrate their professional responsibility (see Chapters 2, 4 and 6). For example, playing cards might be a popular recreational activity that a student develops to promote occupational performance and engagement (see Chapter 2), reporting back to the multidisciplinary team (Higgs and Hunt 1999).

FUTURE DIRECTIONS

Drawing together ideas for the future of occupational therapy education, Mitcham (2014) proposes a conceptual framework based on seeing education as a powerful engine: transmitting, transporting and transforming individuals and society. Locating the engine in a train, she asks what/who is travelling and where is it going? For occupational therapy and mental health, this metaphor suggests there might be students, educators, experts in mental health and all their baggage travelling. The train stops at stations to bring the travellers in contact with mental health issues, people with direct experience, professionals and service settings.

In contrast to pedagogical approaches to occupation, mental health practice requires an interprofessional approach (Shardlow and Doel 2016). In Box 11.6 the concerns and hopes for the future of mental health

---

BOX 11.6
PREPARING FOR WHAT? MENTAL HEALTH PROFESSIONAL ROLES IN THE FUTURE

Rose (2019) investigates the future of mental health professional practice from a sociologist's perspective on psychiatry. In contrast to occupational therapy, psychiatry has still to establish a biopsychosocial approach to mental health. However, there are shared aspects to consider for future practice:

Addressing an apparent epidemic of mental ill-health. While this is often highlighted in mainstream media, Rose argues that it is important to distinguish between distress and disorder (2019). Mental distress is often caused by adverse circumstances which can be addressed directly. Mental disorders require specialist professional interventions. Globally, services for people with mental disorders are under-resourced, placing particular pressures on staff.

Addressing the impact on mental health of neoliberal capitalism. The social and economic determinants for mental health problems affect everyone and so are important to understand.

Diagnosing and treating people. Rose suggests that diagnosis is a problem because definitive signs of mental health problems are difficult to establish, so formulation is a better option (see Chapter 4). However, professional reasoning is essential for creating relationships where formulation can be accurate and implementing interventions effective (see Chapters 3–6). Diagnosis is often a gateway to services, but people do not need one for an occupational therapist to promote their mental health and well-being (Burson et al. 2017).

Evidence-based practice. In relation to medication and other biomedical approaches, Rose is alert to the power of the pharmaceutical industry to fund research, so a critical approach to evidence is important.

Global mental health promotion. Rose suggests it is important to learn from the failures of psychiatry to ground the utopian visions in practice.

Coproduction. The user/survivor moment, according to Rose, is the most important challenge and source of direction for the development of future mental health professionals and services.

---

services are explored using Rose (2019). For students aiming to work in mental health settings, these different ways of seeing the future offer a range of possibilities for developing their professional practice.

Translating the themes in Box 11.6 into a curriculum in the future can be informed by pedagogical research, guided by international and scholarly strategies (Hooper 2016; WFOT 2021). There are challenges for educators with accessing resources to conduct and publish pedagogical research, which is currently dominated by US studies in which few occupational therapists work in mental health services (Broome and Grey 2017; Kemp and Crabtree 2018). Currently there is a focus on student experience, but more investigations into pedagogical approaches are required (Hooper 2016). For example, developing the occupational therapy signature pedagogy could advance knowledge about mental health in curriculum design and delivery (Jensen et al. 2013). Pedagogical research could support innovations in placement education (Patterson et al 2017; Thomas and Penman 2019). Finally, although technological innovation and market-based approaches attract institutional and political attention, there are broader issues to investigate, which could have equal impact on how prepared students are for practice (Barnett 2007). The WFOT strategy for pedagogical research indicates a direction for future investigation (WFOT 2021).

SUMMARY

In this chapter teaching and learning about occupational therapy has been explored with particular reference to mental health. The context for pre-registration education includes mental health in relation to students' direct experiences and motivation for becoming an occupational therapist. Stakeholders include mental health service users who can welcome being involved in curriculum design and programme monitoring as well as teaching. Approaches to teaching and learning are associated with the signature pedagogy and echo approaches to practice, with occupation as a threshold concept forming the base, centre, and focus for being a therapist. As students transform into occupational therapists, they experience challenges which refine and strengthen their professional identity. The effectiveness of this transformative process can be appraised and measured in various ways, including formal assessment, employability, and pedagogical research outcomes.

Effective mental health professional practice is based on awareness of competing discourses, including stigma. Discourses shape personal and professional identities, influencing the actions and thinking of students and educators. Pre-registration education enables successive new generations of students to emerge as occupational therapists and develop occupational therapy as a mental health profession.

QUESTIONS FOR CONSIDERATION

1. Which student identities are most apparent to you in your situation? How and why might they differ in other contexts?
2. Which stakeholder group[s] in Fig. 11.1 has the greatest impact on your current position? Will this change in the future? If so, why?
3. Why is it necessary for the WFOT to set minimum standards for occupational therapy pre-registration education? How are they used?
4. Which aspects of the signature pedagogy for occupational therapy (relational, affective, active contextualized) do you think is most beneficial, influential and/or effective for your learning? See Box 11.1
5. In Box 11.4 what does a scoping review involve? How could the findings of this research inform your approach to education?
6. In Box 11.5 what similar examples have you come across? What effect has it had on your practice and your continuing professional development?
7. Outline the ways in which the different types of stigma occur and how they might be revealed in occupational therapy.
8. Consider the connections between discourses about mental health and your professional and personal identities. How do these connections influence your working relationships with students, educators and colleagues?

REFERENCES

Abdullah, J., Mohd-Isa, W. N., & Samsudin, M. A. (2019). Virtual reality to improve group work skill and self-directed learning in problem-based learning narratives. *Virtual Reality*, 23(4), 461–471.

Adie, L. E., Willis, J., & Van der Kleij, F. M. (2018). Diverse perspectives on student agency in classroom assessment. *Australian Educational Researcher*, 45(1), 1–12.

Advance, H. E. (2020). *Helping HE shape its future*. Available at: https://www.advance-he.ac.uk/about-us.

Alsop, A. (2006). Qualifying as an occupational therapist: An educational journey from ward-based to workplace learning. *British Journal of Occupational Therapy*, 69(10), 442–449. https://doi.org/10.1177/030802260606901002.

American Occupational Therapy Association (AOTA). (2020). *Occupational therapy Code of Ethics*. Available at: https://ajot. aota.org/article.aspx?articleid=2767077.

Arblaster, K., Mackenzie, L., Matthews, L., et al. (2018). Learning from consumers: An eDelphi study of Australian mental health consumers' priorities for recovery-oriented curricula. *Australian Occupational Therapy Journal*, 65(6), 586–597.

Arblaster, K., Mackenzie, L., & Willis, K. (2015). Mental health consumer participation in education: A structured literature review. *Australian Occupational Therapy Journal*, 62(5), 341–362. doi:10.1111/1440-1630.12205.

Atanasova, D., Koteyko, N., Brown, B., & Crawford, P. (2019). Representations of mental health and arts participation in the national and local British press, 2007-2015. *Health*, 23(1), 3–20. https://doi.org/10.1177/1363459317708823.

Barnett, R. (2007). *A Will to Learn. Being a Student in an Age of Uncertainty*. Maidenhead: Open University Press McGraw-Hill Education.

Bentley, A. (2019). A tale of two capitals: A Bourdieusian perspective on counselling in higher education. *British Journal of Guidance & Counselling*, 47(5), 609–618.

Berg, C., Philipp, R., & Taff, S. D. (2019). Critical thinking and transformational learning: Using case studies as narrative frameworks for threshold concepts. *Journal of Occupational Therapy Education*, 3(3). https://doi.org/10.26681/jote.2019.030313.

Bonsaksen, T. (2018). Deep, surface, or both? A study of occupational therapy students' learning concepts. *Occupational Therapy International*, 1–8. https://doi.org/10.1155/2018/3439815.

Bracke, P., Delaruelle, K., & Verhaeghe, M. (2019). Dominant cultural and personal stigma beliefs and the utilization of mental health services: A cross-national comparison. *Frontiers in Sociology*, 4. https://www.frontiersin.org/article/10.3389/fsoc.2019.00040.

Brenner, P. S., Serpe, R. T., & Stryker, S. (2014). The causal ordering of prominence and salience in identity theory: An empirical examination. *Social Psychology Quarterly*, 77(3), 231–252.

Broome, K., & Gray, M. (2017). Benchmarking the research track record and level of appointment of Australian occupational therapy academics. *Australian Occupational Therapy Journal*, 64(5), 400–407. doi:10.1111/1440-1630.12387.

Bryant, W. (2021). Doing more than telling stories. In H. McLaughlin, P. Beresford, C. Cameron, H. Casey, & J. Duffy (Eds.), *The Routledge Handbook of Service User Involvement in Human Services Research and Education*. Abingdon: Routledge.

Bryant, W., Cordingley, K., Adomako, E., & Birken, M. (2019). Making activism a participatory, inclusive and developmental process: A research programme involving mental health service users. *Disability & Society*, 34(7–8), 1264–1288. https://doi.org/10.1080/09687599.2019.1613963.

Bryant, S., & Milstein, E. (2007). Rounds: A 'signature pedagogy' for clinical education? *Social Science Research Network Electronic Journal*. https://doi.org/10.2139/ssrn.1007504.

Burke, B., & Newman, A. (2021). Ethical involvement of service users. In H. McLaughlin, P. Beresford, C. Cameron, H. Casey,

& J. Duffy (Eds.), *The Routledge Handbook of Service User Involvement in Human Services Research and Education*. Abingdon: Routledge.

Burson, K., Fette, C., Orentlicher, M., Precin, P. J., Roush, S. N., & Kannenberg, K. (2017). Mental health promotion, prevention, and intervention in occupational therapy practice. *American Journal of Occupational Therapy*, 71, 1–19.

Carper, B. A. (1978). Fundamental patterns of knowing in nursing. *Advances in Nursing Science*, 1(1), 13–23.

Chapleau, A., & Harrison, J. (2015). Fieldwork I program evaluation of student learning using goal attainment scaling. *American Journal of Occupational Therapy*, 69, 1–8.

Chapman, A., Williams, C., Hannah, J., & Pūras, D. (2020). Reimagining the mental health paradigm for our collective well-being. *Health and Human Rights*, 22(1), 1–6.

Chinn, P. L., & Karmer, M. K. (2008). *Integrated Theory and knowledge Development in Nursing* (7th ed.). St Louis: Mobsy Elsevier.

Clark, F. (1997). Reflections on the human as an occupational being: Biological need, tempo and temporality. *Journal of Occupational Science*, 4(3), 86–92.

Clarke, C., Martin, M., Sadlo, G., & de Visser, R. (2015). 'Facing uncharted waters': Challenges experienced by occupational therapy students undertaking role-emerging placements. *International Journal of Practice-Based Learning in Health and Social Care*, 3(1), 30–45.

Collins English Dictionary, 2021. Available at: https://www.collinsdictionary.com/dictionary/english.

Corrigan, P. W., Markowitz, F. E., & Watson, A. C. (2004). Structural levels of mental illness stigma and discrimination. *Schizophrenia Bulletin*, 30(3), 481–491.

Council of Deans. (2021a). *About*. Available at: https://councilofdeans.org.uk/about/.

Council of Deans. (2021b). *Student Leadership Programme. Home of the #150Leaders*. Available at: https://councilofdeans.org.uk/studentleadership/.

Craik, C. (1995). Stakeholders in the future of occupational therapy. *British Journal of Occupational Therapy*, 58(12), 517–518.

Creek, J. (2010). *The Core Concepts of occupational therapy*. London: Jessica Kingsley.

Crookes, P. A., Else, F. C., & Lewis, P. A. (2020). Signature pedagogies: An integrative review of an emerging concept in nursing education. *Nurse Education Today*, 84, 104206. https://doi.org/10.1016/j.nedt.2019.104206.

Dadswell, R., Williams, B., Bowser, A., & Hughes, F. (2021). A placement replacement module developed through COVID-19: Incorporating spiral learning, case-based learning and simulated pedagogical approaches. *Journal of Occupational Therapy Education*, 5(2).

DeIuliis, E. (2017). *Professionalism across occupational therapy Practice*. Thorofare, NJ: SLACK Incorporated.

Dialectical Behaviour Therapy. (2021). *Self-validation*. Available at: https://dialecticalbehaviortherapy.com/emotion-regulation/self-validation/.

Disability Rights UK. (2021). *Adjustments for Disabled Students.* Available at: https://www.disabilityrightsuk.org/adjustments-disabled-students.

Doel, M., & Shardlow, S. M. (2016). *Educating professionals: Practice learning in health and Social Care.* Abingdon: Routledge.

Egan, B. E., & Cahill, S. M. (2017). National survey to identify mental health topics in entry-level OT and OTA curricula: Implications for occupational therapy education. *Journal of Occupational Therapy Education, 1*(1), 1–14.

Foucault, M. (1974). *The archaeology of knowledge.* London: Tavistock Publications.

Golos, A., & Tekuzener, E. (2019). Perceptions, expectations and satisfaction levels of occupational therapy students prior to and after practice placement and comparison of practice placement models. *BioMed Central Medical Education, 19*(1), 324.

Gomez, INB (2020) Reflections on the role of occupational therapy programmes on the mental health of stakeholders' transition to e-learning during the COVID-19 pandemic, *World Federation of Occupational Therapists Bulletin,* doi:10.1080/14473828.2020.1836791.

Graessle, E. A. (1997). Influences on occupational therapy students' attitudes about mental illness. *Occupational Therapy in Mental Health, 13*(3), 41–61. https://doi.org/10.1300/J004v13n03_03.

Grappone, G. (2018). *The Seven Types of Stigma.* National Alliance on Mental Illness Blogspot. Available at: https://www.nami.org/Blogs/NAMI-Blog/October-2018/Overcoming-Stigma.

Grenier, M.-L., Zafran, H., & Roy, L. (2020). Current landscape of teaching diversity in occupational therapy education: A scoping review. *American Journal of Occupational Therapy, 74*(6), 1–15. https://doi.org/10.5014/ajot.2020.044214.

Gribble, N., Ladyshewsky, R. K., & Parsons, R. (2017). Fluctuations in the emotional intelligence of therapy students during clinical placements: Implication for educators, supervisors, and students. *Journal of Interprofessional Care, 31*(1), 8–17.

Gura, S. T. (2010). Mindfulness in occupational therapy education. *Occupational Therapy in Health Care, 24*(3), 266–273. https://doi.org/10.3109/07380571003770336.

Halter, M. J. (2008). Perceived characteristics of psychiatric nurses: Stigma by association. *Archives of Psychiatric Nursing, 22,* 20–26.

Health and Care Professions Council (HCPC). (2018). *Standards of education and training.* Available at: https://www.hcpc-uk.org/standards/standards-relevant-to-education-and-training/set/.

Health and Care Professions Council (HCPC). (2018). *Service user and carer involvement.* Available at: https://www.hcpc-uk.org/education/resources/education-standards/service-user-and-carer-involvement/.

Health Professions Council of South Africa, 2019. The Minimum Standards for the Education of Occupational Therapists. Available at: https://www.hpcsa.co.za/Uploads/OCP/Policy%20and%20Guidelines/Minimum_Standards_of_OT_Training_Final_22_May_2020.pdf.

Higgins, A., & McGowan, P. (2014). Recovery and the recovery ethos: Challenges and possibilities. In A. Higgins, & S. McDaid (Eds.), *Mental health in Ireland: Policy, practice and Law* (pp. 61–78). Gill & Macmillan.

Higgs, & Hunt. (1999). Rethinking the beginning practitioners: Introducing the 'interactional professional. In J. Higgs, & H. Edwards (Eds.), *Educating Beginning Practitioners: Challenges for health Professional Education.* Oxford: Butterworth-Heinemann.

Hinojosa, J. (2017). How society's philosophy has shaped occupational therapy practice for the past 100 years. *Open Journal of Occupational Therapy, 5*(2).

Hoffman, J., Blessinger, P., & Makhanya, M. (2018). Contexts for Diversity and Gender identities in Higher education: International Perspectives on Equity and Inclusion. In *Innovations in Higher Education Teaching and learning* (1st ed.). Bingley, UK: Emerald Publishing Limited.

Hooper, B. (2016). Broadening the scope and impact of occupational therapy education research by merging two research agendas: A new research agenda matrix. *Open Journal of Occupational Therapy, 4*(3).

Hooper, B., Krishnagiri, S., & Price, P. (2020). The principles of occupation-centred education. In S. Taff, L. Grajo, & B. Hooper (Eds.), *Perspectives on Occupational Therapy Education. Past, Present and Future.* Thorofare, NJ: SLACK Incorporated.

Hora, M. T., Benbow, R. J., & Smolarek, B. B. (2018). Re-thinking soft skills and student employability: A new paradigm for undergraduate education. *Change, 50*(6), 30–37.

Hora, M. T., Smolarek, B. B., Martin, K. N., & Scrivener, L. (2019). Exploring the situated and cultural aspects of communication in the professions: Implications for teaching, student employability, and equity in higher education. *American Educational Research Journal, 56*(6), 2221–2261.

Howarth, J. T., Morris, K., & Cox, D. L. (2018). Challenges of teaching occupation: Introduction of an occupation focused teaching tool. *Journal of Occupational Science, 25*(1), 142–148. https://doi.org/10.1080/14427591.2017.1397535.

Jackson, D. (2019). Students' and their supervisors' evaluations on professional identity in work placements. *Vocations and Learning, 12*(2), 245–266. doi:10.1007/s12186-018-9207-1.

Jensen, G., Peters, C., Pierce, D., Reed, K., & Reed, S. M. (2013). Maturing of the Profession Task group Report to Ad Hoc Committee for future of occupational therapy education. *American Occupational Therapy Association.* Available at: https://www.aota.org/~/media/Corporate/Files/EducationCareers/Educators/Att-5-Maturing-of-the-profession-task-group.PDF.

Johns, C. (2017). *Becoming a Reflective Practitioner.* Hoboken, NJ: Wiley-Blackwell.

Karp, P. (2020). Occupational therapy student readiness for transition to the fieldwork environment: A pilot case study. *Open Journal of Occupational Therapy, 8*(4), 1–14. https://doi.org/10.15453/2168-6408.1719.

Keady, J., & Thompson, R. (2016). The community mental health nurse. In M. Doel, & M. S. Steven (Eds.), *Educating professionals: Practice learning in health and social care.* Abingdon: Routledge.

Kemp, E. L., & Crabtree, J. L. (2018). Differentiating fieldwork settings: Matching student characteristics to demands. *Occupational Therapy in Health Care, 32*(3), 216–229. https://doi.org/10.1080/07380577.2018.1491084.

Kent, F., Glass, S., Courtney, J., Thorpe, J., & Nisbet, G. (2020). Sustainable interprofessional learning on clinical placements: The value of observing others at work. *Journal of Interprofessional Care, 34*(6), 812–818.

Keogh, B., Higgins, A., Devries, J., et al. (2014). 'We have got the tools': Qualitative evaluation of a mental health wellness recovery action planning (WRAP) education programme in Ireland. *Journal of Psychiatric and Mental Health Nursing, 21*, 189–196.

Keptner, K. M. (2019). Relationship between occupational performance measures and adjustment in a sample of university students. *Journal of Occupational Science, 26*(1), 6–17.

Kinsella, E. A., Kirsten, S., Bhanji, S., Shepley, R., Modor, A., & Bertrim, A. (2020). Mindfulness in allied health and social care professional education: A scoping review. *Disability & Rehabilitation, 42*(2), 283–295. https://doi.org/10.1080/09638288.2018.1496150.

Krishnagiri, S., Hooper, B., Price, P., Taff, S. D., & Bilics, A. (2019). A national survey of learning activities and instructional strategies used to teach occupation: Implications for signature pedagogies. *American Journal of Occupational Therapy, 73*(5), 7305205080p7305205081–7305205080p7305205011. https://doi.org/10.5014/ajot.2019.032789.

Krupa, T. (2008). Part of the solution … or part of the problem: Addressing the stigma of mental illness in our midst. *Canadian Journal of Occupational Therapy, 75*(4), 198–207.

Krusen, N. (2015). Student voices following fieldwork failure: A phenomenological inquiry. *International Journal of Practice-based Learning in Health & Social Care, 3*(1), 16–29.

McCombie, R. P., & Antanavage, M. E. (2017). Transitioning from occupational therapy student to practicing occupational therapist: First year of employment. *Occupational Therapy in Health Care, 31*(2), 126–142.

McKenzie, K., Murray, A., Cooper, M., et al. (2020). An exploration of the factors influencing career choice in mental health. *Journal of Clinical Nursing, 29*(19–20), 3764–3773.

Miller, R. A. (2018). Toward intersectional identity perspectives on disability and LGBTQ identities in higher education. *Journal of College Student Development, 59*(3), 327–346.

Mitcham, M. D. (2014). Education as engine. *American Journal of Occupational Therapy, 68*(6), 636–648.

Modelli, A., Candal Setti, V. P., van de Bilt, M. T., Gattaz, W. F., Loch, A. A., & Rössler, W. (2021). Addressing mood disorder diagnosis' stigma with an honest, open, proud (HOP)-based intervention: A randomized controlled trial. *Frontiers in Psychiatry, 10*(11), 582180. https://doi.org/10.3389/fpsyt.2020.582180.

Naidoo, D., van Wyk, J. M., & Dhunpath, R. (2019). Service learning pedagogies to promote student learning in occupational therapy education. *Africa Education Review, 16*(1), 106–124.

Nicola-Richmond, K., Butterworth, B., & Hitch, D. (2017). What factors contribute to failure of fieldwork placement? Perspectives of supervisors and university fieldwork educators. *World Federation of Occupational Therapists Bulletin, 73*(2), 117–124.

O'Brien, A. T., McNeil, K., & Dawson, A. (2019). The student experience of clinical supervision across health disciplines – perspectives and remedies to enhance clinical placement. *Nurse Education in Practice, 34*, 48–55.

Occupational Therapy Board Australia. (2014). *Code of Conduct.* Available at: https://www.occupationaltherapyboard.gov.au/Codes-Guidelines.aspx.

Occupational Therapy Council of Australia Ltd. (2018). *Accreditation Standards for Australian Entry-Level occupational therapy education Programs.* South Perth: Occupational Therapy Council of Australia.

Opoku, E. N., Van Niekerk, L., & Jacobs-Nzuzi Khuabi, L.-A. (2021). Exploring the transition from student to health professional by the first cohort of locally trained occupational therapists in Ghana. *Scandinavian Journal of Occupational Therapy.* https://doi.org/10.1080/11038128.2020.1865448.

Oxford Reference, 2021. Available at: https://www.oxfordreference.com/view/10.1093/oi/authority.20110803095749956

Parutis, V., & Howson, C. K. (2020). Failing to level the playing field: Student discourses on graduate employability. *Research in Post-Compulsory Education, 25*(4), 373–393. https://doi.org/10.1080/13596748.2020.1846312.

Patterson, F., Fleming, J., Marshall, K., & Ninness, N. (2017). Student perspectives of a student-led groups program model of professional practice education in a brain injury rehabilitation unit. *Australian Occupational Therapy Journal, 64*(5), 391–399.

Pescosolido, B. A., Martin, J. K., Long, J. S., Medina, T. R., Phelan, J. C., & Link, B. G. (2010). A disease like any other? A decade of change in public reactions to schizophrenia, depression, and alcohol dependence. *The American Journal of Psychiatry, 167*(11), 1321–1330. https://doi.org/10.1176/appi.ajp.2010.09121743.

Price, P., Hooper, B., Krishnagiri, S., Taff, S. D., & Bilics, A. (2017). A way of seeing: How occupation is portrayed to students when taught as a concept beyond its use in therapy. *American Journal of Occupational Therapy, 71*(4), 7104230010. https://doi.org/10.5014/ajot.2017.024182.

Richards, J., Holttum, S., & Springham, N. (2016). *How do "mental health professionals" who are also or have been "mental health service users" construct their identities?* SAGE Open January-March 2016, 1–14. https://doi.org/10.1177/2158244015621348.

Roberts, M., Hooper, B., & Molineux, M. (2020). Occupational therapy entry-level education scholarship in Australia from 2000 to 2019: A systematic mapping review. *Australian Occupational Therapy Journal, 67*(4), 373–395.

Rodger, S., Thomas, Y., Greber, C., et al. (2014). Attributes of excellence in practice educators: The perspectives of Australian occupational therapy students. *Australian Occupational Therapy Journal, 61*(3), 159–167.

Rose, N. (2019). *Our Psychiatric future.* Cambridge: Polity Press.

Rowan, S., & Alsop, A. (2016). Occupational therapists. In M. Doel, & S. M. Shardlow (Eds.), *Educating professionals: Practice learning in health and social care.* Abingdon: Routledge.

Royal College of Occupational Therapists (RCOT). (2019a). *Learning and Development Standards for Pre-registration education* (revised edition). London: Royal College of Occupational Therapists.

Royal College of Occupational Therapists (RCOT). (2019b). *Degree Level Apprenticeship in occupational therapy (England only).* Available at: https://www.rcot.co.uk/degree-level-apprenticeship-occupational-therapy.

Royal College of Occupational Therapists (RCOT). (2021). *Professional Standards for occupational therapy Practice, Conduct and Ethics.* Available at: https://www.rcot.co.uk/publications/professional-standards-occupational-therapy-practice-conduct-and-ethics.

Sadlo, G. (2016). Threshold concepts for educating people about human engagement in occupation: The study of human systems that enable occupation. *Journal of Occupational Science*, 23(4), 496–509. https://doi.org/10.1080/14427591.2016.1228098.

Schaber, & Candler. (2020). Signature pedagogies and learning designs in occupational therapy education. In S. Taff, L. Grajo, & B. Hooper (Eds.), *Perspectives on Occupational Therapy Education. Past, Present and Future.* Thorofare, NJ: SLACK Incorporated.

Schaber, P., Marsh, L., & Wilcox, K. (2012). Exploring signature pedagogies: Relational learning in occupational therapy professional education. In N. Chick, A. Haynie, & R. Gurung (Eds.), *Exploring More Signature Pedagogies: Approaches to Teaching Disciplinary Habits of Mind* (pp. 188–202). Sterling, VA: Stylus Press.

Schulze, B. (2007). Stigma and mental health professionals: A review of the evidence on an intricate relationship. *International Review of Psychiatry*, 19, 137–155.

Shardlow, S., & Doel, M. (2016). Health and social care: A complex context for professional education. In M. Doel, & S. M. Shardlow (Eds.), *Educating professionals: Practice learning in health and social care.* Abingdon: Routledge.

Shulman, L. S. (2005). Signature pedagogies in the professions. *Dædalus*, 134, 52–59. https://doi.org/10.1162/0011526054622015.

Singapore Association of Occupational Therapists. (2014). *Code of Ethics.* Available at https://www.saot.org.sg/about-us/code-of-ethic.

Stull, L. G., McGrew, J. H., Salyers, M. P., & Ashburn-Nardo, L. (2013). Implicit and explicit stigma of mental illness: Attitudes in an evidence-based practice. *The Journal of Nervous and Mental Disease*, 201(12), 1072–1079. https://doi.org/10.1097/NMD.0000000000000056.

Sullivan, W., Colby, A., Wegner, J. W., Bond, L., & Shulman, L. S. (2007). *Educating lawyers: Preparation for the profession of law.* Stanford, CA: John Wiley and Sons.

Tétreault, S., Bétrisey, C., Gulfi, A., Brisset, C., Kühne, N., & Leanza, Y. (2020). Perceptions, competencies and motivation for study choice: Occupational therapy and social work student perspectives. *International Journal of Practice-based Learning in Health & Social Care*, 8(1), 15–30.

Thomas, Y., & Penman, M. (2019). World Federation of Occupational Therapists (WFOT) standard for 1000 hours of practice placement: Informed by tradition or evidence? *British Journal of Occupational Therapy*, 82(1), 3–4.

Thornicroft, G. (2006). *Shunned: Discrimination against People with mental Illness.* Oxford University Press.

Tomlinson, M. (2017). Forms of graduate capital and their relationship to graduate employability. *Education Training*, 59(4), 338–352.

Tyminski, Q. P., Nguyen, A., & Taff, S. D. (2019). Proposing a metacurriculum for occupational therapy education in 2025 and beyond. *Journal of Occupational Therapy Education*, 3(4). https://doi.org/10.26681/jote.2019.030404.

Walsh, S., & Pollard, N. (2020). Seeing the bigger picture: A post-graduate online learning community facilitates political competence for occupational therapists. *Journal of Further and Higher Education*, 44(7), 971–983.

Waqas, A., Malik, S., Fida, A., et al. (2020). Interventions to reduce stigma related to mental illnesses in educational institutes: A systematic review. *Psychiatric Quarterly*, 91, 887–903. Available at: https://doi.org/10.1007/s11126-020-09751-4.

Wayne, J., Bogo, M., & Raskin, M. (2010). Field education as the signature pedagogy of social work education. *Journal of Social Work Education*, 46(3), 327–339.

Wellard, R., & Edwards, H. (1999). Curriculum models for educating beginning practitioners. In J. Higgs, & H. Edwards (Eds.), *Educating Beginning Practitioners: Challenges for health Professional Education.* Oxford: Butterworth-Heinemann.

Wilcock, A. (1993). A theory of the human need for occupation. *Journal of Occupational Science*, 1(1), 17–24.

Williamson, S. N., Paulsen-Becejac, L., Tong, K., Minette, R., & Forbes-Burford, J. (2020). Embedding graduate employability skills into health and social care course - a scoping review. *World Journal of Advance Healthcare Research*, 4(1), 147–164. Available at: https://www.wjahr.com/admin/assets/article_issue/17122019/1580805454.pdf.

World Federation of Occupational Therapists (WFOT). (2016). *Minimum Standards for the education of occupational Therapists Revised 2016.* Available at: https://www.wfot.org/resources/new-minimum-standards-for-the-education-of-occupational-therapists-2016-e-copy.

World Federation of Occupational Therapists (WFOT). (2021). *Position Statement. Educational Research in occupational therapy.* Available at: https://wfot.org/resources/educational-research-in-occupational-therapy.

12

INTERSECTIONALITY

MARINA MORROW ■ SUSAN HARDIE

INTRODUCTION

Intersectionality is a promising way of seeing the world. Occupational therapists can understand social inequities by exploring people's overlapping and intersecting social locations and experiences, as illustrated in Fig. 12.1. An intersectional framework locates where different social Convention on the Rights of Persons with Disabilities (CRPD) locations come together to explore privilege, oppression, discrimination and, in turn, the impact on mental health. Intersectionality can then be used as a critical tool, investigating what needs to be addressed in occupational therapy with populations, communities, families and individuals. This means carefully considering the barriers to participation and being open to exploring the complex lives of people with mental health issues.

In this chapter we begin by introducing some key concepts to support human rights and social justice based on the understandings of mental health. A series of sections follow, covering:

■ The social determinants of mental health, with particular attention to how mental illness diagnoses have resulted in discriminatory practices and beliefs about people in contact with mental health services;
■ Intersectionality as a way of understanding the complex intersections between different forms of power and social positioning in line with the aims of occupational justice;
■ How mental health reforms shape the complex environment for occupational therapy, including the historical move away from institutional care to community care and the adoption of recovery and well-being models;

INTERSECTIONS

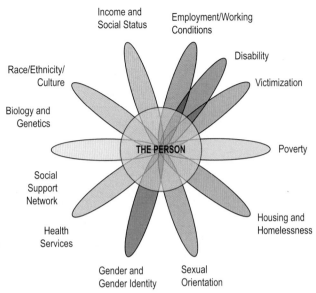

Fig. 12.1 ▪ Intersections.

- Neoliberal government agendas, which reinforce individual models of wellness and self-sufficiency that play into the predominant biomedical view in mental health services and public health;
- How an intersectional framework in occupational therapy can assist practitioners in better understanding and responding to the lives of people (where they live, work and play across their lifespan);
- The United Nations (UN) Convention on the Rights of Persons with Disabilities (CRPD), exploring the activist concept 'Nothing about us without us' and emphasizing the importance of user involvement and coproduction for mental healthcare policy and services which address their needs and concerns;
- Reflexivity and intersectionality to foster the awareness of occupational therapists working with a diverse clientele and to better respond to the power relations inherent in their work;
- Finally, how the principles of intersectionality can be used in practice through the CRPD and peer-driven initiatives.

In this chapter we use the term 'inequity' to refer to 'differences that are unfair or unjust as a result of structural arrangements that are potentially remedial' (Pauly 2008, p. 5). The structural arrangements referred to by Pauly (2008) are social structures, which occur at different levels of society (Crossman 2020).

Occupational Therapy and Mental Health Practice

Occupational therapists face continuously shifting social and economic contexts within their complex and diverse practice situations. All practitioners must realize the importance of, and work to acquire, the knowledge and competencies to engage with these practice realities. At the same time they uphold the profession's core values and principles, including equity, social inclusion, cultural awareness and human rights. This demands that occupational therapists' competencies include engaging in, critically analysing and contributing to 'larger political debates' and dialogues that shape the profession (Richards 2008, p. 26). Townsend (2003) offers a choice:

> Questions about power and justice are often viewed skeptically as being too political. Yet not addressing power and justice is also political; [occupational therapy] can either remain silently compliant with client/consumer injustices and our professional lack of empowerment, or we can take a visible, active stance to advocate for change.
>
> Townsend 2003, p. 85

Engaging with practice realities while upholding values can influence the resources and opportunities available to people who are striving to attain meaningful experiences in their occupations (Hammel 2009). The larger political and policy landscape for addressing mental health issues is concerned with social inclusion, workforce modernization, extended roles and new ways of working, which require a greater breadth of knowledge beyond traditional psychiatry.

Political Contexts

The rights to health and mental health are guaranteed through the UN CRPD, an international, legal commitment that is meant to structure the response of signatory countries (UN n.d.). Despite this, mental health continues to be a neglected area of policy and service delivery with only a small proportion of health budgets typically dedicated to it (between 7% and 11% in countries like Canada, New Zealand and the United Kingdom) (Mental Health Commission of Canada 2012). Additionally, although it is well established that good mental health is dependent on an array of social supports, the field continues to be dominated by a biomedical view (Morrow and Halinka Malcoe 2017; Friedl 2009; Compton and Shim 2015). This view has been described as the 'brain disease model' by Sayce (2015), which locates the origin of all experiences in the brain and favours pharmaceutical solutions, changing brain chemistry and biology. Therefore this view is focused on (neuro)biological frameworks with medical and primarily individualized approaches (Sayce 2015; Beresford 2019).

Occupational therapy can therefore be understood as a profession embedded in larger political, social and cultural contexts. These contexts include complex and often contradictory political environments. For example, in many mental health services there is increased reliance and focus on recovery and on community mental healthcare. Yet there is limited commitment of governments to provide the resources necessary to maintain these supports. There is an international legal environment that upholds the rights of people with disabilities, whereas at the national level, mental health legislation often undermines these rights (Pūras 2017; Brophy et al. 2018). Paradoxically, while research and practical experience show that the social environment is critical to mental well-being, responses continue to be biomedically focused (Morrow 2017; Morrow and Halinka Malcoe 2017). For example, social prescribing, which promotes the use of social resources by people with chronic ill-health, has been named as a medical process requiring a prescription

despite its origins in collaborative development and use of community assets (Dayson 2017; Thew et al. 2017).

The continuing reliance on the biomedical view has restricted development of a mental health system that responds adequately to the stresses caused by the social determinants of mental health (McGibbon 2012; Sayce 2015; Morrow and Halinka Malcoe 2017). Occupational therapy itself can be embedded in complex relationships with a range of professions and organizations dominated by the biomedical view, which influences how occupational therapists use their focus on occupation, social justice and the social causes of mental distress. Clarke (2019) offers the example of hoarding, categorised as a disorder but successfully approached by occupational therapists as a meaningful but risky occupation.

These contexts raise the following important and compelling questions for occupational therapists who are working towards addressing occupational injustices or 'unjust inequities that limit opportunities for participation in society' (Braveman 2009, p. 7):

- How do the frameworks and approaches used by occupational therapists impact existing social and structural inequities associated with mental health and the attainment of meaningful occupation?
- What is the role of occupational therapists with respect to larger political debates about reforms in mental health?
- What does it mean to be a reflexive practitioner and advocate for occupational justice?

There is a long and rich tradition of occupational justice in occupational therapy, which has oriented practitioners towards a social justice framework and meant that professional organizations have engaged in larger political debates (Townsend and Wilcock 2004; Kronenberg et al. 2005; Braveman and Bass-Haugen 2009; Bravemen and Suarez-Balcazar 2009; Townsend and Marvel 2013; Bailliard et al. 2020; see also Chapter 2). This has to be balanced with the day-to-day challenges of occupational therapy practice. Practitioners have to be skilled, knowledgeable and supported in responding to the complexities of practice. Intersectionality offers a framework for thinking about these complexities.

Social and Structural Determinants of Mental Health

To understand intersectionality it is helpful to explore how mental health is affected by social factors, or determinants, revealing inequities. The literature on social inequities and mental health comes from diverse perspectives. In a scoping review of this literature Ingram et al. (2013) identified a range of overlapping explanatory categories for understanding the social context and mental health:

- a social determinants framework;
- equity in the context of access to services;
- specific social locations/processes (e.g., gender and ethnicity);
- critical and feminist literature that challenges psychiatry and the concept of mental illness.

Since this review the literature has continued to grow (Compton and Shim 2015), including policy documents that state mental health equity and social justice as a central goal (Burstow et al. 2014; Morrow and Halinka Malcoe 2017; Daley et al. 2019; Milne and Hamfelt 2019). Occupational therapy scholars have also made important contributions to this literature using a social model of disability and a social justice lens (Townsend 2003; Townsend and Wilcock 2004; Durocher 2017; Bailliard et al. 2020). Collectively, these sources combine to form rich evidence of the intersections between social inequities and mental health, making existing mental health problems worse and contributing to poor mental health. Understanding inequities in these diverse ways highlights different things, as the following examples illustrate.

Social Determinants Framework

Regardless of their origins, experiences of mental health problems take place in the context of family, community and society as a whole, indicating that social determinants of mental health are found in every level of society (Compton and Shim 2015). Social determinants include early life experiences, poverty and access to financial resources, affordable and quality housing, education and access to services, along with forms of intersecting discrimination based on gender, race, ethnicity, sexual orientation, physical ability, age and social status. Social, cultural and historical contexts matter to mental health (Hacking 2002; Shorter 2008; Morrow 2017). These contexts include practices and policies, which improve, reinforce or worsen existing forms of discrimination based on psychiatric diagnoses and social categories such as gender, race, ethnicity, class, religion, ability and sexuality (Ussher 1991, 2011;

Caplan and Cosgrove 2004; Chan et al. 2005; U'Ren 2011; Morrow and Halinka Malcoe 2017). Therefore discrimination is structured through legal, medical and psychological practices and policies. These practices and policies play out in distinct ways for different groups within society.

Social inequities are defined by Whitehead and Dahlgren (2006, p. 2) and by Pauly (2008, p. 5) as the result of structural arrangements which are systematic, socially produced and unfair. They are revealed by differences in health status among and between different social groups as the result of social processes which can be acted on to produce equity. In the mental health field there are similar definitions (Aneshensel 2009; Benbow 2009; Depauw and Glass 2009). Graham (2004) argues that:

> the social factors promoting and undermining the health of individuals and populations should not be confused with the social processes underlying their unequal distribution. This distinction is important because, despite better health and improvement in health determinants, social disparities persist.
>
> *Graham 2004, p. 101*

A social determinants framework for understanding social inequities brings together the key factors in mental well-being and in recovery from mental distress, such as social supports, housing, meaningful activity and adequate income (Mental Health Commission of Canada 2012). Where a person is positioned in society also impacts mental health, that is, the social gradient of health extends to mental health (Marmot et al. 2008; U'Ren 2011). In this example, poverty can both lead to mental health problems and exacerbate them (e.g. Harris 2016).

How a person perceives their social status compared to others is also a mental health stressor. Scholars have also investigated the links between racial discrimination, experiences of migration and mental health (e.g., Morrow et al. 2008) and documented the effects of social inequities such as homelessness, racism, colonialism and poverty on mental health, making existing problems worse and/or creating distress (Boyer et al. 1997; Kirmayer et al. 2001; Mental Health Commission of Canada 2009). The links between trauma, experiences of violence, substance use and mental health influence and inform programs to support people (Harris 2016; Poole and Greaves 2012) and approaches by other health services (Machtinger et al. 2018; Cerny et al. 2019). What these types of scholarship share is an interest in understanding the relationship between socially unequal contexts and mental health.

Shim et al. (2015) argue that although social determinants of physical and mental health are not defined differently, there are reasons to emphasize the different impact. Often social determinants of mental health have been ignored in favour of biomedical and genetic factors. Mental health problems are highly prevalent and linked with disability, often coexisting with or exacerbating physical health challenges (Shim et al. 2015).

Identifying social determinants has raised awareness of how the social environment and policies and politics impact on mental health. However, social determinants frameworks have been criticized for their inability to accurately describe overlapping and intersecting forms of inequity (Morrow et al. 2013). For example, there is an absence of analysis of the many complex ways in which power operates within the mental healthcare system itself and how psychiatric diagnoses can become a form of oppression.

Access to Treatment and Stigma

Social determinants affect how people access health and care services. Many populations are under-served within mental healthcare systems (Marmot et al. 2008). Intense stigma experienced by many individuals in their communities is one reason services are not accessed. Other reasons include the lack of culturally appropriate services and supports. For example, despite the variety of mental health services and supports available, many women, particularly those who are economically disadvantaged, are unable to access appropriate services to address their complex and diverse needs (O'Mahoney and Donnelly 2007). In addition, there are barriers to mental health services for immigrant women due to limited financial resources, language skills, education and mobility (Chiu et al. 2005). Self- and social stigma have also been found to play an important role in women's access to social support and their decisions to access mental health services (Chiu et al. 2005). This problem extends to communities that have been marginalized or historically pathologized by psychiatry, for example, gay, lesbian, bisexual and transgendered people (Bauer et al. 2010; Alencar Albuquerque et al. 2016).

Asian men affected by mental health problems have also been found to have specific experiences of stigma and needs for social supports (Morrow et al. 2019). More medically oriented literature has made the argument that certain groups in society are more vulnerable to mental health problems and are thus at risk of not receiving services and supports (Patterson et al. 2008; Standing Senate Committee on Social Affairs, Science and Technology 2009).

Critical and Feminist Analyses

Critical and feminist analyses challenge psychiatry and the concept of mental illness. These involve investigating how social and structural inequities are built directly into psychiatric diagnostic practices, resulting in discriminatory labels being applied to disenfranchised groups. The practices of psychiatry are then revealed to have historically pathologized some groups of people (e.g., women, racialized people, people living in poverty) over others (Caplan 1995; Baker and Bell 1999; Caplan and Cosgrove 2004; Appignanaesi 2008; Metzl 2009). For example, some psychiatric diagnoses have been disproportionately applied to certain groups (e.g., indigenous and racialized people), and to women's normal life experiences such as the post-partum period and menopause (Ussher 1991, 2011; Metzl 2009; Ussher and Perz 2017). From this perspective, psychiatric diagnoses and labels are seen as a form of inequity (Morrow and Wiesser 2012). This is referred to as 'sanism', (Perlin 2000; Birnbaum 2010; Fabris 2011; Ingram 2011) or in LeFrancois's (2013) terms, 'psychiatrization', which she sees as the practice, or result, of sanism. Sanism and psychiatrization are used to understand the discrimination against people with psychiatric diagnoses but also go further in their aim to unsettle assumptions about rationality, normality and madness. Mad Studies draws thinking about this together, led by people who see themselves as survivors of the psychiatric system (Beresford 2019).

Psychiatric diagnoses are based on symptoms (subjective experiences) and signs (observed by others), which differ dramatically across cultures (Summerfield 2001; Watters 2010; Felman 2018). Although some scholars seek to reinforce the dominance of Western psychiatry, others point to how categorisation of experience is deeply culturally and historically rooted. Still others suggest alternative world views based on long-standing Indigenous traditions and very different modalities of support and care for people (Kirmayer and Valaskakis 2009; Browne, 2017; Clark 2017). Occupational therapists have adopted and utilized a variety of these frameworks in their work (Hammell 2019; Gibson 2020).

Power

The diverse perspectives discussed so far indicate tensions about how to understand and address the connections between social determinants and mental health problems. Some scholars adhere to a biomedical understanding of mental health, seeing the social environment as relevant in the context of treatment and recovery. Others suggest that it is the social environment itself that can contribute to problems. Some question the whole validity of the 'psy' sciences (psychiatry, psychology, criminology) (Chan et al. 2005) and push the boundaries of how we conceptualize differing states of mind/consciousness.

Taken together, however, these diverse perspectives shed light on how power is distributed in society and how this distribution of power extends to mental health services. A biomedical view is powerful in most mental health settings which respond primarily through the provision of services and management of people over and above the social supports that are needed. Combined with the political powers of neoliberalism and the erosion of the welfare state, it has led to systems that ration resources based on the diagnosis and severity of symptoms (Moth 2020). To expand the understanding of such impact and of how social and structural inequities operate in mental health, we propose using an intersectional framework for occupational therapy and mental health (Garcia-Ruiz 2017; Gretschel et al. 2017). Responses to inequities in mental health can be informed and shaped by understanding the social determinants and how they intersect, connect and interact.

INTERSECTIONALITY AND MENTAL HEALTH

Intersectionality is a world view which seeks to reveal the complex interactions among multiple social categories (such as gender, race, class, culture, age, ability and sexuality) with systems and processes of domination and oppression (such as sexism, racism, classism, colonialism, ageism, ableism, sanism and heterosexism). These complex interactions produce experiences of discrimination and privilege simultaneously (Morris and Benjun 2007; Hankivsky and Cormier 2009; Hankivsky 2012; Morrow and Halinka Malcoe 2017). An intersectional framework broadens analysis of the relationships between and among social categories and experiences. This is in contrast to health analyses based on a limited number of categories, like gender and age, or race. The aims of using an intersectional framework are to enhance population health and wellness, seek social justice and address social and health inequities.

Social and structural barriers interact to maintain inequity and occupational injustice. The understanding of these barriers to occupational performance, engagement and participation can be enhanced and clarified using an intersectional framework. Processes and systems of power work to reinforce or reduce discrimination and marginalization within occupational therapy and mental health. For example, occupational therapists facilitating therapeutic groups must not only be aware of how they attend to dynamic processes within the group, but also ensure that therapeutic outcomes from group attendance are shared and considered and possibly protect the space for the group when threatened by service restructuring or relocation. The promise of intersectionality comes from its use as an analytic lens through which inequities can be seen and understood. It also offers a powerful policy and practice framework for working with people and influencing social policy. There is growing attention to the value of intersectional frameworks for practitioners, policy actors and researchers to examine increasingly complex practice realities (see Burman and Chantler 2003; Burman 2004; Morris and Bunjun 2007; Hankivsky 2011, 2012; Rossiter and Morrow 2011; Morrow and Halinka Malcoe 2017; Hankivsky and Jordan-Zachary 2019).

Origins of Intersectionality

Intersectionality has its roots in Black American and Indigenous feminist writing and thinking, emerging primarily during the second wave (i.e., 1970s and 1980s) of the feminist movement in North America (Combahee River Collective 1980; Moraga and Anzaldúa 1981; Hill-Collins 1986, 1990, 2000; Crenshaw 1991). These roots drew on the critique of forms of feminism that focused on gender as the sole or most important form of oppression. Black, Latina and South Asian feminists argued that gender and race could not be understood separately and that, indeed, all forms of oppression/privilege (like patriarchy, white supremacy, class domination) are interconnected, inseparable and prop each other up through professional practice and the use of legislation, policy and ideology. Essentially, they questioned whether women could find solidarity in their shared oppression as women. Intense debates began about diversity and difference and the multiple ways in which oppression affects women. Although the term 'intersectionality' was not coined until the 1990s (Crenshaw 1991), its historic roots are visible throughout these early works.

Traditionally, the expert knowledge of professionals has been seen as superior to knowledge that comes from personal experience. An intersectional framework values personal experience as epistemologically significant, being deeply shaped by oppression and privilege. Therefore a significant form of knowledge and evidence comes from personal experience (e.g., Combahee River Collective 1980; hooks 1984; Hill Collins 1986, 2000). Knowledge about occupation and therapy that arises from people who are marginalized can deeply inform our understanding of the social world and the practices we engage in as professionals (Birken and Bryant 2019; Bryant et al. 2019; see also Chapter 29).

To understand practice and policy issues, an intersectional framework combines with social justice, which frames social and health inequities to be about differential access to power and resources (e.g., Hill-Collins 1990; Burgess-Proctor 2006; Hankivsky and Cormier 2009; Josewski 2017; Morrow and Halinka Malcoe 2017). For example, in the research by Birken and Bryant (2019), to address barriers to participation, the user researcher approached and offered meetings with people, to discuss the project further. As well as having direct experience of the service setting for the study, the user researcher had been involved in previous studies and had overcome her reservations about research. Her approach enabled people who were inpatients in acute mental health and rehabiiltation units to join as participants.

When using an intersectional framework it is assumed that society's resources and power are distributed in inequitable ways which should be challenged and addressed. As Lynn Friedli (2009) indicates,

Levels of mental distress among communities need to be understood less in terms of individual pathology and more as a response to relative deprivation and social injustice, which erode the emotional, spiritual, and intellectual resources essential to psychological wellbeing.
Lynn Friedli 2009, p. 111

Intersectionality has a long history, especially as an activist paradigm and a body of theory, and has increasingly been used in the field of health and mental health as a critical tool within a policy and practice framework (Morrow 2017; Morrow and Halinka Malcoe 2017).

A Critical Tool for Theory and Practice

Used as a critical tool for theories about mental health and about practice (Rossiter and Morrow 2011; Morrow and Halinka Malcoe 2017), an intersectional framework can help us understand how macro structures of power, such as psychiatry and mental health services, operate and impact people's lives. As a framework in mental health, intersectionality tends to focus on gender, race, ethnicity and class and exclude other social categories and processes (e.g., ableism and ageism). The framework has been applied primarily to certain populations (African Americans, South Asians) and mental health problems (depression) (Rossiter and Morrow 2011). This focus on certain social categories and processes and on certain ethno-cultural groups and mental health problems has resulted in less knowledge about a broad range of social categories and mental health issues (Rossiter and Morrow 2011). Some argue, for example, that one of the key forms of oppression in mental health is sanism (Fabris 2011; Ingram 2011; Morrow 2017). Naming sanism challenges assumptions about what constitutes normal behaviour (Fabris 2011; Ingram 2011). The term 'sanism' suggests how the diagnoses and labels of mental illness can result in active forms of discrimination against people, for example, by barring them from making their own medical decisions or from participating in civil society (Perlin 2000; Birnbaum 2010).

Challenging Simple Categories

Despite a growing interest in intersectional approaches in mental health (e.g., Mental Health Commission of Canada 2011), there is still work to be done to move beyond analyses of social categories to analyses of social processes of discrimination and oppression, that is, systems of power and how they operate in mental health. Attention to structural processes is critical for overcoming the limitations of seeing social categories such as age and gender as static and unchanging. This simplification of social categories artificially simplifies complex phenomena by categorising individuals according to broad group membership such as older people with dementia (Warner 2008). Intersectional scholarship explores multiple interlocking forms of oppression and challenges the assumptions that result from simplistic categorisation. Older people experiencing dementia would then include considerations of how their experiences of services and support vary, reflecting different oppressions and privileges. Awareness of multiple interlocking forms of oppression helps researchers, policymakers and practitioners to better understand the complexity of lived experiences and determine the implications of these intersections for service delivery (Burman 2004). This is especially challenging in environments in which rapid psychological assessments are encouraged and in which community-based mental health organizations, which arguably can come to know their clientele well, are under-resourced and over-stretched.

Although intersectional scholarship and practice is complex, it is well-suited to understanding the diverse experiences of people who come into contact with the mental healthcare systems and/or who experience mental distress (Rossiter and Morrow 2011; Morrow and Halinka Malcoe 2017). Intersectionality has the potential to reduce psychiatric stigma and discrimination and increase opportunities for recovery, inclusion and citizenship (Rossiter and Morrow 2011). It is consistent with the goals of occupational justice, namely, to strive to create space in society for the integration of people with mental health problems to engage as full citizens and members of their communities.

One way that intersectionality can be used in practice is by following eight principles, which set out the scope and detail of intersectionality as a framework (Hankivsky 2012). Summarized in Fig. 12.2, Hankivsky (2012, pp. 35–38) identifies the key principles as:

1. **Intersecting categories:** Social categories like gender, race, class, ethnicity, ability and age intersect and interlock, resulting in differing experiences of oppression and privilege;

2. **Multilevel analysis:** Intersectionality is concerned with understanding the impact of oppression and privilege between and across different levels in society (macro, meso and micro), that is, how inequities play out in international/national, provincial and community levels. People engaging with occupational therapy are affected by all these levels;

3. **Power:** Central to intersectionality is attention to how power operates both at the structural and discursive level—through laws, conventions and language—and how processes of power (like sexism and racism) operate to shape experience;

4. **Reflexivity:** Power operates through individuals in their relationships with one another. Researchers and practitioners must remain self-aware and self-critical and commit to ongoing dialogues with those with whom they work. Reflexivity helps us to recognize the power of knowledge that comes from experiences of marginalization and oppression;

5. **Time and space:** Intersectionality recognizes that people's experiences are shaped by where they live and work and that these experiences are not static but continually change with time and context;

6. **Diverse knowledges:** Intersectionality is concerned with the relationship between knowledge and power and how it plays out in creating, producing and sharing knowledge. This means that intersectionality calls on us to respect knowledge that comes from a diverse range of places, including Indigenous knowledge and non- Western forms of knowledge;

7. **Social justice:** Intersectional theorists and activists work for transformation of the social structure and society, so intersectionality foregrounds social justice and is concerned with the equitable distribution of resources in society;

8. **Equity:** Closely tied to social justice is the concept of equity, which is concerned with fairness and the idea that equal treatment does not always result in equity of outcomes.

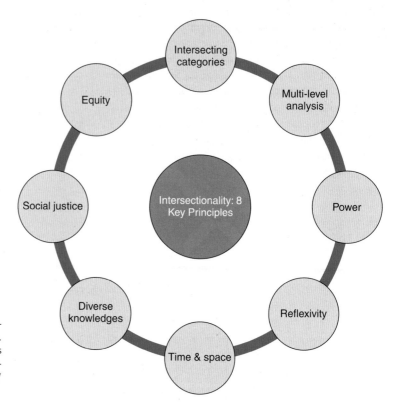

Fig. 12.2 ■ The eight principles of intersectionality. (From Hankivsky (2012). An Intersectionality-Based Policy Analysis Framework. Vancouver: Institute for Intersectionality Research and Policy. http://www.sfu.ca/iirp/index.html)

MENTAL HEALTH REFORMS AND THE COMPLEX PRACTICE ENVIRONMENT

This section begins with a multi-level analysis of the broader context for occupational therapy. There is a particular emphasis on the historical importance of mental health reforms which have resulted in:

- shifts from institutional to community care;
- moves towards recovery-oriented practice and promoting mental health and well-being;
- an emphasis on the involvement of people with lived experience in policy and program development, for example, coproduction.

The focus here is on an inclusive understanding of occupational therapy being concerned with all occupations and activities, which may or may not include paid employment. However, for many people the changing nature of work is particularly relevant. Tensions have arisen from shifting government agendas and neoliberal reforms, affecting equity and social justice by favouring reduced social welfare benefits and emphasizing individual self-sufficiency (Oliver and Barnes 2012). Context is important because occupational therapists are required to adapt to evolving environments, which powerfully challenge and/or support progress towards social and occupational justice.

From the Institution to the Community

Although the closure of institutions has been unfolding for almost five decades in Europe and North America, in some places the closure of large hospitals for people with mental health problems and/or learning disabilities is still relatively new (e.g., the Canadian provinces of British Columbia and Manitoba). With the closures has come a shift to community-based care, which in practice has meant that most places now maintain a wider range of care options from acute psychiatric inpatient care to a range of outpatient programs and housing options (Pilgrim 2005; Hill 2006). Although institutions themselves have not disappeared entirely, particularly in forensic psychiatry, what has changed is that there is now a commitment to ensure that people are supported to live as independently as possible regardless of their level of disability and to respect diverse knowledges of how this might be achieved. This has led to the change and expansion of occupational therapist' roles, shifting from older department-based rehabilitation to flexible approaches which aim to foster recovery and well-being (see also chapters 1 and 22). With this development a space has opened up for increased attention to equity to address limits on opportunities for participation. Concern about social determinants has been reactivated, giving momentum to dialogues in occupational therapy about social justice and health inequities (e.g., Townsend and Wilcock 2004; Kronenberg et al. 2005; Braveman and Suarez-Balcazar 2009; Townsend and Marvel 2013; World Federation of Occupational Therapists 2019; Bailliard et al. 2020).

Occupational Apartheid

The concept of occupational apartheid has been used to describe the inequities that people with disabilities face in gaining access to paid employment and other important occupations (Sy and Ohshima 2019; Washington 2020). Occupational apartheid is an outcome from governance and social policies which structure and control access to occupation and participation (Nilsson and Townsend 2010). The division of labour and the classification of occupations are two key structural factors that contribute to occupational injustice (Nilsson and Townsend 2010). Sy and Ohshima (2019) shared a case story of a former illicit drug user and trader in the Philippines using occupational apartheid as a concept to understand his struggles with access and participation to most occupations necessary for his survival and health. Put slightly differently, Stadnyk et al. (2010) distinguish several forms of occupational injustice (see Chapter 2 for elaborations of these concepts). The contemporary political and economic context is important for understanding how social policies influence these forms of injustice. For example, Washington (2020) explored the implications of occupational apartheid for teenage mothers, using principles of occupational justice to design a parenting programme. The social model of disability is also useful for understanding the current context and is discussed next.

Social Model of Disability

The social model of disability takes issue with bio-medicalism, or medical ideas which view the body as objectively mechanistic and as something that medicine should strive to fix to conform to ideals about what is normal (Oliver 1990). By contrast, the social model of disability points to the fact that disability is experienced within specific social contexts that often engender discrimination and exclusion from society. That is, while people have many physical variations, these alone do not lead to disability; instead, it is society's response to these people that is disabling (Oliver 1990). Shakespeare (2004) reminds us that the concept of social disability arose in Britain in a political context influenced by Marxism and the labour movement. It was tied closely to the disability rights movements of the 80s and 90s. The understanding of disability changed not only because of theoretical developments in the field, but also in response to the political context. The social model of disability has often been used to explain why people with disabilities have been excluded from the labour market and/or used as under-employed forms of reserve labour (Grover and Piggot 2005). From a social model perspective, disability can be reduced or overcome by a social response rather than individual efforts to change. This directly challenges the neoliberal emphasis on individual autonomy. Despite the relevance to occupational therapy's focus on adapting occupations and environments to enable participation, not all occupational therapy education and practice embraces the social model or acknowledges the impact of neoliberalism as discussed in the following section (Heffron et al. 2019).

Neoliberalism

Neoliberal ideologies are currently very powerful, having a substantive impact on how we understand the body, health and disability (Rose 1989; Grover and Piggot 2005; Braedley and Luxton 2010). Neoliberalism is an unfailing belief in market forces, economic liberalization, privatization and free markets. In recent years, the term neoliberalism has come to be used to describe a whole system of governance that critics feel is severely eroding the social welfare state. When translated into policy, neoliberalism promotes:

- individualistic understandings of complex social problems
- the increased use of market mechanisms in health and mental healthcare delivery (managerialism)

■ the development of self-reliance, resilience and volunteerism.

In occupational therapy the influence of neoliberalism can be detected in:

■ the preference for manualized psychosocial interventions, which emphasize individual change,
■ the prevalence of eligibility criteria for services and rigid discharge policies,
■ the emphasis on sign posting to non-statutory services, rather than service provision and
■ global impacts associated with the dominance of Western approaches to health (Hammell 2019).

Consequently, neoliberalism props up the biomedical view, since both are focused at the individual rather than social level (Morrow 2017). One of the cornerstones of neoliberalism is promoting individuals' autonomy from the state so that people are asked to assume the roles and risks of the state. Governments can then avoid recognizing and addressing vulnerability, resulting in problems like increased unemployment and poverty (Cooper and Whyte 2017; Fletcher and Wright 2017). Aldrich and Rudman (2020) have investigated how occupational therapists become 'street-level bureaucrats,' enacting neoliberal policies unless they have realized their potential to resist and question them.

Changes to Health and Welfare Programmes

Although the form that neoliberalism takes differs in different contexts, several recent examples in Canada and the United Kingdom help to illustrate our points. In the Canadian context the shift towards neoliberalism can be traced back to significant social policy changes in the mid-1990s, which were accompanied by massive cuts to health and social welfare programs. Through the 90s some provincial governments (notably British Columbia, Ontario and Alberta) responded by introducing work for welfare programs, tightening access to disability and employment insurance programs, failing to raise social assistance rates to meet climbing costs of living and stressing self-reliance and volunteerism. These changes have had specific implications for people with mental health problems with respect to income security and employment opportunities (Morrow et al. 2009).

In the United Kingdom the shift towards neoliberalism is usually credited to the policies of Margaret Thatcher in the 1980s, supported by her famous statement, 'there is no such thing as society'. This shift has been supported by successive governments and, as in the Canadian example, resulted in new forms of governance, in particular, more regulation and scrutiny of people with disabilities and those living in poverty. In particular, through the introduction of universal credit, which began to be rolled out in 2010, benefits began to be used more explicitly to incentivize paid work. The tying of work to benefits has had particular impact on people with disabilities undergoing repeated reassessment. This process has intensified and has been outsourced to private companies, who are paid for their successes in getting people off of benefits (Jolly 2011).

Universal credit was originally meant to simplify the complex UK social security system and help people transition into work. However, since its introduction, concerns have been raised for people with mental health struggles. For example, a Scottish report found that there were numerous barriers, including difficulties navigating online forms, attending work capability assessments and concerns about the levels of support available (Scottish Association for Mental Health 2019). A national audit of the records in the Department of Work and Pensions found that 69 people had taken their lives because of problems with their benefits, with the actual total likely to be higher but difficult to obtain (National Audit Office 2020). Calls for simplification and refocusing of welfare benefits point out the particular concerns for people with mental health issues (Senior et al. 2020).

In the United Kingdom the Health and Social Care Bill (2012) required that all health services be commissioned by boards who could award contracts to any qualified provider. Critics suggested that rules about competitive tendering may favour private providers (Reynolds and McKee 2012). The more recent bill has streamlined the tendering process, so a qualified provider does not have to go through full competitive tendering to renew a contract (Kings Fund 2021). In this environment, some areas of independent provision have flourished, including Improving Access to Psychological Therapy services, which delivers brief cognitive behavioural interventions, medium and low secure hospitals and out-of-area placements. Galante et al. (2019) noted that outcomes were worse for people displaced from their home area for an out-of-area placement in an independent sector facility.

These changes have occurred alongside welfare state retrenchment and an increasingly intensified governmental discourse that promotes individualism and independence. This context undermines the possibility of understanding people's needs as inter-related. The complex lives and experiences of people with mental health problems could be overlooked in a system that adheres rigidly to individualism, yet ignores the diverse needs of differently situated populations. Neoliberal ideology has influenced economic and social policy in ways that significantly shape how services and supports for people with mental health issues are designed. These practices can hinder people's ability to participate as full and active citizens in occupational and community life and arguably increase occupational marginalization, alienation, deprivation and imbalance.

Occupational Justice as a Critical Response

Although not a direct response to neoliberalism, occupational justice can be seen as a critical response to its impact on people and practices in mental health settings (Townsend and Wilcock 2004). Occupational justice combines the vision of an 'occupationally-just world supported by public health and societal initiatives' (Nilsson and Townsend 2010, p. 57) with an ethical vision of occupational therapy committing to empowerment and social inclusion. Nilsson and Townsend (2010) contend that building a theoretical bridge to practice is essential to 'inspire and empower' professionals. They describe occupational justice as a 'justice of difference', that is, 'a justice to recognize occupational rights regardless of age, ability, gender, social class, or other differences' (p. 58). Their work dovetails with the aims of intersectionality; it is concerned with the root causes of inequities and the structures of power which support them.

Occupational justice has inspired research by occupational therapists investigating experiences of discrimination and inequity (Bailliard et al. 2020). Much of this research is built particularly on one of the eight principles of intersectionality: the belief that lived experience is an important source of knowledge to understand oppression. The contributions and activism of people with lived experience of mental health problems are therefore central to an intersectional framework.

ACTIVISM

'nothing about us without us'

Harpur 2017

One way to use an intersectional framework is to recognize and support the power of collective action. People with lived experience of psychiatry and of institutional living contribute to this by documenting and speaking out about their experiences and by being involved in leading research (e.g., Chamberlin 1977; Burstow and Weiz 1988; Barnes 1991; Capponi 1992, 2003; Blackbridge 1997; Shimrat 2000; Beresford 2005, 2013, see also chapter 1). Historically, they have joined with academic and professional allies as anti-psychiatry activists, to make their lives and experiences visible and with the political aim of changing responses to people experiencing mental distress (e.g., Szasz 1961; Breggin 2008; Metzl 2009; Recovery in the Bin 2016). They have made many of the same claims that disability activists have made, namely, that experiences that do not conform to norms and standards should not all be seen as pathological.

These historic roots of survivor activism continue to be influential, yet the breadth of users and survivors and the scope of their activities have expanded. Today people with lived experience can be supported in making informed choices, which include the choice of disclosure and how to self-identify. Intersectionality points to the importance of locating oneself not only as a way of recognizing power, but also as a means for reclaiming identities that have been marginalized and maligned. Today people involved in activism may choose to use the historic psychiatric survivor label or other terms such as 'user,' 'consumer,' 'survivor,' 'peer,' 'client' and 'patient' (see also Chapter 2). This emphasizes the idea that people with lived experience of mental health issues are human beings with minds bodies and spirits. They may choose to identify as a person, a person with a mental health issue or a person with a diagnosis of a mental illness. The word 'person' is used to raise awareness that people are much more than a psychiatric label: they are people with hopes, dreams and rights who deserve to be treated with dignity and respect equitable to all citizens.

Recurrent Themes from Lived Experience

People with lived experience have been telling their stories about psychiatry and broader health and social services systems, in many different forms. Recurring themes have emerged including:

- poverty,
- lack of stable housing,
- lack or absence of employment,
- food insecurity,
- experiences of violence, discrimination and oppression and
- lack of access to services consistent with recovery, mental health and well-being.

These themes highlight experiences of powerlessness and oppression when mental health is seen as a problem for individuals, with limited attention paid to social and structural inequities. For example, the Diagnostic and Statistical Manual of Mental Disorders, 4th Ed., Text Revision (American Psychiatric Association 2013) is a manual frequently used within psychiatry which acknowledges social determinants of mental health. However, McGibbon (2012) argues that attention to social determinants is so brief that the biomedical view remains most powerful and continues to limit engagement with the economic and political origins of mental health issues.

As survivor activists gain more opportunities to work with others in the disability movement, there is growing awareness of these common themes, as well as distinct differences. A common theme is the shared understanding of the importance of people's active participation in all processes impacting their lives. This understanding is reflected in the phrase 'nothing about us without us' (Harpur 2017), which continues to guide grassroots activism.

User Involvement

Mental health policy has also highlighted the importance of involving people with lived experience in all aspects of governance, planning, service delivery, evaluation, research and leadership. For example, in the first Mental Health Strategy for Canada (Mental Health Commission of Canada 2011) involvement in all aspects of the health, social and other systems impacting on their lives is seen as an essential component of a transformed mental health system grounded in recovery, health and well-being. There are specific recommendations about:

- establishing peer support throughout the mental healthcare system;
- increasing support for peer-run organizations;
- peer research;
- the ongoing grassroots capacity building of leaders within the activist community to bring forth the voices of those they represent.

With support in principle for active participation in national, provincial/territorial and regional mental health plans grounded in recovery, mental health and well-being, the next phase is implementation.

The process of involving people with lived experience, or service users, in working for service development and change is complex and can easily become tokenistic (Fabris 2013). For example, user involvement has often been implemented by the people with both positional and fiscal power, while the activists with actual experience in the movement are excluded. This can result in an individual with lived experience being selected as a 'representative' yet with no connection to other diverse groups of people with lived experience within their locale no knowledge of the needs of others, and no historical knowledge of the activism of people with lived experience. This kind of token representation can stifle the intention to transform how things are done. Individuals representing other people in any capacity must be connected to, and accountable to, a broader collective of individuals in specific locales. Otherwise the benefits of representation grounded in the democratic process will be lost (see Costa et al. 2012; Fabris 2013; Voronka 2017).

There is a risk of token representation in coproduction, which has become popular in UK mental health services. Coproduction is an approach to user involvement in service transformation, sharing power as equals in every stage (Social Care Institute for Excellence (SCIE) 2015). It respects diverse knowledge and encourages multi-level analysis to change services for the benefit of people using services and frontline staff. There are many ways of defining and using it, as discussed by SCIE (2015) and the National Development Team for inclusion (NDTi 2018). However, there is agreement that it involves sharing the power of managers and professionals between everyone who commits to work together for service transformation. Morori and Richards (2017) discuss the challenges for occupational therapists, who might clearly understand the nature of collaborative working, but be less experienced in sharing every aspect of the process with the people receiving their services. Professional and managerial reluctance to share their power has made user-led organizations wary of some coproduction initiatives (NDTi 2016).

International Approaches

Partly in response to these concerns, support to develop peer or user-led innovation has been initiated. Different countries have approached this in different ways. In the late 1980s in the United States, two funded technical assistance centres led to the emergence of peer-led and peer-run organizations (Chamberlin 1977; Harp et al. 1984, 1994). In the United Kingdom there has been a significant investment in supporting the creation of peer support positions throughout the mental health system (Ibrahim et al. 2020). In Australia the decision was made to create a national council of consumers, and subsequently state and regional bodies to foster peer leadership and involvement. In New Zealand users took the lead in developing recovery standards that continue to guide system transformation internationally. In Canada an initial investment was made in fostering grassroots leadership through the Disabled Persons Participation Program. In the early 1990s this funding shifted from departmental core funding to project funding.

Globally, individual activists and collective movements such as Mad Pride work towards the cocreation of a more just and inclusive society. There are many factors that play a role in the development of this collective movement including:

- the leadership of people with lived experience,
- government and organizational policies,
- dedicated resources (e.g., financial, time, space,) and
- opportunities to support grassroots peer-run organizations to fulfil local needs.

As so many factors reside outside user and survivor organizations, the broader psychiatric user and survivor movement has variable development around the world, yet the collective vision is sustained.

Enabling Occupation

The link between the activism of people with lived experience and the work of occupational therapists can be found in the movement towards person-centred practice and the notion of enabling occupation (Townsend 2003). This belief in empowerment through action has been important to occupational therapy throughout the profession's existence. Historically some institutional occupational therapy departments have provided resources for activists, from money for paid (sheltered) work to access to printing and places to meet. Community mental health occupational therapy can bring people together and empower them to become self-supporting. The link between activism and occupational therapy can also be found in scholarship through the increased use of participatory action research (Cockburn and Trentham 2002), especially those studies that employ intersectionality (Morrow et al. 2020). Occupational therapists are well positioned to work side by side with people with lived experience as allies in the struggle for occupational justice.

Reflexivity

Reflexivity is one of the eight principles of intersectionality. It has been described by Kaufman (2012) as a

process of seeing and a process of being. To be reflexive means that we are fully conscious of the lenses through which we view the world. We understand both our situationality and our positionality, our circumstances and our locations.
Kaufman, 2012, p. 2

In contrast to reflection, which might focus on a particular situation, reflexivity involves deeper consideration of recurrent issues and experiences. As Kippax and Kinder (2002) p., 2 indicate, reflexivity:

involves more than an analysis of prior learning of attention to the grounds or justification of one's beliefs and generalizations (content)...what is essential is the taking up an epistemological stance that recognizes multiple positionings and situated knowledge.

An occupational therapy team seeking to build partnerships with survivors and current users would benefit by starting to find out what everyone, including the users, knows from their experience. Rather than offering quick explanations and solutions, being reflexive involves carefully considering together the differences and shared areas of knowledge (Balliard et al. 2020). For reflexivity to be useful it must move beyond acknowledgment of social location to the recognition of how those locations intersect with wider social, economic, cultural, political, historical and structural factors. As such, the purpose of reflexivity is to highlight how power operates in day-to-day encounters in occupational therapy as lived through the intersections of gender, race, class, ability and sexual orientation. If practiced regularly, reflexivity has the potential to review power relations and transform those relations so that the knowledge that comes from lived experience can be valued, respected and acted up on (Bailliard et al. 2020).

IMPLICATIONS AND SUMMARY

Historically, occupational therapy for people with mental health problems has been structured around the needs of the psychiatric hospital system (see Chapter 1). Today many occupational therapists work in both a psychiatric hospital and a community settings, and the focus of their work has shifted. Recognizing the growth of practice, inclusive of and beyond psychiatric care, professional associations dedicate both time and resources to re-examining current roles, responsibilities and practices to fulfill their essential vision of the power of meaningful occupation. Occupational therapists work in complex environments shaped by reforms in mental health and larger political and economic trends such as neoliberalism. There is ongoing tension between the biomedical understandings of mental health and those that are grounded in people's lived experience and an analysis of social and health inequities. In this context occupational therapists are called on to uphold the values of their profession (equity, human rights, social inclusion and cultural awareness) while working to expand their scope of practice and push their thinking about mental health.

As we hope this chapter has demonstrated, an intersectional framework is important for occupational therapists to understand the interlocking nature of oppressions and the underlying systems and processes of power which keep these inequities in place. Intersectionality counters neoliberalism which reinforces individualized frameworks for understanding mental health. In contrast, an intersectional framework pushes the mental health professions to think about how their work is embedded in larger social contexts that are imbued with relations of power. Given that most occupational therapists work at a local level with specific individuals and communities, it can be challenging to find opportunities to be reflexive about their own practice and context. Reflexive practice will assist occupational therapists in responding to the changing nature of their work and in maintaining their goal of addressing inequities that limit participation. This will enable engagement with the larger debates that frame occupational therapy and the mental healthcare system more generally. These debates can be accessed by practitioners in forums and continuing education that are shaped around the broader political needs of people with lived experience and the changing mental health and social policy environment. Occupational therapy is well positioned to further the discussion about mental health and social inequities and to integrate intersectionality into their work.

SERVICE USER COMMENTARY

Intersectionality is an excellent way of looking at the service user through different lenses. By considering the interaction between often competing factors that can worsen or improve a service user's circumstances, the astute occupational therapist will take a holistic but targeted approach to helping the service user.

Many service users will have found that their own intersections (see Fig. 12.1) have been weaponized and used against them by the medical profession and allied health services. For example, a case study during medical training that references a gay male patient almost inevitably leads to a sexual health diagnosis. It is all too easy for the experienced practitioner to make assumptions based on a service user's circumstances and automatically prescribe a routine treatment based on those assumptions alone without considering the unique challenges the service user faces. It has often felt as though the professional is trying to get me to fit into their boxes rather than seeking to understand my situation, challenges, feelings and fears.

Coproduction is increasingly bandied about by health professionals, but I would question whether practitioners understand the true meaning of the word. I've found that service managers will often say a policy or protocol was 'coproduced' with service users, although in reality service users were merely consulted or kept informed instead of having an equal say in its strategic oversight, tactical design and operational delivery. The Ladder of Co-Production (https://www.thinklocalactpersonal.org.uk/_assets/COPRODUCTION/Ladder-of-coproduction.pdf) developed by Think Local Act Personal (TLAP) provides a great model to assess whether an activity is authentically coproduced.

The key challenge presented by coproduction is that it requires health professionals to set aside years of thinking a particular way and their personal prejudices to genuinely regard the service user as their equal with an equal hand in determining the health outcome. Fundamental to this is for the practitioner to examine their own unconscious bias. Coproduction only occurs when the practitioner adopts a flexible mindset and can be comfortable with an outcome that differs from what they might otherwise prescribe. It is impossible for coproduction to thrive in an environment in which the service user perspective is habitually viewed with scepticism.

The social and structural frameworks that inflict inequity on a service user will often present a significant barrier to facilitating a service user's recovery. In my own experience, it is rare that professionals will work beyond their own silo to help me, beyond signposting. When at risk of homelessness a year or so ago, plenty of professionals were able to refer me to the local housing service, but they failed to recognize that the housing service did not have sufficient awareness and understanding of my health condition nor the requisite skills to assist me in using their service. Taking a holistic approach to a service user's needs will naturally involve working across organizations and professional boundaries. Effective occupational therapists are those who not only signpost to, but also actively help service users navigate other organizations' systems.

In short, intersectionality involves proactively identifying and embracing the grey areas in a world that is rarely black and white.

Tim Dee

REFERENCES

Aldrich, R. M., & Rudman, D. L. (2020). Occupational therapists as street-level bureaucrats: Leveraging the political nature of everyday practice. *Canadian Journal of Occupational Therapy*, 87(2), 137–143.

Alencar Albuquerque, G., de Lima Garcia, C., da Silva Quirino, G., et al. (2016). Access to health services by lesbian, gay, bisexual, and transgender persons: Systematic literature review. *BioMed Central International Health and Human Rights*, 16, 2. https://bmcinthealthhumrights.biomedcentral.com/articles/10.1186/s12914-015-0072-9.

American Psychiatric Association. (2013). *Diagnostic and statistical manual of mental disorders* (5th ed.). US: American Psychiatric Association.

Aneshensel, C. S. (2009). Toward explaining mental health disparities. *Journal of Health and Social Behavior*, 50(4), 377–394.

Appignanesi, L. (2008). *Mad, bad and sad: A history of women and the mind doctors from 1800 to the present*. Great Britain: Virago Press.

Bailliard A.L., Dallman A.R., Carroll A., Lee B.D., Szendrey S. Doing Occupational Justice: A Central Dimension of Everyday Occupational Therapy Practice. *Canadian Journal of Occupational Therapy*. 87(2):144–152. doi:10.1177/0008417419898930.

Baker, F. M., & Bell, C. C. (1999). Issues in the psychiatric treatment of African Americans. *Psychiatric Services*, 50(3), 362–368.

Barnes, M. (1991). *Two accounts of a journey through madness (1991) with Joseph Berke*. London: Free Association Books.

Bass-Haugen, J. D. (2009). Health disparities: Examination of evidence relevant for occupational therapy. *American Journal of Occupational Therapy*, 63(1), 24–34.

Bauer, G., Boyce, M., Coleman, T., Kaay, M., Scanlon, K., Travers, R., 2010. Who are trans people in Ontario? Toronto: Trans PULSE E-Bulletin; Report No.: 1(1).

Benbow, S. (2009). Societal abuse in the lives of individuals with mental illness. *Canadian Nurse*, 105(6), 30–32.

Beresford, P., (2003). *It's our lives: A short theory of knowledge, distance and experience*. London: Citizen Press in association with Shaping Our Lives.

Beresford, P., (2005). Theory and practice of user involvement in research: Making the connection with public policy and practice. In L. Lowes, & I. Hulatt (Eds.), *Involving service users in health and social care research* (pp. 6–17). London: Routledge.

Beresford, P. (2013). From 'other' to involved: User involvement in research: An emerging paradigm. *Nordic Social Work Research*, *3*(2), 139–148. https://doi.org/10.1080/2156857X.2013.835138.

Beresford, P. (2019). 'Mad', Mad studies and advancing inclusive resistance. *Disability & Society*. https://doi.org/10.1080/0968759 9.2019.1692168.

Birken, M., & Bryant, W. (2019). A photovoice study of user experiences of an occupational therapy department within an acute inpatient mental health setting. *British Journal of Occupational Therapy*, *82*(9), 532–543.

Birnbaum, R. (2010). My father's advocacy for a right to treatment. *Journal of the American Academy of Psychiatry & the Law Online*, *38*(1), 115–123.

Blackbridge, P. (1997). *Prozac Highway*. Vancouver: Press Gang.

Boyer, M., Ku, J., & Shakir, U. (1997). *The healing journey: Phase II report-women and mental health: Documenting the voices of ethnoracial women within an anti-racist framework*. Toronto: Across Boundaries Mental Health Centre.

Braedley, S., & Luxton, M. (Eds.). (2010). *Neoliberalism and everyday life*. Montreal: McGill Queen's Press.

Braveman, B., & Suarez-Balcazar, Y. (2009). Social justice and resource utilization in a community-based organization: A case illustration of the role of the occupational therapist. *American Journal of Occupational Therapy*, *63*, 13–23.

Breggin, P. R. (2008). *Medication madness: A psychiatrist exposes the dangers of mood-altering medications*. New York: St. Martin's Press.

Brophy, L., Ryan, C. J., & Weller, P. (2018). Community treatment orders: The evidence and the ethical implications. In C. Spivakovsky, K. Seear, & A. Carter (Eds.), *Critical perspectives on coercive interventions* (pp. 42–55). Routledge.

Browne, A. (2017). Moving beyond description: Closing the health equity gap by redressing racism impacting indigenous populations. *Social Science & Medicine*, *184*, 23–26. https://doi. org/10.1016/j.socscimed.2017.04.045.

Bryant, W., Cordingley, K., Adomako, E., & Birken, M. (2019). Making activism a participatory, inclusive and developmental process: A research programme involving mental health service users. *Disability & Society*, *34*(7/8), 1264–1288.

Burgess-Proctor, A. (2006). Intersections of race, class, gender, and crime: Future directions for feminist criminology. *Feminist Criminology*, *1*(1), 27–47.

Burman, E. (2004). From difference to intersectionality: Challenges and resources. *European Journal of Psychotherapy*, *6*(4), 293–308.

Burman, E., & Chantler, K. (2003). Across and between: Reflections on researching "race" gender and mental health. *Feminism & Psychology*, *13*(3), 302–309.

Burstow, B., Lefrançois, B., & Diamond, S. (2014). *Psychiatry disrupted: Theorizing resistance and crafting the (R)evolution*. Montreal: McGill-Queen's University Press.

Burstow, B., & Weitz, D. (1988). *Shrink resistant: The struggle against psychiatry in Canada*. Vancouver: New Star Books.

Caplan, P. (1995). *They say you're crazy: How the world's most powerful psychiatrists decide who's normal*. New York: Perseus Books.

Caplan, P., & Cosgrove, L. (Eds.). (2004). *Bias in psychiatric diagnosis*. Maryland: Roman & Littlefield Publishing.

Capponi, P. (1992). *Upstairs in the Crazy House*. Toronto: Viking Press.

Capponi, P. (2003). *Beyond the crazy house: Changing the future of madness*. Toronto: Penguin Canada.

Cerny, S., Masssssen, A., & Crook, K. (2019). Occupational therapy intervention for survivors of human trafficking. *Occupational Therapy in Mental Health*, *35*(3), 287–299.

Chamberlin, J. (1977). *On our own: A compelling case for patient controlled services; a real alternative to the institutions that destroy the Confident independence of so many*. England: MIND.

Chan, W., Chunn, D., & Menzies, R. (Eds.). (2005). *Women, madness and the law: A feminist reader*. Cavendish, London Portland: Glass House.

Chiu, L., Morrow, M., Ganesan, S., & Clark, N. (2005). Treatment choices by South East asian immigrant women with serious mental illness: A socio-spiritual process. *Translational Psychiatry*, *42*(4), 630–656.

Clarke, C. (2019). Can occupational therapy address the occupational implications of hoarding? *Occupational Therapy International*, *2019*, 5347403.

Clark, N., Walton, P., Drolet, J., et al. (2017). Melq'ilwiye (coming together): Re-imagining mental health for urban indigenous youth through intersections of identity, sovereignty, and resistance. In M. Morrow, & L. Halinka Malcoe (Eds.), *Critical Inquiries for social justice in mental health* (pp. 165–196). Toronto: University of Toronto Press.

Cockburn, L., & Trentham, B. (2002). Participatory action research: Integrating community occupational therapy practice and research. *Canadian Journal of Occupational Therapy*, *69*(1), 20–30.

Combahee River Collective. (1980). *The Combahee River collective statement: History is a weapon*. Available at: http:// historyisaweapon.com/defcon1/combrivercoll.html.

Compton, M., & Shim, R. (Eds.). (2015). *The social determinants of mental health*. Arlington: American Psychiatric Association.

Cooper, V., & Whyte, D. (Eds.). (2017). *The violence of Austerity*. London: Pluto.

Costa, L., Voronka, J., Landry, D., et al. (2012). Recovering our stories: A small act of resistance. *Studies in Social Justice*, *6*(1), 85–101.

Crenshaw, K. (1991). Mapping the margins: Intersectionality, identity politics, and violence against women of colour. *Stanford Law Review*, *43*(6), 1241–1299.

Crossman, A. (2020). The Concept of Social Structure in Sociology. https://www.thoughtco.com/social-structure-defined-3026594.

Daley, A., Costa, L., & Beresford, P. (Eds.). (2019). *Madness, violence and power: A critical collection*. Toronto: University of Toronto Press.

Dayson, C. (2017). Social prescribing 'plus': A model of asset-based collaborative innovation? *People, Place*, and *Policy*, *11*(2), 90–104.

Durocher, E. (2017). Occupational justice: A fine balance for occupational therapists. In N. Pollard, & D. Sakalleriou (Eds.), *Occupational Therapies without Borders* (2nd ed.). Oxford: Elsevier.

Fabris, E. (2011). *Tranquil prisons: Chemical incarceration under community treatment orders.* Toronto: University of Toronto Press.

Fabris, E. (2013). Mad success: What could go Wrong when psychiatry employs us as 'peers. In R. Menzies, G. Reaume, & B. Lefrançois (Eds.), *Mad matters: A critical Reader in Canadian Mad studies* (pp. 130–140). Toronto: Canadian Scholar's Press.

Felman, A. (2018). *Why do signs and symptoms matter? Medical news today.* Available at: https://www.medicalnewstoday.com/articles/161858.

Fletcher, D. R., & Wright, S. (2017). A hand up or a slap down? Criminalizing benefit claimants in Britain via strategies of surveillance, sanctions and deterrence. *Medication Human, 41,* 40–47.

Friedli, L. (2009). *Mental health, resilience and inequalities.* Geneva: WHO. Available at: http://www.mentalhealthpromotion.net/resources/mental-health-resilience-and-inequalities.pdf.

Galante, J. R., Humphreys, R., & Molodynski, A. (2019). Out-of-area placements in acute mental health care: The outcomes. *Progress in Neurology and Psychiatry, 23*(1), 2019.

Garcia-Ruiz, S. (2016). Occupational therapy in a glocalized world. In D. Sakellariou, & N. Pollard (Eds.), *Occupational Therapies without Borders* (2nd ed.) (pp. 185–193). London: Elsevier.

Gibson, C. (2020). When the river runs dry: Leadership, decolonisation and healing in occupational therapy. *New Zealand Journal of Occupational Therapy, 67*(1), 11–20.

Graham, H. (2004). Social determinants and their unequal distribution: Clarifying policy understandings. *The Milbank Quarterly, 82*(1), 101–124.

Gretschel, P., Ramugondo, E., & Galvaan, R. (2017). Factors influencing the role of South African occupational therapists in the occupational therapy intervention design process. In D. Sakellariou, & N. Pollard (Eds.), *Occupational therapies without borders* (2nd ed.) (pp. 302–309). London: Elsevier.

Grover, C., & Piggott, L. (2005). Disabled people, the reserve army of labour and welfare reform. *Disability & Society, 20*(7), 705–717.

Hacking, I. (2002). *Mad travelers: Reflections on the reality of transient mental illnesses.* Boston: Harvard University Press.

Hankivsky, O. (Ed.). (2011). *Health inequities in Canada: Intersectional frameworks and practices.* Vancouver: UBC Press.

Hankivsky, O. (Ed.). (2012). *An intersectionality-based policy analysis framework.* Vancouver: Institute for Intersectionality Research and Policy. Available at: http://www.sfu.ca/iirp/index.html.

Hankivsky, O., & Cormier, R. (2009). *Intersectionality: Moving women's health research and policy forward.* Vancouver, BC: Women's Health Research Network.

Hankivsky, O., & Jordan-Zachary, J. (Eds.). (2019). *The Palgrave Handbook of intersectionality in public policy.* London: Palgrave MacMillan.

Harpur, P. (2017). Nothing about us without us: the un convention on the rights of persons with disabilities. In *Oxford research encyclopedia of politics.* https://oxfordre.com/politics/view/10.1093/acrefore/97.

Harris, M. (2016). Modifications in service delivery for women diagnosed with severe mental illness who are also the survivors of sexual abuse trauma. In M. Harris, & C. Landis (Eds.), *Sexual abuse in the lives of women diagnosed with serious mental illness.* Abingdon: Routledge. E-book https://www.routledge.com/Sexual-Abuse-in-the-Lives-of-Women-Diagnosed-withSerious-Mental-Illness/Harris-Landis/p/book/9781583912744.

Hill, J. (2006). *Mental health today: A handbook.* Brighton: Pavilion Publishing.

Hill Collins, P. (1986). Learning from the outsider within: The sociological significance of black feminist thought. *Social Problems, 33*(6), S14–S32.

Hill Collins, P. (1990). *Black feminist thought: Knowledge, consciousness, and the politics of empowerment.* Boston: Unwin Hyman.

Hill Collins, P. (2000). *Black feminist thought: Knowledge, consciousness, and the politics of empowerment.* New York: Routledge.

Hill Collins, P., & Bilge, S. (2016). *Intersectionality.* Cambridge: Polity Press.

hooks, B. (1984). *Feminist theory: From Margin to center.* Boston: South End Press.

Heffron, J., Lee, D., Vanpuymbrouck, L., Sheth, A. J., & Kish, J. (2019). The bigger picture": Occupational therapy practitioners' perspectives on disability studies. *American Journal of Occupational Therapy, 73,* 2.

Hammell, K. W. (2009). Self-care, productivity and leisure, or dimensions of occupational experience? Rethinking occupational "categories." *Canadian Journal of Occupational Therapy, 76*(2), 107–114.

Hammell, K. W. (2019). Building globally relevant occupational therapy from the strength of our diversity. *World Federation of Occupational Therapists Bulletin, 75*(1), 13–26. https://doi.org/10.1080/14473828.2018.1529480.

Ibrahim, N., Thompson, D., Nixdorf, R., et al. (2020). A systematic review of influences on implementation of peer support work for adults with mental health problems. *Social Psychiatry and Psychiatric Epidemiology, 55,* 285–293. https://link.springer.com/article/10.1007/s00127-019-01739-1#citeas.

Ingram, R. (2011). *Recovery from compulsory sanity.* San Jose, California: Presentation for Society for Disabilities Studies Conference.

Ingram, R., Wasik, A., Cormier, R., & Morrow, M. (2013). *Social inequities and mental health: A scoping review.* Vancouver: Centre for the Study of Gender Social Inequities and Mental Health.

Jolly, D. (2011). *The Government's work capability assessment for disabled people is one of the Toughest in the world – it is not fit for purpose.* Available at: http://eprints.lse.ac.uk/36312/1/blogs.lse.ac.uk-The_governments_Work_Capability_Assessment_for_disabled_people_is_one_of_the_toughest_in_the_world__i.pdf.

Josewski, V. (2017). A "third space" for doing social just research. In M. Morrow, & L. Halinka Malcoe (Eds.), *Critical inquiries for social justice in mental health*. Toronto: University of Toronto Press.

Kings Fund. (2021). The Health and Care Bill: 6 key questions. https://www.kingsfund.org.uk/publications/health-and-care-bill-key-questions.

Kaufman, P. (2012). Scribo ergo cogito: Reflexivity through writing. *Teaching Sociology, 41*(1), 70–81.

Kippax, S., & Kinder, P. (2002). Reflexive practice: The relationship between social research and health promotion in HIV prevention. *Sex Education, 2*(2), 91–104.

Kirmayer, L., Brass, G. M., & Tait, C. L. (2001). The mental health of aboriginal peoples: Transformations of identity and culture. *The Canadian Journal of Psychiatry, 45*(7), 607–617.

Kirmayer, L., & Valasakakis, G. G. (Eds.). (2009). *Healing traditions: The mental health of aboriginal peoples in Canada*. Toronto: University of Toronto Press.

Kronenberg, F., Simó Algado, S., & Pollard, N. (Eds.). (2005). *Occupational therapy without borders: Learning from the spirit of survivors*. Oxford England: Elsevier-Churchill Livingston.

Lefrançois, B. A. (2013). Queering child and adolescent mental health services: The subversion of heteronormativity in practice. *Children & Society, 27*(1), 1–12.

Marmot, M., Friel, S., Bell, R., Houweling, T., & Taylor, S. (2008). Closing the gap in a generation: Health equity through action on the social determinants of health. *Lancet, 372*(9560), 1661–1669.

McGibbon, E. (2012). Oppression and mental health: Pathologizing the outcomes of injustice. In E. McGibbon (Ed.), *Oppression: A social determinant of health* (pp. 123–137). Fernwood Publishing, Winnipeg & Halifax. Available at: http://www.fernwoodpublishing.ca/Oppression/.

Mental Health Commission of Canada. (2009). *Toward recovery & well-being: A framework for a mental health Strategy for Canada*. Calgary, AB: Mental Health Commission of Canada.

Mental Health Commission of Canada. (2012). *Changing directions, changing lives: The mental health Strategy for Canada*. Ottawa: Mental Health Commission of Canada.

Metzl, J. (2009). *The protest psychosis: How schizophrenia became a black disease*. Boston: Beacon Press.

Milne, K., & Hamfelt, A. (2019). *Building an equitable foundation: Removing barriers to access for people with mental health and substance-use related disabilities*. Vancouver: Canadian Mental Health Association.

Momori, N., & Richards, G. (2017). Service user and carer involvement: Co-production. In C. Long, J. Cronin-Davis, & D. Cotterill (Eds.), *Occupational therapy evidence in practice for mental health*. Chichester: John Wiley and Sons Ltd.

Moraga, C., & Anzaldúa, G. (1981). *This bridge called my back: Writings by radical women of color*. Watertown, MA: Persephone Press.

Morris, M., & Bunjun, B. (2007). *Using intersectional feminist frameworks in research*. Ottawa: Canadian Research Institute for the Advancement of Women.

Morrow, M. (2017). Women and madness revisited: Writing against biopsychiatry. In M. Morrow, & L. Halinka Malcoe (Eds.),

Critical Inquiries for social justice in mental health. University of Toronto Press.

Morrow, M., Bryson, S., & Lal, R. (2019). Intersectionality as an analytic framework for understanding the experiences of mental health stigma among racialized men. *The International Journal of Mental Health & Addiction*.

Morrow, M., Frischmuth, S., & Johnson, A. (2006). *Community based mental health services in BC: Changes to income, employment and housing security*. Vancouver: Canadian Centre for Policy Alternatives.

Morrow, M., & Halinka Malcoe, L. (Eds.). (2017). *Critical inquiries for social justice in mental health*. Toronto: University of Toronto Press.

Morrow, M., Reid, C., Landy, A., et al. (2020). Engaging communities: Intersectional feminist participatory action research. In Morrow, M., Hankivsky, O., Varcoe, C., (Eds.). Women's health in Canada: Critical perspectives on theory and policy (2nd ed.). Toronto: University of Toronto Press.

Morrow, M., Smith, J., Lai, Y., & Jaswal, S. (2008). Shifting landscapes: Immigrant women and post partum depression. *Health Care for Women International, 29*(6), 593–617.

Morrow, M., Wasik, A., Cohen, M., & Perry, K. (2009). Removing barriers to work: Building economic security for people with mental illness. *Critical Social Policy, 29*(4), 655–676.

Morrow, M., Wasik, A., Cormier, R., & Ingram, R. (2013). *Social inequities and mental health: A review of the literature*. Vancouver: Centre for the Study of Gender, Social Inequities and Mental Health.

Morrow, M., & Weisser, J. (2012). Towards a social justice framework of mental health recovery. *Studies in Social Justice, 6*(1). 2012. Available at: https://journals.library.brocku.ca/index.php/SSJ/article/view/1067.

Moth, R. (2020). The business end: Neoliberal policy reforms and biomedical residualism in frontline community mental health practice in England. *Competition and Change, 4*(2), 133–153.

National Audit Office, (2020). Information held by the Department for Work & Pensions on deaths by suicide of benefit claimants. Available at: https://www.nao.org.uk/wp-content/uploads/2020/02/Information-held-by-the-DWP-on-deaths-by-suicide-of-benefit-claimants.pdf.

National Development Team for Inclusion (NDTi). (2018). *Co-production in mental health. Not just another guide*. Available at: https://www.ndti.org.uk/resources/co-production-in-mental-health-not-just-another-guide.

Nilsson, I., & Townsend, E. (2010). Occupational justice- bridging theory and practice. *Scandinavian Journal of Occupational Therapy, 17*, 57–63.

Oliver, M. (1990). *The politics of disablement*. Basingstoke: Macmillan.

Oliver, M., & Barnes, C. (2012). *The new politics of disablement*. Basingstoke: Palgrave McMillan.

O'Mahoney, J., & Donnelly, T. (2007). The influence of culture on immigrant women's mental health care experiences from the perspective of healthcare providers. *Issues in Mental Health Nursing, 28*, 453–471.

Patterson, M., Somers, J., McKintosh, K., Shiell, A., & Frankish, J. (2008). *Housing and support for adults with severe addictions and/or mental illness in British Columbia.* Vancouver: Centre for Applied Research in Mental Health and Addiction.

Pauly, B. (2008). Harm reduction through a social justice lens. *International Journal of Drug Policy, 19*(1), 4–10.

Perlin, M. (2000). *The hidden prejudice: Mental disability on trial.* Washington, DC: American Psychological Association.

Perlin, M. (2003). "You have discussed lepers and crooks": Sanism in clinical teaching. *Clinical Law Review, 9,* 683–729.

Pilgrim, D. (2005). *Key concepts in mental health.* London: SAGE Publications.

Poole, N., & Greaves, L. (Eds.). (2012). *Becoming trauma informed.* Toronto: Centre for Addiction and Mental Health.

Pūras, D. (2017). *UN general assembly. Report of the special rapporteur on the right of everyone to the enjoyment of the highest attainable standard of physical and mental health.* Available at: https://reliefweb.int/sites/reliefweb.int/files/resources/G1707604.pdf.

Recovery in the Bin. (2016). *The unrecovery star.* Available at: https://recoveryinthebin.org/unrecovery-star-2/.

Reynolds, L., & McKee, M. (2012). Any qualified provider" in NHS reforms: But who will qualify? *Lancet, 379*(9821), 1083–1084.

Richards, G. (2008). The changing face of occupational therapy in mental health. In E. A. McKay, C. Craik, K. H. Lim, & G. Richards (Eds.), *Advancing occupational therapy in mental health practice* (pp. 17–29). Oxford: Blackwell Publishing Ltd.

Rose, N. (1989). *Governing the soul: The shaping of the private self.* London: Routledge.

Rossiter, K., & Morrow, M. (2011). Intersectional frameworks in mental health: Moving from theory to practice. In O. Hankivsky (Ed.), *Health inequities in Canada: Intersectional frameworks and practices* (pp. 312–330). Vancouver: UBC Press.

Sayce, L. (2015). *From psychiatric patient to citizen revisited.* Basingstoke: Palgrave.

Scottish Association for Mental Health. (2019). *'It was a confusion'. Universal credit and mental health: Recommendations for change.* Available at: https://www.samh.org.uk/documents/ItWasAConfusionReport_ONLINE_VERSION.pdf.

Selena, E., & Washington (2020). Fostering empowerment through occupation: An overview of an urban school-based parenting program. *Journal of Occupational Science, 27*(2), 182–192. https://doi.org/10.1080/14427591.2020.1731844.

Senior, S. L., Caan, W., & Gamsu, M. (2020). Welfare and well-being: Towards mental health-promoting welfare systems. *British Journal of Psychiatry, 216*(1), 4–5. https://doi.org/10.1192/bjp.2019.242.

Shakespeare, T. (2004). Social models of disability and other life strategies. *Scandinavian Journal of Disability Research, 6*(1), 8–21.

Shim, R., Compton, M., Manseau, M., Kaplan, C., Langheim, F., & Powers, R. (2015). Overview of the social determinants of mental health. In M. Compton, & R. Shim (Eds.), *The social determinants of mental health* (pp. 1–23). Arlington, VA: American Psychiatric Association.

Shimrat, I. (2000). *Call me crazy: Stories from the Mad movement.* Vancouver: Press Gang.

Shorter, E. (2008). *Before prozac: The troubled history of mood disorders in psychiatry.* New York: Oxford Press.

Social Care Institute for Excellence (SCIE). (2015). *Co-production in social care. Guide 51.* Available at: https://www.scie.org.uk/publications/guides/guide51/.

Stadnyk, R., Townsend, E. A., & Wilcock, A. (2010). Occupational justice. In C. H. Christiansen, & E. A. Townsend (Eds.), *Introduction to occupation: The Art and science of living* (2nd ed.) (pp. 329–358). Upper Saddle River, NJ: Prentice Hall.

Standing Senate Committee on Social Affairs, Science and Technology. (2009). *Out of the shadows at last: Transforming mental health, mental illness and addiction services in Canada. Final report of the standing senate committee on social Affairs, science and Technology.*

Summerfield, D. (2001). The invention of post-traumatic stress disorder and the social usefulness of a psychiatric category. *British Medical Journal, 322*(7278), 95–98.

Sy, M. P., & Ohshima, N. (2019). Utilising the occupational justice health questionnaire (OJHQ) with a Filipino drug surrenderee in occupational therapy practice: A case report. *World Federation of Occupational Therapists Bulletin, 75*(1), 59–62. https://doi.org/10.1080/14473828.2018.1505682.

Szasz, T. (1961). *The myth of mental illness: Foundations of a theory of personal conduct.* London: Harper & Row.

Thew, M., Bell, F., & Flanagan, E. (2017). Social prescribing: An emerging area for occupational therapy. *British Journal of Occupational Therapy, 80*(9), 523–524.

Townsend, E. (2003). Reflections on power and justice in enabling occupation. *Canadian Journal of Occupational Therapy, 70*(2), 74–87.

Townsend, E., & Marval, R. (2013). Can professionals actually enable occupational justice? *Cadernos de Terapia Ocupacional da UFSCar, 21*(2), 215–228.

Townsend, E., & Wilcock, A. (2004). Occupational justice and client-centred practice: A dialogue in progress. *Canadian Journal of Occupational Therapy, 72*(2), 75–87.

United Nations. (n.d.). Convention on the rights of persons with disabilities (CRPD). Available at: https://www.un.org/development/desa/disabilities/convention-on-the-rights-of-persons-with-disabilities.html.

U'Ren, R. (2011). *Social perspective: The missing element in mental health practice.* Toronto: University of Toronto Press.

Ussher, J. (1991). *Women's madness: Misogyny or mental illness?* Amherst: The University of Massachusetts Press.

Ussher, J. M. (2011). *The madness of women: Myth and experience.* London: Routledge.

Ussher, J., & Perz, J. (2017). Is it normal or PMS? Women's strategies in negotiating and resisting negative premenstrual change. In M. Morrow, & L. Halinka Malcoe (Eds.), *Critical inquiries for social justice in mental health* (pp. 197–228). Toronto: University of Toronto Press.

van Mens-Verhulst, J., & Radtke, L. (2008). *Intersectionality and mental health: A case study IST-travelling.* Available at: http://www.vanmens.info/verhulst/en/wp-content/INTERSECTIONALITY%20AND%20MENTAL%20HEALTH2.pdf.

Voronka, J. (2017). Turning mad knowledge into affective labour: The case of the peer support worker. *American Quarterly, 69*(2), 333–338.

Warner, L. R. (2008). A best practices guide to intersectional approaches in psychological research. *Sex Roles, 59*, 454–463.

Watters, E. (2010). *Crazy like us: The globalization of the American psyche*. New York: Simon & Schuster.

Whitehead, M., Dahlgren, C. (2006). *Concepts and principles for tackling social inequities in health*. Geneva: WHO. https://www.euro.who.int/__data/assets/pdf_file/0010/74737/E89383.pdf.

World Federation of Occupational Therapists (WFOT). (2019). *Position statement. Occupational therapy and human rights (revised)*. Available at: https://wfot.org/resources/occupational-therapy-and-human-rights.

Zinman, S., & The Harp, H. (1994). *Reaching across II: Maintaining our roots*. Sacramento, CA: California Network of Mental Health Clients.

Zinman, S., The Harp, H., & Budd, S. (1987). *Reaching across: Mental health clients helping each other*. Sacramento, CA: California Network of Mental Health Clients.

Section 4 OCCUPATIONS

13 PHYSICAL ACTIVITY

FIONA COLE

INTRODUCTION

This chapter explores physical activity and its proven health benefits. It considers various factors that influence service users' engagement in physical activity (including the meaning ascribed to certain activities) and wider contextual and global factors influencing people's ability to be physically active, such as social and occupational injustices. This occupational perspective aims to develop understanding of the rationale for incorporating physical activity within mental health practice and an appreciation of factors to consider when planning individual and group programmes.

The evidence base for physical activity within contemporary mental health practice is unequivocal.

Research from a wide range of disciplines, including medicine, sports and exercise sciences, psychology and public health, shows that exercise and physical activity are both important aspects of mental health promotion and a therapeutic intervention for people with mental health difficulties (Biddle et al. 2015).

PHYSICAL ACTIVITY, MENTAL HEALTH AND WELLBEING

The value of physical activity in promoting health and wellbeing is firmly on national and global agendas. The World Health Organization (WHO; 2018a) and national governmental organizations such as the

UK's Department of Health, Physical Activity, Health Improvement and Protection (2011) promote the potential preventative and therapeutic influence of physical activity regarding mental health difficulties and long-term physical conditions, such as cardiovascular disease, obesity, diabetes, musculoskeletal problems and cancer. Additionally, such guidance highlights the substantial negative impact (on both individual and population-level health) of an inactive, sedentary lifestyle. Indeed, as the Chief Medical Officer for England (Department of Health (DH) 2010, p. 21) has noted, 'the potential health benefits of physical activity are huge. If a medication existed which had a similar effect, it would be regarded as a wonder drug or miracle cure.'

Occupational therapy's focus on 'doing' and occupational science's specifically occupational perspective of health (Wilcock and Hocking 2015) means occupational therapists are well equipped to enable people to become more physically active, addressing individual and societal health concerns. Occupational therapy also has a strong legacy of using physical activity therapeutically, particularly within psychiatric institutions. This was initially based on the intuitive, practice-based reasoning that activities such as sports, dancing and horticulture improved mental well-being (Wilcock 2001).

The Nature of Physical Activity

Caspersen et al.'s (1985) definition of physical activity as 'any bodily movement produced by skeletal muscles that results in energy expenditure' (p. 126) is still used in guidance from the UK's Chief Medical Officers (Department of Health and Social Care (DHSC) 2019) and WHO (2018a). The emphasis on 'physical activity' (as distinct from 'exercise') in health policy and guidance is significant because it is broader and more inclusive, encompassing not only sports and leisure activities but also the physical activities embedded in day-to-day occupations related to employment, housework, do-it-yourself (DIY), gardening, or travel to school or work, for example (Table 13.1 for terminology and activity examples).

In promoting physical activity, it would seem useful to know 'how much is enough?', but, as with any occupational therapy intervention, the beneficial effect depends on many individual and contextual factors (Pentland et al. 2018). Nevertheless, the health benefits appear to be proportional to the overall amount of physical activity a person does. This is important for therapists using a graded approach to interventions because every increase in activity adds some benefit (DHSC 2019). WHO (2010) guidelines for physical activity are universally recognized and foundational for national policies. For example, in the United Kingdom, to achieve a range of physical and mental health benefits and to reduce the risk of ill-health, the 'headline' figure is that adults and older adults should do at least 150 minutes of moderate-intensity aerobic physical activity a week, and children and young people at

TABLE 13.1
Summary of Activity Terminology

	Definition of Activity	
Physical activity	Any bodily movement produced by skeletal muscles that results in energy expenditure (Casperson et al. 1985; UK Chief Medical Officers 2019). This includes all activities from everyday lifestyle through to competitive sports.	Increasing intensity of effort
Lifestyle physical activity	Activities incorporated into everyday life (e.g., walking or cycling to school, work, or shopping; dog walking; heavy housework or do-it-yourself work; gardening, physically demanding jobs) (Public Health England 2014; WHO 2018).	
Exercise	Activity which is volitional, planned, structured, repetitive and aimed at improvement or maintenance of any aspect of fitness or health (Caspersen et al. 1985; UK Chief Medical Officers 2019) (e.g., swimming, running, gym activities, weight training).	
Sport	Activity which is rule-governed, structured, competitive and requires physical prowess (e.g., athletics, football, hockey). Not all sport is health-enhancing (e.g., darts) (Biddle et al. 2015).	
There is possible overlap between these categories.		

least 60 minutes a day. Additionally, regarding support for individuals to become more active, the UK governments' DHSC (2019) stated 'some is good, more is better' (p. 13). Furthermore, options for achieving this are increased by assurances that benefits accrue from including several periods of activity, each with a duration of approximately 10 minutes. Additional requirements and examples of activities are given in Table 13.2.

Providing options that include the total amount and/or intensity of activity gives more choice when incorporating physical activity into people's daily lives. Moderate intensity physical activity has been found to offer considerable health gains, particularly to those least fit, and is less likely to incur health risks for those unacquainted with exercise (DHSC 2019). Evidence suggests that, for people with severe mental health difficulties, low to moderate intensity physical activities such as walking are preferred and that these can boost confidence and self-efficacy (Subramaniapillai et al. 2016). In the United Kingdom these guidelines were updated in 2019 (DHSC 2019) to reflect emergent

evidence for the health benefits of a very vigorous type of activity known as 'high intensity interval exercise' (HIIT), which includes running upstairs or pedalling extremely fast on a fitness bike in very short bursts. This guidance also emphasized activities for building muscle strength and bone development in children and for countering the natural decline in muscle mass and bone density for those over 50 years old.

Activity targets were deemed to be achievable by many governmental organizations worldwide. However, audits of participation rates and ongoing concerns about population health related to physical inactivity challenge their usefulness. Worldwide 23% of adults and 81% of adolescents (aged 11–17 years) did not meet the global recommendations for physical activity in 2016 (WHO 2018a). In England in 2018, 27% of adults were classed as inactive; that is, they engaged in less than 30 minutes of activity per week and were at risk of ill-health (Health and Social Care Information Centre 2019). Indeed, activity levels may be even lower due to potential underestimation when self-reporting (Kapteyn et al. 2018).

TABLE 13.2
UK Chief Medical Officers' Physical Activity Guidelines (DHSC 2019)

Age Group	Recommended Amounts and Examples of Activity Per Week			
Children and young people	At least 60 minutes spread throughout every day. All activities should increase breathing rate and generate a feeling of warmth (e.g., play, run, skate, skip, climb, dance, physical education at school, cycle, sports and active travel).			
Adults	Moderate intensity physical activity, 150 min/wk. (Increased heart and breathing rates but still able to talk; increased feeling of warmth, possibly sweating). Brisk walking, swimming, cycling, heavier gardening such as digging, dancing, sports such as walking or football.	OR a combination of moderate and vigorous intensities.	Vigorous intensity physical activity, 75 min/wk. (Heart rate feels rapid, breathing fast, difficulty holding a conversation). Running, uphill cycling, aerobic fitness classes, spin cycling, sports such as football, hockey, squash	Strengthening activities for muscles, bones and joints twice weekly. The large muscle groups of the body – legs, hips, chest, abdomen, shoulders and arms – work or hold against a force or weight. Muscles will feel fatigued and, if using structured weight training, then exercised to the point where it is a struggle to complete another repetition. Gym, home exercises, yoga, carrying heavy shopping.
Older adults	As for adults but with additional balance activities to reduce chance of frailty/falls (e.g., tai chi, bowling, dance).			
Adults with disabilities	Moderate intensity activity 150 min/wk. Strengthening and balance activities twice weekly.			
Any activity is better than none, therefore light-intensity activities still contribute to health and mental wellbeing, for example, gardening, housework, do-it-yourself work, walking to school or work.				

Furthermore, Warburton and Bredin (2017) suggested that the physical activity targets may be unachievable for inactive people and thus become a barrier in themselves. This may also apply to people managing mental health difficulties. Their conclusion, and that of the WHO and the UK's DH, is that any physical activity is better than none. These statistics relate to the general population, but within this, there are notable variations. For example, teenage girls, people with disabilities and long-term health conditions, socioeconomically disadvantaged groups and those from some minority ethnic groups have been identified as having lower participation rates (WHO 2018a). Additionally, there is limited data regarding participation rates specifically for people with mental health difficulties. For example, a Sport England (2018a) survey showed that 69% of people who self-identified as having a mental health difficulty said they had done 'no activity' over the previous 28 days. International evidence concurs with a similar percentage of people with major depression not meeting physical activity recommendations and leading more sedentary lives (Schuch et al. 2017). Furthermore, even if targets are met, sedentary behaviour (particularly sitting) is a well-evidenced risk factor for ill-health, particularly cardiovascular disorders and cancer (DHSC 2019). Consequently, a sedentary lifestyle may be additional obstacles to overcome when, for example, experiencing motivational challenges through mental health problems.

Research is more equivocal about the direction of causality between sedentary behaviour and psychological well-being. Although it does seem that people with poor mental health are more likely to choose sedentary pursuits (Biddle et al. 2015; Schuch et al. 2017), the nature of certain sitting activities (e.g., sustained use of computers, excessive screen time surfing the web and participation in chat rooms) may be a risk factor for low mood (Biddle et al. 2015). The influence of social media is a concern, particularly for young people's mental health. A large-scale study by Kelly et al. (2018) reported links between increased time using social media and poor sleep, leading to depressive symptoms, and between online harassment, low self-esteem and poor body image. The complex relationships between types of activity (physical and sedentary) and wellbeing reinforces the need for therapists to understand service users' occupational choices.

For occupational therapists, whose holism leads them to address both physical *and* mental health needs, awareness of the negative health implications of inactivity and the health benefits of activity highlights the value of health promotion. However, some mental health service users caution that, although becoming more active is widely regarded as a sign of personal recovery, service providers' emphasis on 'being active' can feel paternalistic, reflecting a moral belief in the corrective benefits of 'activity' (see Chapter 10). Clearly, there is a risk that rigid adherence to activity guidelines might reinforce this sense of being morally judged, triggering resistance. It also, arguably, conflicts with the person-centredness of occupational therapy. Interpretation of official activity guidelines must therefore take account of individuals' occupational needs, abilities and preferences.

The Health Benefits of Physical Activity

This section examines the relationships between physical activity and mental health and wellbeing but starts with an exploration of physical health issues emphasizing occupational therapy's holism. Evidence tends to be structured according to diagnoses, but occupational therapy does not operate within such delineations, focusing more on tackling problems in living (Szaz 1972).

Physical Health

Improving the physical health of people with enduring mental health difficulties is one of the four recommendations in the UK's Royal College of Occupational Therapists' (RCOT 2018) campaign to promote mental health and wellbeing. This drive responds to data showing increased incidence of serious physical health concerns such as coronary heart and respiratory diseases, type II diabetes and obesity. Significantly, the Scottish government (2017) stated that 'it is unacceptable that people with severe and enduring mental illness may have their lives shortened by 15 to 20 years because of physical ill-health. This is a significant health inequality' (p. 29). Consequently, the Scottish government committed to supporting programmes to increase levels of physical activity so that people live longer, healthier lives.

From a physical health perspective the risk of depression is higher for people with diabetes, hypertension, coronary artery disease, stroke, renal failure and chronic obstructive pulmonary disease (Mitchell 2017). Furthermore, in recognition of the frequent inequality between mental and physical health service provision and the proven links between physical and mental ill-health, the UK's Health and Social Care Act (2012) enshrined the principle of 'parity of esteem,' whereby mental and physical healthcare services should have equal priority.

In short, physical activity can be used to address both physical and mental health difficulties, and occupational therapists have the skills, knowledge, and evidence base to work with individuals across both domains.

Impact on Mood, Self-Esteem and Anxiety

Evidence indicates that there is a 20% to 30% lower risk of developing depression (and dementia) amongst adults who participate in daily physical activity. The National Institute for Health and Care Excellence (NICE 2009) recommended physical activity as an intervention for people with mild to moderate depression, specifying that physical activity programmes should be delivered in groups by a 'competent practitioner' (NICE 2011, p. 13). This NICE quality standard is supported by the UK's RCOT, which states that occupational therapists can fulfil this practitioner role provided they engage in supervision and are flexible regarding collaboration with other physical activity specialists. When assessing an individual's interests with a view to commencing a programme, it should be acknowledged that depression can limit the personal satisfaction derived from activities that the individual once enjoyed. It may also influence individuals' accounts of what they once liked doing, even when previous enjoyment was considerable. Graded re-engagement can thus be a powerful intervention because the experience of doing something is often different to the idea, or memory, of doing it.

Biddle et al. (2015) concluded that physical activity can be used to promote physical self-worth and other positive physical self-perceptions related to body image, competence and fitness, for example, which may be beneficial for people with low mood and low self-esteem. These self-perceptions strongly correlate with individuals' subjective sense of mental wellbeing and quality of life. Conversely, perceptions of inadequacy in performing physical activities can lower self-esteem,

highlighting the importance of grading and/or pacing to establish the 'just right challenge' (Yerxa 1998) that is integral to occupational therapy.

Regarding work with people experiencing anxiety, Remes et al.'s (2016) systematic review concluded that, globally, anxiety is the most prevalent mental health condition, especially in the west, and is also a risk factor for other conditions such as mood disorders, substance misuse and physical problems, particularly cardiovascular disease. Being physically active can reduce anxiety symptoms and promote additional psychological benefits such as improved self-esteem and self-efficacy (Kandola et al. 2018). Additionally, since anxiety and depression often coexist, the authors emphasized the overall influence of physical activity on mood and wellbeing. Physical activity may have a small to moderate effect on non-clinical anxiety (that is, for individuals not needing mental health services) and may also reduce long-term vulnerability to anxiety (Biddle et al. 2015). Additionally, low levels of physical activity (Stubbs et al. 2017) and high levels of sedentary behaviour (Teychenne et al. 2015) are associated with increased prevalence of anxiety, suggesting that physical activity has a preventative effect. Both reports are inconclusive about the mechanisms underlying these effects, but an occupational therapist may interpret these positive influences on anxiety as being due to improved occupational performance and engagement in meaningful activities (Creek 2010; Townsend and Polatajko 2013; Roberts and Bannigan 2019).

This standpoint is essential in distinguishing an occupational perspective of physical activity's positive impact on health, which may be minimized or even omitted from purely physiological perspectives. It is important that this holistic (as in 'whole system') perspective is maintained by occupational therapists when collaborating with other professionals to deliver physical activity-orientated programmes.

The educational aspect of the therapist's role may be particularly important regarding the physiological consequences of physical activity, such as breathing changes, perspiration and increased heart rate, which can be similar to the experience of anxiety itself. These experiences may be distressing if not understood or expected. Therefore guidance on the intensity of physical exercise needs to be carefully tailored to avoid misinterpretations that exercise aggravates anxiety

(Lam et al. 2016). Again, careful grading of the activities' intensity within an occupational therapy programme is the key to maintaining participation.

COGNITIVE HEALTH AND ACTIVE AGING

For older people, increasing physical activity improves cardiovascular fitness, strength, and physical function. It also reduces aspects of cognitive decline (including the risk of dementia), lowers susceptibility to falls and can improve self-esteem and mood (Park et al. 2014). Livingston et al. (2017) reported that older adults who exercise are more likely to maintain cognition than those who are inactive and that high levels of exercise are the most protective against cognitive decline. The authors also noted the link between the number of depressive episodes in older people and the risk of dementia, highlighting the significance of physical activity in preventing and managing these conditions. Therapists working in mental health or frailty and falls services may frequently encounter older people who have fallen and have physical rehabilitation needs and associated anxieties. Guidelines are clear about the role of physical activity in reducing the risk of falls and in regaining strength, balance and coordination (DHSC 2019).

Additionally, occupational therapists' skills in enabling participation in meaningful activities such as social groups involving physical activity may also improve people's confidence and address anxieties about returning to activity after a fall.

LIVING WITH PSYCHOSIS

Psychoses can have a major impact on individuals' occupational functioning and quality of life, and, although medication is commonly prescribed to address positive symptoms, such as delusions, hallucinations and thought disorders, it has little influence on (and may even exacerbate) negative symptoms such as lethargy, flattening of affect, social withdrawal and general lack of interest in activities.

Gorczynski and Faulkner (2010) concluded that exercise significantly improved negative symptoms and that clinicians should encourage service users to become more active. Holley et al. (2011) reviewed qualitative studies on the role of physical activity on psychological well-being, finding improvements in perceptions of autonomy, competence, social interest, psychological and physical health and overall self-concept. Similar outcomes were confirmed from an occupational therapy football programme for people living with psychosis (Moloney and Rohde 2017) in addition to the impact on wider occupational functioning such as re-engagement with valued life roles. People living with psychosis may also experience depression and anxiety so the beneficial effects of physical activity in relation to these difficulties, as noted above, may equally apply.

People living with psychosis often face stigma and social, occupational and economic deprivation that may preclude access to community resources. Smyth et al. (2011) reported that weight gain associated with neuroleptic medication may also cause individuals to feel more self-conscious and uncomfortable when out in public. These factors compound the difficulties of managing health-related lifestyle issues, such as poor diet, smoking and physical inactivity. A graded approach within occupational therapy that first builds confidence in the home (for example, via one of the many free online exercise, yoga or dance videos) could then progress towards more social and/or community-based activities.

POPULATION HEALTH AND SUSTAINABILITY WITHIN OCCUPATIONAL THERAPY

A public or population-level perspective of health within occupational therapy has been espoused since the emergence of occupational science (see Wilcock 1998), yet its potential has yet to be fully realized, despite repeated calls for an occupational perspective of health promotion (see Wilcock and Hocking 2015).

At a societal level, a more physically active population contributes to the wider sustainability agenda because communities will tend to have reduced fossil fuel use, cleaner air, reduced congestion and safer roads (WHO 2018b). WHO promotes physical activities such as walking, cycling, active recreation, sports and play as contributing to the United Nations 2030 Agenda for Sustainable Development (United Nations 2015) and a more equitable, sustainable and prosperous world. Furthermore, the World Federation of Occupational Therapists encourages therapists and students to use their knowledge about occupations to address such environmental sustainability challenges. For example, Turcotte and Drolet (2020) asserted that because climate change is mainly due to human occupation, therapists should be 'change agents in reshaping the interactions between people, their occupations, and environments' (p. 171). If encouraging individuals and groups to be physically active within their communities also positively influences other changes such as reducing fossil fuel use (through walking or cycling), sourcing locally produced food and reusing/recycling, then this is an important contribution to global issues. As the Global Advocacy Council for Physical Activity (GAPA 2010, p. 370) states,

Physical activity promotes well-being, physical and mental health, prevents disease, improves social connectedness and quality of life, provides economic benefits and contributes to environmental sustainability.

Concepts such as social connectedness, quality of life and environmental sustainability—as noted in the Toronto Charter for Physical Activity (GAPA 2010) above—are becoming increasingly prominent within occupational therapy. Many group or collective occupations can be facilitated using physical activities that promote social connectedness and a sense of belonging that add to the positivity of the overall experience (Kantartzis 2017).

Additionally, Gerlach et al. (2017) assert that individualism within practice assumes that people have autonomy over their occupations, but socio-economic, political and funding contexts may preclude access to services for certain groups of people, limiting their occupational choices. For example, Hartley et al. (2017) identified that government policies restricting access to work and study contributed to social exclusion of asylum seekers from mainstream community activities. These wide-ranging and systemic issues are consistent with the drive within occupational therapy to respond to global movements of people and population level needs (Wilcock and Hocking 2015). Significantly, in Hartley et al.'s (2017) study, engagement in physical activity, such as going to a subsidized gym or walking, benefitted mental and physical health, built social capital and became a means of structuring time; an important consideration in relation to occupationally deprived living.

These global developments present challenges, arguably, to the orthodoxy of conventional 'individualist' occupational therapy with its focus on independence. For students and practitioners alike this perspective presents an opportunity to future-proof professional reasoning and ensure knowledge and skills continue to be valued and relevant. For example, Hammell (2009) has challenged the often-cited classification of occupations as being either self-care, productivity or leisure. She has, instead, recommended consideration of occupations that foster belonging and collaboration and those valued for their social context and potential to strengthen social roles, thus contributing to the well-being of the person and others. It could be said that events raising money for charities, for example, in the United Kingdom, the Race for Life, the Great North Run, the London Marathon and innumerable others, motivate people to become physically active, facilitate social connectedness and promote a sense of social contribution and belonging.

INFLUENCING MENTAL HEALTH AND WELLBEING THROUGH PHYSICAL ACTIVITY

Although evidence for the positive effects of physical activity on mental health is conclusive, the precise biochemical and physiological mechanisms underpinning this phenomenon are still the subject of much debate. Occupational therapists may find it helpful to have some basic knowledge in this area should service users be interested, such as the pleasurable effect of increased endorphins during exercise and physiological changes affecting serotonin receptors, which positively influence mood and/or anxiety.

Kandola et al. (2019) summarized the effects of physical activity relating to improved neuroplasticity in regions of the brain adversely affected by depression, anti-inflammatory properties and improved functioning of the neuro-endocrine system. For a detailed discussion regarding the mechanisms associated with the efficacy of physical activity, see Ekkekakis (2013) and Biddle et al. (2015).

Clearly, a holistic, whole person-centred perspective has a broader focus than simply exploring explanatory biochemical/physiological mechanisms for reducing the symptoms of mental health problems. To appreciate an occupational perspective it is especially important to understand the relationships between psychosocial factors and wellbeing within the contexts of diverse environments.

Psychosocial and Socio-Economic Influences

Importantly, being more physically active, rather than fitness itself, has been shown to improve short-term and long-term mental well-being (DHSC 2011). Since it is not essential to focus on the aerobic or strength effects of training, individuals therefore have greater choice of options to be physically active, with likely benefits including a sense of achievement, satisfaction and self-determination and greater self-confidence in physical abilities (Biddle et al. 2015). Again, this supports an occupational therapy perspective in that engagement in meaningful activities involves a feeling of choice or control, a sense of challenge (and of challenge being met) and an awareness of personal agency (Pentland et al. 2018).

This concept of engagement is important to understand when working with people to establish physical activity goals; that is, it is essential to explore not just the 'doing' of the activity but how individuals think and feel about it and what the whole experience means to them (Hasselkus 2011). It is essential that all features of engagement are considered; those relating to the person, the occupation and the context for the activity (Pentland et al. 2018), thereby activating the full range of psychosocial mechanisms which influence wellbeing. Knowledge of these phenomena and of their complex interactions underpins occupational therapists' harnessing of physical activity as a wholly transformative experience for service users in mental health practice.

Physical activity levels are also influenced by inequalities in opportunity (Public Health England 2014). From a global perspective, girls; women; older adults; those of low socio-economic status or rural communities and people with long-term health problems have fewer opportunities to access safe, affordable and appropriate programmes and places in which to be physically active (WHO 2018a). Such occupational injustices (Hocking 2017) may also be relevant and even exacerbated, where individuals move and settle in different cultures, such as refugees and asylum seekers might do. Difficulties with communication and in gaining employment can have a severe impact on financial independence and can also affect self-esteem, mood and motivation to participate in physical activities (Hartley et al. 2017).

This kind of occupational injustice also applies to the expanding population of homeless people and others with mental health difficulties living in poverty (Illman et al. 2013; Boland 2019). Lower levels of physical activity are associated with low socio-economic status, long-term health conditions, social exclusion and marginalization, geographical isolation (such as in rural communities) and limited access to resources (WHO 2018a). Clearly, this highlights the importance of practitioners' cultural sensitivity when supporting people to participate in activities as part of an overall awareness of the environmental context.

Environmental Influences

Occupational therapists recognize the physical and social environments as determinants in people's occupational engagement. Consequently, exploring the interaction between 'place' and 'activity' is important in understanding people's physical activity aspirations. Similarly, practitioners' consideration of social and environmental influences may enable them to identify and overcome barriers and challenges that individuals may face as they become more physically active.

Exercising in groups or with a supportive family member or friend can enhance attitude and mood, reflecting people's fundamental need for interpersonal attachment. For example, Carless and Douglas (2008) explored how social support was important for men with severe mental health problems when initiating and maintaining exercise. Significantly, a lack of social support was highly correlated with physical inactivity amongst participants who were diagnosed with bipolar disorder or schizophrenia.

A substantial body of literature highlights the value of physical activity in promoting wellbeing, such as by bringing people together socially; fostering feelings of connectedness, belonging, inclusion, mutual acceptance and support; and underlining the value of shared experiences. For example, Borges da Costa (2016) explored the meaning of circle dance to participants and demonstrated its impact on their mental wellbeing through it being both an individual and a shared occupation, particularly regarding the key element of it being performed in a circle, which developed social relationships, belonging, a sense of community and social integration. Similarly, social environmental influences are evident in Alexandratos et al.'s (2012) review of exercise in general, in Mynard et al.'s (2009) study on Australian football rules, in Feighan and Roberts' (2017) analysis of identity and the meaning of cycling, in Christie and Cole's (2017) study of conservation work and in Whatley et al.'s (2015) exploration of community gardening. Significantly, both Christie and Cole (2017) and Whatley et al. (2017) noted that the social context for the activity was characterized by blurred boundaries between staff and participants due to the collaborative nature of the activities, which felt more inclusive. The democratizing nature of the activities whereby people expressed shared interests through non-stigmatizing occupations was similarly noted in reviews of horticulture-based interventions by York and Wiseman (2012) and Genter et al. (2015). Nature-based interventions are discussed in Chapter 19.

Although certain physical activity-based occupations are highly suitable for fostering community integration and inclusiveness through the creation of move-on pathways into the mainstream of society, for example, it is important to remember that some service users prefer, and (arguably) need, to be engaged within supportive mental health settings. Socially inclusive practice must accommodate individuals at all points on a social inclusion continuum, ranging from those with high level support needs to those able to attend community-based groups (Parkinson et al. 2011).

BECOMING PHYSICALLY ACTIVE AND MAINTAINING INVOLVEMENT

The initiation, maintenance, and resumption of many health-promoting behaviours, including being physically active, is rarely easy, especially when compounded by the effects of mental health difficulties. Complex biological, psychological, social, cultural and environmental factors influence participation (Biddle et al. 2015), highlighting the challenge of understanding each individual's unique support needs to enable engagement.

Motivating Factors for Change

Biddle et al. (2015) suggest that intrinsic motivation is vital to sustaining involvement in exercise; that is, doing something for its own sake because of the in-built incentives, and in the absence of external (extrinsic) rewards or pressures. Enjoyment, social contact, satisfaction and sense of achievement motivate engagement, as do feelings of self-control or self-determination, as described earlier. In contrast, *extrinsic* motivation usually occurs through pressures originating outside the individual's control, such as paternalistic or authoritarian messages telling people to exercise because they are overweight or because 'it's good for you.' Nonetheless, if these external pressures were to be removed, it is likely that people's motivation would decline in the absence of any intrinsic interest. Indeed, as occupational therapists are aware, the value that individuals ascribe to an activity influences their commitment to it (Creek 2010). The challenge for therapists is therefore to work with the individual to identify intrinsically motivating factors that prompt engagement. This may require ingenuity because, for example, people with depression may have difficulty recalling the intrinsic motivator of enjoyment because of a loss of pleasure in life (Glowacki et al. 2017; Mental Health Foundation 2018).

Enabling 'Doing': Differentiating Between Participation and Engagement

Service users may wish to increase participation in physical activity because a particular form of exercise meets their needs and carries personal meaning and value. Considering the categories of self-care, productivity and leisure (Townsend and Polatajko 2013) for example, a particular physical activity may fall into one or more of these. A dancer may engage in Pilates exercises as a self-care activity to improve flexibility and control, a postal worker may build up walking tolerance to return to work and a group of friends may go cycling for leisure at the weekend. These (physically active) occupations have intrinsic value and carry social, cultural, symbolic and spiritual significance for the individuals concerned (Creek 2010).

According to Pierce (2001), valuing the individual's subjective experiences of occupation and the context in which it takes place helps to differentiate between occupation and activity. Understanding this distinction can be influential because person-centred goals (regarding *occupations*) can focus on overcoming occupational performance difficulties; the individual's drive to engage being comparatively strong because of the significance the occupation has in their lives. However, regarding more generic physical activity, which (because it is not an occupation) may not carry the same personal meaning, the degree of motivation to overcome barriers to participation is likely to be less. An individual may still wish to participate to some degree because they are aware of potential benefits or perhaps because participation will enable them to achieve other occupational goals (for example, walking or cycling to work), but this is a different kind of motivation. Essentially, echoing Pierce's (2001) terminology, this chapter therefore differentiates between participation in a physical activity and engagement in a physically active occupation.

With this distinction in mind, occupational therapists are attuned to the ambiguity in the term 'physical activity.' For some people a 'physical activity' is indeed merely an activity; that is, 'a structured series of actions or tasks that contribute to occupations' (Creek 2010, p. 74). An example of this might be walking to the university to engage in the occupation of attending a lecture. For others, 'physical occupations' would be a more accurate term, as used to describe playing in the university netball team, for example. An exploration of these nuanced perspectives is warranted because it can assist therapists to collaborate with service users in setting goals.

Recognizing the participation/engagement distinction implicitly involves therapists' professional reasoning regarding the role of choice in what people do. On the one hand, because an active lifestyle confers inherent health benefits, people in the United Kingdom are urged to achieve weekly physical activity levels recommended by the government (DHSC 2019). In this context the choice to be physically active—a dimension of occupation that is so fundamental—may be minimal. Becoming more active in this way may feel like an obligation, in other words. On the other hand, many people make occupational choices to cycle, dance, swim or garden, for example, because of the value, meaning and purpose they ascribe to it; that is, due to the nature of the occupation itself.

A Lifestyle Approach to Participation

Lifestyle change is fundamental to occupational therapy and, for those whose occupational identity does not include being physically active but who nevertheless want to improve their mental and physical well-being, a lifestyle approach to participation can be adopted. Incorporating physical activity within everyday routines (see Table 13.1) avoids the necessity of finding time and resources to do additional, specific exercise-orientated activities. A key aim for lifestyle physical activities is that participation becomes habituated within daily routines (Lee and Kielhofner 2017a). The vignette in Box 13.1 describing Claude's walking illustrates this.

The UK's Chief Medical Officers (DH 2011) recommended a lifestyle approach such as this because 'for most people, the easiest and most acceptable forms of physical activity are those that can be incorporated into everyday life. Examples include walking or cycling instead of travelling by car, bus or train' (p. 17).

A whole-person occupational therapy approach addressing people's lifestyles is supported by evidence from other disciplines indicating that physical activity within an overall healthier lifestyle (that is, low alcohol

---

BOX 13.1

CLAUDE: A LIFESTYLE APPROACH TO PARTICIPATION

Claude is 35 years old and has been living with schizophrenia since his late teens. He lives independently with community mental health team support. His occupational goals are to return to college and resume his interest in computer science, which was interrupted with the onset of psychosis. Claude also wants to improve his overall health and wellbeing and acknowledges a need for more physical activity.

However, Claude is not interested in exercise as such, and his attempts at participating in an exercise referral scheme (see Rowley et al. 2018) were unsuccessful because he felt he did not fit into the group sessions within the sports centre environment and could not overcome his associated anxieties about attending. The occupational therapist, in collaboration with Claude, recognizes that a lifestyle approach to incorporating walking within his day-to-day activities might be more realistic.

The therapist's professional reasoning suggests that, whilst walking has only minimal intrinsic value for Claude, it still enables him to improve his health and wellbeing and contribute to achieving wider occupational goals. Incorporating walking into Claude's occupational engagement (in shopping and going to college, for example) enhances his subjective sense of wellbeing and contributes to his overall recovery.

It is anticipated that, ultimately, Claude may come to enjoy walking for its intrinsic value, as an added benefit, but this is not the initial intervention goal.

consumption, not smoking, good sleep quality and diet) is associated with enhanced wellbeing (Haapasalo et al. 2018; Martin et al. 2020). Furthermore, this occupation-focused approach is shown to work well in promoting physical activity for people living with psychosis, where activity goals must be realistic and instrumental in helping individuals pursue meaningful occupations in their lives (Holley et al. 2011).

An Occupational Approach to Engagement

The vignette in Box 13.2 details a contrasting occupational approach to physical activity used with Katrina who is intrinsically motivated through her enjoyment of physical activity for its own sake. It illustrates some important considerations, namely, how a negative physical self-perception can be a barrier to participation in activities where one's body is publicly visible (Biddle et al. 2015) and how a cognitive-behavioural approach to increasing physical activity may complement an occupational approach which, on its own, may be insufficient. It may be necessary, for example, to foster a lift in a person's mood as a prelude to their engagement (Cole 2010).

Supporting Technologies

Whilst digital media and energy-saving technologies may contribute to sedentary lifestyles (Teychenne et al. 2015), these resources can also support people to become more physically active. Organizations such as the NHS in the United Kingdom, Public Health England and international researchers such as Schoeppe et al. (2016) have acknowledged the potential of fitness watches, smart phones and health apps to encourage, motivate, reward and increase physical activity (Romeo et al. 2019).

There are various perspectives regarding how these technologies may be incorporated within an occupational therapy programme. Most simply, apps can be an extension of activity diaries, as used with Katrina (Box 13.2). The immediacy and convenience of an app which records a person's activity and then asks 'how was it?' or 'how did you feel?', or shows a map of a walk, perhaps, can provide feedback that can be referred to later if motivation is low. Alternatively, apps can support the application of core skills, such as grading and pacing of activities (College of Occupational Therapists (COT) 2015) when working towards physical activity goals. For example, the UK NHS's 'Couch to 5k' podcast app (NHS 2020) (listened to on headphones whilst active three times weekly over nine weeks) coaches people from a few minutes of walking to running 5 km. Music, instructions and an encouraging voice talking directly to the listener support their participation and progress.

The value of apps varies according to people's needs. Alerts can be set on devices to remind and prompt

---

BOX 13.2

KATRINA: AN OCCUPATIONAL APPROACH TO ENGAGEMENT

Katrina is 35 years old, married, with two children (aged 8 and 10) and has intermittently experienced depression throughout her adult life. This has been exacerbated by a 6-month absence from work due to chronic back pain, initially triggered by an incident in her job as a home care support worker. In addition to low mood, Katrina is increasingly anxious about meeting people and is becoming socially isolated at home.

The occupational therapist uses the Model of Human Occupation (Taylor 2017) and the Occupational Self-Assessment (OSA; Baron et al. 1998) because it allows people to indicate personal values and set priorities for therapy (Kramer et al. 2017). This helps Katrina who, when depressed, feels powerless and unable to change. She wants to reintroduce physical activity into her lifestyle to enjoy it for its own sake and to help with managing her back pain but, although she recalls being a good swimmer as a young adult, Katrina feels she cannot overcome her volitional challenges to resuming swimming, which include an increasingly negative body image.

The therapist uses short and long-term physical activity goals graded from light gardening, walking her children to school, joining a peer-led walking group, to ultimately attending a women-only swimming session. These are integrated within a cognitive behavioural approach focused on enabling Katrina to challenge negative thoughts about herself and her abilities to develop her sense of achievement and self-efficacy. In an activity diary, Katrina plans and records what she does and the associated thoughts and feelings, thus linking engagement in occupation with its impact on mood and anxiety.

The programme is evaluated through noting Katrina's goal attainment, a repeat of the OSA and informal feedback to the therapist. Experiences of success, enhanced self-worth and confidence motivate Katrina to engage in other meaningful occupations. Valuing the support of others, she also reflects on her progress and achievements to peers within the walking group (Mawani et al. 2020), encouraging others to pursue their activity goals. Over time, as her mood and physical functioning improve, Katrina commences a graded return to work programme with support from her employer and the occupational therapist.

activity. Apps such as 'Active 10' (Brannan et al. 2019) support physical activity by encouraging and recording at least one 10-minute brisk walk a day. Others such as Strava (www.strava.com 2020) 'track' activity whilst providing feedback on performance. These trackers alone may be rewarding enough to reinforce individuals' sense of achievement and self-efficacy (Romeo et al. 2019). Additionally, the sharing of activities with 'friends,' 'followers' and online communities has also become an integral part of the activity, providing social reinforcement. Stragier and Mechant (2013) have considered how online peers play an important role in what they characterize as a 'new dimension to physical activity' (p. 1), noting that feedback, information-sharing and belonging to an online community can be positive influences on participation. Brown (2011) suggested that client-centred practice must take account of people's familiarity and confidence in using technologies and reinforced the importance of bespoke activity analysis and grading when using commercially available digital resources. Brown (2011) also recommended that occupational therapists consider whether individuals are 'digital natives' (p. 313) (that is, people who have grown up with such technologies and are familiar with them). Similarly, Fischl et al. (2017) noted the particular challenge for some older adults who have neither access to, nor the capacity for, digital technologies, which may therefore limit their use. Therapists who are not digital natives may also need to develop their own competencies as with any other practice development. This is also an opportunity for therapists to empower technologically confident service users by validating their expertise; acknowledging this as something that the therapist can also learn from.

The ease of access to free apps makes them a valuable resource, but risks should be recognized. For example, excessive 'online living' may have an isolating effect, and posting a sporting achievement online may create a burdensome expectation, presenting an image to the world which subsequently becomes difficult to sustain, ultimately exacerbating mental distress.

Some activities can be either solitary or social depending on the context and purpose. A run to clear one's head after a stressful day may be a private experience, but joining a running group such as England Athletics' 'Run Together' (https://runtogether.co.uk/2020) may achieve similar health benefits with the bonuses of social contact and real-time encouragement and support. There is a personal balance to be struck between a walk/run with headphones whilst listening to a 'Couch to 5k' podcast or to music, for example, and actual interaction with people. Schoeppe et al. (2016) concluded that multicomponent interventions (for example, personal telephone and/or social support or text messaging) could be more effective than apps alone, concurring with health behaviour change approaches that advocate multiple strategies to achieve longer-term benefits (Rebar and Taylor 2017). Additionally, Romeo et al. (2019) have indicated that apps have been most effective in the short term, up to 3 months, for example.

Reflection on these issues above underlines the value of occupational therapy's collaborative approach to enabling occupational engagement and self-management and highlights the opportunities available to embrace technological developments within professional practice.

ENABLING PHYSICAL ACTIVITY IN PRACTICE

As discussed in Chapter 15, group work is integral to occupational therapy, and group activities can be particularly helpful in enabling physical activity. As already noted the social context for an activity may contribute significantly to the sense of wellbeing people derive from it. Additionally, the support of others and a shared commitment to regular, planned group sessions can be important in overcoming motivational barriers to engagement.

Negotiating a consensus with service users regarding needs and goals (COT 2015), as illustrated in relation to Claude and Katrina (Boxes 13.1 and 13.2), is important when planning physical activity groups. A variety of aims may emerge, such as engaging in physical activity taster sessions, incorporating physical activities into habituated lifestyles, weaving physical activity (as a secondary goal) into groups which address other needs (such as social interaction), developing transferable and vocational skills (such as organizational and leadership skills) and, of course, engaging in physically active occupations for their intrinsic value.

Collaboration with service users is a well-established occupational therapy core skill (COT 2015), yet the power dynamics of relations between service providers and service users is widely acknowledged to be unequal (Beresford 2018). Indeed, Castillo and Ramon (2017) highlighted service users' concern about 'being done to rather than worked with, sometimes leaving them doubting their own perspective' (p. 176). In contrast, coproduction has emerged as a means of enabling a more equal sharing of power and decision-making between service users as 'experts by experience' and health professionals as 'experts by qualification,' each bringing distinct but equally essential knowledge, skills and resources to the care-planning process (Mayer and McKenzie 2017, p. 1185).

Working *with* people is embedded within occupational therapy practice, however, coproduction takes service users' involvement a step further than merely hearing and valuing their voices. It advocates for service user roles (including paid employment) in both the design and production of services (Norton 2019). Whiteford (2020) analysed the potential of coproduction and codesign for ensuring that occupational therapy addresses issues of diversity in power-sharing partnerships, settings and approaches. In relation to physical activity, Matthews et al. (2017) suggested that codesign could bring about suitable and sustainable physical activity provision for inclusive mental health practice. Tremendous opportunities exist to utilize service users' skills. For example, horticultural knowledge may be useful for a gardening/allotment group, familiarity with local geography may inform a walking or cycling group, or sporting expertise can be applied in coaching sports sessions. This kind of peer involvement can be a powerful source of practical and emotional support to others (Tweed et al. 2020).

Examples of Individual and Group Activities

Earlier sections of this chapter discussed the positive influences of physical activity, highlighting that the activity need not be particularly vigorous and that any activity is better than none. Therefore many opportunities exist to collaborate with people in identifying activities of interest that will help motivate participation. Activity choices are highly individualized and further research is required into particular activity types. Nevertheless, an occupational therapist can utilize service users' expertise in knowing their own health and occupational preferences to identify the activities that are most likely to be beneficial or which ones are, at least, worth trying. What follows is an overview of the evidence of benefits from certain types of activity which may assist occupational therapists' work with service users.

Walking

Walking has the advantages of requiring minimal organization and no specialist skill or equipment and incurs

no cost. It can effectively be habituated within a person's lifestyle as noted with Claude (Box 13.1). Walking is easily graded and paced to accommodate an individual's level of fitness and abilities. It has been shown to promote wellbeing through a sense of achievement, purpose and enjoyment. A widely-known comment attributed to Hippocrates, that walking is 'man's best medicine' (Stamatakis 2018) effectively sums this up. Reviews of evidence into group walking programmes consistently identify the social element as being a strong motivator and influence on positive emotional experiences and belonging (Wensley and Slade 2012; Raine et al. 2017; Swinson et al. 2020).

Subramaniapillai et al. (2016) explored physical activity for people diagnosed with bipolar affective disorder and schizophrenia, concluding that walking was most preferred and suggesting that physical activity preferences of low to moderate intensity are consistent with those of the general population. In addition to the potential health benefits of walking itself, there is also the potential to harness the synergistic impact on wellbeing of accessing outdoor green spaces (see Chapter 19) within an intervention that is economical to deliver in both in-patient and community settings (Krzanowski et al. 2020).

Mass Participation Events

Mass participation sporting events have the potential to allow people to try out physical activity, usually in a spirit of social engagement, with their friends and/or to raise money for charity. A very popular and global example is 'parkrun' (https://www.parkrun.com/), which has individual and public health potential for encouraging regular physical activity (Stevinson et al. 2015). Although elite level sportspeople can take part in these 5 km runs, the goal is to increase wide-ranging participation and engagement rather than sports performance as such. There are no costs, special equipment or age restrictions, and a single one-off online registration gives indefinite access to the runs and electronic timing via an individual barcode. In contrast with other annual mass participation events, parkruns happen every weekend throughout the year, which promotes habituated participation. Stevinson et al. (2015) reported that receiving online run times provides extrinsic motivation, which improves participation.

The importance of intrinsic motivation was discussed earlier, and Feighan and Roberts (2017) identified that some cyclists in their study had a less competitive focus towards achievement and were intrinsically motivated by a collective sense of pride as they crossed an event finish line together. This demonstrates that both intrinsic and extrinsic factors may influence motivation to engage and achieve. Individual motivating factors can be accommodated within the collective experience because, for example, parkrun involves running as an individual but also with others, instilling a sense of belonging to a mass participation event, including social support. Furthermore achievement is underpinned by self-efficacy (Lee and Kielhofner 2017b); that is, confidence in one's own ability to succeed in a situation.

Links between self-efficacy and physical activity are well-established because confidence is important in maintaining participation (Biddle et al. 2015). It appears that parkrun attracts participants from diverse backgrounds including those known to have found it challenging to engage in, such as women, people who are overweight or obese and those with poorer health (Cleland et al. 2019). Therefore the relaxed ethos and inclusivity embedded in parkrun could be important to emphasize when setting goals for increased physical activity within occupational therapy.

Other Activities

Clearly, the variety of options for engaging in physical activities and occupations is tremendous. Pentland et al. (2018) recommended that, from an occupational therapy perspective, service users' engagement was optimized if there was choice of activity, a willingness to explore and manage risks, an opportunity to develop and maintain skills and the motivation to remain engaged. For therapists, the issues discussed previously (regarding motivation, environments, participation and engagement) need to be incorporated into professional reasoning. Evidence is widespread, both within occupational therapy and beyond, for many activities such as cycling (Feighan and Roberts 2017; Schnor et al. 2019), football (Friedrich and Mason 2018; Pettican et al. 2021), walking football (Lamont et al. 2017), swimming and blue exercise (White et al. 2016; MacIntyre et al. 2019), adventure therapy (Jeffrey and Wilson 2017; Rogerson et al. 2019) and dance (Borges da Costa 2016).

Sustaining Engagement

Social inclusion is fundamental to mental health, so integration with community resources should be an aim of physical activity-based interventions to facilitate sustainable engagement beyond the occupational therapy intervention stage.

Fortunately, in addition to a multitude of local public and privately organized sports and leisure centre activities, many health promoting programmes exist such as Green Gyms (Lister et al. 2017) and Walking Works (Walking for Health Team 2014). Many also offer volunteering opportunities. For example, individuals may train as voluntary walk leaders or undertake vocational qualifications through horticultural organizations or through groups such as The Conservation Volunteers (https://www.tcv.org.uk/) who manage the Green Gyms, and associated social prescribing projects whereby people can be referred for physical outdoor conservation activities.

Parkrun (see earlier) also has a volunteering system whereby people contribute to the sustainability of their local run (Stevenson et al. 2015). This enables individuals to remain occupationally engaged when injured or otherwise unable to run. Volunteering is congruent with occupational therapy and occupational science philosophies which acknowledge the positive impact of work (paid or unpaid) on health (Wilcock and Hocking 2015) and on mental health recovery and social inclusion (Farrell and Bryant 2009). Box 13.3 illustrates how occupational therapy and community organizations can collaborate to tackle social exclusion and occupational injustice in enabling physical activity for people with mental and other health difficulties.

CONCLUSION

This chapter has explored extensive evidence for the benefits of physical activity to health, specifically focusing on mental wellbeing. Physical activity is prominent in all health agenda from both treatment and prevention perspectives, yet it is evident that participation and engagement (as discussed in this chapter) are complex phenomena involving multifarious physical, psychosocial and environmental factors. Occupational therapy, with its holistic focus on 'doing' and its professional reasoning capable of engaging with complexity is uniquely placed to meet these challenges within contemporary health and social care environments.

BOX 13.3
SPORT FOR CONFIDENCE

Sport for Confidence (https://sportforconfidence.com/) is a social enterprise concerned with enabling inclusive and accessible sport and physical activity opportunities for marginalized groups, such as people with mental health difficulties. This is achieved by placing occupational therapists and specialist sports coaches into leisure centres to run inclusive sports sessions and ensure the mainstream leisure centre environment is as accessible as possible. Sport for Confidence considers it to be an occupational injustice (see Hocking 2017) that people with mental health difficulties are deterred or prevented from participating in health-promoting occupations (such as sport and physical activity) due to conditions outside of their control.

The premise of 'inclusive sport' (Sport for Confidence's central approach) is that people with or without a disability or a long-term health condition can participate in sport together. This may involve some adjustments and modifications to playing rules, but such an approach avoids the segregation that can be perpetuated by specialist sports projects' orientation to particular marginalized groups or health conditions. It provides people with the opportunity to participate in sport with friends, family members and neighbours as active citizens in their own community.

Sport for Confidence staff plan and deliver the inclusive sport sessions to meet the needs of whoever chooses to participate, and their work is regarded as an exemplar within both sport and health strategy (Chief Allied Health Professions Officer's Team 2017; Sport England 2018b). Their occupational therapists also work with other national organizations such as Sport England to promote the ethos of inclusive and accessible sport and physical activity opportunities.

SERVICE USER COMMENTARY

I liked this chapter, but I have to balance my enjoyment of it with the anger I sometimes feel when I hear people talk of how, in despair, they seek help when life is 'right on the edge' and they need something so much and are told of the value of 'a walk' and the help that exercise gives to a troubled and desperate mind. Such advice can feel patronizing, dismissive and alienating, and I suppose, in some ways, this chapter contains elements of this in places.

But I do get that ideal regarding activity. I remember long walks along the beach in the winter when the wide skies, the clouds, the sea, the scent of seaweed and the sound of the oyster catchers soothed my rushing desperate thoughts and mellowed my loneliness; just to feel the wind, to watch the sand hissing along the beach, meant I felt more part of things, less closed in than in a room where it was unlikely the phone would ring or friends would come by.

The chapter also made me think of going to the gym when I was an inpatient. I had said I needed exercise, but I loathe treadmills and weights; especially when all you do is stare at the wall in front of you and wonder who will be your escort to take you back to the isolation of constant observations on the ward. I do remember one of the assistants; she nattered, chattered, and filled the room with laughter. She knew everyone and was pleased to see them and, despite her laughter, knew in her heart the bleakness of our lives. She had indeed experienced it herself. In a reluctant way I began to look forward to those daily excursions to the gym and the comments we made to each other; the shy and lovely warmth of that patient from rehab on crutches who had been on a section for so many months and eventually found release, to our dismay, when she managed to escape and take her own life, and who I still think of warmly for what she gave to us.

While I was an inpatient I was allowed off the ward for walks under escort. I loved the walks to the duck pond in the woods (where the dead tree had been carved into so many different animals) and occasionally up in the hills in the mist with the gorse bushes, the cairn and the ancient fort and the delight that we got lost and were late back from my allotted time away from the dead air of the ward where we had to mingle and sit. I also loved the rare occasions when I was taken by car across the city to the woods for a walk and we would visit this grove by the waterside where the bushes and the trees were festooned with rags and clothes, placed there with wishes for I know not what; healing, love, a myriad of things.

Lastly, one thing I really loved as an inpatient was getting together with an occupational therapist to do weekly nature walks hosted by a local environmental charity; walking in woods, by water, in the hills and by the sea; talking and learning about the plants, the birds and the mammals; and settling down at the end to drink tea brewed on a makeshift fire, to eat flapjacks, to feel free from boundaries and 'professionalism,' free from labels, free from restrictions, relishing conversations with not the slightest hint that this was 'a therapy,' much more that this was something we could enjoy as people, delighting in the sun and the clouds, forgetting the darkness of life and the tedious hours, pausing to eat a blackberry and look at the heron colony; a time to look at life brightly when some of us did not think this was possible.

Graham Morgan

QUESTIONS FOR CONSIDERATION

1. Why is physical activity important?
2. Why would an occupational therapist distinguish between physical activity and physical exercise? Is this distinction important?
3. What are the global recommendations, as outlined by WHO, for physical activity?
4. Why is it important to be aware of both the physical and mental health of mental health service users?
5. When approaching a client with limited mobility or a disinclination to be active, what kind of activity could you suggest for them that is sustainable, encouraging and easy to develop?
6. What work can be done to make safe, affordable and appropriate programmes of physical activity more accessible to service user groups who are commonly excluded from these opportunities?
7. What benefits will Claude (see Box 13.1) gain from increasing the amount of walking he undertakes? Considering his interests and goals, might there be any other possible physical activities you could suggest?
8. What techniques might you employ to reassure and encourage Katrina (see Box 13.2) to resume swimming or other physical activities?

Acknowledgements

The author acknowledges the invaluable contribution of Dr Anna Pettican, Occupational Therapist, Sport for Confidence & Post-Doctoral Researcher, University of Essex, United Kingdom.

REFERENCES

Alexandratos, K., Barnett, F., & Thomas, Y. (2012). The impact of exercise on the mental health and quality of life of people with severe mental illness: A critical review. *British Journal of Occupational Therapy, 75*, 48–60.

Baron, K., Kielhofner, G., Iyenger, J., Goldhammer, V., & Wolenski, J. (1998). *Occupational Self-Assessment (OSA) Manual.* Chicago: University of Illinois.

Beresford, P. (2018). A failure of national mental health policy and the failure of a global summit. *British Journal of Mental Health Nursing, 7*(5), 198–199.

Biddle, S. J. H., Mutrie, N., & Gorely, T. (2015). *Psychology of physical activity. Determinants, Well-being and Interventions* (3rd ed.). London: Routledge.

Boland, L., & Cunningham, M. (2019). Homelessness: Critical reflections and observations from an occupational perspective. *Journal of Occupational Science, 26*(2), 308–315.

Borges da Costa, A. L., & Cox, D. L. (2016). The experience of meaning in circle dance. *Journal of Occupational Science, 23*(2), 196–207.

Brannan, M., Foster, C., Timpson, C., et al. (2019). Active 10: A new approach to increase physical activity in inactive people in England. *Progress in Cardiovascular Diseases, 62*(2), 135–139. Available at: https://www.sciencedirect.com/science/article/abs/pii/S0033062019300350.

Brown, T. (2011). Are you a digital native or a digital immigrant? Being client centred in the digital era. *British Journal of Occupational Therapy, 74*(7), 313.

Carless, D., & Douglas, K. (2008). Social support for and through exercise and sport in a sample of men with serious mental illness. *Issues in Mental Health Nursing, 29*, 1179–1199.

Caspersen, C., Powell, K., & Christenson, N. (1985). Physical activity, exercise, and physical fitness: Definitions and distinctions for health-related research. *Public Health Reports, 100*, 126–131.

Castillo, H., & Ramon, S. (2017). Work with me: Service users' perspectives on shared decision making in mental health. *Mental Health Review Journal, 22*(3), 166–178.

Chief Allied Health Professions Officer's Team. (2017). *Allied health Professions into Action Using Allied health Professionals to Transform health.* Care & Wellbeing. NHS England.

Christie, M. A., & Cole, F. (2017). The impact of green exercise on volunteers' mental health and well being: Findings from a community project in a woodland setting. *The Journal of Therapeutic Horticulture, 27*(1), 17–33.

Cleland, V., Nash, M., Sharman, M. J., & Claflin, S. (2019). Exploring the health-promoting potential of the "parkrun" phenomenon: What factors are associated with higher levels of participation? *American Journal of Health Promotion, 33*(1), 13–23.

Cole, F. (2010). Physical activity for its mental health benefits: Conceptualising participation within the model of human occupation. *British Journal of Occupational Therapy, 73*, 607–615.

College of Occupational Therapists (COT). (2015). *Entry Level occupational therapy Core Knowledge and practice Skills.* London: College of Occupational Therapists.

Creek, J. (2010). *The Core Concepts of occupational therapy. A Dynamic Framework for practice.* London: Jessica Kingsley Publishers.

Department of Health (DH). (2010). *On the State of Public health: Annual Report of the Chief Medical Officer 2009.* London: Department of Health.

Department of Health. (2011). *Physical activity, health Improvement and Protection. Start active, Stay active: A Report on physical*

activity from the Four Home Countries' Chief Medical Officers.
London: Department of Health.

Department of Health and Social Care (DHSC). (2019). *UK Chief Medical Officers' physical activity Guidelines.* London: DHSC.

Duncan, E., & Fletcher-Shaw, S. (2020). The cognitive-behavioural frame of reference. In E. Duncan (Ed.), *Foundations for Practice in Occupational Therapy* (6th ed.) (pp. 141–151). Edinburgh: Elsevier.

Ekkekakis, P., & Cook, D. B. (2013). *Routledge Handbook of physical activity and mental health.* London: Routledge.

England, S. (2018a). *Active Lives Survey.* Available at: https://activelives.sportengland.org.

England, S. (2018b). *Working in an active Nation: The Professional Workforce Strategy for England.* London: Sport England.

Farrell, C., & Bryant, W. (2009). Voluntary work for adults with mental health problems: A route to inclusion? A review of the literature. *British Journal of Occupational Therapy, 72*(4), 163–173.

Feighan, M., & Roberts, A. (2017). The value of cycling as a meaningful and therapeutic occupation. *British Journal of Occupational Therapy, 80*(5), 319–326.

Fischl, C., Asaba, E., & Nilsson, I. (2017). Exploring potential in participation mediated by digital technology among older adults. *Journal of Occupational Science, 24*(3), 314–326.

Freidrich, B., & Mason, O. (2018). Qualitative evaluation of a football intervention for people with mental health problems in the north east of London. *Mental Health and Physical Activity, 15*, 132–138.

Genter, C., Roberts, A., Richardson, J., & Sheaff, M. (2015). The contribution of allotment gardening to health and wellbeing: A systematic review of the literature. *British Journal of Occupational Therapy, 78*(10), 593–605.

Gerlach, A., Teachman, G., Laliberte-Rudman, D., Aldrich, R., & Huot, S. (2017). Expanding beyond individualism: Engaging critical perspectives on occupation. *Scandinavian Journal of Occupational Therapy, 25*(1), 35–43.

Global Advocacy Council for Physical Activity. (2010). The Toronto charter for physical activity. A global call for action. *Journal of Physical Activity and Health, 3*, S370–S373.

Glowacki, K., Duncan, M., Gainforth, H., & Faulkner, G. (2017). Barriers and facilitators to physical activity and exercise among adults with depression: A scoping review. *Mental Health and Physical Activity, 13*, 108–119.

Gorczynski, P., & Faulkner, G. (2010). Exercise therapy for schizophrenia. *Cochrane Database of Systematic Reviews, 5.*

Haapasalo, V., de Vries, H., Vandelanotte, C., Rosenkranz, R., & Duncan, M. J. (2018). Cross-sectional associations between multiple lifestyle behaviours and excellent well-being in Australian adults. *Preventive Medicine, 116*, 119–125.

Hammell, K. W. (2009). Self-care, productivity, and leisure, or dimensions of occupational experience? Rethinking occupational "categories". *Canadian Journal of Occupational Therapy, 76*(2), 107–114.

Hartley, L., Fleay, C., & Tye, M. (2017). Exploring physical activity engagement and barriers for asylum seekers in Australia coping with prolonged uncertainty and no right to work. *Health and Social Care in the Community, 25*(3), 1190–1198.

Hasselkus, B. (2011). *Meaning of Everyday Occupation* (2nd ed.). Thorofare, NJ: Slack Inc..

Health and Social Care Act, 2012. Available at: https://www.legislation.gov.uk/ukpga/2012/7/contents/enacted.

Health and Social Care Information Centre. (2019). *Health Survey for England 2018.* NHS Digital.

Hocking, C. (2017). Occupational justice as social justice: The moral claim for inclusion. *Journal of Occupational Science, 24*(1), 29–42.

Holley, J., Crone, D., Tyson, P., & Lovell, G. (2011). The effects of physical activity on psychological well-being for those with schizophrenia: A systematic review. *British Journal of Clinical Psychology, 50*(1), 84–105. Available at: https://bpspsychub.onlinelibrary.wiley.com/doi/abs/10.1348/014466510X496220.

Illman, S. C., Spence, S., O'Campo, P. J., & Kirsh, B. H. (2013). Exploring the occupations of homeless adults living with mental illnesses in Toronto/explorer les occupations d'adultes sans-abri atteints de maladies mentales vivant à Toronto. *Canadian Journal of Occupational Therapy, 80*(4), 215–223.

Jeffery, H., & Wilson, L. (2017). New Zealand occupational therapists' use of adventure therapy in mental health practice. *New Zealand Journal of Occupational Therapy, 64*(1), 32.

Kandola, A., Ashdown-Franks, G., Hendrikse, J., Sabiston, C., & Stubbs, B. (2019). Physical activity and depression: Towards understanding the antidepressant mechanisms of physical activity. *Neuroscience & Biobehavioral Reviews, 107*, 525–539.

Kandola, A., Vancampfort, D., Herring, M., et al. (2018). Moving to beat anxiety: Epidemiology and therapeutic issues with physical activity for anxiety. *Current Psychiatry Reports, 20*(8), 63.

Kantarzis, S. (2017). Exploring occupation beyond the individual: Family and collective occupation. In D. Sakellario, & N. Pollard (Eds.), *Occupational Therapy without Borders. Integrating Justice with Practice* (2nd ed.) (pp. 19–28). Edinburgh: Elsevier.

Kapteyn, A., Banks, J., Hamer, M., Smith, J.P., Steptoe, A., Van Soest, A., Koster, A. and Wah, S.H. (2018). What they say and what they do: comparing physical activity across the USA, England and the Netherlands. *Journal of Epidemiology & Community Health, 72*(6), 471–476.

Kelly, Y., Zilanawala, A., Booker, C., & Sacker, A. (2018). Social media use and adolescent mental health: Findings from the UK millennium cohort study. *EClinicalMedicine, 6*, 59–68.

Kramer, J., Forsyth, K., Lavedure, P., et al. (2017). Self-reports: Eliciting clients' perspectives. In R. Taylor (Ed.), *Kielhofner's Model of Human Occupation* (5th ed.) (pp. 248–274). Philadephia: Wolters Kluwer.

Krzanowski, J., Mortimer, F., & Stancliffe, R. (2020). *Green walking in mental health recovery: A guide.* Centre for Sustainable Healthcare.

Lam, L., Mak, A., & Lee, S. (2016). Physical activity to calm your 'nerves. In L. Lam, & M. Riba (Eds.), *Physical exercise Interventions for Mental Health* (pp. 79–95). Cambridge: Cambridge Press.

Lamont, E., Harris, J., McDonald, G., Kerin, T., & Dickens, G. L. (2017). Qualitative investigation of the role of collaborative football and walking football groups in mental health recovery. *Mental Health and Physical Activity*, 12, 116–123.

Lee, S. W., & Kielhofner, G. (2017a). Habituation: Patterns of daily occupation. In R. Taylor (Ed.), *Kielhofner's Model of Human Occupation* (5th ed.) (pp. 57–73). Philadelphia: Wolters Kluwer.

Lee, W. E., & Kielhofner, G. (2017b). Volition. In R. Taylor (Ed.), *Kielfhofner's Model of Human Occupation* (5th ed.) (pp. 38–56). Philadelphia: Wolters Kluwer.

Lister, C., Reid, S., Musgrove, M., & Speirs, C. (2017). Pro-active minds green gym launch. *Journal of Public Mental Health*, 16(2), 88–90.

Livingston, G., Sommerlad, A., Orgeta, V., et al. (2017). Dementia prevention, intervention, and care. *Lancet*, 390(10113), 2673–2734.

MacIntyre, T., Walkin, A., Caloguiuri, G., et al. (2019). Immersion, watersports and blueways and the blue mind. In A. A. Donnelly, & T. E. MacIntyre (Eds.), *Physical Activity in Natural Settings. Green and Blue exercise* (pp. 210–225). London: Routledge.

Martín, M. N., Caballero, F. F., Moreno-Agostino, D., et al. (2020). Relationship between subjective well-being and healthy lifestyle behaviours in older adults: A longitudinal study. *Aging & Mental Health*, 24(4), 611–619.

Matthews, E., Cowman, M., & Denieffe, S. (2017). Using experience-based co-design for the development of physical activity provision in rehabilitation and recovery mental health care. *Journal of Psychiatric and Mental Health Nursing*, 24(7), 545–552.

Mawani, F. N., & Ibrahim, S. (2020). Building roads together: A peer-led, community-based walking and rolling peer support program for inclusion and mental health. *Canadian Journal of Public Health*, 112, 142–151.

Mayer, C., & McKenzie, K. (2017). "…it shows that there's no limits": The psychological impact of co-production for experts by experience working in youth mental health. *Health and Social Care in the Community*, 25(3), 1181–1189.

Mental Health Foundation. (2018). *Depression*. Available at: https://www.mentalhealth.org.uk/a-to-z/d/depression.

Mitchell, A., Hardy, S., & Shiers, D. (2017). Parity of esteem: Addressing the inequalities between mental and physical health care. *BJPsych Advances*, 23, 193–205.

Moloney, L., & Rohde, D. (2017). Experiences of men with psychosis participating in a community-based football programme. *Indian Journal of Occupational Therapy*, 45(2), 100–110.

Mynard, L., Howie, L., & Collister, L. (2009). Belonging to a community-based football team: An ethnographic study. *Australian Occupational Therapy Journal*, 56(4), 266–274.

National Institute for Health and Care Excellence (NICE). (2009). *Depression in Adults: Recognition and Management [CG90]*. NICE.

National Institute for Health and Care Excellence (NICE). (2011). *Depression in Adults*. NICE: Quality Standard.

NHS. (2020). *Couch to 5k week by week*. Available at: https://www.nhs.uk/live-well/exercise/couch-to-5k-week-by-week/.

Norton, M. (2019). Implementing co-production in traditional statutory mental health services. *Mental Health Practice*, 4(3).

Park, S. H., Han, K. S., & Kang, C. B. (2014). Effects of exercise programs on depressive symptoms, quality of life, and self-esteem in older people: A systematic review of randomized controlled trials. *Applied Nursing Research*, 27(4), 219–226.

Parkinson, S., Lowe, C., & Vecsey, T. (2011). The therapeutic benefits of horticulture in a mental health service. *British Journal of Occupational Therapy*, 74(11), 525–534.

Parkrun. Available at: https://www.parkrun.com/

Pentland, D., Kantartzis, S., Giatsi Clausen, M., & Witemyre, K. (2018). *Occupational therapy and complexity: Defining and describing practice*. London: Royal College of Occupational Therapists.

Pierce, D. (2001). Untangling occupation and activity. *American Journal of Occupational Therapy*, 55(2), 138–146.

Public Health England. (2014). *Everybody active, every day. An evidence-based approach to physical activity*. London: Crown Copyright.

Raine, R., Roberts, A., Callaghan, L., Sydenham, Z., & Bannigan, K. (2017). Factors affecting sustained engagement in walking for health: A focus group study. *British Journal of Occupational Therapy*, 80(3), 183–190.

Rebar, A. L., & Taylor, A. (2017). Physical activity and mental health; it is more than just a prescription. *Mental Health and Physical Activity*, 13, 77–82.

Remes, O., Brayne, C., Van Der Linde, R., & Lafortune, L. (2016). A systematic review of reviews on the prevalence of anxiety disorders in adult populations. *Brain and Behavior*, 6(7), e00497.

Roberts, A. E., & Bannigan, K. (2018). Dimensions of personal meaning from engagement in occupations: A metasynthesis. *Canadian Journal of Occupational Therapy*, 85(5), 386–396.

Rogerson, M., Kelly, S., Coetzee, S., Barton, J., & Pretty, J. (2019). Doing adventure. The mental health benefits of using occupational therapy approaches in adventure therapy settings. In A. A. Donnelly, & T. E. MacIntyre (Eds.), *Physical Activity in Natural Settings. Green and Blue exercise* (pp. 241–255). London: Routledge.

Romeo, A., Edney, S., Plotnikoff, R., et al. (2019). Can smartphone apps increase physical activity? Systematic review and meta-analysis. *Journal of Medical Internet Research*, 21(3), e12053.

Rowley, N., Mann, S., Steele, J., Horton, E., & Jimenez, A. (2018). The effects of exercise referral schemes in the United Kingdom in those with cardiovascular, mental health, and musculoskeletal disorders: A preliminary systematic review. *BioMed Central Public Health*, 18(1), 1–18.

Royal College of Occupational Therapists (RCOT). (2018). *Getting my life back: Occupational therapy promoting mental health and wellbeing in England*. London: RCOT.

Schnor, H., Linderoth, S., & Midtgaard, J. (2019). Experiences with participation in a supervised group-based outdoor cycling programme for people with mental illness: A focus group study. *International Journal of Environmental Research and Public Health*, 16, 528.

Schoeppe, S., Alley, S., Vam Lippevelde, W., et al. (2016). Efficacy of interventions that use apps to improve diet, physical activity and sedentary behaviour: A systematic review. *International Journal of Behavioral Nutrition and Physical Activity*, 13(1), n/a.

Schuch, F., Vancampfort, D., Firth, J., et al. (2017). Physical activity and sedentary behaviour in people with major depressive disorder: A systematic review and meta-analysis. *Journal of Affective Disorders, 210,* 139–150.

Scottish Government. (2017). *Mental health Strategy: 2017–2027.* Edinburgh: Scottish Government.

Smyth, G., Harries, P., & Dorer, G. (2011). Exploring mental health service users' experiences of social inclusion in their community occupations. *British Journal of Occupational Therapy, 74,* 323–331.

Stamatakis, E., Hamer, M., & Murphy, M. (2018). What Hippocrates called 'man's best medicine': Walking is humanity's path to a better world. *British Journal of Sports Medicine, 52,* 753–754.

Stevinson, C., Wiltshire, G., & Hickson, M. (2015). Facilitating participation in health-enhancing physical activity: A qualitative study of parkrun. *International Journal of Behavioral Medicine, 22*(2), 170–177.

Stragier, J., & Mechant, P. (2013). *Mobile fitness apps for promoting physical activity on Twitter: The #RunKeeper case.* Available at: https://biblio.ugent.be/publication/3129098.

Strava. (2020). Available at: www.strava.com.

Stubbs, B., Koyanagi, A., Hallgren, M., et al. (2017). Physical activity and anxiety: A perspective from the world health survey. *Journal of Affective Disorders, 208,* 545–552.

Subramaniapillai, M., Arbour-Nicitopoulos, K., Duncan, M., et al. (2016). Physical activity preferences of individuals diagnosed with schizophrenia or bipolar disorder. *BioMed Central Research Notes, 9*(1), 340.

Swinson, T., Wenborn, J., & Sugarhood, P. (2020). Green walking groups: A mixed-methods review of the mental health outcomes for adults with mental health problems. *British Journal of Occupational Therapy, 83*(3), 162–171.

Szaz, T. S. (1972). *The Myth of mental Illness.* London: Paladin.

Taylor, R. (2017). *Kielhofner's Model of Human Occupation* (5th ed.). Philadephia: Wolters Kluwer.

Teychenne, M., Costigan, S. A., & Parker, K. (2015). The association between sedentary behaviour and risk of anxiety: A systematic review. *BioMed Central Public Health, 15*(1), 1–8.

Townsend, E. A., & Polatajko, H. J. (2013). Enabling occupation II: Advancing an occupational therapy Vision for health. In *Well-being, & Justice through Occupation: Official Practice Guidelines for the Canadian Association of Occupational Therapists* (2nd ed.). Ottowa: Canadian Association of Occupational Therapists.

Turcotte, P.-L., & Drolet, M.-J. (2020). Occupational therapists must declare the climate emergency. *Canadian Journal of Occupational Therapy, 87*(3), 171–172.

Tweed, M., Rogers, E., & Kinnafick, F. (2020). Literature on peer-based community physical activity programmes for mental

health service users: A scoping review. *Health Psychology Review, 15*(2), 287–313.

United Nations General Assembly. (2015). *Transforming Our World. The 2030 Agenda for Sustainable Development.* United Nations. Available at: https://www.un.org/ga/search/view_doc. asp?symbol=A/RES/70/1&Lang=E.

Walking for Health Team (2014). *Walking works: making the case to encourage greater uptake of walking as a physical activity to reduce the burden of long-term health conditions on the NHS.* London: The Ramblers.

Warburton, D. E., & Bredin, S. S. (2017). Health benefits of physical activity: A systematic review of current systematic reviews. *Current Opinion in Cardiology, 32*(5), 541–556.

Wensley, R., & Slade, A. (2012). Walking as a meaningful leisure occupation: The implications for occupational therapy. *British Journal of Occupational Therapy, 75,* 85–92.

Whatley, E., Fortune, T., & Williams, A. (2015). Enabling occupational participation and social inclusion for people recovering from mental ill-health through community gardening. *Australian Occupational Therapy Journal, 62,* 428–437.

White, P., Bell, S., Elliott, L., Jenkin, R., Wheeler, B., & Depledge, M. (2016). The health benefits of blue exercise in the UK. In J. Barton, R. Bragg, C. Wood, & J. Pretty (Eds.), *Green exercise: Linking Nature, Health and Well-being* (pp. 69–78). London: Routledge.

Whiteford, G. E. (2020). Sylvia Docker memorial lecture: Together we go further—service co-design, knowledge co-production and radical solidarity. *Australian Occupational Therapy Journal, 66*(6), 682–689.

Wilcock, A. A. (1998). Occupation for health. *British Journal of Occupational Therapy, 61*(8), 340–345.

Wilcock, A.A., 2001. Occupation for Health. Vol. 1 A Journey From Self-Health to Prescription. British Association and College of Occupational Therapists, London.

Wilcock, A. A., & Hocking, C. (2015). In *An Occupational Perspective of Health* (3rd ed.). Thorofare, NJ: Slack.

World Health Organisation (WHO). (2010). *Global Recommendations for physical activity and health.* Geneva: WHO.

World Health Organisation (WHO). (2018a). *Global Action Plan on physical activity 2018–2030: More active People for a Healthier World.* Geneva: WHO.

World Health Organisation (WHO). (2018b). *Sustainability Agenda 2030.* Geneva: WHO.

Yerxa, E. (1998). Health and the human spirit for occupation. *American Journal of Occupational Therapy, 52,* 412–418.

York, M., & Wiseman, T. (2012). Gardening as an occupation: A critical review. *British Journal of Occupational Therapy, 75,* 76–84.

14

LIFE-LONG LEARNING

JUANITA BESTER ■ DEBORAH HARRISON

CHAPTER OUTLINE

INTRODUCTION

Occupational therapy supports people to learn new knowledge and skills through engagement with occupations. It could be argued that occupational therapists teach and facilitate learning in every interaction with the people they work with. There are some situations, however, in which teaching or education is a dominant element of occupational therapy and when intervention tools are specifically selected with that aim. This chapter explores this approach. It examines how occupational therapists incorporate teaching and education into their interventions and facilitate life-long learning and personal development. It also discusses a broad definition of learning and explores different approaches, including its importance for good mental health and well-being and the role that learning plays in recovery from mental health problems. It covers

young adults who have completed their formal education, mature adults and old age adults. The chapter acknowledges that learning and development continue throughout life and discusses the necessity of learning as a tool to improve mental health and well-being. It also explores how learning and education empower people to achieve their potential in life and to build resilience to cope with challenges, underpinned by concepts drawn from occupational science. It also acknowledges some challenges that people face when learning.

The ways in which we talk about people doing education-based occupations will vary (see also Chapter 2), for example, learners, clients, patients, prisoners or participants. This is related to the context in which the learning takes place, and therefore different words are used in different parts of the chapter. The chapter begins by considering the importance of learning for mental well-being and occupational justice. Then the use of learning as a means to achieve mental well-being is introduced; the frames of reference that inform the use of learning as a therapeutic tool are considered, as well as the specific learning techniques that may be employed. Finally, opportunities for facilitating access to learning in the broader community are described.

LEARNING TO PROMOTE MENTAL HEALTH AND WELL-BEING

This section discusses the promotion of good mental health, well-being and the prevention of mental ill-health. It uses a broad definition of learning as life-long personal development outside the classroom and acquiring new life skills. It uses the 'Five Ways to Wellbeing' as a framework for occupational therapy in this area. This section also examines social inclusion and life-long learning, making conceptual links with occupational science.

Mental Health Promotion Using the 'Five Ways to Wellbeing'

A useful framework for occupational therapists who are working to support mental health promotion is the 'Five Ways to Wellbeing' developed from research carried out by the New Economics Foundation (Aked et al. 2008). Although this is a generic framework not designed for a specific profession, it aligns closely with an occupation-based approach to mental health promotion.

The five ways are to connect, be active, take notice, learn and give. Learning includes engaging in work and educational activities that may be simple, such as learning new words, reading the news, or, more complex, starting a new class. The 'Five Ways to Wellbeing' arose from the 'Foresight, mental capital and wellbeing' project which considered how to improve everyone's mental capital and mental well-being through life. The concept of thriving, not just surviving, has resonance for occupational therapists who aim to support people to reach their full potential in life. Evidence from the project suggested that a small improvement in well-being can help to decrease some mental health problems and help people to flourish.

The concept of mental capital is useful in understanding the elements of a person's capabilities occupational therapists might identify and develop to promote good mental health. It includes a person's both cognitive as well as emotional resources. Cognitive ability considers how flexible and efficient they are at learning; the emotional resources can be identified as emotional intelligence, such as their social skills and resilience in the face of stress. A person's mental capital therefore conditions how well they are able to contribute effectively to society and experience a high personal quality of life. The word capital naturally sparks association with ideas of financial capital and it might be challenging for occupational therapists to think of a person's capabilities in this way. If the concept is used, however, to recognize that people vary in how many resources they start with, and also to note that those resources can be built on and 'banked' for a rainy day, then it becomes more natural to think of the mind in this way.

The importance of promoting positive mental health for the general population is a consistent message throughout the 'Mental capital and well-being' project, that the 'Five Ways to Wellbeing' have relevance for everyone. The project concludes that if a small change in the average level of well-being across the population could be achieved, then this would produce a large decrease in the percentage living with identified mental health problems and improve the lives of people who have sub-clinical disorders. These people are not fulfilling their full potential and are identified as 'languishing.'

Throughout the 'Mental capital and wellbeing' project, interventions are proposed to promote positive mental health and well-being for people across the life span. In the United Kingdom the commitment of occupational therapists to promote good health is captured in the Allied Health Professionals (AHP) Public Health Strategy published by the AHP Federation with Public Health England (Public Health England 2019). It outlines the key role that AHPs can play in the public health of the nation. 'AHPs must be recognized as an integral part of the public health workforce, with responsibility for designing and delivering improvements to healthcare and reducing health inequalities.'

Access to Learning, Social Inclusion and Occupational Justice

Facilitating the engagement of people with learning and education throughout the lifespan promotes social inclusion by providing opportunities to participate more fully in society. There is therefore a natural fit with facilitating engagement with education and the philosophy of occupational science, in particular occupational justice (see also Chapter 3). Sagan (2008) provides an interesting analysis for an occupational scientist in the context of learning because she explores the concept of identity. She found that through learning there is a change in identity and a process of leaving behind the past and an opening up of new possibilities. These ideas of being through doing and transformation through doing have a strong resonance with occupational science.

Occupational deprivation arises from barriers within communities that exclude people from full participation in everyday activities. In the learning domain, for example, occupational deprivation may be evident when young people cannot access schooling because of armed conflict where they live or because of their gender, in the case of girls in some parts of the world. Occupational justice identifies inequalities in participation in occupations; for example, deprivation in learning occupations occur when children are growing up in poverty and their access to both recreational activities and formal education might be challenging for them.

It is important that occupational therapists critically reflect on their role in facilitating access to education and learning for marginalized groups. For many people globally, life is focused on survival rather than thriving. Ratima and Ratima (2005), in discussing practice in a marginalized context, remind occupational therapists to tailor their ways of working to meet the needs and preferences of particular populations.

An example of an occupational therapist in the United Kingdom meeting the needs of a marginalized group is Osborne (2018) who works with a charity supporting people living in food poverty. The charity realized that providing food parcels did not fully meet the needs of the population and identified that a number of life skills also needed addressing. An allotment project has been developed so people can learn how to grow their own fruits and vegetables, and sessions on money management skills are provided. Osborne (2018) comments that occupational therapists need to be aware of the direct effects of food poverty on a person's role, values and occupations.

A population of young people who can experience disadvantage are those growing up in military families. Evidence is emerging that the frequent moves in housing and schooling, along with the uncertainty and anxiety of having a parent deployed overseas, can have a negative impact on well-being (Cunitz et. al., 2019). A charity in the United Kingdom (Surf Action) teaches surfing to military children, funded by the Royal British Legion and the Armed Forces Covenant Trust. The children learn about safety in the ocean as well as the actual skills involved in surfing. Anecdotal evidence from these groups suggests that the children find the surfing very beneficial, increasing their confidence and resilience. Evaluation of the impact of participation in surfing clubs on children in the civilian population who face challenges in life (e.g., mental health difficulties and physical disability) has demonstrated that the activity promotes well-being (Godfrey et al. 2015). These surfing activities might not be delivered directly by an occupational therapist (e.g., in the United Kingdom they are provided by trained volunteers), but having an awareness of these opportunities is important so that children can be referred to them and encouraged to attend.

Life-Long Learning: A Developmental Approach to Learning

Life-long learning is the purposeful and continuous acquisition of skills and knowledge throughout the lifespan. Within the 'Five Ways to Wellbeing,' life-long learning is specifically identified as having a role to play in promoting good mental health and helping people build resilience to cope with mental health problems. The other four ways to well-being can also encompass doing new things and learning, which, in turn, promotes change and development. Learning happens in a wide variety of ways and can include reading books, learning from the internet, joining a club or society. Anytime a person tries doing something new, it involves learning, for example, using a new app on a mobile phone, driving a car, cooking a meal or doing a new creative or craft activity.

An innovative project in the United Kingdom taught American military personnel and their families archaeology skills at a former World War II airbase. Carvell (2018), an occupational therapy student, volunteered with the project and found that the participants enjoyed learning skills completely unrelated to the 'day job'; they valued connecting with the local community and exploring their shared history. Her subjective impression, based on conversation with the participants, was that this learning boosted their well-being. A small qualitative study confirms that there are biopsychosocial benefits to engaging with archaeology (Finnegan 2016) in this example for military veterans as well as serving personnel. This aligns well with the aims of the 'Five Ways to Wellbeing' as, in addition to learning new skills, participants make connections in a social context and spend time outdoors getting involved in a physical activity. Occupational therapists might not readily consider archaeology as an activity they could engage their service users with, but this research suggests that exploring innovative learning environments could be beneficial.

Once formal education is finished, adults who are resilient are able to continue to learn and develop and will need to do so in the workplace. It is necessary to have basic skills, for example, numeracy, literacy and information technology as well as flexibility and motivation to continue learning new skills to adapt to continually changing work demands. Continued learning and personal development helps to build confidence, self-esteem, and resilience. Setting achievable goals is helpful and supports people to adapt to life changes and challenges. Coaching (see below) might be relevant in this context.

Continued learning throughout the lifespan enhances self-esteem and encourages social interaction and a more active life. Anecdotal evidence from the well-respected UK charity Mind (2019) suggests that the opportunity to engage in work or educational activities particularly helps to lift older people out of depression. The practice of setting goals, which is related to adult learning in particular, has been strongly associated with higher levels of well-being (Mind 2019). As people age and might leave paid employment, continued learning and development is important. It reduces loneliness and depression and might slow onset of dementia or make people more resilient to cope with the changes (Mind 2019).

LEARNING INTERVENTIONS FOR RECOVERY

In the context of occupational therapy for recovery, learning can mean gaining information or understanding, acquiring skills, changing the way things are valued and to problem solve. To ensure that learning is happening optimally for people engaging with occupational therapy, it is important to have a working knowledge and understanding of key learning theories underpinning the interventions. Learning is a complex process that is supported by physical, emotional, cognitive and environmental factors. These factors can be used together to understand the reasons for ineffective learning.

- Physical reasons – Learning may be compromised if there is damage to the physical capacity to learn and/or to perform, for example, following a traumatic brain injury or loss of sight.
- Motivational reasons – Feelings of anxiety or insecurity and motivational problems can lead to ineffective learning.
- Cognitive reasons – A lack of foundational skills may affect the learner's readiness to learn, for example, cognitive ability or perceptual problems/deficits.
- Environmental reasons – Learning may be ineffective if there is a failure of communication between therapist and person, limited opportunities or conditions for learning or if the tools and materials needed for learning are not available.

Theoretical Understanding of Learning

In this section the focus is on the behaviourist, cognitivist, social, humanistic and constructivist learning approaches as five examples of theoretical approaches that influence the way learning is used as means and end in occupational therapy. A brief overview of each of these five is followed by a summary (Table 14.1).

Behavioural Approach

In this approach the focus is on observable change in behaviour that is shaped by the environment through positive or negative reinforcement. Positive reinforcement strengthens a desired behaviour, while negative reinforcement diminishes or stops an unwanted behaviour. A behavioural approach is suitable for the development of basic and more advanced behavioural skills. Basic behavioural skills can be defined as the execution of simple tasks and activities (e.g., brushing of teeth). The goal of basic behavioural skill development is to get the person to a predetermined level of competence in the task. For example, a person with moderate intellectual disability might learn to use their mobile phone to be able to call their parents independently.

TABLE 14.1

Summary of Five Learning Theories and Approaches

Learning Orientation	Behaviourist	Cognitivist	Social	Humanist	Constructivist
Theorists	Pavlov, Watson, Thorndike, Skinner	Piaget	Bandura	Maslow, Rogers, Knowles, Freire	Dewey, Piaget, Lave, Vygotsky
Focus of Orientation	Client has to master steps of a task in a sequential manner.	The focus is on the client as a 'learner' and not on the external environment.	Learning happens through the interaction between the person, the learning environment and the desired behaviour.	Learning is viewed as a personal act to fulfill one's potential.	Learning happens when meaning and understanding is constructed through experiences.
Goal of Learning	To change behaviour in a predetermined direction.	To develop the client's capacity and skills to become more self-directed.	To obtain an internal reward (e.g., sense of accomplishment, confidence or satisfaction after performing the behaviour).	To facilitate the learner to become autonomous and self-directed.	To deepen the understanding and meaning of experiences.
Role of Therapist	Therapist structures/ manipulates the environment to elicit a specific response from the learner/client.	Therapist facilitates cognitive processing by helping the learner/client 'learn how to learn.'	Therapist models new roles, guides behaviours and provides opportunities to practice new roles and behaviours.	Therapist facilitates growth and development of the learner/ client.	Therapist encourages critical reflection and discusses meaning with learners.
Strategies	-Chaining (backward and forward) -Token economy -Behaviour charts -Behaviour contracts	-Reflection -Concept maps -Homework tasks	-Role modelling -Demonstration -Self-regulation	-Adult teaching and learning principles -Self-directed learning -Role playing	-Scaffolding -Developmental readiness/task demands -Whole task learning
Techniques	-Prompting -Cueing -Shaping -Reinforcing -Coaching	-Transference of skills	-Robot technique (stop-think-do) -Goal setting -Time scheduling	-Self-evaluation -Taking responsibility -Brainstorming	-Mnemonics to assist recall -Concept/mind maps -Examples -Written instructions -Hand-outs

To achieve this, the task of making a call needs to be analysed into observable behavioural components. This approach is useful with people with learning disabilities (e.g., attention deficit hyperactivity disorder (ADHD)), traumatic brain injury or intellectual disability and pervasive developmental disorders (e.g., Asperger's or autism spectrum disorders).

An advanced behavioural skill can be described as the performance of an occupation, which includes a number of tasks and activities simultaneously. When developing advanced behavioural skills, collaborative decision-making between the person and the occupational therapist is important so that the goal and how success will be measured is very clear to all. What needs to be learnt and practised for occupational performance is made explicit. For example, a person living with agoraphobia may set a goal to stay inside the library for 15 minutes and borrow two books while practising an abdominal breathing technique.

There are a number of other strategies that are also used in the behavioural approach. Chaining is a strategy used to teach somebody a task that needs to be completed in sequential order. The task is broken down into each of its sequential components, and the person learns each component in sequential order. Forward chaining starts with the first step of the task, while in backward chaining the therapist may complete all of the initial steps in a task and then the person only completes the final steps. Grading is determined by the amount of prompting a person needs to complete the task, starting with full prompting and then gradually reducing the amount of prompting needed (Meadows 2011; Najdowski 2017).

Behavioural or reward charts are another important strategy typically used with young children to reward a specific positive behaviour. After a certain number of small rewards, the person achieves a larger reward. Similarly, in a token economy a person learns to regulate and self-monitor their behaviour through the allocation of tokens for a range of positive behaviours. The items or activities that motivate the person are identified at the beginning of the process, and the number of tokens that needs to be earned to receive the reward is agreed upon.

Behavioural contracts are another strategy in which the person and occupational therapist agree to the desired behaviours as well as the consequences of negative behaviours. These contracts, which are less common in contemporary practice, can be useful when working with people who are struggling to develop the social behaviours considered to be appropriate in their social context. This approach is more successful if the person is motivated to engage in the process and wants to work within a clearly defined set of parameters to achieve their specific goals (National Center on Intensive Intervention 2015; Stainbrook et al. 2019).

Cognitive Approach

The focus of this approach is on the person and how they gradually construct a model of reality for themselves. Learning in this orientation is about the discovery of meaning so that the person can understand the structure of knowledge. The person uses their cognitive abilities such as insight, information processing, perception and memory to transfer meaning to other situations. In essence the person acquires knowledge and develops skills that can be used in various situations. Reflection is considered an essential tool to help with the discovering of meaning for the client/learner. Learning can be seen as a process of acquiring, storing and retrieving of information.

A cognitive approach to learning involves developing the skills to be able to learn, what works best for the person and how they learn as an individual. This approach might include trying out a number of different methods of learning, like making mind maps, cue cards, reflective journals or mnemonics for learning a list of items.

Social Learning

Social learning as an approach focuses on observation and modelling as the main methods of learning. Learning occurs as a result of the interaction with and observation of others within a social context. This can include learning from other group members as well as from the occupational therapist. People integrate new knowledge and skills through role modelling and practising of observed behaviours. There are three models of observational learning: i) an actual person performs an occupation (live model); ii) the learner is exposed to detailed descriptions of an occupation (verbal instruction model) and iii) either a real person or fictional character demonstrates the occupation (e.g., movies, books, television, radio, etc.) (symbolic model). For example, when learning conflict management skills, an occupational therapist may use role play (live model) or draw on example from popular soap operas (symbolic model).

Role training is another important strategy in which a person learns a specific skill, for example, going for a job interview and acting in an appropriate way for that situation, by enacting an interview situation in a safe environment with feedback from peers and the occupational therapist.

Humanistic Approach

Within the humanistic approach the emphasis is on the natural desire or motivation of a person to learn and ultimately reach their full potential. Key features of learning within this theory include i) personal involvement of the learner, ii) self-initiated learning and iii) self-evaluation of learning through which the person becomes self-directed.

An occupational therapist might use this approach when working with people with anxiety to identify the coping strategies a person uses effectively and the triggers that might lead to re-admission and how to prevent this. The therapist employing this learning orientation needs to model behaviour, be explicit about how a group activity will enable the person to achieve their goals, promote interaction between group members so that people learn from each other and promote autonomy by giving individuals choice and control. In this approach, the occupational therapist acts as a facilitator of learning rather than as a teacher of knowledge.

Constructivist Approach

This approach is built on the assumption that learning is a process of building an understanding based on constructing meaning from the learner's own experiences. This process is dependent on the existing knowledge structure of the learner, and new information is given meaning through this existing knowledge framework. The new knowledge is linked with existing knowledge, and the result is a more integrated knowledge framework. Learning is viewed as a continuous and lifelong process. For example, in social skills training, the starting point would be to identify what a person already does that leads to conflict, or reduces conflict, in a situation. New conflict management techniques are then learnt that build on the person's existing skills. Impoverished or restricted environments which limit the scope for exploration and experimentation can severely constrain the learning process. For example, children living with parents who are substance dependent may not have the opportunity to learn positive coping strategies and so become more at risk of becoming substance dependent themselves at a younger age. An occupational therapist's focus when using a constructivist approach is on creating an environment in which learning can happen together (Kaufman 2003; Aliakbari et al. 2015).

Learning Interventions

This section will explore learning interventions that support people who live with mental health challenges. Some of these sit within a recovery-based approach (see Chapter 4). The concept of recovery is relevant to the discussion here because recovery involves people taking on meaningful roles within their communities and society and building a stronger sense of personal identity. Engagement with learning occupations can be an important part of this personal development. Learning occupations can be encountered by people living with mental health problems in a variety of ways:

1. Learning encountered through structured therapy, for example, cognitive behaviour therapy (CBT) and psychoeducation;
2. Learning through creative arts groups or life skills activities in the context of a mental health service. This includes Recovery Colleges;
3. Learning in non-traditional educational settings like an art group, creative writing group or reading group. This can be specific to mental health service users (often service user led) or general community groups;
4. Learning through mainstream adult learning contexts, for example, evening classes, further education colleges and higher education institutions. Support can be provided at different levels up to and including providing one-to-one support in and out of the classroom. The role of occupational therapists in these settings may either include facilitating access or ensuring that accommodations to support learning are in place. There may be an emerging role within student services in higher education.

Cognitive Behavioural Techniques

CBT is an evidence based, structured psychological intervention that addresses unhelpful thought patterns and changes behaviour. It is used by a range of mental health professionals in the form of structured packages of therapy, often six to eight weekly sessions for groups. Occupational therapists often draw on CBT by applying its techniques in a range of interventions including anxiety management, assertiveness training, treatment of eating disorders, pain management, management of chronic fatigue syndrome and social skills training (Donaghy et al. 2008; Goldingay et al. 2020). It is also possible to deliver CBT via telerehabilitation, which may also include telephone contact with a therapist. Research has demonstrated that it is very effective, although this is probably specific to a certain service user group and assumes that people have access to the internet (Paxlingab et al. 2011).

There is a strong educational component when using cognitive behavioural techniques, for example, service users learn the CBT 'model' and the connections between thoughts, feelings and their behaviours. They are taught about automatic thoughts and how to notice them, also learning ways of recording and challenging these. Participants develop a toolbox of coping mechanisms to help them to overcome their difficulties and set graded goals for themselves. Occupational therapists can empower their service users to reach their occupational goals by teaching within this framework. They can also work very effectively with the behavioural components by ensuring that goals are graded and achievable for the service user.

There is a long-running debate about whether occupational therapists should use CBT in their work. Some argue that they should not because it is not an occupation-based technique and it detracts from the specialist, profession-specific skills. Others will argue that occupational therapists have the skills to use CBT as part of their therapeutic 'toolbox.' Some occupational therapists, however, use it extensively. The difficulty is that CBT is a very common intervention delivered in mental health services, and sometimes it is used without question and without awareness of its underlying theories and philosophy. A balanced view would be that occupational therapists can use CBT if it meets the person's occupational goals, but they need to do it in a reflective way, always keeping occupation as the central focus (Duncan 2006).

Psychoeducation

Psychoeducation involves educating a person living with a mental illness about the symptoms, treatments and prognosis of their illness (Zhao et al. 2015). It is delivered as a structured educational package of up to 12 weeks, often in groups, and may include providing information in leaflets or other media. It is often used with people who have schizophrenia, but is also used with other conditions such as affective disorder and eating disorders. Psychoeducation was originally developed as a family therapy intervention; it was based on the 'stress-vulnerability' model of schizophrenia and a systems approach to family work aimed to reduce criticism and blame within the family.

The key principles of psychoeducation are:

- Service users and their families are helped by having factual information about the illness and the treatment.
- Service users are informed that the service user has a defined illness and needs to take medication to improve.
- Service users are taught coping strategies, especially for relapse prevention.

The educational elements of psychoeducation may include briefing individuals about their mental health diagnosis and medication, problem solving training, communication training and self-assertiveness training (Bauml et al. 2006). There is a strong element of cognitive and behavioural therapy in psychoeducation, and it strongly supports the medical treatment of mental illness. It can utilize group therapy principles in its delivery. Any information given about a condition and treatment might be called 'psychoeducation' but might not embrace all the key principles described above.

Psychoeducation does align with some elements in recovery approaches and occupational science, for example, it instills hope. It also addresses identity but in a way that labels the person clearly with their diagnosis. A meaningful life is not specifically addressed but assumed. Control, however, is a key difference with psychoeducation. It requires acceptance of the diagnosis and adherence to medication. For occupational therapists working with people living with mental health problems, it offers some promising elements, that is, education and empowerment, problem solving approaches and a positive view that 'recovery' is possible. However, there are some challenges. For example, the content of psychoeducation is based on the medical model, and success may be equated with taking medication. This might go against the wishes or beliefs of the service user and their family. It also does not acknowledge (in its pure form) the 'expert by experience.' An occupational therapist working within this approach needs to be reflective about these elements and negotiate a way of working that sits comfortably within their values and commitment to occupation-centred practice (see Chapter 2). Educating and empowering service users are both essential goals.

Psychoeducation can be delivered by different professionals working together. Eaton (2002), an occupational therapist on an acute mental health ward in the United Kingdom, delivered psychoeducation working with a psychologist and a staff nurse. This intervention may be viewed as more occupation-centred than other psychoeducation approaches, because it focussed on participants' needs rather than symptoms and medication. It also explicitly provided opportunities for social interaction beyond receiving information only. Eaton concludes that occupational therapists, with their knowledge of group processes and activity, are well placed to deliver psychoeducational interventions.

The research evidence base for psychoeducation is ambivalent. Buaml et al. (2006) made strong claims for its effectiveness from the literature and their own randomized controlled trial. Xia et al. (2011), in a Cochrane Review, found that psychoeducation for schizophrenia 'does seem to reduce relapse, readmission and encourage medication compliance, as well as reduce the length of hospital stay'; but the evidence is weak. Zhao et al. (2015) in another Cochrane Review found that 'brief psychoeducation of any form appears to reduce relapse in the medium term, and promote medication compliance in the short term,' but this is based on mainly low to very low quality evidence from a limited number of studies, and more research is needed.

Coaching

Coaching is training or development in which a person, the coach, supports a learner in achieving specific personal or professional goals. Setgouchi et al. (2020) describe it as a key enablement skill in occupational therapy. It is time-limited and goal-specific. Coaching addresses motivation using a positive approach and is unconditionally accepting of the person being coached. In their integrative review of the use of coaching in occupational therapy, Kessler and Graham (2015) identify an educational component as one of the common features across different practice settings.

Coaching is an approach that can be used both to promote mental health and support people who are in recovery. In health promotion an occupational therapist might be working with people to set well-being goals, and this can include physical exercise targets to boost overall health. For people living with long-term conditions like arthritis and chronic fatigue syndrome, a coaching approach can assist with physical and psychological progress by setting achievable goals for daily activities. It is also a very helpful way of working to address workplace stress and to assist with achieving career goals. An example of how coaching is used, recovery from mental ill-health is supporting people to return to education and/or the workplace, assisting their transition and reintegration. Coaching may also be delivered in a variety of ways, including telerehabilitation and the use of mobile applications (apps) as a tool (Setoguchi et al. 2020).

Kessler and Graham (2015), in a review of the use of coaching in occupational therapy, found that occupational therapists have begun to use coaching as a therapeutic tool to promote client-centredness in their practice. They also found, however, a lack of a clear definition of what constituted coaching and a lack of robust evidence of the effectiveness of these interventions. They concluded that more research using clear descriptions of the coaching approach and employing more robust research methods is needed to better inform clinical practice.

Working with People with Low Literacy Levels and Learning in a Second Language

The fourth goal of the United Nations 2030 Agenda for Sustainable Development is quality education, with literacy as a key target of this goal (United Nations Educational, Scientific and Cultural Organization (UNESCO) 2017). According to the UNESCO report, low levels of literacy are unfortunately still prevalent in middle and low-level income countries, specifically in Asia and Sub-Saharan Africa (UNESCO 2017). The multicultural contexts in which occupational therapists work globally also means that people are not always fluent in the predominant language. Both low literacy and communicating in a second language cause barriers to learning and occupational deprivation. People with low literacy levels may organize their thoughts more slowly and are not as comprehensive in their observation of stimulus material. They may also read every letter of a word and one word at a time, which influences their ability to fully comprehend what they have read. People with low literacy levels may also struggle to understand abbreviations, have a more limited vocabulary, make limited use of adjectives and may think in a more concrete way. If they do not understand information, they are less likely to ask for clarification. They also tend to rely on or give basic or nonspecific information and do not make connections between pieces of information (United States Department of Health and Human Services 2015b).

It is not only people with low levels of functional literacy that have difficulty with health literacy. Health literacy is defined as 'the degree to which individuals have the capacity to obtain, process, and understand basic health information and services needed to make appropriate health decisions' (United States Department of Health and Human Services 2015a). A number of factors can influence health literacy including the environment, low vision and hearing loss, cognitive impairment and multiple chronic health conditions (Smith and Gutman 2011). Health literacy affects people's ability to navigate the healthcare system, including filling out complex forms and locating providers and services. People with low levels of health literacy may find it difficult to share personal information, such as their health history, with providers. They may also find it difficult to engage in self-care occupations such as taking medication or managing their mental health. They may also experience inadequate knowledge of health issues, increased readmissions, medication mistakes, higher healthcare costs, decreased health status and limited access to preventative services (Smith and Gutman 2011).

Occupational therapists have an obligation to the people that they serve to ensure that all educational materials and training are adjusted to match the clients' health literacy abilities (American Occupational Therapy Association 2011; Smith and Gutman 2011). Therefore the potential learning barriers have to be identified and health literacy strategies established with the aim of improving the health of the individual, group or population.

Three strategies to improve the usability of health information are:

1) Ensure that the information is appropriate for the users by identifying the intended users of the health information and services and know their barriers to health literacy; evaluate users' understanding before, during and after the introduction of information and services and acknowledge cultural differences and communicate information with respect.
2) Adapt both the design and the readability levels of texts to ensure that they are easy to read.
3) Speaking clearly and listening carefully are essential, along with scheduling enough time to discuss information and engaging the audience. Ask open-ended questions and provide information in the persons' home language or make use of a medically trained interpreter. Occupational therapists can check for understanding through the use of the teach-back method. After explaining a plan or concept, ask the person to repeat back the plan or concept in their own words so that it can determined if the communication was clear enough (Roett and Wessel 2012; United States Department of Health and Human Services 2015a, 2015b).

Further strategies to improve the layout and design of health literacy materials are presented in Box 14.1.

When creating written materials to support learning such as handouts or worksheets, it is useful to assess the readability of the text for the intended audience.

Ensuring Readability

The FOG readability index (Gunning 1952) is a good tool to determine the readability of a piece of text. Readability refers to the use of plain language and whether the written material is presented on the functional literacy level of the people it is intended for. The steps to follow to determine the FOG index are presented in Box 14.2.

BOX 14.1
STRATEGIES TO IMPROVE HEALTH LITERACY MATERIALS

White spaces	Create clearly separated short chunks of text. Ensure that pages have margins and spaces between paragraphs.
Line spacing	The spacing between lines is important to ensure easier reading. If they are too close, the reader can drop lines; if they are too far apart, the reader might not be sure whether the lines relate to each other.
Font choice and size	The font choice needs to be clear (e.g., Arial, Plantin or Helvetica). Font size is dependent on the potential user and the purpose of the text.
Uppercase and lowercase letters	Use a combination and avoid the overuse of uppercase as persons with lower literacy levels tend to read lowercase easier.
Organizing the information	The most important points come first and the number of messages should be limited. To indicate the importance of a part of the text, use bold type or boxing. Breaking down complex information into understandable chunks will help to make written communication look easy to read. Use simple, plain language, and define technical terms.
Use the active voice	Places the focus on the action needed from the person.

BOX 14.2
CALCULATING THE FOG READABILITY INDEX

Step 1	Choose a paragraph from the text (120 words)
Step 2	Count the number of words and the number of sentences Determine the average length of sentences (ALS) ALS = Number of words/Number of sentences
Step 3	Determine the number of polysyllables (three or more) Ignore past tense words with three or more syllables Percent difficult words (PDW) PDW = Polysyllables/Number of words x 100
Step 4	FOG = (ALS + PDW) x 0.4 = Legibility level of text (e.g., 13 = Grade 12 + 1 year)

LEARNING AS ENDS: OCCUPATIONAL THERAPISTS FACILITATING ACCESS TO LEARNING

Social Prescribing

Social prescribing links patients in primary care with sources of support within the community. It provides general practitionerss and other health practitioners with a non-medical referral option that can operate alongside existing treatments to improve health and well-being (Kings Fund n.d.) (see Chapter 6).

Social prescribing has the potential to engage many more people with their local communities and to support them when engaging with and learning new activities. Social prescribing might provide a wide range of services, not all of which would be regarded as primarily education based or facilitating learning, for example advice about housing, debt or benefits. However, it might also deliver opportunities to learn new skills or engage in different activities, for example, creative arts groups, cooking skills or team sports. This could support people to learn something they have never done before or to take up an activity they engaged with as a child in school but not as an adult.

Recovery Colleges

Recovery Colleges deliver comprehensive, peer-led education and training programmes within mental health services. Sommer et al. (2017) describe the Recovery College as an innovative way of educating people with mental health problems, their carers and mental health professionals. Recovery Colleges should be run like any other college, providing education as a route to recovery, not as a form of therapy (NHS Confederation 2012). When attending a Recovery College, students access education and training programs that assist them with their recovery and develop their skills and confidence to live well (Research into Recovery 2019)

There is a small body of largely positive research evidence into the outcomes of Recovery Colleges. Qualitative research in Australia (Sommer et al. 2018) found that they had the potential to facilitate both personal recovery gains and organizational transformation towards recovery-focused service provision. Participants in this study were positive about their involvement in the Recovery College. Four themes emerged from their thematic analysis: connection with others, hope for the future, the importance of the lived experience and changing attitudes and systems. Bourne et al. (2018) found that students in the United Kingdom used mental health services less after attending a Recovery College. Students who attended the Recovery College showed significant reductions in occupied hospital bed days, admissions, admissions under section and community contacts in the 18 months post compared with the 18 months before registering. Reductions in service use were greater for those who completed a course than those who registered but did not complete a course. Stevens et al. (2018), in an evaluation of arts-based courses in a UK Recovery College, also found statistically significant increases in self-reported mental well-being following course attendance. At follow-up, 17 of 24 students reported improved mental well-being, and some spoke of increased social inclusion and continuing to use skills learned in the course to maintain well-being.

The role of occupational therapists and their relationship to Recovery Colleges is not defined in the literature. The colleges' defining feature is that they are peer-led. In many locations occupational therapists will be facilitating the involvement of people with the colleges and supporting their engagement but not being directly involved in the design and delivery of the programmes. An occupational therapist working within a community mental health team might, for example, facilitate the attendance of a service user at a Recovery College by making them aware of the existence of the college and encouraging their attendance.

Within an in-patient mental health setting, the occupational therapist can provide a link to the Recovery College provision in the community as preparation for discharge and to support the recovery journey. Softley and Marrows (2019) describe how they provide

'bite-size' courses in acute mental health wards in the local area, having benefits for staff and service users. The full day courses provided by the Recovery College are difficult for people who are acutely unwell to engage with, but the shorter sessions provided on the ward are a good introduction. As well as being a positive experience for the participants (called students in this context), the sessions raised awareness of the Recovery College with the wards.

Learning in Non-Traditional Educational Settings

There are many initiatives within local communities, often provided by charities or non-profit organizations, which provide opportunities to learn new occupations in a social context. Some of these are targeted at the general population with the aim of promoting well-being. Others are specifically designed to support the recovery of people who have mental health problems. Increasingly, however, these artificial boundaries are being broken down and the activities are open to all. People from all parts of the community are encouraged to 'have a go' at activities they have not done before. Singing groups and community choirs are an example of this kind of initiative. These are often the groups and activities accessed via social prescribing (see above).

An example of a non-traditional educational setting provided for armed forces veterans living with post-traumatic disorder is a care farm (Walker et al. 2017). The farm provided an opportunity to learn new skills, both practical and interpersonal, in a sociable environment. Participants had the opportunity to learn agricultural and land management skills, along with food preparation and cooking for the group. Occupational therapy students who worked as volunteers on the farm observed that the veterans increased their self-esteem as they felt a sense of achievement, learning skills in a supportive environment (Walker et al. 2017). The student volunteers recognized that this was not a traditional setting for occupational therapists to work in, but they felt that the occupational therapy role in mental health could be extended into this kind of learning environment.

Facilitating Access to Adult Education

When supporting a service user in recovery, an occupational therapist should explore further education as a potential route to help the person to reach their life goals. This might be a graded approach, possibly engaging in a short, online course first to build confidence, then perhaps attending an evening class that is not assessed. Service users who want to return to paid employment might have specific qualifications that they need to acquire, and the occupational therapist can identify these and encourage the person's engagement.

A number of barriers for people with mental health problems to accessing education have been identified. These include factors internal to the person such as their symptoms, fear of disclosure of their diagnosis and their knowledge of their mental health condition as well as external factors (Hartrey et al. 2017). These external factors may include the beliefs and attitudes of the institution (Hartrey et al. 2017), lack of local support, financial problems, transport, the stress of attending college and completing assessments. Conversely, there are a number of benefits of involvement in adult continuing education for people with mental health difficulties (James and Talbot-Strettle 2008). For example, it can provide qualifications for work and facilitate leisure opportunities, social interaction and community participation.

Supported education, particularly learning in mainstream further education colleges in groups specifically for people with mental health difficulties and supported by mental health staff, has been found to be useful. A supported education service in Australia found positive outcomes and made a good case for the involvement of occupational therapists in providing this service (Best et al. 2008).

Attending further or higher education has been shown to be useful for military veterans in their transition from military life to being a civilian, a process that can be challenging for some. Gregg et al. (2016) found that veterans are able to make use of their military experiences and begin to construct a civilian identity in the college environment. Occupational therapists working with the veteran population when setting goals for transition should consider attendance at a college or university as a positive step towards civilian life. Support can be given to the veteran with identifying an appropriate programme to meet their longer-term goals and to assist with the application process.

Occupational therapists should take into account the challenges of participating in higher education when working with people to achieve that goal. A World Health Organization mental health survey found that approximately one third of first-year university students screened positive for a mental health problem (Auerbach et al. 2018). Many of these problems started in early to late adolescence and continued when students started higher education. Quinn et al. (2014) found that students with Asperger's syndrome face challenges in higher and further education related to the person, environment and occupation. Their study described an occupational therapy service that aimed to enhance the interplay between the student and their occupation within the college environment. It was found that goals and concerns shift according to students' progress with their course, and they recommended that services employ a student-centred, flexible approach responsive to the particular concerns of these students. Goodman (2019) outlined the case for occupational therapists providing mental health services for students attending university and shared current examples. She states that occupational therapy 'has the potential to address unmet student needs, particularly in regard to developing healthy habits and routines, supporting meaningful engagement, setting and meeting goals, managing time and stress, encouraging social and community participation, enhancing academic and study skills, providing disability supports and accommodations, promoting self-advocacy and strengthening life skills.'

SUMMARY

Education is very much in the heart of occupational therapy and might be disregarded as a distinct approach in its own right. This chapter has shone a light on the theoretical foundations for interventions that have an educational focus and described a number of ways that this can enhance mental health promotion and support people in recovery. Occupational science provides the rationale and inspiration to support people in learning and developing across every life stage so they can thrive in everyday life, doing the things they need to do and want to do to build healthy and meaningful lives.

SUGGESTED QUESTION OR POINT FOR CONSIDERATION

1. Why is lifelong learning important for occupational therapists?

2. How do the 'Five Ways to Wellbeing' tie into occupational approaches to mental healthcare?

3. Suggest examples of the physical, motivational, cognitive and environmental reasons for ineffective learning in your practice setting.

4. How might you determine which learning approach would be the most relevant and effective for a service user?

5. Analyse and evaluate the arguments for the use of CBT by occupational therapists.

6. In comparison to psychoeducation, how might you determine what constitutes 'coaching?'

7. Besides adaptations for written material (outlined in Box 14.1), what other ways could an occupational therapist make healthcare more accessible for those with poor literacy skills and support learning?

8. Suggest an intervention that occupational therapists could develop to address mental health difficulties in higher education.

SERVICE USER COMMENTARY

Occupational therapy drew on my love of learning. Since 1994 I had collected various diagnoses and lost my job, profession and other life opportunities. I was socially isolated due to symptoms of severe mental illness for many years. However, I continued to research my diagnoses and career options, pursuing challenges but with little success.

In 2020 I benefitted from occupational therapy, which changed my life. During the initial assessment I told Sarah, the occupational therapist, that I am like a sponge soaking up knowledge even though I could not concentrate for long on reading. I should have been an easy patient as I had discovered and used informal strategies such as creative activities, learning languages and cold-water swimming, as well as self-directed learning about my diagnoses. I kept busy and distracted from feeling lonely and bitter, while harbouring a vague hope of being lifted out of the disability poverty trap by earning an income. But despite my enthusiasm and persistence, I could not see things through. I got bored, discouraged, relapsed or had other serious life stressors to deal with. I was unsupported and felt aimless, being suicidal in 2020. I was overwhelmed by everyday life and the invisible barriers to accessing services.

While waiting for occupational therapy I found I could listen to self-help podcasts if I wore headphones and did a practical task at the same time (Chatterjee 2019; Fogg 2019). This inspired me to change one small thing, celebrate my success and try not to dwell on failure. My natural competitiveness kicked in and I set myself targets. Little did I realize how these approaches to change are rooted in occupational

therapy. Sarah's assessment covered my routine, environment, motivation and skills. She noticed my organizing and problem-solving difficulties and recommended further assessment of ADHD and autistic traits. I had wondered but these diagnoses had never been mentioned before. It was hugely empowering to discuss my problems with maintaining focus, motivation, procrastination and forgetfulness without feeling a failure or being ignored. I'd never experienced person-centred care like this. It wasn't easy to learn that I was an equal partner in this intervention, along with Sarah and a support worker, Fiona, who she supervised.

Together we gradually learned what worked for me. It was hard to be honest as I often felt like I'd failed, not meeting expectations. Sarah said that if a strategy didn't help, it was more her failure than mine. Slowly I rebuilt my self-esteem as I was guided to explore and experiment with knowledge and activities. Learning about proprioception was a lightbulb moment. Sarah knew that I would hyperfocus on learning about it as something new and interesting. The strange things I do made sense, such as not noticing when I'm hungry, thirsty, cold, overheating, have a full bladder or need a shower. As a 52-year-old woman, I'd found these things too shameful to talk about before. With relief, I learned it wasn't my fault and I wasn't lazy but my brain didn't recognize my body's signals. I understood why I could spend 6 hours gardening without breaks but could rarely manage to remember important appointments.

I learned about hyperfocus and hyperfixation and realized I'd been using these to escape and pass time. I had been

SERVICE USER COMMENTARY—cont'd

reclusive and productive but rarely achieving much. I understood why I felt exhausted despite little physical activity or outside stimulation: my brain was constantly working overtime. Learning about proprioception explained how physical outdoor activities in my youth had helped to manage my ADHD symptoms by giving me dopamine fixes along with cognitive and social benefits. Then injury and health issues meant I'd become a couch potato, putting on nearly 20 kg, staying indoors and sinking into depression.

In occupational therapy I learned to take proprioceptive breaks, setting alarms to counter my time-blindness and using music and citrus smells to focus. I spent 5 minutes doing proprioceptive exercises every half an hour, such as sweeping my back yard and getting natural sunlight, which is a very calming activity for me.

Sarah saw me as me. I am unreliable, prone to emotional outbursts and sensitive to rejection. But I'm also highly creative, knowledgeable, enthusiastic, empathetic and outraged by society's inequalities. Sarah helped me accept that these are positive qualities to celebrate. She encouraged me to continue to learn, to have a voice and to see my strengths by guiding me without being patronizing or coercing. Thanks to occupational therapy I've started to learn who I am, what makes me tick and that I am not socially unacceptable. I have become my own occupational therapist by using what I've learned, sometimes subconsciously, in compensatory strategies. Occupational therapy has been the most useful, supportive, accessible and productive mental health intervention I've ever had, changing my life. I'm now exploring educational and career opportunities in occupational therapy. I'm finally beginning to find and like myself.

JASMINE SCOTT*

Pseudonym agreed with the author. The names of the occupational therapist and support worker are used with permission.

REFERENCES

Aked, J., Marks, N., Cordon, C., & Thompson, S. (2008). *Five ways to wellbeing. Communicating the evidence.* Available at https://neweconomics.org/2008/10/five-ways-to-wellbeing.

Aliakbari, F., Parvin, N., Heidari, M., & Haghani, F. (2015). Learning theories application in nursingeducation. *Journal of Education and Health Promotion, 4*(2), 1–13. https://doi.org/10.4103/2277-9531.151867.

American Occupational Therapy Association (AOTA). (2011). AOTA's societal statement on health literacy. *American Journal of Occupational Therapy, 65*(6_Suppl. l.), S78–S79. https://doi.org/10.5014/ajot.2011.65s78.

Auerbach, R. P., Mortier, P., Bruffaerts, R., et al. (2018). The WHO world mental health surveys international college student project: Prevalence and distribution of mental disorders. *Journal of Abnormal Psychology, 127*(7), 623–638.

Bauml, J., Frobose, T., Kraemer, S., Rentrop, M., & Pitschel-Walz, G. (2006). Psychoeducation: A basic psychotherapeutic intervention for patients with schizophrenia and their families. *Schizophrenia, 32*(Suppl. 1), S1–S9 Bull.

Best, L. J., Still, M., & Cameron, G. (2008). Supported education: Enabling course completion for people experiencing mental illness. *Australian Occupational Therapy Journal, 55*, 65–68.

Bourne, P., Meddings, S., & Whittington, A. (2018). An evaluation of service use outcomes in a Recovery College. *Journal of Mental Health, 27*(4), 359–366.

Carvell, K. (2018). Archaeology as a meaningful occupation for military personnel. *Occupational Therapy News, 26*(9), 24–26.

Donaghy, M., Nicol, M., & Davidson, K. (Eds.). (2008). *Cognitive-behavioural interventions in Physiotherapy and occupational therapy.* Edinburgh: Elsevier.

Duncan, E. (Ed.). (2006). *Foundations for practice in occupational therapy* (4th ed.) Edinburgh: Elsevier.

Eaton, P. (2002). Psychoeducation in acute mental health settings: Is there a role for occupational therapists? *British Journal of Occupational Therapy, 65*(7), 321–326.

Finnegan, A. (2016). The biopsychosocial benefits and shortfalls for armed forces veterans engaged in archaeological activities. *Nurse Education in. Today's Office, 47*, 15–22.

Godfrey, C., Devine-Wright, H., Taylor, J., 2015. The positive impact of structured surfing courses on the wellbeing of vulnerable young people. *Community Practitioner, 88*(1), 26–29.

Goldingay, S., Stagnitti, K., Robertson, N., Pepin, G., Sheppard, L., & Dean, B. (2020). Implicit play or explicit cognitive behaviour therapy: The impact of intervention approaches to facilitate social skills development in adolescents. *Australian Occupational Therapy Journal, 67*(4), 360–372.

Goodman, L. (2019). *Occupational therapy: An Untapped resource in student mental health and well-being.* Thrive Global on Campus. Available at https://thriveglobal.com/stories/occupational-therapy-an-untapped-resource-in-student-mental-health-and-wellbeing/.

Greg, B. T., Howell, D. M., & Shordike, A. (2016). Experiences of veterans transitioning to postsecondary education. *American Journal of Occupational Therapy, 70*(6), 1–8.

Gunning, R. (1952). *The technique of clear writing.* Toronto: McGraw-Hill.

Hartrey, L., Denieffe, S., & Wells, J. S. G. (2017). A systematic review of barriers and supports to the participation of students with mental health difficulties in higher education. *Mental Health & Prevention, 6*(3).

James, K., & Talbot-Strettle, L. (2008). *I'd turn up even if I won the lottery! Research into the factors that impact on attendance, retention and achievement of learners with mental health difficulties.* Quality Improvement Agency.

Kaufman, D. M. (2003). ABC of learning and teaching in medicine: Applying educational theory in practice. *British Medical Journal*, *326*(7382), 213–216. https://doi.org/10.1136/bmj.326.7382.213.

Kessler, D., & Graham, F. (2015). The use of coaching in occupational therapy: An integrative review. *Australian Occupational Therapy Journal*, *62*(3), 160–176.

Kings Fund, n.d. Available at: http://www.kingsfund.co.uk/.

Meadows, T. (2011). *Backward & Forward chaining - I love ABA!* Available at https://www.iloveaba.com/2013/09/backward-forward-chaining.html.

Mind. (2019). *Five ways to wellbeing*. Available at http://www.mind.org.uk/workplace/mental-health-at-work/taking-care-of-yourself/five-ways-to-wellbeing/.

Najdowski, A. C. (2017). Principles behind the lessons. In *Flexible and focused* (pp. 7–21). Elsevier. https://doi.org/10.1016/b978-0-12-809833-2.00002-9.

National Center on Intensive Intervention. (2015). *Behavior contracts*. Available at https://intensiveintervention.org/sites/default/files/Behavior_Contracts_508.pdf.

NHS Confederation. (2012). *Community support*. Available at https://www.nhsconfed.org.

Osborne, H. (2018). Occupational therapists working in food banks. *Occupational Therapy News*, *26*(11), 36–37.

Paxlingab, B., Almlöva, J., Dahlinc, M., et al. (2011). Guided internet-delivered cognitive behavior therapy for generalized anxiety disorder: A randomized controlled trial. *Cognitive Behavior Therapy*, *40*(3), 159–173.

Public Health England. (2019). *A strategy to develop the capacity, impact and profile of Allied health professionals in public health 2015-2018*. Available at http://www.ahpf.org.uk/files/AHP%20Public%20Health%20Strategy.pdf.

Quinn, S., Gleeson, C., & Nolan, C. (2014). An occupational therapy support service for university students with Asperger's syndrome (AS). *Occupational Therapy in Mental Health*, *30*(2), 109–125.

Ratima, M., & Ratima, M. (2005). Practice in an indigenous context. In G. Whiteford, & V. Wright-St Clair (Eds.), *Occupation & practice in context*, 230–241. Marrackville: Elsevier.

Research into Recovery, 2019. Available at: https://www.researchintorecovery.com.

Roett, M. A., & Wessel, L. (2012). Help your patient "get" what you just said: A health literacy guide. *Journal of Family Practice*, *61*(4), 190–196.

Sagan, O. (2008). The loneliness of the long anxious learner: Mental illness, narrative biography and learning to write. *Psychodynamics in Practice*, *14*(1), 43–58.

Secker, J., & Gelling, L. (2006). Still dreaming: Service users' employment, education and training goals. *Journal of Mental Health*, *15*(1), 103–111.

Secker, J., Grove, B., & Seebohm, P. (2001). Challenging barriers to employment, training and education for mental health service users: The service users perspective. *Journal of Mental Health*, *10*(4), 395–404.

Setoguchi, M., Motruk, S., Frank, V., & Kessler, D. (2020). A review of mobile applications to enhance coaching in occupational therapy. *British Journal of Occupational Therapy*, *83*(9), 549–560.

Smith, D. L., & Gutman, S. A. (2011). Health literacy in occupational therapy practice and research. *American Journal of Occupational Therapy*, *65*(4), 367–369. https://doi.org/10.5014/ajot.2011.002139.

Softley, E., & Marrows, L. (2019). Exploring recovery together. *Occupational Therapy News*, *27*(7), 28–30.

Sommer, J., Gill, K., & Stein-Parbury, J. (2018). Walking side-by-side: Recovery Colleges revolutionising mental health care. *Mental Health and Social Inclusion*, *22*, 18–26.

Stainbrook, A., Blumberg, S., & Juarez, P. (2019). *Token economy - Tips and resources for teachers*. Available at https://vkc.vumc.org/assets/files/tipsheets/tokeneconomytips.pdf.

Stevens, J., Butterfield, C., Whittington, A., & Holttum, S. (2018). Evaluation of arts based courses within a UK Recovery College for people with mental health challenges. *International Journal of Environmental Research and Public Health*, *15*, 1170.

United Nations Educational, & Scientific and Cultural Organization (UNESCO). (2017). More than one-half of children and adolescents are not learning Worldwide. *The UNESCO Institute for Statistics (UIS)*, *67*(46), 25.

United States Department of Health and Human Services. (2015a). *Quick Guide to health literacy Fact Sheets strategies* Available at https://healthliteracycentre.eu/wp-content/uploads/2015/11/Quick-guide-to-health-literacy.pdf.

United States Department of Health and Human Services. (2015b). Health literacy online: A guide to Simplifying the user experience. *Office of Disease Prevention and Health Promotion*. Available at https://health.gov/our-work/health-literacy/health-literacy-online.

Walker, G., Anderson, B., Thody, M., et al. (2017). Supporting veterans with their transition. *Occupational Therapy News*, *25*(4), 42–44.

Xia, J., Merinder, L. B., & Belgamwar, M. R. (2011). Psychoeducation for schizophrenia. *Cochrane Database of Systematic Reviews* (6).

Zhao, S., Sampson, S., Xia, J., & Jayaram, M. B. (2015). Psychoeducation (brief) for people with serious mental illness. *Cochrane Database of Systematic Reviews* (4).

15

CLIENT-CENTRED GROUPS

MARILYN B. COLE

INTRODUCTION

In recent years the focus of healthcare has generally shifted from illness-orientation to wellness-orientation (Pitts and MacIntyre 2016) accompanied by a paradigm shift in occupational therapy (Pizzi and Richards 2017). This gives group work added impetus, thereby promoting mental health for many populations across occupational therapy practice. In many mental health settings groups may be the prevailing or standard form of intervention and not simply used for treating several persons at once. A growing body of evidence supports the central role of social connections and participation in health and longevity (Holt-Lunstad et al. 2010; Cole and Macdonald 2015; Haslam et al. 2018). Occupational therapy group interventions have the potential to maximize the therapeutic power of member interactions for social learning and emotional support, adding to the effectiveness of a broad range of goals. To support such practice, this chapter provides an overview of group leadership, dynamics, and the design of occupational therapy group interventions in mental health practice. Additionally, it reviews and gives examples of evidence of group efficacy.

THEORIES SUPPORTING OCCUPATIONAL THERAPY GROUP WORK

Several theoretical developments validate occupational therapy's use of group interventions. First, the emergence of social identity theory affirms the importance of social learning in groups. Jettan et al. (2017) found that 'to the extent that group memberships provide individuals with meaning, support and agency (i.e., a positive sense of social identity), health is positively impacted' (p. 1). Additionally, complexity theory helps to explain the simultaneous levels of thinking required to design and lead effective groups, while client-centred principles shape the overall leadership approach of Cole's seven-step structure.

Social Identity and Reasoning

Research on the impact of social identity (Jettan et al. 2017) implies that well-designed group interventions can have a powerful therapeutic effect on participants' physical and mental health, especially if participation strengthens a member's social identity, which relates to one's membership and roles in social groups (Sani 2012). For example, nurses, accountants, and builders are social identities associated with work groups, while parents, children, and home maintainers are social identities associated with family groups. These examples might also be considered 'occupational roles' because they imply specific sets of tasks. How well we perform these tasks in our own and others' judgment has a significant impact on our self-worth.

Social identities also include self-categorization, or 'the tendency of people to perceive themselves and others in terms of particular social categories' (Ellemers 2019); for example, Hispanic, Jewish, elderly

or disabled. Kellezi et al. (2018) found that even self-categorization within marginalized groups still offers a buffer against environmental threats (in this study, immigration detainees), giving individuals a sense of having peer social support.

Social reasoning in occupational therapy requires practitioners to view social roles and occupations as inseparable and to approach occupational performance within the client's social contexts (Cole 2016). Acknowledging each client's unique social identities within a therapeutic group and providing opportunities to enact them through occupations takes advantage of the health-giving power of social support and connectedness.

For mental health service users, occupational therapy group leaders can build and support positive social identities of group members by incorporating client-centred principles such as inclusiveness, nonjudgmental acceptance, respect, and genuineness. Following Cole's seven steps (described later) can maximize the group's potential for interaction, self-disclosure and mutual support and provide an appreciation of the therapeutic value of occupation to enable continued participation in the social groups that make up members' lives.

The Complex Nature of Groups

Group dynamics and occupational performance are complex phenomena. Combine them within a therapeutic group, and the number of interacting variables can be mind-boggling. Complexity theory bridges the gap between order (the scientific method, objective reality) and disorder (chaos theory, subjective realities). As applied to group dynamics it acknowledges the existence of multiple factors influencing group behaviours and outcomes, some of which are, by definition, unpredictable. Yet, some theoretical principles can be harnessed to increase the probability of positive outcomes; namely, Yalom's therapeutic factors of universality, altruism and cohesiveness (Yalom and Leszcz 2005) or Bandura's concept of self-efficacy (2004), reviewed later in this chapter.

Clark (2010) used the metaphor of 'high-definition occupational therapy: HD OT' (p. 848) to illustrate the complexity of occupational therapy practice. In a high-definition picture we can zoom in for a better look at the detail of a person's face, the position of a tennis ball regarding the foul line or a car's number plate, but then we can broaden the scope to take in the bigger picture, the multiple contexts within which the action takes place. Likewise, in complexity theory, reductionism and holism can coexist. For example, in applying theory, occupational therapists do not have to choose between a frame of reference, such as biomechanics (notably reductionist) and an occupation-based model, such as The Model of Human Occupation (Taylor 2017). Both views of the person are helpful, and one does not exclude the other. This helps to explain how an occupational therapy group leader can consider each member individually and simultaneously attend to the needs of the group as a whole.

Professional Reasoning in Groups

Acknowledging complexity paves the way to understanding the multiple levels of thinking that occur, often simultaneously, when facilitating an occupational therapy group. Schell and Schell (2018) describe the multiple types of reasoning representing the science, art and ethics of occupational therapy. These may be thought of as the therapeutic equivalent of multitasking, shifting attention from one level to another as needed to address the real-time situations of an interacting, ongoing group. While this may seem challenging, expert clinicians do it automatically.

For novice group leaders much of this reasoning can be done at the planning stage. Cole's seven steps remind group planners to incorporate multiple levels of generalization, beginning with a concrete shared experience and moving through discussions of feelings, responses to one another, possible meanings of their collective experience and the potential applications for each individual in his or her own life. When planning groups it is first necessary to consider the typical challenges of a service user population and published evidence about the effectiveness of certain interventions. Then, in matching the activity to the group members, the leader will analyse and grade the activity demands and select an environment with appropriate characteristics. A frame of reference and/ or occupation-based model of practice may guide the selection and adaptation of the group activity and environmental characteristics. Considering the issues typical of persons with specific disabilities such as those associated with stroke, attention deficit hyperactivity disorder or schizophrenia, these levels of thinking might be labelled diagnostic, procedural or scientific. This aligns with the medical model (focusing on symptoms or disability areas) according to Schell and Schell (2018).

However, when therapists begin to interact with group members, they may need to adapt their original group design to accommodate the fact that each member has their own life story (narrative reasoning) and life circumstances and to reflect the mission, values and practical limitations of the setting (conditional reasoning). Group members' immediate problems and concerns must also be addressed early on to promote their interest in the activity and engagement in the group process (pragmatic reasoning) (Schell and Schell 2018).

The first thing a leader must do is establish a therapeutic group culture that includes respect, genuineness, open self-disclosure and non-judgmental acceptance (group values and ethics). Group leaders then engage in interactive reasoning and therapeutic use of self to communicate empathy, encourage participation, facilitate interaction, promote trust between members and move the group towards a state of cohesiveness; the ideal conditions of all working groups.

Most mental health occupational therapists understand the efficacy of well-facilitated groups. Students, however, need to first practise group leadership by facilitating groups of their peers so that the steps become second nature and their own personal style can develop.

Client-Centred Principles in Groups: An Overview

Regardless of health challenges or disabilities, most people seek to recover roles or develop new or adapted roles in society when these are lost. Facilitating engagement in occupations can support people's participation in desired social roles. When people understand the connection between occupational therapy group interventions and their own goals for social participation, their motivation to engage in group activities usually increases (Cole 2018). This connection is central to the client-centred focus of groups in occupational therapy.

Client-centred groups follow the principles of client-centred practice as originally defined by Carl Rogers (1961), such as non-judgmental acceptance (empathy for people with diverse viewpoints), conveying genuineness, respect (recognizing individuals' inherent expertise and problem-solving capacity) and client directedness (enabling clients to choose the direction of therapy). Townsend and Polatajko (2013) updated the evidence for central concepts of client-centred practice, such as power sharing, communication, choice and hope. An additional quality drawn from positive psychology programs is the therapists' communication of empathetic understanding (Cherry 2017).

Boyt-Schell et al. (2014) defined client-centred practice as an 'approach ... that incorporates respect for and partnership with clients as active participants in the therapy process' (p. 1230). When group members collaborate with the occupational therapy leader in setting goals and priorities, the client-centred therapeutic partnership extends to the group as a whole.

Based on occupational therapy's appreciation of the environment as a context for performance, therapeutic groups provide a supportive social and cultural context within which people can experiment with new behaviours and learn to interact more effectively with others.

COLE'S SEVEN STEPS OF GROUP FACILITATION

For the new practitioner Cole's (2018) seven steps establish the basics of therapeutic group facilitation. This prototype can then be adapted as the therapist integrates further knowledge of particular health problems, models of practice and frames of reference, human developmental stages and health/social care settings. The steps address the full range of needs, including those of highly functional group members and, as such, are appropriate for students to practise with their peers also.

Step 1: Introduction

The session begins with stating one's name, the name of the group and one's role as the group leader. To assist the group members in learning each other's names, in addition to stating names around the circle, members can tell the group something unique about themselves, such as where they are from, what most interests them about the group and even something as simple as their favourite colour. What is shared should match service user factors such as cognitive level, disability and age. Names should be repeated at the beginning of

each session not only as an introduction, but also as a way to acknowledge the importance of each member's presence, a gesture which promotes self-identity and participation.

For many groups, a warm-up activity (up to five minutes usually) is recommended. It can capture group members' attention (diverting them from whatever they came to the group thinking about) and prepare them for the activity to come. For example, choosing picture cards with facial expressions expressing different moods may be a useful warm-up for a group role-play to promote self-expression. A warm-up can be energizing or calming. For example, a series of stretches may stimulate an early morning group, while a short relaxation exercise might counteract agitation. Warm-ups may be formal or informal. When members know each other well, an informal chat about how they are feeling may suffice.

Another function of the introduction is to set the mood. The group leader conveys this through facial expressions, body language and tone of voice, as well as with words. The mood of the group should match the goals and content. If the activity of the day is light-hearted the introduction can be upbeat (with humour, smiles and a playful exercise perhaps), while a more serious tone may be needed for topics such as work readiness or coping with loss.

Explaining the purpose clearly is essential. It should occur after the greetings and warm-up, when members are alert and attentive. The goals and methods should be clarified using everyday language. When people understand why they are being asked to take part in a group activity they tend to participate more readily.

In groups which focus on learning, sometimes introductory educational concepts are outlined. For example, a cultural awareness group may begin with a definition of culture and some exploration of group members' perceptions of different aspects of culture. When member discussion is included, this may replace the warm-up since it serves a similar purpose.

The final component of the introduction is a brief outline of the session. For example, saying 'we will be drawing for 15 minutes, then for the next 30 minutes we will share our drawings and discuss their meaning with the group.' This serves several purposes. First, the time limit provides a guideline for how detailed and complex individuals' drawings should be. Second, it tells them that what they draw will be discussed openly with the group, so they can manage their own self-disclosure accordingly. Third, it highlights that the point of the drawing is not to demonstrate artistic ability, but to clarify some aspect of the self and to communicate its meaning through discussion. Research has shown that the initial guidelines, including purpose and structure set forth in the first meeting, have a lasting influence on subsequent sessions (Gersick 2003).

Step 2: Activity

The activity provides the means or method for accomplishing group goals. In our prototype this portion of the group lasts from 10 to 20 minutes and must generate enough raw material to sustain a meaningful discussion for the next 30 to 40 minutes. Activity selection is a complex process, based on the therapist's knowledge of theory and research, activity demands, service user factors and health conditions. A simplified method of selection will be outlined here, with the expectation that the novice group leader will refine it based on experience. This selection process includes activity analysis and synthesis, consideration of timing, goals, the physical and mental capacities of members and the skill of the leader.

Most activities will need to be adapted for use with groups. This is accomplished through activity analysis and synthesis. Activity analysis refers to 'breaking up an activity into the components that influence how it is chosen, organized and carried out in interaction with the environment' (Creek 2010, p. 25). The occupational therapist identifies the component parts and sequences to derive the skills required for an activity's performance, thus allowing the therapist to evaluate its therapeutic potential. Activity synthesis refers to 'combining activity components and features of the environment to produce a new activity that will enable performance to be assessed or achieve a desired therapeutic outcome' (Creek 2003, p. 50). The outcome of this complex matching process between member abilities, skills and preferences and the components of an activity determines the activity selection.

The timing of groups informs activity choice. Most group sessions last from 30 to 90 minutes, averaging about an hour. If discussion is emphasized, the activity itself should take up no more than one-third of the session. In addition, members of the group need to be able to engage with the activity simultaneously within the same environment.

Therapeutic goals will also guide activity selection. In client-centred practice, service users' goals are prioritized and group leaders aim to form groups of people who have similar goals and priorities. Ideally, therapists should hold a group discussion of goals and priorities, as well as activity preferences, before finalizing the group design. However, not all participants are capable of this level of collaboration. In such cases, the occupational therapy leader relies on pre-group interviews with individual members, carers and/or significant others to identify goals.

The physical and mental capacities of members will be a primary consideration in selecting any activity, and formal or informal assessment of service users' occupational performance should inform this. Interventions work best with groups of people with similar functional abilities. For example, Claudia Allen (Allen 1999; Earhart and McCraith 2019) defined six cognitive levels and 52 modes of performance, giving occupational therapy one of its most well-researched and detailed sets of assessments of cognitive ability. Each level (especially 2–5) defines guidelines for task selection, analysis and adaptation, cueing (assisting) during task performance and adapting the environment for maximum functioning. Allen (2005) suggested grouping people of similar Allen cognitive level.

Group leaders also consider their own experience and select group activities based on familiarity, comfort level and past effectiveness.

Step 3: Sharing

The activity should have a definite end. At that point, materials used during the activity are removed from view and the product is shared. The group leader may model sharing with their own example (such as their drawing or writing) or may ask for a volunteer to start. The best way to ensure everyone gets a turn is to proceed around the circle, a norm which becomes automatic after the first few sessions. For activities which include group discussion as a common component, the sharing step is unnecessary.

Step 4: Processing

This addresses the question, 'How did you feel about the activity, the leader and each other?' Feelings are discussed first to prevent them from interfering with the subsequent discussion. The group leader generates the discussion by asking open-ended questions. For example, asking, 'What was hard about communicating non-verbally?' enables members to express feelings of frustration, inadequacy or objection to the activity requirements; 'Whose drawing most relates to you?' encourages group interaction and emotional feedback responses.

Step 5: Generalizing

This addresses the question, 'What did you learn?' Abstract reasoning is needed to derive a few general principles from the data of the group activity. Again, group leaders facilitate generalizing by asking open-ended questions, such as, 'What were some common triggers of stress we shared?' or 'Which coping strategies are good or bad?' Ideally, the general principles discovered by the group will closely align with the group's goals.

Step 6: Application

To learn to be effective, group members need to understand how the principles learned apply to their own lives. The group leader asks questions that facilitate this connection, such as, 'What part of today's activity will you take home with you?' or 'How can you use social skills in your life outside of the group?' Each group member interprets the group experience in their own way, so this application step is an opportunity to verbalize the meaning of the group experience regarding individual goals. Therefore group leaders must ensure every member contributes to the discussion about applications and, if possible, gives a specific example. Assigning homework or keeping journals can reinforce the application of learning outside the group.

Step 7: Summary

A summary of the session reviews each of the seven steps and reinforces the main principles learned. Preferably, members should help summarize. Group leaders end by thanking members for participating and by sharing their own positive feedback on the group experience. Plans for the next session and reminders for application can be added as a final note.

PRINCIPLES OF GROUP LEADERSHIP

Group leadership is generally regarded as a formal position that carries certain responsibilities such as selecting members, setting goals, designing method and structure and providing guidance during the sessions. Dunbar (2009) defines leadership as 'a process that involves a significant degree of complexity through interactive and relational operations to meet the goals of individuals or groups' (p. 2). Research shows that there is no single preferred style of small group leadership. The consensus is that optimal leadership changes to meet varying needs and circumstances (Adams and Galanes 2018).

Mosey (1986) suggested a multilevel approach to the leadership of occupational therapy groups, defining five developmental levels for assisting people in learning group interaction skills (Table 15.1). Mosey's groups recapitulate (repeat) the normal sequence in which children learn to interact in groups. More recently, Donohue (2013, 2017, 2018) has validated Mosey's developmental group theory using structured observation with children's groups and mental health groups. Donohue's (2013, 2018) 'Social Profile' is a useful assessment tool for evaluating both individuals' and groups' need for social and communication skill development as a prerequisite for social participation.

Three Styles of Occupational Therapy Group Leadership

Occupational therapy group leadership may be understood as a continuum that encompasses directive, facilitative and advisory styles. No single style is better than the others; suitability to the particular context is always the key. Choice of style is informed by factors such as participants' abilities and maturity and goals of the task and theoretical approach (Table 15.2).

Directive Leadership

Directive leadership exerts the most influence over the group. It should be used when client groups require considerable direction to benefit from the group activity, such as for people functioning at a low cognitive level or lacking motivation, and for addressing goals that require education, learning and the practise of skills. Groups using a sensory integrative model

	TABLE 15.1	
	Mosey's Developmental Group Leadership	
Group Level	**Occupational Therapy Leader Role**	**Activity Examples**
Parallel (directive leadership)	Providing task, structure and emotional/social support for members.	Imitative group exercises, painting or other creative tasks, simple crafts.
Project/associative (modified directive leadership)	Providing some choices of task, encouraging interaction around task issues and awareness of others. The leader continues to provide support.	Structured learning groups, Allen's Level 3–4 craft groups.
Egocentric – cooperative (facilitative leadership)	Members choose the task. The therapist facilitates interaction and assists members in meeting social and emotional needs.	Task-oriented groups, insight-oriented verbal groups, self-exploration and communication-focused groups.
Cooperative (advisory leadership)	Relationships and socialisation take precedence over task accomplishment. Members provide social/emotional support for each other. The therapist acts as an advisor, provides resources as needed and assists with problem-solving or conflict resolution.	Playing beach volleyball, having a birthday party, group outings.
Mature (participatory leadership)	Members lead. The therapist participates as an equal comember, using modelling, therapeutic self-disclosure and social learning to influence outcomes.	Fund-raising events, self-help groups.

Reprinted from Mosey, A.C. (1986). *Psychosocial Components of Occupational Therapy.* Raven Press; New York: Donohue, M.V. (2017). Evaluation of social participation. In Sladyk, K., Jacobs, K., MacCrae, N. (Eds.), *Occupational Therapy Essentials for Clinical Competence* (3rd ed.). Thorofare, NJ: Slack.

require directive leadership in continually grading and adapting the activity according to member responses. The term 'directive' should not be confused with, authoritative' or 'autocratic'.

Facilitative Leadership

Facilitative leadership is sometimes compared with a democratic approach and, as such, may be the most familiar to occupational therapists. The term 'facilitation' means 'to make easier.' Group leaders use a variety of techniques to enable group participation, encourage communication and self-disclosure and to reinforce problem-solving and social learning. Facilitation is the preferred style when group members have no cognitive difficulties and when the goal is to develop self-awareness and insight. Sometimes facilitation involves shared leadership, allowing group members to take on leadership responsibilities. Gordon (1955) has called this a 'group-centred approach' to leadership.

Advisory Leadership

Advisory leadership exerts the least amount of authority over the group and is reserved for mature and highly motivated groups where participants can structure and organize the group themselves. An advisor intervenes only when members run into difficulty in solving a problem, require additional resources or expertise or need assistance with conflict resolution. Advisory leadership is appropriately used in a consulting role when working with community groups.

Group Leadership Skills

Facilitating Interaction

When a group begins, members tend to look to the leader for direction, and care must be taken not to set up a pattern of communicating only through the leader. When asked a direct question, the leader can defer to another member, asking, 'What do you think?' or 'What would you do in Mary's situation?' Observing

TABLE 15.2			
Occupational Therapy Leadership Continuum			
Factors Influencing Leadership Style	Directive Leadership	Facilitative Leadership	Advisory Leadership
Power factors (extent of control over the group and its members)	Greatest influence. Providing structure, task and support.	Medium influence. Encouraging group participation in decisions and support for each other.	Least influence. Intervening as needed only.
Group maturity	Low. Little connection between members.	Medium. Interrelationships are inconsistent.	Highly cohesive.
Service user factors (mental and physical abilities)	Low cognitive level. Psychological issues create barriers to group interaction.	Medium cognitive level. Capable of some reasoning and insight.	High cognitive level. Highly motivated.
Task factors	Productivity-oriented, non-verbal interaction, psycho-educational goals.	Learning-oriented, self-awareness- or insight-oriented.	Socialisation-oriented, problem-oriented.
Theoretical factors	Sensory motor and cognitive disability approaches.	Psychodynamic and cognitive-behavioural approaches.	Developmental and systems-oriented approaches.
Group focus	Task achievement skill training.	Interpersonal learning, communication or relationship goals.	Problem-solving, wellness or prevention goals.

who responds most often, the group leader looks for ways to involve the less verbal members and to make sure all have an equal opportunity to participate. Silence may raise anxiety levels for some members, but jumping into every silent moment should be discouraged. Sometimes silence allows members to consider a discussion point and formulate their own contribution. When asking a discussion question be sure that several, if not all, members have an opportunity to answer before moving on. Never assume that one or two members speak for the group as a whole. Only when every member has contributed can a true consensus on any issue be reached.

Setting Limits

When members deviate from the group task or goal, the group leader needs to redirect them. In therapy groups various techniques are used for managing inappropriate behaviours that interfere with successful group outcomes. This is best accomplished using the least possible amount of authority. For example, when one member monopolizes the group, the group leader can interrupt by asking the other members, 'How does it make you feel when John does all the talking?' This invites the group members to share the responsibility for setting limits. A good rule of thumb is to never do for the group what the members can do for themselves.

Communicating Empathy

This is one of the best ways to build trust among members; a necessary step in developing group cohesiveness. Empathy is an understanding of each participant's emotions and unique point of view. The group leader needs a broad vocabulary of feelings to convey an accurate understanding of how people might feel about themselves, the task or each other. For example, 'You must be terrified of crowds if you're going to so much trouble to avoid them' might be an empathic response to someone who has shared an episode of agoraphobia. Such statements serve a number of purposes. First, they acknowledge the group member's feelings with non-judgmental acceptance, encouraging further self-disclosure. Second, they give other members permission to verbalize their own emotions. Third, they model for the group an empathic way to respond to one another.

In summary, 'effective leaders are complex information processors who are sensitive to the subtle qualities of individuals and the group environment' (Barge 2003, p. 200). Group leaders should remain flexible and adjust their style according to the group's developmental level, members' psychological or cognitive maturity, the theoretical approach being used and the goal of the group activity.

UNDERSTANDING GROUP DYNAMICS

Groups are a good example of complex systems. Complex systems (chaos) theory compels us to avoid oversimplifying group interactions, which are the result of many individual elements and contexts (Adams and Galanes 2018). As in chaos theory, the complex interplay of group interactions with contextual factors makes group outcomes unpredictable. The application of occupational therapy models of practice can help define these transactions, thereby increasing the odds of positive group outcomes (Cole and Tufano 2020). For example, the Person-Environment-Occupation Model (Baptiste 2018) or Kielhofner's Model of Human Occupation (Taylor 2017) can help the group leader to make appropriate connections between the client factors and the environmental factors that may either facilitate or act as barriers to their occupational performance. In current practice it is not uncommon to combine such models with particular frames of reference, such as sensory integration (Ayres 1979; Lane et al. 2014) or the dynamic model of cognition (Toglia et al. 2014), when designing group interventions for specific populations. Experienced group leaders learn to combine theoretical evidence with the unfolding narratives of members and situations to provide relevant group experiences (Cole 2018).

Group Dynamics as Therapy

Group dynamics have been widely researched for many years across numerous disciplines. This section reviews some key findings. Yalom's (Yalom and Leszcz 2005) therapeutic factors, derived from summarizing many research studies over decades (Table 15.3), offer insight into the healing power of groups and are frequently cited. For example, Restek-Petrovic et al. (2014) found that in groups of people with psychosis,

the installation of hope, cohesiveness and existential factors ranked highest in importance. Hauber et al. (2019) applied Yalom's factors in groups with high-risk adolescents, showing that cohesion, interpersonal learning, guidance and identification were most effective for recovery. These researchers also updated Yalom's ideas by adding four more factors: self-esteem, turning point, resilience and epistemic trust, further defined in Table 15.3.

Group Process

Group process may be best understood by what it is not: it is not content. Content includes what is said and done by group members. Process refers to social structures, symbolic meanings, transference and countertransference, communication patterns, non-verbal communication and emotional responses that often lie beneath one's conscious awareness. Yalom and Leszcz (2005) describe group process as a focus on the interrelationships of members in the 'here and now,' that is, during the session itself. They describe a self-reflective loop with both an experiencing and a reflecting component. In simple terms, the group participates in a shared experience and then reflects on its meaning through group discussion. Cole's seven steps incorporate this concept using short structured tasks on which to reflect through analysis of processing (feelings), generalizing (thoughts/ideas) and application (behaviours). Through the analysis process, group members may develop an awareness of how their own behaviours affect others and what must be changed to engage in more meaningful relationships with other people.

Because of the subtle yet complex qualities of group process, group leaders become skilled at observing and facilitating process only through experience. Consequently, supervision is necessary for students to become fully aware of these very powerful yet often invisible forces within groups.

Group Culture (Norms)

Group norms are an 'unspoken and often unwritten set of informal rules that govern individual behaviours in a group' (Business Dictionary 2022). They are customary ways of doing things within a group culture, which is based on group members' shared attitudes, beliefs, customs, and both written and unwritten rules (Business

TABLE 15.3	
Irvin Yalom's Therapeutic Factors of Groups	
Therapeutic Factor	**Brief Interpretation for Occupational Therapy Groups**
Instillation of hope	Even in anticipation of group membership clients are inclined to believe that change is possible through the group experience.
Universality	Through group sharing and interaction members learn, often with great relief, that they are not alone.
Altruism	With coaching and modelling members become aware that they have much to offer each other and that offering help to others can benefit themselves as well.
Imparting information (guidance)	Groups offer a practical means of educating those with similar issues, but often the most useful information comes from the group members sharing advice, ideas and solutions.
Corrective recapitulation of the primary family group (family re-enactment)	Maladaptive learning from one's own imperfect family can be openly explored and modified within an emotionally safe group environment and through altered perceptions of reality.
Development of socialising techniques	According to Bandura's (1977, 2004) social learning theory, people learn appropriate social behaviours through observation of others. Groups offer multiple opportunities to do this.
Imitative behaviour	When group members observe that certain behaviours have positive consequences for others, they tend to imitate those behaviours.
Interpersonal learning	Groups offer multiple opportunities for giving and receiving feedback from others. Through feedback, members develop a more accurate self-perception and reality-orientation.
Group cohesiveness	Cohesiveness is a preferred state in which the group members accept and support one another and freely self-disclose.
Catharsis	Emotional expression of previously hidden emotionally-charged issues or experiences can have a healing effect.
Existential factors	Many spiritual concerns, such as the meaning of one's life, the acceptance of anxiety as a part of living and an awareness of one's own mortality can be clarified through group interaction.
Self-esteem	A sense of worth within the group, self-confidence.
Turning point	Member pointing out a crucial moment of change in the therapy group.
Resilience	Belief that one can cope with stressful life events.
Epistemic trust	Able to trust and learn from other people.

From Yalom, I., Leszcz, M. (2005). *The Theory and Practice of Group Psychotherapy* (5th ed.). New York: Basic Books; Hauber, et al. (2019).

Dictionary 2022). According to Adams and Galanes (2018), 'the whole process of communication among group members is "rule-governed"' (p. 100). Explicit norms (or rules) are verbalized by the group leader at the outset, such as the venue and timings, the expectation for participation and the importance of confidentiality and mutual respect. Non-explicit norms are not verbalized or written down but assumed (Adams and Galanes 2018) and may include, for example, social conventions, such as, 'If you don't have something good to say, don't say anything,' which may incline members to avoid conflict, resulting in the censorship of negative emotions or responses. Therapists should discourage social norms which inhibit the free expression of emotion while preserving a culture of respect and genuineness. Group leaders sometimes need to model the constructive expression of negative emotions or feedback. For example, 'Sometimes you come across as rude' can be stated more positively as 'when you use sarcasm it makes me (or others) feel defensive and I'm not sure

TABLE 15.4 Therapeutic Norms of Occupational Therapy Groups	
Group Norm	**Occupational Therapy Example**
Open self-disclosure	Sharing personal drawings with the group, including both positive and negative aspects of self-identity.
Group interaction	Members ask each other questions about their drawings and offer empathetic responses.
Focus on process	Open discussion of feeling responses to the task after sharing, including what was hardest and easiest and why.
Give feedback to others	Members discuss what they like and do not like about each other's behaviour, stating dislikes constructively.
'Receive feedback thoughtfully	Therapist uses empathy to help members explore both positive and negative responses to feedback.
Verbalize concrete application of group learning for each member	Members use an 'ideal person' drawing to define qualities they admire in a friend. They agree that each will identify and have a conversation with one such friend during the coming week.

From Yalom, I., Leszcz, M. (2005). *The Theory and Practice of Group Psychotherapy* (5th ed.). New York: Basic Books.

that's the response you're looking for.' It is suggested that students practise doing this with each other before attempting to model it for service users.

Norms can be therapeutic or non-therapeutic. Group members speaking to the leader but not to each other is a non-therapeutic norm. Once established, group cultural norms can be very persistent. Therefore group leaders should never hesitate to redirect the group at the first sign of trouble. Therapeutic norms (Table 15.4) promote group cohesiveness, while non-therapeutic norms hinder group development.

Group Roles

Roles in groups may be assigned or voluntary. In health and/or social care teams, for example, managers supervise staff according to a predetermined organizational structure, with each assigned role (or job description) specifically defined. In the classic study by Benne and Sheats (1948) three types of non-explicit or voluntary roles were identified: task roles, group maintenance roles and individual (or problematic) roles, as confirmed by Adams and Galanes (2018).

Task roles include initiator, information/opinion-seeker and -giver, elaborator, coordinator, orienter, evaluator critic, energizer, recorder and procedural technician. These roles help a group to accomplish its task. Group maintenance roles influence the relationships among members: encourager, harmonizer, compromiser, gate keeper/expediter, standard setter, group (process) observer and commentator and follower. Members of a mature group voluntarily take on a variety of roles; or, put another way, a member's comfort with a variety of roles is regarded as a sign of maturity. Group roles may be understood as a form of shared leadership. When members take on task and maintenance roles, they can accomplish the group's goal with minimal intervention from the leader (advisory leadership). When members are unable or unwilling to undertake roles, the leader steps in (directive leadership). Facilitative leadership falls somewhere in between these two opposites, as the group leader enables members to take on some roles while retaining others, in the group's best interests.

Problem Behaviours of Members

Some group roles can disrupt or interfere with group functioning and integrity and may be seen as problem group behaviours. Benne and Sheats (1948) referred to these as individual roles. Attention-seeking roles such as dominator, aggressor, recognition-seeker, special interest pleader and self-confessor divert the group to irrelevant issues unless redirected by the leader.

Empathy and group member involvement are possible strategies for meeting the member's need for attention/recognition while allowing member feedback to expose the effect of their individually-centred behaviours. Likewise, the blocker, help-seeker and elitist roles (adopted by individuals who feel they deserve special treatment) use self-centred behaviours to meet their own emotional needs at the expense of the group. For example, a blocker's silence or stubborn resistance

		Beginning of the Group -- End of the Group				
Theorist	**Year***	**1**				
Bion	1961	Flight		Fight		Unite
Schutz	1958	Inclusion		Control		Affection
Tuckman & Jensen	1977 2010	Forming	Storming	Norming	Performing	Adjourning
Yalom	1985	Orientation		Conflict	Cohesiveness	Maturity
Poole	1983 2003	Multiple sequences, cycles, breakpoints, activity tracks				
Gersick	1984	First meeting	Phase 1	Midpoint transition	Phase 2	Conclusion

TABLE 15.5

Summary of the Emergence of Influential Group Development Models

*Year refers to the earliest introduction of each specific group development theory to show when each model emerged and how earlier models influenced later ones.
Reprinted from Cole, M. (2018). Group Dynamics in Occupational Therapy: The Theoretical Basis and Practice Application of Group Intervention (5th ed.) (p. 34). Thorofare, NJ: SLACK Incorporated. Reprinted with permission from SLACK Incorporated.

to self-disclosure may cause other members to feel judged or criticized. Help-seekers actively seek help but reject it, angering advice-giving members. Elitists remain cynical and uninvolved, also provoking resentment among members. These difficult behaviours must be dealt with by the occupational therapy leader to preserve the group's integrity. When one member's behaviour continues to block the group's development, that member should be removed from the group and treated individually. The group leader should never sacrifice the group's well-being because of one member.

Group Development

Theories of group development have changed dramatically over time (Table 15.5). Until the mid-1980s there was a relative agreement that all groups evolved through predictable stages of development. Phase theorists, such as Tuckman (1965), Bion (1961), Schutz (1958) and Yalom (1985), all defined an initial phase marked by a dependence on the leader and a search for structure and purpose. Subsequently, the group encountered a conflict phase during which the leader, task and/or group structure was challenged. All theorists concurred that conflict must be resolved for the group to reach cohesiveness. Continued growth involved the free expression of both positive and negative emotions, moving the group towards cohesive maturity, the final and ideal group stage.

Tuckman's (1965) model has undergone the most extensive revision as currently applied with work teams in business, also known as 'team development' (Abudi 2010). Tuckman's final stage, entitled 'adjourning,' includes a team self-assessment after each work task ends so that group members can improve the process of working together in future tasks. Ravi and Tuckman's (2016) study of the organizational literature concluded that a combination of Tuckman's and Gersick's models have the most relevance in natural, everyday environments and in corporate ones.

Gersick (2003) studied eight diverse work teams to discover how their function changed over time. She changed the focus of group development from looking at typical behaviours to exploring the mechanisms of change; considering both internal and environmental contingencies. She found the first half of a group's actual meeting time was an inertial (non-directional) movement, the direction of which is set during the first meeting. This places great importance on the initial meeting at a time when the group's culture may be easily shaped. Groups then undergo a midpoint transition during which the direction of the group is revised. The group acknowledges earlier problems and faces the reality of limited time left to complete its task. The ideal outcome gives way to a more realistic one, and both content and process adapt to accommodate this altered goal. Progress may spur ahead to reach a markedly accelerated conclusion.

The influence of context on groups not addressed by phase theorists is significant in Gersick's (2003) model. Context influences group development at three critical points: design of the group, the first meeting and the midpoint transition. Adams and Galanes (2018) refer to 'Gersick's two-phase model' (p. 93), recognizing the two distinct periods occurring before and after the midpoint. Newer theorists add a non-linear systems perspective including three processes: input, throughput and output. The presence of feedback at every juncture allows groups to learn from past mistakes or misfortunes and, ultimately, to improve outcomes (Hurt 2012).

In client-centred occupational therapy groups, when members take on more leadership responsibility, we are more likely to see the kind of dynamics reported by Gersick (2003). Group leaders should acknowledge the importance of initial planning and establishing therapeutic norms assertively during the first meeting. With economic pressures in healthcare, more therapeutic groups will be time limited. Consequently, occupational therapy group leaders should anticipate the midpoint transition and use it as an opportunity to redirect and refine goals, correct non-therapeutic norms and provide the resources needed to increase the likelihood of positive outcomes.

Ending Groups Therapeutically

Separation issues affect groups which have met over a long period and need to be considered as the end approaches. As in life, when relationships end, some people are better at letting go and moving on than others. When a group has six or more sessions preparation for the end should begin two weeks beforehand, with comments or questions during the session, summary. This gives group members time to think about their goals and what still needs to be done. When the group leader encourages open expression of both positive and negative feelings, members can have the added benefit of feedback from both the therapist and each other. Reviewing the group's activities can help the group to summarize what was learned. Finally, the occupational therapy group leader shares their own perspective, reinforcing positive outcomes. For those members who typically cope negatively with loss (anger, depression, withdrawal, re-emergence of symptoms), a positive group termination provides a model for future endings in life.

DESIGNING GROUP INTERVENTIONS

Careful planning is essential. The written group plan, or group protocol, serves as a guide for group sessions and may also be used to promote the group. This section reviews the main components of a group protocol: needs assessment, member selection, group goal-setting, choosing a frame of reference, logistics (group size, time, setting), session outlines, supplies and cost and outcome criteria.

Needs Assessment

An occupational therapy needs assessment can be made using case notes and/or by gathering information from referrers, significant others (such as carers) and service users themselves (through surveys or interviews). Focus groups, comprising representatives of the target population, or others knowledgeable about them, can employ group process to assess the needs and priorities of potential group members (Cole 2018). In client-centred practice, the participants' collective occupational priorities form the basis for defining group goals.

Member Selection

Designing a written group protocol can guide member selection by outlining the group's inclusion and exclusion criteria. Therapists select group members with common abilities and/or challenges, and the purpose of group membership should be discussed with each member prior to the initial session.

Group Goal-Setting

Collective goal-setting is ideally accomplished in an initial group meeting with potential members and will inform group design and the selection of appropriate activities. Themes are combined with occupational therapy modalities in creating titles for groups, for example, 'Art for Social Skills,' 'Mental Problem Solving for Work Readiness,' or 'Movement for Health.' Each title includes both goals and methods in a different occupational therapy frame of reference (see below). The group protocol should include at least five therapeutic goals, with a rationale for each.

Theory-Based Groups

Selecting the most appropriate occupational therapy model(s) of practice and frame(s) of reference is integral to therapists' professional reasoning. These should be identified within the group protocol and briefly justified for use with the specific populations and goals described. For example, the psychodynamic frame of reference may guide the application of creative media with goals involving self-awareness, insight, effective expression or control of emotion and development of skills for maintaining satisfying interpersonal relations. A group entitled 'Art for Social Skills' suggests using art to raise member self-awareness as a basis for forming trusting relationships with others.

'Mental Problem Solving for Work Readiness' suggests the use of cognitive-behavioural exercises to build vocational skills. The cognitive-behavioural frame of reference may guide the use of learning or the practise of skills and be applicable to communication/memory games or problem-solving tasks related to members' work-readiness goals such as stress management, assertiveness, time management and the modulation of maladaptive occupational patterns such as compulsions or addictions.

'Movement for Health' applies sensory motor principles, such as biomechanics or sensory integration, in designing movement activities for the group. Depending on the importance of repetition and skilled movement, the activity portion of the group may be extended to two-thirds and discussion time diminished correspondingly if participants have limited capacity to verbalize. For example, Ross's five stage groups (Cole 2018) use the principles of sensory integration with a structure similar to Cole's seven steps, emphasizing non-verbal communication. Ross's groups work on goals such as increasing attention and alertness for people with minimal cognitive functioning. Cole (2014) described the advantages of physical exercise such as sports, yoga, zumba and relaxation for mental health clients; most of which easily lend themselves to making the connection between physical and mental well-being in groups (See also Chapter 13). However, the creative use of movement, such as in dance therapy, might be better understood using a psychodynamic frame of reference.

Group Logistics: Size, Timing and Setting

While the group leader may create a smaller group when more therapist assistance is anticipated, most therapeutic groups should not exceed eight members (Cole 2018). A similar recommendation is made for business managers: Axtell (2018) notes that 'the most productive meetings contain only five to eight people' (p. 1). He also suggests 'there is a tipping point beyond which the quality of the conversation begins to erode' (Axtell 2019, p. 2). Wang and Evans (2019) reviewed the size of business teams, noting an overall pattern: large diverse teams which dominate in industry, science and sports excel at solving problems that build on existing and popular ideas. But small teams are more likely to 'disrupt conventional thinking by generating new directions' (p. 5). This implies that therapeutic change might be more likely in a smaller sized group; but how small? In business there is a popular saying that 'if you can't feed a team with two pizzas, it's too large' (Wang and Evans 2019, p. 6). Another similarity between therapeutic groups and corporate teams is that both function best when they work through their individual, functional, and hierarchical differences towards a common plan (Katzenbach and Smith 2011).

As noted earlier, most group sessions last about an hour, although this is adaptable according to the activity selected and members' attention span. The time and place for a group to meet may depend on contextual factors, such as the availability of equipment, the need for privacy and freedom from distractions or the use of community resources.

Session Outlines

Outlines for each session should follow the format in Box 15.1. Activity descriptions should be clear and detailed enough for another occupational therapist to follow and lead the group as you intended. At least three open-ended discussion questions should be included for Steps 4 to 6 (see Cole's seven steps described earlier). Points for summary should be anticipated, even though they will change as the actual session unfolds. Planning at least six sessions is suggested when writing a group protocol.

BOX 15.1
GROUP SESSION OUTLINE USING COLE'S SEVEN STEPS

Title of group (overall theme)

Title of session (today's activity)

Number in sequence (e.g., Session 3 of 8 total)

Goals addressed

Timeframe (e.g., warm up – 5 min, activity – 15 min, etc.)

Supplies (list and include number needed)

Description

Warm-up

Activity instructions

Processing questions (at least three open questions)

Generalizing questions (at least three open questions)

Application questions (at least three open questions)

Points for summary

Supplies and Cost

Supplies and costs can be estimated from the session outlines. This information will be needed for marketing the group to service managers and/or community partners. Cost will depend upon the number of members, the average cost of items needed and what resources might be available free of charge.

Outcome Criteria

Occupational therapists use outcome criteria to evaluate interventions by measuring goal achievement. Pre- and post-group assessments may determine what has changed. To assess progress during each session, a check sheet or rating scale may be designed. Occasionally, published assessment tools may fit specific group goals, and these may be incorporated into the sessions. For example, role assessments (Hemphill and Urish 2019) may be incorporated into a retirement planning group for anticipating changes in role status, or Toglia and White's (2019) weekly calendar planning activity may be used in a mental health recovery group for determining levels of self-awareness, learning and executive functioning.

GROUP EFFECTIVENESS: THE EVIDENCE

Group therapy is a 'popular and effective format for psychological intervention, and both anecdotal and empirical data consistently point to group dynamics as the primary driver of its benefits' (Cruwys et al. 2019, p. 1). Ezhumalai et al. (2018) cite ample evidence of the overall effectiveness of group therapy, making a distinction between group work (focused on growth and development) and group therapy (focused on increasing health and recovery). These authors, offering group therapy to groups of 8 to 12 members with substance abuse disorders in India (led by psychiatrists, social workers, nurses and occupational therapists), found that group engagement resulted in members' reduced symptoms, better social functioning and declining relapse rates; changes which remained relatively stable over time (Ezhumalai et al. 2018). Several psychology studies used group interventions with cognitive techniques, such as cognitive remediation and emotion skills training (Tchanturia et al. 2014), reminiscence for male veterans (Chueh and Chang 2013) and narrative enhancement (Roe et al. 2013). These findings emphasize the importance of therapeutic use of self, group dynamics and skilled leadership for occupational therapy group leaders.

Self-Efficacy in Groups

According to Bandura (2004), 'human health is a social matter, not just an individual one' (p. 143). Self-belief, or self-efficacy, plays a central role in building good health habits and maintaining social relationships. However, this is a problem area for many people with mental health difficulties. For example, Clarke et al. (2014) found improving self-efficacy is a key element in reducing anxiety and depression.

Occupational therapy group leaders can strengthen self-efficacy by having members practise different group roles. Members of a group can focus on expressing emotions and empathizing with one another while doing activities together. A group leader can model effective responses and problem-solving, as well demonstrate how to correct misunderstandings and resolve conflicts.

Occupational Therapy Group Evidence

A systematic review of evidence for the effectiveness of 'activity-based groups' for mental health populations proclaimed a lack of high-level evidence (randomized controlled trials) and a need for 'large scale rigorous research' (Bullock and Bannigan 2011, p. 257). However, if one looks beyond mental health practice, specifically, and considers quasi-experimental and qualitative methodology, there is a wealth of evidence for the value of group interventions. For example, occupational therapy group interventions for people who had experienced a stroke were shown to be more effective than individual therapy, demonstrating significant increases in both occupational performance and satisfaction (Mehdizadeh et al. 2017) (see Table 15.6 for further evidence).

Probably the best-known evidence of occupational therapy group effectiveness comes from the University of Southern California Well Elderly Study (Clark et al. 1997, 2012), a nationwide randomized controlled trial using multiple pre- and post-measures of health and well-being. This nine-month occupational therapy programme for community-living older adults combined individual and group work, citing an earlier edition of Cole's seven steps (2018) in outlining the structure and leadership for their group interventions. Clark et al. (1997) described the intervention as 'an OT group, a social activity group and a non-treatment control group,' resulting in 'significant benefits for the OT preventive treatment group ... across various health, function, and quality of life domains' (p. 1321). Craig and Mountain (2007) conducted similar groups in the United Kingdom, with equally positive results, namely:

- a sense of validation by the older person's peer group
- reduced isolation, social support, and friendships
- new skills practised in a supportive environment
- generation of ideas through mutual listening and group problem-solving
- modelling in which other members acted as role models.

A follow-up study by Mountain and Craig (2011) attributed these benefits to an increase in self-efficacy that resulted from members doing activities with others and 'translat(ing) skills developed within the safety of the group into real world experiences' (p. 57). In both studies, participants had maintained gains in occupational participation, health and well-being in a six-month follow-up measure after the programme ended.

CONCLUSION

This chapter has reviewed how occupational therapy group interventions contribute much to client-centred mental health practice and also suggests how group interventions can address psychosocial needs for a broad range of populations outside traditional mental health settings (see Table 15.6).

A carefully designed group (using Cole's seven steps), the application of appropriate theory, prudent selection of members and service user participation in goal selection all contribute to the positive outcomes indicated. Additionally, group leaders need an understanding of group dynamics, as well as good leadership skills, including writing a clear, concise group protocol, attentiveness to unfolding group dynamics and the skilled facilitation of member involvement using the techniques described.

In short, this chapter has shown how group work continues to be a dynamic and cost-effective tool for both evaluation and intervention in occupational therapy.

TABLE 15.6
Group Examples in the Occupational Therapy Literature

Group/Population	Brief Description	Citation
Lifestyle re-design groups with community-living older adults	Small groups of community-dwelling seniors met 2 h/wk for 9 months following pre-set modules – e.g., using public transport. The occupational therapy groups improved members' health and well-being and reduced healthcare costs.	Mandel et al. (1999) Mountain and Craig (2011); Clark et al. (2012)
Women recovering from substance abuse at an alcohol and drug abuse centre	A programme of weekly, craft-based self-development/life skills occupational therapy groups promoting recovery through the re-definition of self, meaningful activity, greater personal control and mutual support. A survey (n = 893) showed high satisfaction (97.3%) and engagement. The groups used a person-environment-occupation model and Cole's seven steps.	Peloquin et al. (2018)
Sensory-focused play and attachment for children and foster parents	A group programme facilitated by occupational therapy students on fieldwork placement for 30 child/foster parent pairs using sensory-focused play and relaxation to promote regulation of emotion and attachment. Positive outcomes in self-regulation, attachment, social interaction and relationships with significant others.	Sanders et al. (2016)
People experiencing negative psychotic symptoms as inpatients	An occupational therapy group programme for four to six inpatients with negative symptoms (e.g., anhedonia, or inability to experience pleasure). Between 10 and 12 task-based 'feelings and doings' sessions encouraged members to anticipate positive emotions and self-efficacy through shared activities, social interaction and peer support.	Revheim et al. (2016)
A community mobility program for older adults	A 4-week programme modelled on Clark et al.'s (2012) Well Elderly study promoted community mobility for seven non-driving elders via education, assistive devices, peer support and alternative transport strategies. Outcomes indicated increased mobility, awareness, confidence and social participation.	Mulry (2016)
Psychological well-being in childhood cancer survivors through self-expression	A programme of five 'Discover Your Awesome' sessions for three adults regarded as trauma survivors (childhood PTSD) following childhood cancer. The 90-minute sessions used collage, painting to music, photography, scrapbooking and casting/painting face masks. Outcomes showed enhanced psychological well-being.	Briskey et al. (2017)
Gardening for people with severe mental health problems	A gardening group program for 20 adults with severe mental health problems, led by occupational therapy students and community mental health centre staff, showed (using qualitative and quantitative data) that building/caring for a garden can facilitate mental health recovery.	Smidl et al. (2017)
Empowering girls for success through an adventure-based program	A 10-week programme for seven adolescent girls (10–13 years old), led by occupational therapy students partnered with a university 'adventure program,' used team-building and adventure-based activities (e.g., zip wire, assault course) to build social interaction and self-concept. Qualitative assessments showed positive outcomes in both areas.	Lauer et al. (2017)
Song writing for goal attainment for homeless men with mental health problems	A programme of eight bi-weekly song-writing group sessions for four men in a homeless men's transitional shelter, led by occupational therapy students, music teachers and music therapists, supported members attainment of personal goals by expressing deep-seated emotional issues through musical performance.	Raphael-Greenfield, Westover and Winterbottom (2017)

Continued on following page

TABLE 15.6		
Group Examples in the Occupational Therapy Literature _(Continued)_		
Group/Population	Brief Description	Citation
Dance as exercise and a meaningful activity for adults with Parkinson disease	A community-based therapeutic exercise programme, led by occupational therapy students and drawing on research-based evidence that Argentinian Tango can benefit balance/gait, fatigue and Parkinson disease–associated quality of life, offered dance classes to people with the disease. Participants reported that the classes helped maintain functional abilities and provided social support.	Lathrop et al. (2016)
Pilot for group-based occupational therapy for people who have had a stroke	Stroke patients participated in six group sessions involving crafts, mobility exercises and cooking, with significant increases in functioning and satisfaction levels.	Mehdizadeh et al. (2017)
Health and wellness group for older adults	An 11-week 'feed your mind, body, and soul' group for 10 older adults, led by occupational therapy students on fieldwork experience, addressed cognition and mindfulness (via brain games and activities), sensory experiences, physical fitness and yoga, nutrition, social participation and leisure engagement. Positive outcomes are reported anecdotally.	Hoffman (2018)

QUESTION FOR CONSIDERATION

1. Why is _social identity_ important to mental health service users?
2. How might you convey the principles of client-centred practice to a service user group? What language would be most accessible?
3. What _inappropriate behaviours_ should an occupational therapist anticipate in a group setting?
4. Do you believe that group-based occupational therapy is better suited to particular groups, such as particular age groups or those with specific mental health difficulties?
5. What are the benefits to group members of a cohesive working group?
6. List examples of implied social norms, and suggest whether they may need to be explicitly discussed and discouraged in a group therapy setting.
7. How can an occupational therapy group leader facilitate positive social learning when members have 1) cognitive impairments, 2) trust issues, 3) histories of trauma or 4) problems with communication?
8. Outline a themed group session with short points for activities and discussion questions for each of Cole's seven steps.

SERVICE USER COMMENTARY

It is always inspiring to hear from a profession so keen to support people's exploration of the life they want for themselves. Occupational therapists do this more than most, perhaps, and this chapter conveys that enthusiasm. One observation might be, however, that the view of professionals about what helps people, particularly from a 'wellness' perspective, is not necessarily the view of the individuals themselves – those with lived experience – and is often considered neoliberalist, reductionist and ableist by user-led groups such as Recovery in the Bin.

Occupational therapy prides itself on being client-centred, but I wonder if this chapter might lean more towards a directive approach. Having participated in and cofacilitated several occupational therapy groups, the biggest difficulty I have with this chapter is that the power seems to inherently lie with the facilitator or 'leader' (as they are repeatedly called here).

For me the power of group interventions, as opposed to didactic teaching, lies within the group. Although this chapter refers to 'ideally' gaining consensus on group goals, it does not focus sufficiently on coproduction or collaboration. For instance, if a group's aim is to strengthen members' social identity, is it not counterintuitive to prescribe and direct what that social identity should be? Would it not be more beneficial to facilitate members' joint exploration and learning of themselves? It is not merely 'ideal' to do this, it is paramount. To feel empowered, one must hold some element of power.

Regarding the emphasis on group task, it may be worth remembering that it is individuals' subjective experience of a group activity that is important, not prescribed occupations chosen by the 'leader.' Arguably, the most important part of a group intervention is group members' interactions; the collective understanding of experience and the social learning and emotional support that springs from them. The task is secondary to these therapeutic processes.

The chapter states that members should share and disclose, but who holds the power if members feel coerced into sharing information they might not want to? The priority must not be simply self-disclosure but cocreation of a group environment in which it feels safe to share pain and vulnerability. Genuine connection and validation of experience can be liberating and life changing, but we often forget the potential for re-traumatization of other members and/or the individual who is disclosing, not to mention people feeling exposed. Trauma-informed practice is not about pressuring people to disclose. The focus on the leader being the role model sounds useful, but the modelling of effective behaviour or skills can come more powerfully from the group if given the space to do so.

Another aspect of the chapter that really struck me was the shaming, blaming and pejorative language used to describe members' 'problematic' behaviours. No thought appeared to be given to how the group leader may be equally problematic. Perhaps understandably, practitioners may react negatively to an 'aggressor,' but it would be worth including more empathic explanations as to why people may take on particular group roles like that. Labelling people personalizes problems rather than seeing them as part of a dynamic. I would hate to come to a 6-week group feeling unsafe and be expected to share my vulnerabilities with a bunch of strangers while a therapist labelled me as a 'blocker.' It would be useful to think about the reactions/responses elicited in the 'leader' and how they can respond more thoughtfully. I suspect this chapter will help therapists who want to remain 'in control.' It would be great to validate those practitioners who want to share power, decision-making and responsibility.

Finally, regarding groups in residential settings (including hospitals), please remember that while the therapist goes home at the end of the day, anything that is shared within the group stays with us. It is not compartmentalized in 'the group' but shared with every person we live with. Sometimes this can be useful, but in high turnover environments like acute wards, the discomfort to benefit ratio is too high to make sharing beneficial. There might be things you too would keep from your friends and colleagues. Please don't expect us to share what we would prefer to keep inside with those we don't know, trust and perhaps don't even like.

Hollie Berrigan

REFERENCES

Abudi, G. (2010). *The Five Stages of Team Development: A Case Study*. Available at: http://www.projectsmart.co.uk/the-five-stages-of-team-development.php.

Adams, C., & Galanes, G. (2018). *Communicating in groups* (10th ed.). McGraw Hill Education.

Allen, C. K. (1999). *Structures of the Cognitive Performance Modes*. Ormond Beach, FL: Allen Conferences, Inc.

Allen, C. K. (2005). *Personal communication*.

Axtell, P. (2018). The most productive meetings have fewer than 8 people. *Harvard Business Review*, 1–3.

Ayres, A. J. (1979). *Sensory Integration and the Child*. LA: Western Psychological Services.

Bandura, A. (2004). Health promotion by social cognitive means. *Health Education & Behavior*, 31(2), 143–164.

Baptiste, S. (2017). The person-environment-occupation model. In J. Hinojosa, P. Kramer, & C. B. Royeen (Eds.), *Perspectives on Human Occupation: Theories Underlying Practice* (2nd ed.) (pp. 137–159). Philadelphia, PA: F.A. Davis.

Barge, J. K. (2003). Leadership as Organising. In R. Hirokawa, R. Cathcart, L. Samovar, et al. (Eds.), *Small Group Communication: Theory and Practice: An Anthology* (8th ed.). Los Angeles, CA: Roxbury Publishing.

Benne, K., & Sheats, P. (1948). Functional roles of group members. *Journal of Social Issues, 2*(4), 123–135.

Bion, W. (1961). *Experiences in groups and Other Papers.* New York: Basic Books.

Boyt-Schell, B., Gillen, G., & Scaffa, M. (2014). Glossary. In B. Boyt-Schell, G. Gillen, & M. Scaffa (Eds.), *Willard & Spackman's occupational therapy* (12th ed.). Philadelphia, PA: Lippincott Williams & Wilkins.

Briskey, C., Powderly, E., Richardson, E., & Atkinson, M. (2017). Discover your awesome: Promoting psychological well-being in childhood cancer survivors through self-expression. *Occupational Therapy Practice, 25,* 22–24.

Bullock, A., & Bannigan, K. (2011). Effectiveness of activity-based group work in community mental health: A systematic review. *American Journal of Occupational Therapy, 65,* 257–266.

Business Dictionary. (2022). Definitions. Available at: https://businessdictionary.info/.

Cherry, K. (2017). *Three key qualities of client centered care.* Available at: www.positivepsychologyprogram.org.

Clark, F. (2010). High definition occupational therapy: HDOT. *American Journal of Occupational Therapy, 64*(4), 848–854.

Clark, F., Azen, S., Zemke, R., et al. (1997). Occupational therapy for independent-living older adults: A randomized controlled trial. *Journal of the American Medical Association, 278,* 1321–1326.

Clark, F., Jackson, J., Carlson, M., et al. (2012). Effectiveness of a lifestyle intervention in promoting the well-being of independently living older people: Results of the well Elderly 2 randomised controlled trial. *Journal of Epidemiology & Community Health, 66*(9), 782–790.

Clarke, J., Proudfoot, J., & Birch, M. R. (2014). Effects of mental health self-efficacy on outcomes of a mobile phone and web intervention for mild-to-moderate depression, anxiety and stress: Secondary analysis of a randomised controlled trial. *BioMed Central Psychiatry, 26.* https://doi:101186/s12888-014-1. http://www.biomedcentral.com/1471-244x/14/272/abstract.

Cole, F. (2014). Physical activity for mental health and wellbeing. In W. Bryant, J. Fieldhouse, & K. Bannigan (Eds.), *Creek's occupational therapy and mental health* (5th ed.) (pp. 205–223). London: Churchill Livingstone, Elsevier.

Cole, M. B. (2016). Social reasoning in occupational therapy: Integrating social theories. In M. Cole, & J. Creek (Eds.), *Global Perspectives in Professional Reasoning* (pp. 145–164). Thorofare, NJ: Slack, Inc.

Cole, M. B. (2018). *Group Dynamics in occupational Therapy* (5th ed.). Thorofare, NJ: Slack.

Cole, M., & Macdonald, K. (2015). *Productive Aging: An Occupational Perspective.* Thorofare, NJ: Slack.

Cole, M. B., & Tufano, R. (2020). *Applied Theories in occupational Therapy* (2nd ed.). Thorofare, NJ: Slack.

Craig, C., & Mountain, G. (2007). *Lifestyle Matters: An occupational Approach to Healthy Aging.* Milton Keynes: Speechmark Publishing.

Creek, J. (2003). *Occupational Therapy Defined as a Complex Intervention.* London: College of Occupational Therapists.

Cruwys, T., Steffens, N. K., Hasla, S. A., Hornsey, M. J., & Skorich, D. P. (2019). *Psychotherapy Research,* 1–14.

Donohue, M. V. (2013). *Social Profile Manual.* Bethesda, MD: AOTA Press.

Donohue, M. V. (2017). Evaluation of social participation. In K. Sladyk, K. Jacobs, & N. MacCrae (Eds.), *Occupational therapy Essentials for Clinical Competence* (3rd ed.). Thorofare, NJ: Slack. Available at: www.Social-Profile.com.

Donohue, M. V. (2018). Social Profile assessment of social participation in children, adolescents, and adults. In B. J. Hemphill-Pearson, & C. K. Urish (Eds.), *Assessment in occupational therapy mental health* (3rd ed.). Thorofare, NJ: Slack.

Dunbar, S. (2009). *An occupational perspective on leadership.* Thorofare, NJ: Slack, Inc.

Earhart, C., & McCraith, D. (2019). Cognitive disabilities model: Allen cognitive level screen-5 and Allen diagnostic module. In B. Hemphill-Pearson, & C. Urish (Eds.), *Assessments in occupational therapy mental health: An Integrative Approach* (2nd ed.) (pp. 255–284). Thorofare, NJ: Slack.

Ellemers, N. (2019). Social identity theory. In *Encyclopedia Britannica, Inc.* Available at: http://www.britannica.com/topic/social-identity-theory.

Gersick, C. G. (1984). *Life cycles of ad hoc task groups: Time, transitions and learning in teams.* New Haven, CT, USA: Unpublished doctoral dissertation. Yale University.

Gersick, C. G. (2003). Time and transition in work teams. In R. Hirokawa, R. Cathcart, L. Samovar, et al. (Eds.), *Small Group Communication: Theory and Practice: An Anthology* (8th ed.) (pp. 59–75). Los Angeles, CA: Roxbury.

Gordon, T. (1955). *Group centered leadership: A Way of Releasing the Creative Power of groups.* Oxford, England: Houghton Mifflin.

Haslam, S. A., McMahon, C., Cruwys, T., Haslam, C., Jettan, J., & Steffens, N. (2018). Social cure, what social cure? The propensity to underestimate the importance of social factors for health. *Social Science & Medicine, 198,* 14–21.

Hemphill, B., & Urish, C. (2019). Role assessment used in mental health. In B. Hemphill-Pearson, & C. Urish (Eds.), *Assessments in occupational therapy mental health* (pp. 565–578).

Hoffman, L. (2018). Health and wellness group for older adults: Focusing on mind, body, and soul. *Occupational Therapy Practice, 18,* 28–30.

Holt-Lunstat, J., Smith, T., & Layton, B. (2010). *Social relationships and mortality risk: A meta-analytic review.* Available at: http://www.okisneducube,rg.artucke.ubfi%3Adiu%2F10.1371%2Fjournal.pmed.1000316.

Hurt, A. (2012). The punctuated-Tuckman: A conceptual model for the integration of Tuckman, PEM, and systems group developmental theories. *Leadership and Organizational Management,* 143–152.

Jettan, J., Haslam, S. A., Cruwys, T., Greenaway, K., Haslam, C., & Steffens, N. (2017). Advancing the social identity approach to health and well-being: Progressing the social cure research agenda. *European Journal of Social Psychology, 47,* 1–5 https://doi:10.1002/ejsp.2333.

Katzenbach, J. R., & Smith, D. K. (2011). The discipline of teams. In *Building Better Teams.* Boston, MA: Harvard Business Review Press.

Kellezi, B., Bowe, M., Wakefield, J., McNamara, N., & Botsworth, M. (2018). Understanding and coping with immigration detention: Social identity as cure and curse. *European Journal of Social Psychology, 49*, 333–351.

Lane, S., Roley, S. S., & Champagne, T. (2014). In B. Boyt-Schell, G. Gillen, & M. Scaffa (Eds.), *Sensory integration and processing* (pp. 816–868). Philadelphia, PA: Lippincott, Williams & Wilkins.

Lathrop, K., Malsch, A., Massart, R., Goloff, S., Bebeau, D., & Pickett, K. (2016). Dancing the tango: Promoting exercise as meaningful activity for adults with Parkinson disease. *Occupational Therapy Practice, 21*, 17–19.

Lauer, K., Bathurst, T., & Richardson, E. (2017). Ropes and low elements: Empowering girls for success through an adventure-based program. *Occupational Therapy Practice, 9*, 19–21.

Mandel, D., Jackson, J., Zemke, et al. (1999). *Lifestyle Redesign: Implementing the Well Elderly Program*. Bethesda, MD: American Occupational Therapy Association.

Mehdizadeh, M., Hassani Mehraban, A., & Zabediyannasah, R. (2017). The effect of group-based occupational therapy of stroke survivors: Pilot trial, neuro-occupational view. *Basic and Clinical Neuroscience, 8*(1), 69–76. Available at: http://dx.crossref.org/10.15412/J.BCN.03080109.

Mosey, A. C. (1986). *Psychosocial Components of occupational Therapy*. New York: Raven Press.

Mountain, G., & Craig, C. (2011). The lived experience of redesigning lifestyle post-retirement in the UK. *Occupational Therapy International, 18*(1), 48–58.

Mulry, C. M. (2016). Promoting productive aging using an innovative community mobility program. *Special Interest Section Quarterly (SIS), 1*(I), 18–19.

Peloquin, S. M., Ciro, C. A., & Patterson, T. (2018). Population centered groups for women recovering from substance abuse: Satisfaction, engagement, and lessons learned. *Occupational Therapy in Mental Health, 34*, 138–150.

Pitts, D., & McIntyre, E. (2016). Health promotion and wellness for persons with psychiatric disabilities. In T. Krupa, B. Kirsh, D. Pitts, & E. Fossey (Eds.), *Bruce & Borg's Psychosocial Frames of Reference* (4th ed.) (pp. 245–264). Thorofare, NJ: Slack.

Pizzi, M., & Richards, L. G. (2017). Promoting health, well-being, and quality of life in occupational therapy: A commitment to a paradigm shift for the next 100 years. *American Journal of Occupational Therapy, 71*, 7104170010. https://doi.org/10.5014/ajot.2017.028456.

Poole, M. S. (1983). Decision development in small groups II: A study of multiple sequences in group development. *Communication Monographs, 50*, 206–232.

Poole, M. S. (2003). A multiple sequence model of group decision development. In R. Hirokawa, R. Cathcart, L. Samovar, et al. (Eds.), *Small Group Communication: Theory and Practice: An Anthology* (8th ed.) (pp. 76–82). Los Angeles, CA: Roxbury.

Raphael-Greenfield, E., Westover, L., & Winterbottom, L. (2017). Songwriting as an occupation: A medium for occupational goal attainment for homeless men with mental illness. *Occupational Therapy Practice, 30*, 21–23.

Ravi, B. S., & Sumathi, G. (2016). Study on theory of group development: Groups and teams. *IOSR: Journal of Business and Management, 18*(2), 58–61.

Revheim, N., Han, S., Plattotham, M., Buschbacher, K., & Tremeau, F. (2016). Feelings and doings group: An innovative approach for negative symptoms. *Special Interest Section (SIS) Quarterly Practice Connections: A Supplement to OT Practice, 1*(1), 12–13.

Rogers, C. (1961). *On Becoming a Person*. Boston, MA: Houghton Mifflin.

Sanders, H., Sears, A., & Apodaca, J. (2016). Sensory-focused play and attachment: Interdisciplinary collaboration in treatment foster care. *Special Interest Section (SIS) Quarterly Practice Connections: A Supplement to OT Practice, 1*(I), 2–3.

Sani, F. (2012). Group identification, social relationships, and health. In Y. Jetten, C. Haslam, & S. A. Haslam (Eds.), *The Social Cure: Identity, health, and Well-Being* (pp. 21–38). East Sussex: Psychology Press.

Schell, B. B., & Schell, J. W. (2018). *Clinical and Professional Reasoning in occupational Therapy* (2nd ed.). Philadelphia, PA: Wolters Kluwer, Lippincott, Williams & Wilkins.

Schutz, W. (1958). The interpersonal underworld. *Harvard Business Review, 36*(4), 123–135.

Smidl, S., Mitchell, D. M., & Creighton, C. L. (2017). Outcomes of a therapeutic gardening program in a mental health recovery center. *Occupational Therapy in Mental Health, 33*, 374–385.

Taylor, R. (2017). *Kielhofner's model of human occupation* (5th ed.). Philadelphia, PA: Wolters Kluwer.

Toglia, J., Golitz, K., & Goverover, Y. (2014). In B. Boyt-Schell, G. Gillen, & M. Scaffa (Eds.), *Cognition, perception, and occupational performance* (pp. 779–815). Philadelphia, PA: Lippincott, Williams & Wilkins.

Toglia, J., & White, S. (2019). Weekly calendar planning activity. In B. Hemphill-Pearson, & C. Urish (Eds.), *Assessments in occupational therapy mental health* (pp. 219–238).

Townsend, E., & Polatajko, H. (2013). *Enabling occupation II: A Canadian perspective*. Ottawa, ON: CAOT Publications ACE.

Tuckman, B. (1965). Developmental sequence in small groups. *Psychological Bulletin, 63*, 384–389.

Tuckman, B., & Jensen, M. A. (1977). Stages of small group development revisited. *Group & Organization Studies, 2*, 419–427.

Tuckman, B., & Jensen, M. A. (2010). Stages of small group development revisited. *Group Facilitation, 10*, 43–48.

Wang, D., & Evans, J. (2019). Research: When small teams are better than big ones. *Harvard Business Review*, 1–7. Available at: https://hbr.org/2019/02/research-when-small-teams-are-better-than-big-ones.

Yalom, I., & Leszcz, M. (2005). *The Theory and Practice of Group Psychotherapy* (5th ed.). New York: Basic Books.

16 CREATIVE ACTIVITIES

JULIE WALTERS ■ DINAH LAPRAIRIE ■ HELEN MASON

CHAPTER OUTLINE

INTRODUCTION

Everyone, irrespective of age, gender or culture can be creative through their occupations (Reynolds 2009). Being creative is inherent in the performance of many activities and occupations that are an integral part of everyday life. Creativity, like occupation, is central to being human (Blanche 2007). On this premise, creativity can be seen to positively influence health and well-being (Horghagen 2014; Perruzza and Kinsella 2010) and is amenable to being harnessed in therapeutic interventions.

From the start, the occupational therapy profession used handicrafts and other practical activities to assist in the management of and recovery from physical and mental health problems and trauma (Wilcock 2002). The use of crafts went out of fashion in the middle of

the 20th century, both in society at large and in occupational therapy. However, in recent years, there has been a renewed interest in making things by hand (Greenlees and Jones 2011), together with an increased understanding of the health potential of different forms of activity (APPGAHW 2017).

Key Terms Used in the Chapter

This section explains how several key terms—occupation, meaning, activity, creativity, creative activity, making and maker—are used by the authors to explore the use of creative activities in occupational therapy.

Occupational therapy discourse has sought to distinguish between the terms 'activity' and 'occupation' (e.g., Polatajko et al. 2004). For occupational therapists, 'occupation' has been defined as 'a group of activities that has personal and socio-cultural meaning, is named within a culture and supports participation in society' (Creek 2012, p. 25). Examples of occupations include housekeeping, parenting, gardening and banking.

The term 'meaning' refers to 'the social and symbolic significance of participation at any one moment' (Shove et al. 2012, p. 23). The socio-cultural and personal meanings of an activity derive from the occupations to which the activity contributes; therefore meaning will change at different times and in different contexts. The term 'meaningful' is used to indicate that something is significant or full of meaning. 'The *meaningfulness* of an *activity* [authors' italics] is to be found in the fact that it links together the motives and goals of the individual, thus fulfilling the need that lies behind the motive' (Fortmeier and Thanning 2002, p. 134).

An 'activity' is 'a structured series of actions or tasks that contribute to occupations' (Creek 2012, p. 25). Some of the activities that contribute to the occupation of housekeeping, for example, include food shopping, cooking, washing up, house cleaning, laundering, ironing and bed-making; although these may also be considered as occupations in their own right, depending on the context.

The term 'create' comes from the Latin word 'creare' meaning to bring into being, beget, give birth to or cause to grow (Merriam-Webster.com Dictionary 2020). Creativity is the process of creating something new or original that is of worth or value to the creator or others (Pöllänen 2013).

'Creative activity' is action that allows for individual expression or interpretation. Creative activities may be art-based (e.g., visual arts, theatre arts, music, poetry), or they may encourage reinterpretation or new thinking (e.g., working out a solution to a practical problem, designing a garden or critiquing a film). It is possible to approach many of the activities of daily life creatively and use them as vehicles for self-expression (Hasselkus 2002).

People may specifically express their creativity through the action of making something, such as painting, silk screen printing, scrapbooking, sculpting, designing a web page, knitting, or video and film making. To make is to 'produce by combination of parts or ingredients . . . construct, frame [or] fashion'

(Shorter Oxford English Dictionary 2007). 'Making' means producing, constructing or composing. Some crafters and hobbyists identify themselves as makers or artisans. A 'maker' is 'anyone that uses their abilities to create, whether it be mechanical, electrical, musical, visual, or anything else' (Gantt 2013). An artisan is a skilled worker or craftsperson.

How this Chapter Is Organized

This chapter begins with a brief history of the use of arts and crafts in occupational therapy followed by a summary of some of the main benefits of engaging in creative activities. The second section discusses some of the principles and skills used by occupational therapists who employ creative activities in their work, including three examples of creative approaches. The chapter ends with three case studies that illustrate ways in which creative activities are used in therapeutic practice.

CREATIVITY AND MAKING

This section begins by describing how some of the values of the Victorian arts and crafts movement were adopted by the emerging profession of occupational therapy and still influence practice today. It then outlines some of the therapeutic benefits of creative activity: mastery, self-expression, learning, connection and sensory stimulation.

The Arts and Crafts Movement

The multiple, beneficial effects of creating with the hands were well understood by practitioners of the Victorian arts and crafts movement, which was a major influence on the founders of the occupational therapy profession (Griffiths and Corr 2007; Hocking 2008; Laws 2011). William Morris and John Ruskin, who led the arts and crafts movement in the United Kingdom, celebrated people as playful, creative, inspired and unruly beings who are to be valued as autonomous makers, alive with the desire to make and share things (Hocking 2008; Gauntlett 2018).

The first occupational therapy practitioners used carefully chosen crafts to engage the interest of their patients and develop or redevelop their skills. For example, Elizabeth Brodie, the Lady Superintendent of the Glasgow Royal Mental Hospital, wrote:

*Work for the mentally afflicted should be regarded
from a therapeutic rather than an economic
viewpoint [...] Not all patients find their interest
in the lighter crafts. Some find it in the garden, in
the sewing room, in the laundry and in the kitchen
[...] It has been suggested that a patient should not
be utilized at his own trade, but [...] there does
not in general seem to be any good reason for this
argument. The boot-maker, for instance, who is good
at his job, would find his greatest joy in turning out a
boot worthy of his best efforts.*

Brodie 1925, pp. 73–74

Between the first and second World Wars, work was
undertaken by the American Occupational Therapy
Association (AOTA) to classify and analyse crafts; a
skill which was central in the occupational therapist's
repertoire between the wars (AOTA 1928, as cited in
Creighton 1992). For example, Creighton (1992) notes
'the report included guidelines for analysing crafts in
terms of joint motion and muscle strength' (p. 47).

In the second half of the 20th century the use of crafts
as therapeutic media went out of fashion but the ideals
of the arts and crafts movement survived. This can be
seen in the similarity between these two passages, written by Morris in 1884 and Mary Reilly in 1962:

*'[A] man at work, making something that he feels will
exist because he is working at it and wills it, is exercising
the energies of his mind and soul as well as of his body'*

Morris 1884, p. 3

*[M]an, through the use of his hands, as they are
energized by mind and will, can influence the state of
his own health.'*

Reilly 1962, p. 18

In the 1960s an American occupational therapy
writer, Gail Fidler, suggested that what makes occupational therapy unique in the health professions is the
use of activities or objects as part of the therapeutic
process (Fidler and Fidler 1963). Throughout the 1960s
and 1970s, the use of crafts came to be understood in
terms of psychodynamic and humanistic approaches
(Thompson and Blair 1998).

However, in the early 1980s occupational therapy experienced a crisis of confidence, owing to the
dominance within health and social care of a positivis-
tic, bio-medical discourse, and the profession's wish to
adopt this epistemology to enhance its scientific credibility (Creek 2009; Turner 2011). Making does not fit
comfortably within a bio-medical paradigm, nor do
psychodynamic and humanistic theories that rely on
subjectivity to demonstrate efficacy (Thompson and
Blair 1998). In addition, engaging with crafts has historically been associated with the female and domestic.
It has, arguably, been a challenge for a largely female
profession to transcend this stereotype and use crafts
with pride and confidence (Pollard and Walsh 2000).

The Benefits of Creativity and Making

In the early 21st century people are re-discovering the
health and social benefits of engaging in arts activities,
play and creativity in their daily lives (APPGAHW
2017). The do-it-yourself interest of the early 2000s
has transformed itself into many forms; hobbyists are
self-identifying as makers, crafters and artisans. Maker
culture brings people together, in person or online,
to solve practical and social problems through skills
application, often using technology. Crafting continues to include traditional activities, such as crochet or
willow-weaving, but the maker movement has placed
more value on time-intensive, artisanal qualities. It is
said that this focus is a reaction to the pervasiveness
of media and technology, much like the arts and crafts
movement, when artists and makers reacted to the
industrial revolution by returning to simpler, more
meaningful ways of making products and art.

Making in occupational therapy can be used to
achieve many goals. The therapist can use the opportunity of a creative activity to have discussions with the
service user about mistakes and learning and about the
perseverance and dedication needed to master a craft.
For example, practising scales on a piano develops
muscle memory; pulling apart a few rows of knitting
to correct the pattern shows dedication to the quality of the product; waiting for paint on canvas to dry
before touching up the image requires patience; repro-
gramming a computer can improve a process. Once
they achieve proficiency and confidence, individuals
may find themselves attempting new, creative ways
of interpreting and modifying their work, learning
when to break the rules to create something better and
innovative.

Some of the benefits of creativity and making that are discussed here include mastery, self-expression, learning, connection and sensory stimulation/regulation. Many of these benefits may be embedded in one another and/or coexist within the same act of making.

Mastery

To master creative skills an individual must learn from failure and uncertainty and develop the ability to persevere. This mastery, or comprehensive knowledge and expertise, leads to making becoming part of someone's identity; for example, 'I am an artist,' 'I am a singer,' 'I am a maker.'

Creative activities are so numerous and varied that they can accommodate a wide range of abilities with the possibility of advancement to new levels of mastery as the individual becomes more fluent in their chosen art form or craft. The occupational therapist selects or grades activities to provide just the right level of challenge to capture the person's interest without it looking too difficult. The complexity of the challenge or project can be increased as the individual's mastery develops.

There is self-esteem and pride in accomplishment, completion and mastery; it may inspire the individual to consider a new vocation or convince them they have the abilities to engage in occupation elsewhere—transferring a revitalized sense of self-efficacy to other contexts perhaps.

Self-Expression

Creative activities may be used as opportunities for self-expression, either through art or craft making. For example, Müllersdorf and Ivarsson (2016), in their survey of Swedish occupational therapists, found that many used creative activities to 'facilitate the clients' thinking, feeling and doing' (p. 372) to support the clients' self-expression and to thereby become more creative human beings. For example, a therapist facilitating a child to draw an 'explosion monster' allows the child to express anger, which can be helpful in finding an external outlet for the emotion. This is especially relevant to people who struggle to express themselves verbally due age or level of development, for instance. It is unsurprising, therefore, that creative activities are used to augment talking-based therapies such as cognitive behavioural therapy (Zandt and Barrett 2017) and cognitive analytical therapy (Turner 2016).

Zandt and Barrett (2017) provide guidance for practitioners working in child mental health in using creative activities to support externalization of emotions, thoughts and feelings through music, colour, movement or crafts, as noted earlier. For example, a therapist facilitating a child to draw an 'explosion monster' allows the child to express anger, which can be helpful in finding an external outlet for the emotion.

The Kawa River model is another way self-expression can be facilitated using creative activity. Developed by Japanese and Canadian occupational therapists, it allows service users to express their life journey using the visual, metaphorical symbolism of a river's flow (Iwama et al. 2009)

Essentially, the occupational therapist works with the preferences and desires of the service user or group to find the most appropriate creative medium for self-expression. This has the potential to transform the 'illness experience,' as the first author found in her engagement with digital storytelling (Walters 2018).

Learning

Creative and making activities can be used to enable learning and reflection. Psychologists and learning theorists, building on the pioneering work of William James (1899/ 2008), suggest that learning happens more effectively when people are active in making tangible objects in the real world. This phenomenon has been studied by constructivist and constructionist scholars such as Piaget and Cook (2013) and Papert and Harel (1991) and is influential in both child and adult education.

Nelson's (2006) reflections on how knowledge is created in practice have highlighted the work of phenomenologist Merleau-Ponty (1908–1961); in particular, the notion that understanding arises from an encounter between the person, the world they are part of, and their actions within it so that 'experience is perceived through the body and its immersion in the world' (Nelson 2006, p. 110). In other words, experiential learning challenges the idea of mind-body separation and sees true 'knowing' as something that arises through a transaction between ourselves, what we are doing and in what context the action takes place through the lived body.

These philosophies give rise to the phenomenon of The Maker Lab (Flores 2016) in which teachers allow a 'joyous convergence of wonder, discovery, problem solving, creation and collaboration' (p. xi) in the science classroom through practical making activities and projects. Thus the act of making supports learning because it both creates and shares knowledge. For example, Hardy and Sumner (2017), in their work facilitating digital storytelling with people experiencing mental health difficulties, identified the personal transformation that can occur when a person is supported to make and share a digital story about their life experience.

Connection

The emotional and symbolic language of arts and crafts offers a powerful conduit to communication and connection. Making is connecting. 'Through making things and sharing them in the world, we increase our engagement and connection with our social and physical environments' (Gauntlett 2018, p. 10). Making within a group provides an opportunity to be affirmed and supported, contributing to a sense of well-being, acceptance and intrinsic worth. An example of this can be seen in Case Study 16.2.

Well-being is a complex, multifaceted concept (Hammell and Iwama 2012; Fieldhouse and Bannigan 2014). In addition to identifying well-being as a state of contentment or harmony with one's physical and mental health, the authors also recognize emotional/spiritual health, self-worth, a sense of belonging and relationships, personal and economic security and opportunities to engage in meaningful and purposeful occupations as important and necessary dimensions. Similarly, the influential Foresight report (Foresight 2008) on mental capital and well-being defines mental well-being as, 'a dynamic state, in which the individual is able to develop their potential, work productively and creatively, build strong and positive relationships with others, and contribute to their community' (p. 10).

Occupational therapists use crafts and other creative activities to bring people together and reduce social anxiety. This may be regarded as an expression of Wilcock's d + b³ notion (Wilcock 2007) in which 'doing' (when it is truly occupational) not only will reinforce a strong sense of the do-ers' identity (being), but it will also evoke in them a sense of the transformative power of occupation (becoming) and facilitate connection to other people (belonging). Making can

also enhance the therapeutic relationship between the occupational therapist and the service user or help a person and their loved one find things to talk about.

Sensory Stimulation/Regulation

The variety of media and techniques available for creative activity can stimulate the senses in different ways so that people are exposed to the beauty in the world as experienced through sound, smell, taste, touch, sight and motion.

Through engaging in creative activities service users have opportunities to learn about their own sensory preferences and begin to develop ways to adjust, compensate or regulate their own body and feelings (Biel 2014). When engaging in the art of creating something with the hands (e.g., knitting or painting) or in whole body making (e.g., gardening, dance or drama), participants can learn to regulate and ground themselves through engagement in a meaningful activity (Heller 2003). For some, this experience is even described as meditative in nature (Cohen et al. 2006, pp. 85–86; Rosenbaum 2019).

OVERARCHING CONSIDERATIONS WHEN USING CREATIVE ACTIVITIES IN OCCUPATIONAL THERAPY PRACTICE

This section sets out two overarching considerations that intersect with occupational therapy practice in the area of creative activities, namely activism and trauma-informed practice. It then describes some of the skills and principles that underpin the use of creative activities as therapeutic media. It includes three examples of specific creative approaches used by occupational therapists, specifically re-animation, storytelling and play.

Activism

Activism is policy and/or vigorous action intended to bring about political or social change (Bryant et al. 2019). At its core, activism is about raising awareness and challenging injustice. It may take various forms, including joining protest marches, signing petitions, writing letters, boycotting companies and holding local meetings to raise awareness and plan action.

While these actions may fall outside of the day-to-day activities of occupational therapy, the socio-political positioning of people with mental health problems is important, especially for those who have intersecting identities in which racism, colonialism and ableism have a significant impact on their health. Creative activities that speak to the personal-political space can support someone in expressing their needs and offer opportunities to participate in bringing about change.

All disability arts movements react against the message that the body is the problem and that disability should be met with charity and paternalism. They challenge the idea that art is an elitist, able bodied occupation and promote disabled people as producers of art and culture, not just consumers or audience members. Artists in the movement are also using their art and their disability to subvert systems that are rife with barriers, with calls to 'crip,' or creatively disrupt, the arts; that is, to frame art practice in relation to disabilities based on notions of desirable possibilities, not limitation (Reid 2020). As Myers (2019) puts it,

To 'crip' the arts is to embrace the ways that disability can disrupt the status quo and lead with difference. By 'cripping,' or subverting, the language used within the arts, exclusionary or patronizing tropes related to disability can be dismantled, allowing access and inclusion to be standardized, terminology to be reclaimed, artists and audiences to be empowered and proper representation to be achieved.

Myers, 2019, p.

Occupational therapists must be aware that these movements are taking place and that there is value in creating art outside of the therapeutic context; an 'occupation,' as distinct from 'occupational therapy.' Therapists are not needed in these person-led movements; however, the creative activities within them can overlap and intersect with the work of the practitioner and their service users. The practitioner may want to adapt activities to recognize the work of activism and, when appropriate, encourage participation outside of the therapeutic context. What follows are two examples of creation as activism.

Craftivism is an approach that uses craft as a tool for activism. For some time, making activities of all kinds has been escaping the confines of the domestic domain and is being performed in new ways and for new purposes (Corbett 2017). Craftivism has been described as a tool for gentle protest that allows the maker time to think slowly and carefully about the issue being raised. Youngson (2019) urges occupational therapists to engage in craftivism and, while highlighting our Arts and Crafts historical roots, offers that craftivism could be used to enable the profession to 'consider our wider role in social transformation and reflect on how we could deploy the occupation of craftivism as one way to highlight occupational injustices and promote the value of the profession in meeting occupational challenges' (p. 384).

Recovery in the bin (RitB) is a critical theorist and activist collective of mental health survivors and supporters based in the United Kingdom, whose creative satire of the mental healthcare 'system' is presented in a long-running blog and zine, or non-commercial self-published print-work (RitB 2020). The group was formed in 2014 by people who felt they had been abandoned by 'recovery.' Their work has been cited in academic publications. For example, Newman-Taylor et al. (2019) used it in teaching and training of health professionals and informs debate about mental health practice. The RitB zine is shown in Fig. 16.1.

Trauma-Informed Practice

Trauma-informed practice recognizes that many mental health problems have their foundation in early trauma (van der Kolk 2014). It is a process through which services move, beginning with awareness of the prevalence of trauma and leading to trauma-informed practice becoming the organizational norm (Missouri Department of Health and Partners 2014). The principles of trauma-informed care include safety, trustworthiness and transparency, peer support, collaboration and mutuality, empowerment, voice and choice and acknowledgement of cultural, historical and gender issues (Centers for Disease Control and Prevention 2018).

Van der Kolk (2014) highlights the importance of understanding that trauma is a 'whole body experience.' Trauma may arise from abuse or interrupted developmental opportunities or from sources that are not obvious.

An important aspect of working in a trauma-informed way is helping the service user to feel relaxed and safe within the therapeutic space. Creative activities, if meaningful and directed by the person, can achieve this, whereas more traditional approaches such as meditation may inadvertently be uncomfortable or triggering for the person. For example, inviting the service user to

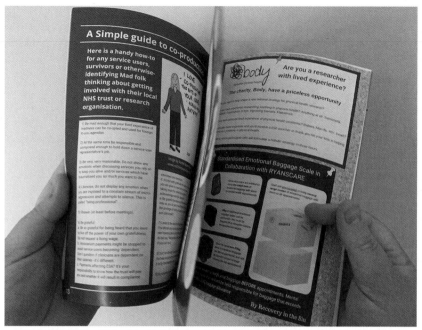

Fig. 16.1 ■ **Recovery in the Bin 'zine.** (Edited by Nell Aitch and featuring illustrations by Rachel Rowan Olive and others. Used with permission.)

bring their choice of relaxing music or creative making activity into the therapy session may offer an alternative way of enabling relaxation (Cohen 2017).

It is recommended that all therapists working with relaxation attune to the person they are working with and be curious; this enables the practitioner to adjust and come alongside the person and identify any challenges (Cohen et al. 2017; Malchiodi 2020). Where difficulties relating to specific trauma are identified, it may be appropriate to refer on to other professionals, for example, an art psychotherapist (Malchiodi 2020). By being trauma-aware, the occupational therapist can assist the professional team working with the service user to identify triggers and gain awareness of how different activities are impacting on the person.

SKILLS AND PRINCIPLES UNDERPINNING CREATIVE ACTIVITIES AND THERAPEUTIC MEDIA

Getting Started with Creativity

Not all occupational therapists are confident in their own creativity or see themselves as makers, but all occupational therapists will understand the power of making as a way of working with service users. The media or techniques chosen do not have to be original but can be other people's ideas adapted to the particular situation (see Case Study 16.3, for example).

For those therapists who feel under-confident in their own artistic skill, working with an artist or a creative arts therapist can build the therapist's confidence in using a new medium and greatly enhance the user experience. Therapists and artists can work together, for example, by creating fun spaces where the activity is specifically adjusted to achieve therapeutic aims in an engaging and motivating way.

Activity Analysis

Activity analysis is 'a process of dissecting an activity into its component parts and task sequence to identify its inherent properties and the skills required for its performance, thus allowing the therapist to evaluate its therapeutic potential' (Creek 2003, p. 49) and to apply professional reasoning to adapt the activity to become a therapeutic intervention. Activity analysis reveals the intrinsic properties of a making process; that is, the sequence and pattern of the activity, the abilities required for its performance and how it might be adapted and graded to meet particular needs.

Activity analysis is therefore key to understanding creative media and how to utilize them in therapy. By the careful design of making activities, occupational therapists can create opportunities for people to gain confidence and self-belief through the acquisition of skills. Activity analysis informs how a craft can be chosen, adapted and utilized in a specific context for an individual service user. This enables the occupational therapist to select activities that both meet therapeutic goals and engage the service user's interest as well as provide the right level of structure for the individual. If someone is anxious about trying creative activities, it can be helpful to provide more structure and a more concrete goal to start with, gradually reducing the amount of structure as the person becomes more confident. The structure may be inherent in the activity used—for example, patchwork is more structured than free painting—or the structure may be in the way the session is organized. For example, the first session of a creative writing group could involve a short description of a building that people know—something impersonal, in other words—while a later session might invite them to describe their own feelings (Creek 2008). As the group develops, members may progress to choosing their own topics.

Creative Media and Approaches

Occupational therapists use many creative media and approaches. Three examples—re-animation, storytelling and play—are described here to illustrate this rich variety.

Re-Animation

The re-animation approach (Mason 2011) was developed by occupational therapist (and chapter co-author) Helen Mason from her work in child and adolescent mental healthcare in the United Kingdom. It is used by practitioners and academics in the United Kingdom and elsewhere to complement their practice. The approach uses specifically selected animated activities—for example, stop motion, claymation, zoetrope (see later)—to engage and work with people at three levels: 'just for fun,' therapy work and performance animation. The first two levels are mainly used with individuals experiencing specific health problems and/or trauma and the third with communities.

Re-animation techniques and tools have a wide range of applications, such as early childhood development, family therapy, mental health recovery and community development. The way that the approach is applied in practice will vary, depending on the person or group it is used with, the clinical or artistic background of the practitioner and the context of the intervention.

A simple example of an animation technique is the zoetrope, a method originating in the 19th century (Fig. 16.2A). Sequential images are placed on the inside of a drum, which is then spun; slats on the outside of the drum enable the viewer to look through to the inside of the drum to see the revolving images which, when the drum spins quickly, creates the illusion of movement. With advances in digital technology a similar effect can be created using a strip of boxes (Fig. 16.2B). Each of the images is photographed and when they are displayed in sequence using animation software similar to a spinning zoetrope, the illusion of movement is created. An example of the use of zoetrope animation in therapy is given in Case Study 16.2.

Storytelling

Storytelling can be utilized in occupational therapy in a large number of ways, and life story work may involve a variety of different creative media, for example, the digital tools involved in digital storytelling (Lambert and Hessler 2018). Whatever the creative media used, the process of assisting someone to adapt an aspect of their life experience into a narrative structure can be transformative for the individual. It can allow a reframing or

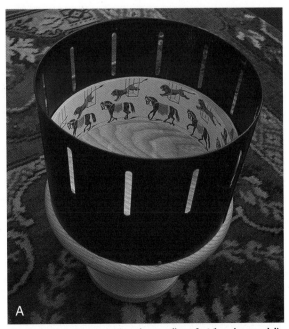

Fig. 16.2 ▪ A, Zoetrope (modern replica of a Victorian model).

re-storying of experience (see also the Self-Expression section above). The way the individual chooses to share what they have made is a further opportunity to connect with others and to be heard and understood.

Storytelling may also be used in ways that are not reliant on memory and instead focus on the use of imagination. Arts-based storytelling intervention, TimeSlips (2020), focuses on the strengths and assets of persons living with dementia in long-term care settings. The approach 'involves facilitators using surreal, staged visual images to encourage participants to respond in a spontaneous, improvisational manner as part of a storytelling group' (Vigliotti et al. 2019, p. 163). Approaches such as TimeSlips give participants the opportunity to find meaning and creative expression in the present and can be used when life story work or reminiscence is not possible.

Vigliotti et al. (2019) evaluated a TimeSlips intervention over a six-month period and found positive benefits for people with mild, moderate and severe dementia. The study demonstrated 'how the arts can uniquely reach people with advanced memory loss

and therefore support quality of life' (Vigliotti et al. 2019, p. 169). As shown in Case Study 16.1, storytelling interventions have the potential to reduce agitation and anxiety and to increase positive staff–resident interaction.

Play

Engaging people's capacity for playfulness is an important occupational therapy skill that involves creativity. Play is universal across all cultures and is important throughout the lifespan. For children, it is said to be the primary vehicle for creativity (see Chapter 17 Play).

The conditions of play include taking a make-believe stance to reality, imagination, repetition, competition, cooperation, voluntary intent, fun and pleasure (Reilly 1974). These conditions 'provide safety for risk-taking, promote ... a no-nonsense ethics about failure..., reduce discouragement and strengthen courage as a response mode' (Reilly 1974, p. 60). Playfulness and fun can involve and include everyone in the therapy setting: residents, carers, staff and volunteers. It can transform ward

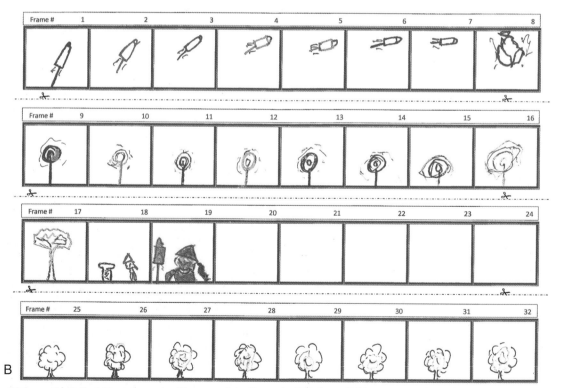

B

Fig. 16.2, cont'd ■ **B, A Zoetrope strip.** (Photograph by Dunn, A. (2004). Available at www.andrewdunnphoto.com CC BY-SA 2.0, https://commons.wikimedia.org/w/index.php?curid=1169107.)

culture, decrease behaviours that challenge and reduce staff sickness and burnout, which, obviously, would have an indirect impact on quality of care. An example of a playful activity is described in Case Study 16.1. Occupational therapists can facilitate playfulness by creating a physical and temporal space for play, choosing creative media and techniques that are culturally and age appropriate and modelling playful behaviour.

Ethics and Safety

Working creatively does not mean abandoning structure. There are particular ethical and safety issues to be considered. These include applying ethical principles (e.g., around self-disclosure), using media safely, adhering to the laws on copyright and staying within the scope of the occupational therapist's practice.

Applying Ethical Principles

The ethics of working with creative media are no different from those of occupational therapy in general, although they may be applied differently. Ethics provide a sound basis for developing policies on issues such as:

- sharing service users' work or images of their work in the public arena (e.g., on social media). For example, the project described in Case Study 16.3 involved people's personal comments being on public display and photographed to create a permanent record. Participants had to be made aware of this before taking part;
- storing, retaining and destroying work produced by service users as part of their therapy;
- ensuring that the techniques, materials and tools used are culturally appropriate for each service user's identity and life stage.

Using Media Safely

Occupational therapists must follow local guidelines and strategies for assessing and managing the risks associated with using creative media. Examples of risks include working with sharp tools and toxic substances such as glue, accidents during physical activities such as dance and unintentionally evoking distressing memories and/or associations.

Following Copyright Guidance

When working in healthcare organizations, charities or companies offering creative activity to support people's recovery, the occupational therapist should review copyright policy regarding who owns artwork created in therapy. It should not be assumed that policy always allows full intellectual property rights to be owned by the service user. Care should also be taken to establish the usage rights of creative media such as photographs, video and music when planning creative activities.

Staying Within the Scope of Your Practice

State-registered occupational therapists are required to work within their scope of practice as defined by their registration body. For example, the UK standards of proficiency for occupational therapists state that registered occupational therapists must 'know the limits of their practice and when to seek advice or refer to another professional' (Health and Care Professions Council 2013, p. 7). Where occupational therapists lack skills and experience with creative media, they should seek out collaborations with artists or creative arts therapists to ensure that the techniques are being used competently and safely.

Professional Development

As noted earlier, occupational therapists are skilled in the use of various therapeutic and creative media. However, to grow and advance their practice, they must continue to expand their skill base and might choose to undertake further training in particular media or approaches; perhaps a short course or a university programme leading to a formal qualification in a creative arts therapy, such as art or drama. Post-registration training may be useful in trauma-informed ways of working, such as trauma-focused cognitive behavioural therapy, in sensory approaches such as Ayres (1979) sensory integration, or regarding psychodynamic theories of attachment. Keeping up to date with scientific advances, for example, the expanding knowledge of neuroscience, can assist therapists in justifying the need for further training and development.

Similarly, practitioners can benefit from nurturing their own creative interests, perhaps by taking a knitting or upholstery course. This not only extends the repertoire of therapeutic media they can draw on but may support their own health and well-being at the same time.

Some of the principles and skills outlined above are illustrated in the three case studies that follow.

Creative Activities on an Inpatient Dementia Assessment Unit

This case study illustrates how the introduction of art and imaginative techniques on an inpatient dementia assessment unit (see Chapter 23) reduced patients' agitation and improved staff morale.

THE SETTING

A 17-bed inpatient dementia assessment unit received a concentration of admissions of individuals with violent and abusive behaviours which staff found challenging and which impacted negatively on staff sickness absence, recruitment and retention. This created a number of problems on the unit, such as:

- overuse of agency staff who did not know residents well;
- deprioritization of ward-based therapeutic activities, including reduced multidisciplinary team engagement in activities provided by the occupational therapists and activity coordinator;
- a reactive staff response to patients' agitation and behaviours which staff found challenging.

THE CREATIVE ACTIVITIES PROJECT

An innovation fund within the organization enabled a service re-design project led by the occupational therapists. The aim was to influence ward culture by increasing the opportunities for service users to participate in meaningful creative activities.

The choice of activities was framed by the Pool Activity Levels tool (Pool 2012), a widely used framework for activity-based care for people with cognitive issues including dementia. The project involved all staff on the unit. Activities were selected and graded by occupational therapists to engage service users and provide just the right challenge. Examples of the creative activities are shown in Boxes 16.1 and 16.2.

Activities were also embedded into themed activity days (Box 16.3), designed to highlight the connection between person-centred care, creative activity and improved service user outcomes to all members

---

BOX 16.1
THEMED RUMMAGE BOXES

Small boxes are filled with everyday items that staff can use to stimulate communication and reminiscence, individually or in groups. Themes might include childhood toys, photographs of people at work or household items. Exploring tactile and physical items can stimulate memory and, for some people, increase verbal communication. Those who are not able to communicate verbally can still interact through sharing tactile experiences.

BOX 16.2
PLAYLIST FOR LIFE

Evidence indicates that music is deeply attached to memories and emotions and can therefore induce feelings of well-being (Garabedian and Kelly 2018). The Playlist for Life activity builds a personal playlist of songs or pieces of music for each person living with dementia. The UK charity Playlist for Life suggests on its website that a playlist for life consists of all the songs or pieces of music that make up the soundtrack of a person's life. These are the tunes that give that 'flashback-feeling' whenever they are heard; that take you back to another time, person or place (Playlist for Life 2019). Caregivers build the playlist through exploring the person's life story to gather the music that is most deeply attached to their memories and emotions. This can then be recorded in any convenient format and played to stimulate memories and communication, thus reducing distress and enhancing quality of life. The playlist can also be used to increase physical activity and movement through dance, which can increase strength and balance and contribute to reduced falls.

---

of the multidisciplinary team. Family and carers were also invited to these days so that they could join in with their loved ones.

During these themed activity days some participants engaged fully, others required one-to-one support to join in while some just observed. For those not physically engaged in the activity, there were opportunities for visual, tactile and auditory stimulation; for reminiscence and to express emotions connected with the theme of the day.

Continued on following page

CASE STUDY 16.1

Creative Activities on an Inpatient Dementia Assessment Unit (Continued)

BOX 16.3
THEMED ACTIVITY DAYS

A TRIP TO SPAIN

Staff and service users wore some form of traditional Spanish dress and enjoyed themed food and drink, such as paella and non-alcoholic sangria. Postcards depicting places in Spain were handed around, and photographs were projected onto the walls. Spanish music was played to evoke the atmosphere of being in another country.

A VISIT TO THE SEASIDE

The atmosphere of a British coastal resort was evoked by eating foods that stimulated olfactory, gustatory and visual senses with the potential to evoke culturally relevant memories, such as fish and chips and ice cream. Service users were also invited to do things that evoked memories of the seaside, such as wearing handkerchiefs on their heads with knots tied at the corners or sitting in an old-style deck chair which was brought into the unit for the day. Photographs of local coastal resorts were handed around and projected onto the walls, and an audio-recording of seagulls and waves crashing onto the shore was played.

ARMISTICE DAY

A culturally relevant, seasonal event around Armistice Day involved a group making remembrance poppies that were displayed as a tribute to those who died in the first and second World Wars. Participants, including service users and their relatives, used card (cutting/sticking), fabrics (with a strong tactile stimulus) or knitting and sewing to make the poppies. Staff guided and supported different levels of engagement by selecting the method that provided the right level of challenge for the individual.

PROJECT OUTCOMES

The project offered staff new, easy-to-understand and imaginative ways of relating to service users. It transformed the culture of the unit in that many staff would naturally engage and spend time with service users rather than waiting to react to a need or be asked to speak with the person as a specific task. One of the unanticipated outcomes of the project was that ward staff found the activities personally engaging and relevant to them, too, which also increased staff–service user interaction.

Other positive outcomes included a consistent downward trend in the need for agency staff and in the number of violent or aggressive incidents on the unit. For example, while the project was taking place, there were 70 such incidents compared with 248 on another ward that was not part of the service re-design project. Significantly, the hospital chose to invest in the redevelopment of care pathways and looked to conduct further research into this new approach.

REFLECTIONS

Careful selection of a variety of tools, such as the Pool Activity Levels and TimeSlips, enabled an expert tailoring of creative engagement for each individual. The emotional and symbolic language of the arts can be used to stimulate the imagination, enabling a way of connecting people through creativity. This stimulation can be provided through the act of making and through sound, movement, words, images, dance and storytelling.

CASE STUDY 16.2

A Coproduced Animation Project Connecting Service Users and Staff to a Cultural Event

This case study illustrates the impact of a collaborative, coproduced animation project on staff–service user relations within an adult mental health secure unit (see Chapter 26).

THE SETTING

The project took place in an inpatient forensic secure unit (run by a UK charity) serving approximately 900 adults with complex and challenging mental health needs. The unit had various creative therapy departments, including music and visual arts. The creative media department (part of the occupational therapy department) promoted service users' self-expression and life skills development through a range of creative activities including graphic design and illustration, film and photography, animation, audio-recording, 3D design, printing and sculpture.

Cultural events and holidays were frequently used by the occupational therapy department as opportunities for social events aimed at developing service users' social skills and enhancing staff–service user relations through collaborative working. One year, service users indicated that they would like to celebrate Bonfire Night (an event held in the United Kingdom each November 5th to commemorate a failed attempt to blow up the Houses of Parliament in the 17th century). Hitherto, the constraints of a locked ward had made this celebration impracticable on the unit (one of the key features of Bonfire Night being a firework display). Fireworks were not allowed on hospital grounds, and service users did not have leave to go outside the hospital to watch public displays.

THE BONFIRE NIGHT ANIMATION PROJECT

The occupational therapy staff (after consultation with service users) initiated a coproduced project to celebrate Bonfire Night using animation. Given the safety issues regarding real fireworks, an animated screening of fireworks would enable service users to create their own social event in the main hall of the hospital, including traditional refreshments such as hot dogs and hot chocolate.

Several of the occupational therapy media production team had received training in the re-animation approach™ (Mason 2011) described earlier. Staff used the 'just for fun' level of re-animation to engage service users and staff from across the hospital in creating an animated film of fireworks. The zoetrope animation technique was chosen because it is effective for animating fireworks, and its ease of use could maximize engagement by staff and service users across a wide range of abilities. For those participants with performance anxiety or low levels of functioning, simple marks made in the strip of boxes could create pleasing effects when music was added. More confident participants could focus on creating their own firework display. Being paper-based, the activity could be offered on the wards to accommodate service users subject to the Mental Health Act (1983 and 2007) leave restrictions. Fig. 16.3 is an example zoetrope strip (before sequencing) used in the animation. An example of a more ambitious animation is described in Box 16.4.

The project provided opportunities for meeting graded therapeutic goals through the technical challenge of editing the animations and through the experience of organizing, attending and running a community event; one that brought staff and service users together socially.

Over 50 staff and service users contributed with illustrated explosions and pyrotechnics for the display. One service user took on the role of director/producer and another volunteered to assist staff in sequencing the material to create approximately two minutes of film. This was later expanded by staff and service users to eight minutes, using additional animation techniques and software. The finished animation (Fig. 16.3) is an example of some stills from the final Bonfire Night animation as projected. It was looped, burned onto a DVD and projected onto a large screen in the hospital's main conference room as part of the Bonfire Night event. Copies of the DVD were circulated to all wards so that services users who did not have permission to leave the ward could still participate in the event.

PROJECT OUTCOMES

Reactions to the project were overwhelmingly positive and the project was repeated annually for five years until superseded by a real firework display. Coproduction practices evolved over time. Each subsequent year a service user volunteer, with control over visual content and access to footage from previous years, has worked with staff to cocreate an annually growing and evolving display.

While this was a hospital-wide event, the animation work with the service user who created 'Guy Fork' opened up additional therapeutic avenues. A second film called 'What the Fork?' was planned in individual therapy sessions (see Box 16.4). Other therapists picked up the theme within psychology sessions, leading to a creative exchange regarding how to manage anxiety through story-making with the 'Guy Fork' character.

REFLECTIONS

This collaborative animation method enabled occupational therapists to engage a wide range of service users, regardless of their diagnosis, technical ability or leave status. The film-making project, informed by coproduction principles, promoted service users' pro-social behaviour, engaged their creativity, fostered a sense of mastery and offered active roles as contributors to a widely appreciated and inclusive social and cultural event.

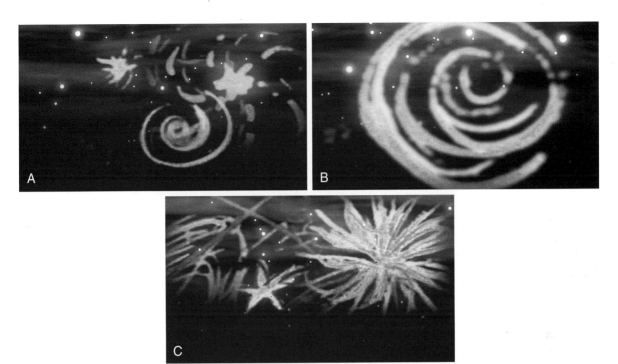

Fig. 16.3 ■ A-C, Zoetrope stills (used in Bonfire Night animation – see Case Study 16.2).

BOX 16.4
'GUY FORK' ANIMATION

One service user working at the performance level of the re-animation approach™ (Mason 2011) produced a custom-animated introduction to the display that starred a character of their own creation, 'Guy Fork,' who provided safe guidance on the use of fireworks. The name 'Guy Fork' is a playful reference to the lead conspirator in the Bonfire Night celebration, Guy Fawkes; the joke being that the animated puppet was made from a plastic fork.

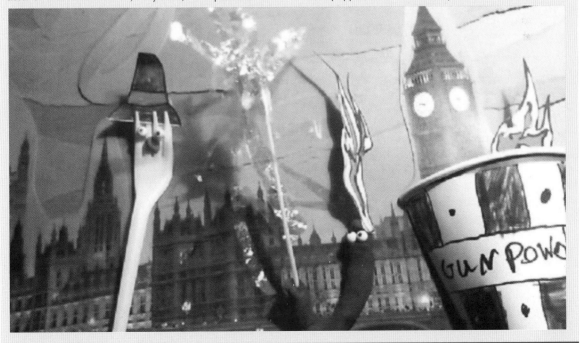

CASE STUDY 16.3

Using a Chalkboard as a Creative Response to Mental Distress

This case study highlights a creative community arts-based project which challenged participants to identify valued goals and hopes for living.

BACKGROUND

The Northern Initiative for Social Action (NISA) is an occupation-based, consumer-run, non-profit organization in Canada (www.nisa.on.ca). Members have developed opportunities for themselves and others to engage in activities that propel their own personal recovery journeys rather than being passive recipients of services (Rebeiro et al. 2001). The programme at NISA is peer-led and is for anyone who has used or is using mental health services or who self-identifies as having lived experience of mental health problems. People with this lived experience also manage and decide the strategic direction of the organization on the basis that individuals with lived experience are uniquely qualified to support each other and have the insight and ability to determine how best to move through their own mental health recovery.

Within NISA, a long-running artists' group (open to beginners and professional artists alike) used a range of media to encourage self-expression regarding the lived experience of mental health problems and to educate society through exhibiting these works in community settings. Artwork produced by group members was also shown in the permanent exhibition held at the organization's premises.

The project described here arose from discussions in NISA's Alternatives to Suicide support group and was facilitated using skills and knowledge available within the artists' group. Working together, these two groups developed a creative intervention regarding suicidal thinking and how to promote strategies for living.

THE 'BEFORE I DIE' WALL PROJECT

Group members were inspired by US-based artist Candy Chang's installation of a participatory chalkboard painted on the wall of an abandoned building in her neighbourhood. It had been prompted by her need to respond to the death of a loved one (Chang 2013) and featured the stencilled prompt 'Before I Die I want to . . .'. Passers-by could use the chalk provided to share their hopes and dreams in the face of their own mortality. In her 2012 TED talk, Chang said:

> . . . the neglected space became a constructive one, people's hopes and dreams made me laugh out loud, tear up, and they consoled me during my own tough times. It's about knowing that you are not alone, it's about understanding our neighbours in new and enlightening ways. It's about making space for reflection and contemplation, and remembering what really matters to us as we grow and change.

> *Chang 2012*

Chang's work resonated with the group's aims of self-expression and education. Following Chang's (2013) how-to' guide, members created their own 'Before I Die 'wall on two 4-ft × 4-ft boards as shown in Fig. 16.4AB. The chalkboard took less than a day to create with paint and stencil, and the completed work featured at a local arts festival.

RESPONSES

At the local arts festival, people were invited to share their hopes for a well-lived life on the wall, in chalk. The boards were subsequently erased and filled in many times over and featured in other events. Photo documentation preserved the responses. These ranged from the simple, 'Before I die I want to eat hummus,' to the existential, 'Before I die I want to live and be happy,' to the fantastic, 'Before I die I want to float in air.' Some responses spoke to the social position of the individual, as in 'Before I die I want to be first,' while some referenced people's

Continued on following page

CASE STUDY 16.3

Using a Chalkboard as a Creative Response to Mental Distress (Continued)

self-perception, as seen in 'I want to be confident.' Other responses told stories of the past, of regret, perhaps: 'Before I die I want to hold my first-born again,' while others allowed the writer's dreams of the future to take hold, naming places they wanted to visit. Some people even let out their secret thoughts, with 'Before I die I want to be a nude model' or 'I want to marry my ex.' The most common response spoke to a general feeling that the current direction of their life was not satisfying: 'Before I die I want to live.'

In coaching their peers and festival attendees through participation, the project organizers noted that some people initially needed to be challenged to turn their thinking away from death, to consider life and what made it meaningful.

REFLECTIONS

Membership organizations such as NISA give people opportunities to express themselves and connect as individuals rather than as 'service users.' Such community spaces offer opportunities for peer support and self-organization, enabling creative responses to mental distress and life's difficulties, which is both an important aspect of recovery and a spur to developing professional art skills.

The 'Before I Die' wall project offered participants an empowering opportunity to step outside of the everyday challenges of life; to dream and to hope. It shows that creative activities need be neither original nor expensive to be effective.

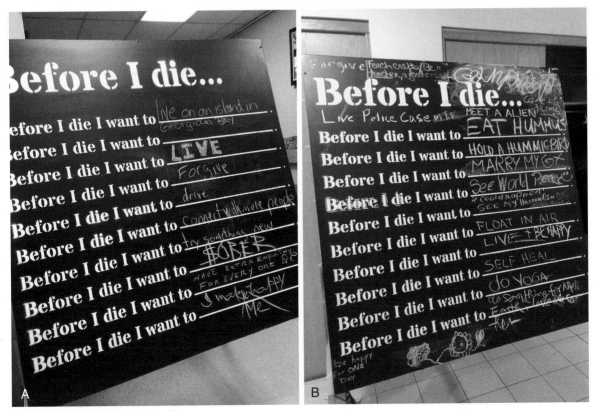

Fig. 16.4 ■ A-B, 'Before I Die' wall.

CONCLUSION

This chapter has highlighted the therapeutic value of creative activity, particularly of making, and has considered this in the context of the history of the occupational therapy profession. This valuable legacy places the profession in a good position to connect with a general resurgence of interest in crafts in contemporary contexts and to utilize this interest in supporting the well-being of individuals and communities. The chapter has also discussed some of the skills and principles that support this, giving case examples of creative activities used in real life practice.

Occupational therapists understand how to select and adapt activities to suit individual preferences and needs; they are also aware that the type of activity chosen is less important than its capacity to stimulate and engage people, whether they be service users, staff or visitors. This way of working is about creating opportunities for joy; for experimentation; for play; for making; connecting, remembering, engaging and, perhaps, producing something that means something. Working in a creative way brings hope and it makes coming to work energizing because both service users and staff are being acknowledged and celebrated as human beings. This is the magic of creativity, of making.

Whether creative activity is employed for vocational rehabilitation, to develop a sense of achievement through the creation of a product or for exploring or regulating emotions and connecting socially through making, creative activities are a treasure in the occupational therapist's toolbox, both historically and in the modern day.

Acknowledgements

The authors would like to thank the following for their input to this chapter: Jennifer Creek, Carol Duff, Carol Rogers, David Saunders and Jacky Tyson.

QUESTIONS FOR CONSIDERATION

1. What are the benefits of hands on activities?
2. How do arts and crafts stimulate physical and mental action?
3. Could there be negatives to failure in the arts? For example, for those who aren't naturally artistic?
4. How could an occupational therapist keep the service user focussed on learning from failure and reflecting on it?
5. Are there situations where socio-political action does fall inside occupational therapy?
6. What are some of the dangers of a 'recovery in the bin' attitude?
7. On theme days would it have been appropriate for the team to provide alternate activities or could that undermine the meaning of the creative activities?
8. How could the success of the bonfire night animation be replicated with another celebration?
9. Would there be benefits to preserving the mural in another way for individuals? Are photos suitable for the significance of the activity?

SERVICE USER COMMENTARY

This reflection is based on my experience of creative activity in occupational therapy during my day-patient treatment for anorexia nervosa. It includes additional thoughts from the perspective of my subsequent role as an occupational therapy student.

For a number of years I lost my identity to anorexia nervosa. When I started treatment for this I received enhanced cognitive behavioural therapy as an outpatient. However, I tended to intellectualize my thoughts and feelings and made few improvements. I was then offered intensive day-patient

Continued on following page

SERVICE USER COMMENTARY (Continued)

treatment instead. It was here that I received twice-weekly occupational therapy.

One of the weekly occupational therapy sessions was dedicated to meal preparation, food shopping and/or cooking. The other session typically took the form of an art-based group activity but occasionally included activities such as gardening or yoga. The sessions were semi-structured, with the occupational therapist deciding on a general activity and then we, as service users, would decide on the materials we used and the individual designs we would create.

My first occupational therapy session was a turning point for both my recovery and my decision to train as an occupational therapist. We were creating hand-painted coasters using tiles. I enjoyed painting, it was something that I believed I was good at, but I felt very apprehensive and reluctant to participate as I was given no time to prepare, plan or perfect my design. And then there was the issue of the paintbrushes: they were all well-used and 'frizzy'; they would not allow for perfection, let alone precision. Sensing my discomfort, the occupational therapist said, 'It's not about the outcome, it's about the process.' At the time, I didn't believe her, but before I knew it, an hour had passed, and my hand-painted coasters were finished. They were imperfect, but she was right: it was not about the outcome. That was the first hour in a long time that I had not thought about my illness. This was particularly poignant as the session took place after meal-time, a time which would usually have been very distressing for me.

This experience resonates strongly with two key topics discussed in this chapter. First, I was able to regulate my emotions and ground myself through creative activity and flow. This is described in the section on the benefits of creativity and making for sensory stimulation/regulation. Importantly, this was not unique to the particular session described above but something I continued to experience and practise throughout my treatment and beyond. Second, I felt strong resonances with the section discussing the benefits of creativity for communication and connection. Whilst engaging in creative activity I was able to build a good therapeutic relationship with my occupational therapist; a key relationship in my recovery. I started to talk about things other than my illness and began to take steps towards reforming my identity.

Since leaving day-patient treatment I consider creative activity the most valuable treasure in my toolbox. It has been vital in helping me regulate my emotions, reform my identity and maintain my recovery. It is something that I have carried with me to inform my own practice as I embark on the journey towards becoming a qualified occupational therapist.

Helen Drucker

REFERENCES

All-Party Parliamentary Group on Arts, Health and Wellbeing (APPGAHW) (2017). *Creative health: The Arts for health and Wellbeing.* All-Party Parliamentary Group for Arts, Health and Wellbeing Inquiry Report. Available at https://www.culturehealthandwellbeing.org.uk/appg-inquiry/.

Ayres, A. J. (1979). *Sensory Integration and the Child.* LA: Western Psychological Services.

Biel, L. (2014). *Sensory Processing Challenges: Effective Clinical Work with Kids and Teens.* New York: Norton and Company.

Blanche, E. I. (2007). The expression of creativity through occupation. *Journal of Occupational Science, 14*(1), 21–29. https://doi.org/10.1080/14427591.2007.9686580.

Brodie, E. (1925). Occupational therapy: A series of papers read at a meeting of the Scottish division held at the Glasgow royal mental hospital on Friday, May 2, 1924: III. *Journal of Mental Science, 71*(292), 59–80.

Brooks, R., & Dunford, C. (2014). Play. In W. Bryant, J. Fieldhouse, & `K. Bannigan (Eds.), *Creek's Occupational Therapy and Mental Health* (5th ed.) (pp. 277–293). Edinburgh: Churchill Livingstone Elsevier.

Bryant, W., Cordingley, K., Adomako, E., & Birken, M. (2019). Making activism a participatory, inclusive and developmental process: A research programme involving mental health service users. *Disability & Society, 34*(7–8), 1264–1288. https://doi.org/1 0.1080/09687599.2019.1613963.

Centers for Disease Control and Prevention (CDC). (2018). *Infographic: 6 Guiding Principles to a Trauma-informed Approach.* Available at https://www.cdc.gov/cpr/infographics/6_principles_trauma_info.htm.

Chang, C. (2012). Before I die I want to... [Video]. In *TED Global 2012 conference* Available at https://www.ted.com/talks/candy_chang_before_i_die_i_want_to.

Chang, C. (2013). *Before I Die.* New York: St. Martin's Press.

Cohen, J. A., Mannarino, A. P., & Deblinger, E. (2017). *Treating Trauma and Traumatic Grief in Children and Adolescents* (2nd ed.). New York: Guilford Press.

Corbett, S. (2017). *How to be a Craftivist: The Gentle Art of Protest.* London: Unbound.

Creek, J. (2003). *Occupational therapy Defined as a Complex Intervention.* London: College of Occupational Therapists.

Creek, J. (2008). Creative activities. In J. Creek, & L. Lougher (Eds.), *Occupational Therapy and Mental Health* (4th ed.) (pp. 333–343). Edinburgh: Churchill Livingstone Elsevier.

Creek, J. (2009). Something lost and something gained. *Occupational Therapy in Mental Health, 14*(9), 45–51.

Creek, J. (2012). *The Core Concepts of Occupational therapy: A Dynamic Framework for Practice.* London: Jessica Kingsley.

Creighton, C. (1992). The origin and evolution of activity analysis. *American Journal of Occupational Therapy, 46*(1), 45–48. https://doi.org/10.5014/ajot.46.1.45.

Fidler, G. S., & Fidler, J. W. (1963). *Occupational therapy, a Communication Process in Psychiatry*. New York: Macmillan.

Fieldhouse, J., & Bannigan, K. (2014). Mental health and wellbeing. In W. Bryant, J. Fieldhouse, & K. Bannigan (Eds.), *Creek's Occupational Therapy and Mental Health* (5th ed.) (pp. 15–26). Edinburgh: Churchill Livingstone/Elsevier.

Flores, C. (2016). *Making Science: Reimagining STEM Education in Middle School and beyond*. Torrance, CA: Constructing Modern Knowledge Press.

Foresight (2008). Mental Capital and wellbeing: Making the Most of Ourselves in the 21st century. In *Final Project Report. UK Government Office for Science* Available at https://www.gov.uk/government/publications/mental-capital-and-wellbeing-making-the-most-of-ourselves-in-the-21st-century.

Fortmeier, S., & Thanning, G. (2002). *From the Patient's Point of View: An Activity Theory Approach to Occupational therapy*. Copenhagen: Ergoterapeutforeningen.

Gantt, C. (2013). *What is a Maker? What it Really Means to be a 'Maker'*. Available at https://www.tweaktown.com/articles/5301/what-is-a-maker-what-it-really-means-to-be-a-maker-/index.html.

Garabedian, C. E., & Kelly, F. (2018). Haven: Sharing receptive music listening to foster connections and wellbeing for people with dementia who are nearing the end of life, and those who care for them. *Dementia*, 19(5), 1657–1671. https://doi.org/10.1177/1471301218804728.

Gauntlett, D. (2018). *Making is Connecting: The Social Power of Creativity, from Craft and Knitting to Digital Everything* (2nd ed.). Cambridge: Polity Press.

Greenlees, R., & Jones, M. (2011). Foreword. In D. Charny (Ed.), *Power of Making* (p.5). London: V&A Publishing and the Crafts Council.

Griffiths, S., & Corr, S. (2007). *The use of creative activities with people with mental health problems: a survey of Occupational therapists. British Journal of Occupational Therapy*, 70(3), 107 https://doi. org/10.1177/030802260707000303.

Hardy, P., & Sumner, T. (2017). Chapter 7: Digital storytelling with users and survivors of the UK mental health system. In M. Dunford, & T. Jenkins (Eds.), *Digital Storytelling: Form and Content* (pp. 57–69). London: Palgrave Macmillan.

Hasselkus, B. R. (2002). *The Meaning of Everyday occupation*. Thorofare, NJ: Slack.

Health and Care Professions Council. (2013). *Standards of Proficiency: Occupational Therapists*. London: HCPC.

Heller, S. (2003). *Too Loud Too Bright Too Fast Too Tight: What to Do if You Are Sensory Defensive in an Overstimulating World*. New York: Quill/HarperCollins.

Hocking, C. (2008). The way we were: Romantic assumptions of pioneering occupational therapists in the United Kingdom. *British Journal of Occupational Therapy*, 71(4), 146–154. https://doi.org/10.1177/030802260807100405.

Horghagen, S. (2014). *The Transformative Potential of Craft and Creative Occupations for People in Vulnerable Life Situations*. Doctoral Thesis. Trondheim: Norwegian University of Science and Technology.

Iwama, M., Thompson, N., & Macdonald, R. (2009). The Kawa model: The power of culturally responsive occupational therapy. *Disability & Rehabilitation*, 31(14), 1125–1135.

James W. (1899/2008). *Talks to Teachers on Psychology*. Rockville, MD: ARC Manor.

van der Kolk, B. (2014). *The Body Keeps the Score: Mind, Brain and Body in the Transformation of Trauma*. New York: Penguin Random House.

Lambert, J., & Hessler, B. (2018). *Digital Storytelling: Capturing Lives, Creating Community* (5th ed.). New York: Routledge.

Laws, J. (2011). Crackpots and basket-cases: A history of therapeutic work and occupation. *History of the Human Sciences*, 24(2), 65–81. https://doi.org/10.1177/0952695111399677.

Malchiodi, C. A. (2020). *Trauma and Expressive Arts therapy: Brain, Body and Imagination in the Healing Process*. New York: Guilford Press.

Mason, H. (2011). The re-animation approach: Animation and therapy. *Journal of Assistive Technologies*, 5(1), 40–42. https://doi.org/10.5042/jat.2011.0102.

Mental Health Act, 1983. UK Gov Department of Health. HMSO.

Mental Health Act, 2007. UK Gov Department of Health. HMSO.

Merriam-Webster Dictionary. (2020). *Merriam-Webster Inc.* Available at https://www.merriam-webster.com.

Missouri Department of Health and Partners. (2014). *Missouri Model: A Developmental Framework for Trauma-informed Approaches*. Available at https://dmh.mo.gov/media/pdf/missouri-model-developmental-framework-trauma-informed-approaches.

Morris, W. (1884). *Useful Work versus Useless Toil, reprinted 2008*. London: Penguin, 1–29.

Müllersdorf, M., & Ivarsson, A. (2016). What, why, how – creative activities in occupational therapy practice in Sweden. *Occupational Therapy International*, 23, 369–378.

Myers, C. (2019). *On the Complexity of Cripping the Arts*. Canadian Art. Available at: https://canadianart.ca/features/on-the-complexity-of-cripping-the-arts/.

Nelson, R. (2006). Practice-as-research and the problem of knowledge. *Performance Research*, 11(4), 105–116. https://doi.org/10.1080/13528160701363556.

Newman-Taylor, K., Maguire, T., & Bowen, A. (2019). Why are we not measuring what matters in mental health in the UK? The case for routine use of recovery outcome measures. *Perspect. Public Health*, 139(4), 181–183 https://doi.org/10.1177/1757913919851414.

Papert, S., & Harel, I. (1991). *Constructionism*. New York: Ablex Publishing Corporation.

Perruzza, N., & Kinsella, E. A. (2010). Creative arts occupations in therapeutic practice: A review of the literature. *British Journal of Occupational Therapy*, 73(6), 261–268. https://doi.org/10.4276/030802210X12759925468943.

Piaget, J., & Cook, M. (2013). *The Construction of Reality in the Child*. London: Routledge.

Playlist for Life, n.d. Available at: https://www.playlistforlife.org.uk/.

Polatajko, H. J., Davis, J. A., Hobson, S. J. Landry J. E., Mandich A., Street S. L., Whippey E., Yee S. (2004). Meeting the responsibility that comes with the privilege: introducing a Taxonomic code for understanding occupation. *Canadian Journal of Occupational Therapy/Revue Canadienne D'Ergothãrapie*. 71 (5): 261–264.

Pöllänen, S. (2013). The meaning of craft: Craft makers' descriptions of craft as an occupation. *Scandinavian Journal of Occupational Therapy*, 20(3), 217–227. https://doi.org/10.3109/11038128.2012.725182.

Pollard, N., & Walsh, S. (2000). Occupational therapy, gender and mental health: An inclusive perspective? *British Journal of Occupational Therapy*, 63(9), 425–431. https://doi.org/10.1177/030802260006300904.

Pool, J. (2012). *The Pool Activity Level (PAL) Instrument for Occupational Profiling: A Practical Resource for Carers of people with cognitive Impairment* (4th ed.). London: Jessica Kingsley.

Rapaport, D., Schafer, R., Gill, M. M., & Holt, R. R. (1968). *Diagnostic Psychological Testing*. Madison, CT: International Universities Press.

Rebeiro, K. L., Day, D. G., Semeniuk, B., O'Brien, M. C., & Wilson, B. (2001). Northern initiative for social action: An occupation-based, mental health program. *American Journal of Occupational Therapy*, 55, 493–500. https://doi.org/10.5014/ajot.55.5.493.

Recovery in the Bin (RitB). (2020). *Recovery in the Bin [Blog post]*. Available at https://recoveryinthebin.org/.

Reid, J. (2020). *Cripping the Arts: It's about Time*. Available at https://canadianart.ca/features/cripping-arts-time/.

Reilly, M. (1962). Occupational therapy can be one of the great ideas of 20th century medicine: 1961 Eleanor Clarke Slagle lecture. *American Journal of Occupational Therapy*, 16(1), 1–9.

Reilly, M. (1974). Defining a cobweb. In M. Reilly (Ed.), *Play as Exploratory Learning: Studies of Curiosity Behaviour* (pp. 57–116). Newbury Park, CA: Sage.

Reynolds, F. (2009). Creative occupations: A need for in-depth longitudinal qualitative studies (editorial). *British Journal of Occupational Therapy*, 72(1), 1.

Rosenbaum, J. L. (2019). Art and mindfulness behind bars. *The Prison Journal*, 99(4) 3S–13S. Available at: https://doi.org/10.1177/0032885519860524.

Shorter Oxford English Dictionary. (2007). *Shorter Oxford English Dictionary* (6th ed.). Oxford: Oxford University Press.

Shove, E., Pantzar, M., & Watson, M. (2012). *The Dynamics of Social Practice: Everyday Life and How it Changes*. Newbury Park, CA: Sage.

Thompson, M., & Blair, S. E. E. (1998). Creative arts in occupational therapy: Ancient history or contemporary practice? *Occupational Therapy International*, 5(1), 49–65.

TimeSlips. (2020). Available at: https://www.timeslips.org/.

Turner, A. (2011). The Elizabeth Casson memorial lecture 2011: Occupational therapy – a profession in adolescence? *British Journal of Occupational Therapy*, 74(7), 314–322.

Turner, J. B. (2016). *Development and evaluation of a pictorial metaphor technique in cognitive analytic therapy*. Doctoral. Sheffield Hallam University.

Vigliotti, A. A., Chinchilli, V. M., & George, D. R. (2019). Evaluating the benefits of the TimeSlips creative storytelling program for persons with varying degrees of dementia severity. *American Journal of Alzheimer's Disease & Other Dementias*, 34(3), 163–170. https://doi.org/10.1177/1533317518802427.

Walters, J. (2018). Chapter 12: Healing journeys: Digital storytelling with service user educators. In P. Hardy, & T. Sumner (Eds.), *Cultivating Compassion: How Digital Storytelling is Transforming Healthcare*. London: Palgrave Macmillan/Springer. pp.199–211.

Wilcock, A., 2002. Occupation for health, Volume 2: A Journey from Prescription to Self Health. London: College of Occupational Therapists.

Wilcock, A. (2007). Occupation and health: Are they one and the same? *Journal of Occupational Science*, 14(1), 3–8. https://doi.org/10.1080/14427591.2007.9686577.

Youngson, B. (2019). Craftivism for occupational therapists: Finding our political voice. *British Journal of Occupational Therapy*, 82(6), 383–385. https://doi.org/10.1177/0308022619825807.

Zandt, F., & Barrett, S. (2017). *Creative Ways to Help Children Manage BIG Feelings: A Therapist's Guide to Working with Preschool and Primary Children*. London: Jessica Kingsley.

17

PLAY

ROB BROOKS ■ CAROLYN DUNSFORD

CHAPTER OUTLINE

INTRODUCTION

Play is recognized as a universal right for every child in the United Nations Convention on the Rights of the Child (Article 31). Children have the right to rest and leisure, to engage in play and recreational activities appropriate to their age and to participate freely in cultural life and the arts. Participating fully in cultural and artistic life should be respected and promoted through the provision of appropriate opportunities for cultural, artistic, recreational and leisure activities. Attention should be given to the broader historical, social-economic and political structures that have the potential to create occupational injustices that preclude participation in play (Gerlach et al. 2014).

Participation in play contributes to children's sense of happiness (Moore and Lynch 2018) and influences their mental health and overall development. Play is the context for the development of childhood friendships and enables children to learn about and develop occupational roles (Bundy 2012). Play deprivation can have a profound, negative effect on development, social competence and mental well-being and result in an increased incidence of mental disorders, such as anxiety, depression and attention deficit hyperactivity disorder (ADHD) (Brown and Patte 2013). The presence of a mental health condition in either the child or parent can also affect the development of play occupations, having further effects on the child's mental health. In paediatric occupational therapy and mental health literature and practice there has been a shift from the developmental significance of play and adaptation towards themes of socialisation, play assessment, play as a primary occupation and play as an intervention and outcome of occupational therapy (Lynch and Moore 2016).

Occupational therapists believe that participation in meaningful occupations can promote health and well-being (World Federation of Occupational Therapists 2009). Children and young people may engage in productive occupations, such as paid work, school-related activities or household activities as directed by an adult (d'Entremont et al. 2017). Self-care occupations, such as toileting and bathing often reflect culturally shared expectations and performance but, again, are required or enforced by adults. Play, on the contrary, is chosen freely, is enjoyable and is self-directed.

The delineation between the constructs of play and leisure has not been adequately defined, and they are often lumped together as a single construct. Very young children are not usually considered to have leisure occupations, and play is generally seen as the province of children. However, playing can be a meaningful occupation for adults as well. There is a shift from play to leisure activities with increasing age. Leisure is defined by the American Occupational Therapy Association (AOTA) as a non-obligatory activity that is intrinsically motivated and engaged in during discretionary time (AOTA 2017). Townsend and Polatajko (2013) believed that the purpose of leisure is enjoyment, for example, socialising; creative expressions; outdoor activities and games and sport. Passmore (1998) described three types of leisure: achievement, social and time out:

- **Achievement leisure:** This involves challenging and demanding activities such as playing sports or music. Achievement leisure is thought to impact on self-efficacy beliefs and self-esteem.
- **Social leisure:** The primary purpose of social leisure is to be with others, and this supports competencies with relationships and social acceptance.
- **Time out leisure:** The purpose of time out leisure is relaxation which can have positive benefits in terms of providing rest; however, too much time out leisure can have a negative effect as it is socially isolating and generally less demanding.

While leisure occupations sit within the taxonomy of occupations for young people and adults, the notion of play can be seen as the primary occupation for young children. There is no universally accepted definition of play, and it could be argued that defining an activity as play can only truly be done by the player themselves; however, it has been suggested that there are some critical characteristics which delineate play from other occupations (Rigby and Rodger 2006). These include intrinsic motivation, process not product orientated, pretending, not governed by external rules and requiring active participation of the player (Rigby and Rodger 2006). Lynch and Moore (2016, p. 519) described play as a 'subjective experience of joy and fun, that comes from engaging in freely chosen, intrinsically motivated, self-directed meaningful occupations.' Bundy (1991) echoed the defining aspects of play as being intrinsically motivated and internally controlled, but she added that it should also be free from objective reality. Creativity can be explored through play and expressed through a wide range of occupations throughout life, but for young children play is the primary vehicle for creativity.

Environment and Play

Participation in play requires interaction with and is shaped by the physical, social, cultural, economic and political environments (Ziviani and Rodger 2006; Moore and Lynch 2018). As well as facilitating play, the environment can be a barrier; it is necessary to consider the environmental context at different levels including individual, family, neighbourhood, community and society (Table 17.1).

Children are often most aware of their physical environment, and this has been of interest to researchers for some time. The design of the outdoor play environment has been found to be an influencing factor on play. Playground designs can include traditional playgrounds (slides, swings, seesaws), contemporary playgrounds (aesthetically pleasing timber connected to provide space for social interaction and graded challenges) and free play areas (unstructured natural environments) (Stanton-Chapman et al. 2018). It has been found that contemporary play areas create more complex play, including rockets, boats, castles and bridges. Whilst playgrounds are generally seen as being conducive to children's play, for some children with disabilities, including autism and intellectual disability, playgrounds lack accessibility and restrict play acting as a form of occupational injustice (Prellwitz and Skär 2016). Play in natural environments has been found to promote social and emotional well-being and

TABLE 17.1	
Environmental Influences on Play Occupations	
Environment	**Definition/Example**
Physical environment	The natural environment such as the terrain and climate; the built environment including the design of buildings and objects within it such as toys
Social environment	Expectations and attitudes of social support including family, friends and caregivers
Cultural environment	Societal norms including beliefs, customs, social behaviours, attitudes and expectations
Economic environment	Availability of resources such as finances at both a local and societal level
Organizational environment	Structures that mediate resources including the government, policies and managers

attention (Kemple et al. 2016). Play is, however, not always limited to areas specifically constructed for play participation. In less economically prosperous countries studies have identified the street as an informal place claimed by children for play (Bartie et al. 2015; Brackmann et al. 2017). Street play has been characterized by young people as a social and fun experience that is free from the supervision of adults (Berinstein and Magalhaes 2009; Njelesani et al. 2011).

A further aspect of the physical play environment is the availability and use of toys, objects, or materials (Smith 2010). Whilst the use of objects in play is universal, the types of objects are culturally informed and reflect available resources. The nature of play objects in many western societies can include children's sized kitchen utensils, stoves, irons and ironing boards, toy phones, dress up clothes and toy miniatures. European-American children's play has also been found to be inspired by the use of superhero toy miniatures influenced by children's movies (Johnson et al. 1999). Cross-cultural examples of children's play objects include Yucatec Mayan children in Mexico using objects such as rocks, leaves and fruit from the natural environment (Gaskins 2015) and children in Zanzibar using coconut shells and sticks to pretend to cook over an open fire (Berinstein and Magalhaes 2009).

The social, economic and political environment can restrict occupational choice and result in reduced play opportunities (Galvaan 2012). For example, in countries with political conflict, designated areas for children to play in may have been damaged; we are also only just beginning to understand how the functioning and development, including play of young people, are impacted by their experiences of violence (Barber 2015). In many cultures, the family environment has undergone significant changes with parents working from home, caregiving by grandparents, increased structured play and less free-time, financial pressures and parental separation and reconstituted families (Darlington and Rodger 2006). Parents' and caregivers' mental health status can also lead to reduced play opportunities for children and young people. For example, persistent maternal depression has been associated with less time spent reading with a child, taking outings and trips to the park and playing indoors (Frech and Kimbro 2011). It is important when working with children and families to appreciate the family context and use family-centred practice. Family-centred practice has, at the centre of it, the beliefs that the family is the constant in the child's life, knows their child best, wants the best for their child and will know the child in a way that a therapist will never be able to. This approach favours a collaborative parent-therapist partnership in which the therapist has technical expertise and the parents are experts on their child (Rodger and Keen 2017).

Culture and Play

Play is universal yet culturally determined and contextualized, representing the values, beliefs, ethics, history and society that the individual belongs to (Ramugondo 2012; Roopnarine 2015). Play both maintains and develops a culture's identity, and what is seen as play by one culture may not be by another. Through play, children learn to master their environment, learn society's rules, practice skills, rehearse adult roles and understand cultural norms, symbols and attitudes (Drewes 2009). With the changing ecology of childhood, if is imperative that occupational therapists become conversant with the meaning and relevance of play in diverse cultures (Berinstein and Magalhaes 2009). There is a growing body of evidence to suggest that there are cultural differences in children's play across Mexico, Africa, Asia, China, India, Korea, Japan, the United States and Europe as well as in indigenous populations (Gerlach et al. 2014; Roopnarine 2015). Haight et al. (1999) examined the differences in European-American and Chinese children's play themes. They found that European-American children's play emphasized individuality, independence and self-expression, while Chinese children's play emphasized harmonious social interaction obtained through obeying, respecting and submitting to elders as well as adherence to rules and cooperation. Cultural influence on play has also been reported by Ramugondo (2012) in an ethnographic study of three generations in one South African family. In this study attention was drawn not only to the persistence of play themes across generations that reflected religious events and folklore, but also to the critical influence of technology that reduced opportunities for shared intergenerational play opportunities.

Further cultural values can be seen in the link between play and gender. Early literature from Sutton-Smith et al. (1963) identified boys playing with soldiers, cowboys, spacemen and hunting toys, while girls played dolls, dress-up, school and actresses. Paley (1986) identified a nursery as a place where sexual stereotypes begin. At age three play is alike for sexes: everyone cooks, policemen dress the baby and sweep the floor. By four years old, girls prefer to be mothers and boys prefer to be monsters and superheroes. In a more recent study of play among migrant farmworkers of Mexican origin it was found that when migrant parents have less gender-specific roles working in the fields, this is reflected in gender-neutral play of their younger children (Mathur 2015).

THEORETICAL UNDERSTANDINGS OF PLAY

A theory is an explanation or understanding of a natural phenomenon; just as there are numerous definitions of play, there are multiple and diverse theories of play. Classical understandings of play from the 19th and early 20th century were predominantly grounded in sociological and psychological theory and attempted to explain the existence and purpose of play (Stagnitti 2004).

Classical Play Theories

There are three classical theories of play: surplus energy, practice and recapitulation.

- **The surplus energy theory** arose from the work of Spencer (1878) and proposed that children were not responsible for their own survival and that they had left over energy which was directed into play.
- **The practice theory of play** was formulated by Groos (1901). Groos posited the idea that play existed in children so that they could practise instinctive behaviours necessary for survival. Groos also recommended forms and functions of play, that is, experimental play, including sensory and motor activities, and socioeconomic play, including fighting, chasing, social and family games.
- **Recapitulation theory** refers to rehearsing activities of the child's ancestors (Hall 1920). Hall viewed the function of play as cathartic rather than mastery and that during play, children played out the history of mankind. For example, the throwing, running and hitting of cricket reflect a summary of hunting activity.

These classical theories of play have been widely critiqued but form the basis from which the contemporary study of play has evolved.

Contemporary Play Theories

Contemporary accounts of play developed after the 1920's have been drawn from a range of knowledge bases but have often endeavoured to explain the role of play in child development. There are too many modern theories of play to discuss in detail in this chapter, but the main ones were developed by Freud (1961) who believed play had a role in children's personality and emotional development, Piaget (1936) who proposed a theory of intellectual development through play and Mead (1934) who postulated that, through play, children learn social rules. These theories have served to further our understanding of child development and form important foundation knowledge for occupational therapists working with children and young people (Case-Smith 2015).

OCCUPATIONAL THERAPY AND PLAY

In the early years of the occupational therapy profession the 'play spirit' was considered essential for worthwhile life (Slagle 1922). Reflecting the prevailing trend in occupational therapy during the mid-20th century for a more medical and reductionist approach, Knox

(2010) described how 'Play in the early years of occupational therapy was used for a variety of purposes such as diversion, development of skills and remediation' (p. 543). In the late 20th century occupational therapy scholars started to reclaim play itself as an essential part of occupational therapy (Crepeau et al. 2009). Play is a primary occupation of childhood and is seen as having a unique value for its own sake beyond acquiring skills (Lynch and Moore 2016). Play has to be child rather than adult directed, whereas occupational therapists often direct play activities to enable acquisition of specific skills such as making choices or developing fine motor dexterity (Lynch et al. 2018).

Occupational therapy theory tends to group occupations into the broad categories of self-care, productivity, play and leisure. The Canadian model of occupational performance and engagement has a category of leisure which it describes as being for enjoyment such as socialising, creative expressions, outdoor activities and games and sport (Townsend and Polatajko 2013). The model of human occupation has a play and leisure category described as activities undertaken for their own sake (Taylor 2017). It has been suggested that these categories focus on the purpose of the occupation but do not capture its meaningfulness (Hammell 2004). Hammell suggested we should consider the schema of doing, being, becoming and belonging (Wilcock and Hocking 2015). By 'doing' play, children acquire new skills and explore their environment. The experience of 'being' during play could, for example, include a connection to people and nature and has the potential to build self-esteem which is integral to mental health. Play can engender a sense of 'belonging' to different social groups such as family, peers and wider society. Through play, children and young people can learn how to develop mastery over their environment, and this gives it the potential to be a powerful therapeutic medium. 'If play is the vehicle by which individuals become masters of their environments, then play should be the most powerful of therapeutic tools' (Bundy 1991, p. 61).

Leisure occupations have been shown to have a significant and positive relationship with mental health, including self-efficacy beliefs for adolescents (Passmore and French 2003). In adolescents with disabilities, participation in leisure activities is positively associated with fun, freedom and fulfilment (Powrie

et al. 2015). It has also been suggested that there may be a correlation between depression and participation in play and leisure activities, with engaging in active leisure activities having a potential protective factor against depression (Desha and Zivianni 2007). When children and young people are involved in setting goals for occupational therapy intervention they frequently identify participation in specific play or leisure activities as a desired goal (Costa et al. 2016).

Developing as a Player

Children develop the role of player alongside the roles of daughter/son, sibling, friend and student. The term 'player' refers to a child's engagement in different types of play over time, which reflects the context, for example, parallel play with a peer at the sand pit or constructional and solitary play with blocks at home (Rigby and Rodger 2006). Through the role of player, a child engages with family and peers, learns to problem solve and uses their imagination. The role of player unfolds throughout childhood and adolescence as developing physical, cognitive and psychosocial skills enable them to expand their play repertoire.

The development of play and the occupational role of player begins with the sensorimotor exploration of children's own bodies. First, children discover their hands and feet. Then they start to explore their immediate environment and learn that they can cause things to happen around them and will repeat actions to elicit pleasurable responses. Functional play enables children to explore the purpose of objects and their relationship to them. Social play initially occurs alongside others with cooperative play and turn taking emerging during the second year. The number of other children they can play with increases with age.

Once in school, peer relationships become important and friendships develop. Children learn to regulate their behaviour and consider others. They engage in games with increasingly complex rules and have competitive relationships. Learning the behaviours associated with different occupational roles is part of the socialisation process, and children develop social skills through play. As children grow older they widen the number of occupational roles they have, including formal roles with specific expectations such as being a member of a sports team. A number of studies have considered how children and adolescents spend their time. Rees (2017) examined how children aged 12 to 16 years old used their time across 16 countries including low-, middle- and high-income countries. A large variation was found across some play and leisure occupations. For example, 3% of children in Ethiopia and 7% in Nepal used a computer outside of school whilst this figure was 67% in Estonia and 69% in Malta. Regarding organized leisure activities, 5% of children participated in these activities in Poland and Estonia, but the figure was 21% in Malta and 29% in South Africa. Time use studies are useful in providing some guidance around typical occupational balances for children and young people.

Development of player role behaviours can be a vehicle for testing and experimenting with different roles in preparation for adult life (Case-Smith 2015). There is a whole range of occupations involved in parenting a child, and being a playmate for ones' child could be viewed as one of the occupational roles. Parents and carers need to learn how to play with their children and facilitate play as an occupation through providing suitable opportunities. A variety of factors can influence a parent or carer's ability to offer occupational opportunities for their child including their own mental health status, experiences of being looked after as a child, parenting style and financial and time resources (Jaffe and Cosper 2015). Occupational therapists can enable parents and carers to learn how to play with their child and provide appropriate play and leisure opportunities. This enables the child to explore their occupational role as a 'player', which is discussed further later in this chapter.

Occupational Play Theories

Occupational therapists have challenged the assumptions and relevance of existing play theories (see above). Occupational science has facilitated an occupational perspective of play which embraces complexity and participation (Stagnitti 2004). Occupational therapists acknowledge a range of theoretical understandings about play but identify the limitations of interpreting play only through its physical, cognitive and psychosocial components. In accordance with this view, Humphry (2005) reported that there has been an over-reliance on play theories that provide an organismic subsystem view. Occupational therapists need to appreciate the multiple understandings of play which consider the occupational nature of people. An occupational perspective of play requires an evolutionary, ecological and humanist approach (Wilcock and Hocking 2015). The use of occupational science helps occupational therapists to consider play as a dynamic interaction between the child, their environment and the occupation. Occupational therapists have begun to develop a holistic understanding of play from an occupational perspective. An example of this is the concept of playfulness.

Playfulness Theory

Bundy, an occupational therapist, proposed an interactionist perspective called 'playfulness,' which is 'the disposition or tendency to play' (Cordier and Bundy 2009, p. 46). In this theory there are four key concepts:

1. **Intrinsic motivation** refers to an element of the activity itself, not an external reward that motivates involvement; participation occurs because of enjoyment rather than an outcome.
2. **Internal control** concerns the control that players have over their play which can be as close or as far from object reality as they want which describes the concept of being free of constraints.
3. **Freedom from the constraints of reality** means how close to object reality the play will be.
4. **Framing** refers to the ability of players to read social cues and interact.

In her model, Bundy also utilized the environment, suggesting that this can either impede or facilitate play with optimal environments being safe, allowing adaptation, promoting involvement and supporting motivation and mastery (Cordier and Bundy 2009). Playfulness can be disturbed when any of the key elements are not present or when the environment does not support play. Factors intrinsic to the child, such as mental health problems, can also affect playfulness. For example, children with autism can have difficulty with the suspension of reality and are therefore susceptible to deficits in playfulness (Skaines et al. 2006).

OCCUPATIONAL DEVELOPMENT IN CHILDREN AND YOUNG PEOPLE

Children and young people's play occupations occur within their own unique context through a dynamic interaction between the person, the play occupation and the environment (Law et al. 1996; Wiseman et al. 2005). Children engage in different types of play (exploratory, functional, social, pretend/symbolic, dramatic, constructive, imaginative, creative, rough and tumble, games with rules and sports related). Current theories describe child development as emerging from the dynamic interaction of multiple systems and subsystems within the child such as biomechanics, central nervous system, physiology, cognition, motivation, experiences; as well as the environment (i.e., physical, social, cultural) and the child's occupations (Thelan 1995; Case-Smith 2015). Developmental changes in motor, cognitive and psychosocial domains interact dynamically with the child's experiences to influence their play development. However, occupational therapists need to understand development in a way that goes beyond milestones and developmental norms to development of the knowledge and skills required to enable children to fulfil their occupational roles. Play needs to be viewed from the child's unique perspective that is shaped by their environment and culture. Occupational therapists should also consider all aspects of the environment as important when understanding children's play. Home, neighbourhood and community environments have a significant impact on play; in high-income countries the expansion of sedentary play activities, increased urbanization, demise of playgrounds, growth of apartment living and concerns about safety all influence play choices. Writing about the loss of a neighbourhood pond in Canada, Manuel (2003) used an occupational science perspective to describe how the physical pond environment facilitated play occupations including ice skating, frog catching and fishing. Manuel also highlighted the impact of the social and cultural environment including neighbourhood skating parties and community spectators. In low- and middle-income countries and those in conflict or experiencing disaster, concerns are about access to safe play environments and time for children to play. In low-socio economic rural communities the absence of conventional play equipment and environments has, however, not been found to hinder play because children are innovative and create their own games (Bartie et al. 2015).

There are a number of proposed models or theories of child occupational development.

Humphry (2005) has proposed the model of processes transforming occupations (PTO) as a way to understand how children's occupations (rather than abilities) develop. The PTO can be applied to children's occupations which are described as 'activities that children find interesting or pleasurable and want to do or do because others manifest value in their doing so' (Humphry 2005, p. 38). The PTO applies dynamic systems theory to play, meaning that a child's intrinsic capacities (physical, cognitive and psychosocial skills) self-organize into a performance pattern for that play situation; these intrinsic capacities are interdependent and dynamic and so should not be separated (Humphry 2002). The focus is on the interaction of the child, the environment and the occupation which reflect the occupational meaning. The PTO has three clusters which can be used to explain participation in play occupations:

1. **Construction of occupational opportunities:** This first cluster considers the influence of community, societal and cultural environments. Communities have shared cultural practices which are reflected in the nature of children's play, for example, the use of manufactured toys.
2. **Social transaction in developing occupation:** This second cluster refers to the idea that being involved in a co-occupation contributes to the development and adaptation of the occupation. Two children bring different performance patterns and skills to a joint play occupation, such as playing dress-up, which creates a new co-constructed occupation and new meaning.
3. **Self-organizing processes underlying transformations in occupation:** This final cluster applies dynamic systems. Intrinsic capabilities within the child are assembled to enable occupational performance for that play occupation. These capabilities are reorganized as an occupation changes, but repeated use through occupation enables enhanced performance.

The process for establishing children's occupations (PECO) (Wiseman et al. 2005) is a further example of a theory of occupational development in young people. The PECO was developed from a qualitative study of young people's engagement in occupations and similarly focuses on the development of occupations rather than the development of the individual. The authors described two themes which emerged from 12 in-depth interviews. The first theme includes the reasons why children do the things they do (opportunities, resources, motivations, parental views and values), and the second theme identifies a process by which children's occupations become established (innate drive, exposure, initiation, continuation, transformation, cessation and outcomes). The PECO was developed from an exploratory study but offers an initial representation of how and what influences the development of occupations in young people. Case-Smith (2015) has admirably presented the development of children's occupations in the book chapter 'Development of children's occupations.' Table 17.2 gives a quick reference guide to play occupations at different ages.

Occupational development is supported or constrained by other developmental components such as movement, cognition and psychosocial abilities.

- **Movement** is an integral part of many play activities. There is a wide range of individual variability in the emergence of motor milestones. Cross-cultural differences in motor milestones have been reported (Bardid et al. 2015; Haga et al. 2018), therefore charts featuring the ages at which children achieve certain skills should be viewed with caution when making developmental assessments.
- **Cognitive development** includes intelligence, attention and problem solving, all of which can be explored during play. As children's understanding of the world increases, their play becomes more complex. As they develop emotional intelligence, they are able to link behaviours with feeling and develop 'theory of mind,' which enables them to place themselves in another's position.
- **Psychosocial development** includes dealing with emotions, social cognition and self-management. A child with poor social skills finds it difficult to join in games with their peers, which reduces the opportunities for physical play and social interaction. A child's development of temperament includes confidence and motivation, with a confident child being more likely to be motivated to try a new task and risk failure than a child who lacks confidence.

Infancy (Birth–2 Years)

In the first six months sensorimotor play predominates and social play is focussed on attachment and bonding, which often co-occurs with self-care occupations. The infant starts to learn to regulate their emotions with self-soothing behaviours such as non-nutritive sucking and responding to parents' soothing behaviours (Case-Smith 2015). Attachment theory was proposed by Bowlby (1969), a psychiatrist, and refers to the emotional bond between a child and their caregiver. The relationship between attachment and occupation is discussed by Whitcomb (2012) who highlights the need for co-occupation, particularly between mother and child, as a facilitator to attachment. Sensorimotor play develops into functional play with toys being used for their purpose. Interest in picture books emerges. The child expresses their emotions through verbalizations to indicate whether they are enjoying play or not, and they will repeat actions that give them pleasurable experiences many times. By the end of the first year they can play 'give and take,' showing an emerging ability to take turns. They play contently when their parents are in the room and will interact briefly with other infants. As the child's motor skills develop, they are able to explore their environment using crawling and rolling initially. They engage in simple pretend play such as eating or sleeping, in parallel play and basic peer interactions. As they approach their second birthday they start showing more interest in their peers and begin to take turns. Initially, toys are used for their functional purpose, but between 12 to 18 months simple pretend play starts to emerge. By the age of two the child can perform multiple related actions together. The play environment in these early years is usually home or childcare based with interaction taking place primarily with parents, family members and a small number of others which may include a paid carer. Outside play is weather dependent and in extreme climates may be challenging for young children.

Early Childhood (2–5 Years)

For many children early childhood is the time when their social contacts widen as they mix with similar aged peers, friends and family members. At 2 to 3 years old their play is primarily parallel but associated to what is happening around them. They are able to cooperate with others, play in small groups and understand taking

TABLE 17.2	
A Developmental Guide to Play	
0–6 months	Sensorimotor play predominates Social play focused on attachment and bonding Repeats actions for pleasurable experiences Coos, squeals, smiles, laughs
6–12 months	EXPLORATORY Sensorimotor play evolves into functional play FUNCTIONAL Uses toys according to functional purpose Looks at picture book SOCIAL Attachment relating to parent Plays give and take Interacts briefly with other infants Plays contently when parents are in the room
12–18 months	EXPLORATORY Explores all the spaces in the room using rolling and crawling FUNCTIONAL Simple pretend play directed towards self (pretend eating/sleeping) Imitative play from immediate model SOCIAL Begins peer interactions Parallel play Shares toys with parent
18–24 months	FUNCTIONAL Performs multiple related actions together SOCIAL Participates in parallel play Imitates parents and peers Group play Watches other children Begins to take turns Enjoys solitary play (e.g., colouring, building) PRETEND/SYMBOLIC Inanimate objects perform actions (dolls eating, dancing, hugging) Pretends objects are real/symbolize other objects Matches pictures to real things
24–36 months or 2–3 years	SOCIAL Associative parallel play predominates Cooperative play, takes turns Interest in peers, enjoys having companions Begins cooperative play and in small groups Shy with strangers, especially adults Makes messes Matches red and yellow (3 years) PRETEND/SYMBOLIC Uses toys to represent animals or people Plays out drama with animals or imaginary friends CONSTRUCTIVE Drawing and puzzles Imitates adults, using toys

Continued on following page

TABLE 17.2
A Developmental Guide to Play (Continued)

3–4 years	**SOCIAL** Participates in role play and dressing up Tells stories Continues with pretend play that involves scripts with imaginary characters Enjoys clowning Sings whole songs Role play based on parents' roles **CONSTRUCTION** Takes pride in products Shows interest in goal of art activity Constructs complex structures **GAMES WITH RULES** Begins group games with simple rules Engages in organized play with prescribed roles Participates in organized gross motor game
4–5 years	**SOCIAL PLAY** Understands taking turns Will take turns with 8–9 other children Plays with 2–3 children for 20 minutes in cooperative activity (e.g., project or game) **PRETEND/DRAMATIC PLAY** Dressing up Pretend play with scripts/imaginary characters **CONSTRUCTION PLAY** Takes pride in products Interested in goal of art activity Constructs complex structures **GAMES WITH RULES** Begins group games with simple rules Organized play with prescribed roles **SPORTS** Pedals tricycle turning corners Climbs on playground equipment, swinging from arms or legs
5–6 years	**SOCIAL** Plays with 4–5 children on cooperative activity without constant supervision **PRETEND/DRAMATIC PLAY** Acts out part of story, playing a part or using puppets **CONSTRUCTION PLAY** Builds complex structures (Lego) Plans and builds using simple tools (inclined plane, fulcrum, lever, pulley) **GAMES WITH RULES** Explains rules of game/activity to others Board games **SPORTS** Swings on swing Rides bicycle Can jump rope by self Skates forward 3 metres Hits ball with bat or stick Walks or plays in waist-high water in swimming pool Hangs 10 seconds from horizontal bar, bearing own weight on arms

Continued on following page

TABLE 17.2
A Developmental Guide to Play *(Continued)*

6–10 years	SOCIAL
	Play includes talking and joking
	Peer play predominates at school and home
	Has best friend
	Plays with consistent friends
	Is part of cliques
	Cooperative, less egocentric
	Tries to please others
	Less impulsive and able to regulate behaviour
	Has competitive relationships
	GAMES WITH RULES
	Card games
	Computer games
	Has collections
	May have hobby
	SPORTS
	Cooperative and competitive play in groups/teams
	Winning and skills emphasized

turns. At 3 to 4 years they will tell stories and sing whole songs. By 4 to 5 years they can take turns with eight or nine other children. They will play with a group of two to three children for up to 20 minutes cooperatively on a project or game. Towards the end of this stage children can play group games with simple rules. In early childhood symbolic or pretend play emerges with the child showing imagination through play (Case-Smith 2015). Toys are used to represent animate objects, and children will act out stories with real or imagined friends. Constructive play starts to emerge including drawing, painting, building and doing puzzles. By the age of 4 years they start to take interest in the end product of their creative activities and can build complex structures.

Middle Childhood (6–10 Years)

Play during middle childhood includes construction, crafts and hobbies, games with rules, media and technology use (e.g., tablets, digital video discs and computers), organized sport and social and dramatic play. During constructive play children build complex structures with blocks or interlocking shapes including puzzles. Crafts and hobbies include drawing and collecting things such as stamps, cards and stickers. The games with rules that are played include playground, computer, board and card games that require abstract thinking. Media and technology use is common amongst this age group such as watching TV, using game consoles, listening to music and using the

internet. Organized sporting activities are influenced by local cultures such as whether football or rugby is popular. Participation in sport has been found to have an overall positive effect on children's health and behaviour (Felfe et al. 2016). Social play includes talking and joking with peers and simply hanging out. During this time children's play takes on more social and cooperative forms compared to younger children's play.

Adolescence and Adulthood

Adolescents describe leisure time as providing enjoyment, freedom of choice and 'time out' (Passmore and French 2003). Young people have described leisure occupations as giving them enjoyment and satisfaction, as well as opportunity for relaxation and recovery (Widmark and Fristedt 2018). A lack of leisure can, however, be associated with feelings of boredom. Boredom is associated with higher risks of leaving school early, misusing drugs or alcohol and youth-offending activities (Wegner and Flisher 2009). Sexual play emerges with puberty. In early adolescence same-sex friendships are the most common and eventually evolve into one to one relationships and the selection of intimate partner(s) (Vroman 2015). The top four interests of youth with and without disabilities are listening to music, hanging out with friends, watching television and talking on the phone (Law 2002). Young adults play, and leisure includes establishing occupational balance, socialising, dating, team sports and exploring and pursuing interests. In middle adulthood leisure is often focussed around the immediate family with interests and hobbies generally established.

Although an appreciation of play as a catalyst for child development is important knowledge for occupational therapists, the issue of play as an occupation is our unique perspective. As such this chapter examines the role of play in occupational therapy and considers play as an occupation, the development of the occupational role of the player and occupational theories of play. Having considered theory, the focus shifts to practice, which involves an examination of the range of play assessments available to occupational therapists, the play interventions used by occupational therapists and the impact of play on specific conditions.

PLAY-CENTRED OCCUPATIONAL THERAPY

Play is the primary occupation of children and young people, making it a domain of concern for the occupational therapist. Play should be imbedded in occupational therapy assessment, intervention and outcome measurement. Through the facilitation of play, occupational therapists can assist children and young people to achieve positive mental health and well-being.

Play Assessments

An assessment of play may be made for a number of reasons including establishing a baseline of performance, showing change over time, supplementing subjective observations and assisting with treatment planning as outcome measures or for research (Brown and McDonald 2009). The reason for the assessment should guide

the therapist's assessment tool selection. It is important that assessments are considered carefully and an informed evaluation of psychometric properties, such as validity, reliability and clinical utility, is conducted. As many assessments were developed using limited normative samples, occupational therapists should appraise whether an assessment is culturally appropriate. There is a range of assessment tools available which specifically examine play or leisure occupations including the Symbolic and Imaginative Play Developmental Checklist (Stagnitti 1998), the Test of Playfulness (ToP; Bundy et al. 2001), the Revised Knox Preschool Play Scale (Knox 1997), the Kids Play Profile (Henry 2000), the Preteen Play Profile (Henry 2000), the Adolescent Leisure Interest Profile (Henry 2000), the Children's Assessment of Participation and Enjoyment (CAPE) and the Preferences for Activities of Children (King et al. 2004). Table 17.3 shows a range of available play assessments and their uses; two occupation-based play assessments are discussed in further detail.

Child-Initiated Pretend Play Assessment

The Child-Initiated Pretend Play Assessment (ChIPPA) was developed by Stagnitti (2007) in Australia, although it has now been developed for other cultures and languages (Pfeifer et al. 2011; Golchin et al. 2017). This norm-referenced standardized assessment of spontaneous pretend play is suitable for ages 3 to 7 years and 11 months. The ChIPPA takes between 18 and 30 minutes to administer and requires the therapist to construct a Wendy house before sitting with the child to complete a conventional-imaginative play session followed by a symbolic play session. The items for the first session comprise common play items including dolls, a tea set, animals and a truck. The second

TABLE 17.3	
Play Assessments for Occupational Therapists	
Reason for Assessment	**Example of Play Assessment**
Establish a baseline of performance	Revised Knox Preschool Play Scale (Knox 1997)
Show change over time	ToP (Bundy 2001)
Assist with treatment planning	The Symbolic and Imaginative Play Developmental Checklist (Stagnitti 1998)
Outcome measure	Child-Initiated Pretend Play Assessment (Stagnitti 2007)
Research	Penn Interactive Peer Play Scale (Fantuzzo and Hampton 2000)

session utilizes unstructured items such as a tin, a piece of wood, a stone and a cloth. The assessment is child-centred and non-directive and is scored by recording every action the child uses and assigning a code (Stagnitti 2009). Analysis of the codes shows the play process, themes and repetitions which highlight typical or deficient pretend play. A number of studies have been completed to evaluate the reliability and validity of the ChIPPA (Stagnitti et al. 2000; Stagnitti and Unsworth 2004; Uren and Stagnitti 2009).

Test of Playfulness

The ToP (Skard and Bundy 2007) provides an objective measure of engagement in play activity. It is based on Bundy's model of playfulness (1991) and evaluates free play for children 6 months to 14 years of age. The ToP is administered by observing the child in a familiar natural environment for 15 to 20 minutes, both indoor and outdoor if possible and appropriate. It has 24 items that reflect the domains of intrinsic motivation, internal control and freedom to suspend reality. The examiner rates the extent, intensity and/or skillfulness of the observed behaviours. Overall playfulness is determined by the combined scores in each domain (Skard and Bundy 2007). The ToP has been established as a valuable and reliable outcome measure in a variety of contexts, for example, with children who are human immunodeficiency virus–positive in South Africa (Ramugondo et al. 2018) and children with autism spectrum disorders in Australia (Vousden et al. 2019). Alongside the ToP, clinicians use the Test of Environmental Supportiveness (TOES) (Bundy 1999), a 17-item observation measure of environmental elements that influence playfulness. When used together, the ToP and TOES provide a comprehensive play assessment for children with and without disabilities (Hamm 2006) and can assist clinicians in planning interventions that modify the environment to support play (Bundy et al. 2009).

Play Interventions for Occupational Therapists

As well as progress with play assessments for occupational therapists, there have also been developments in play interventions. Play interventions use play as therapy with either play outcomes or non-play outcomes. The latter has historically been used by occupational therapists working in mental health settings often using non-directive play interventions or with additional training play therapy. Play therapy makes use of play to help a child play out feelings and problems and experience growth (Cooper 2009). It draws on theory from developmental psychology and is often used with children who have been traumatised or abused (Brown 2018). Play therapy is not an occupation-based intervention, but due to the paucity of alternatives, has often defined occupational therapists' role in mental health settings.

Increasingly, occupational therapists have been adopting play-centred practice that incorporates occupation-based or occupation-focused play interventions (Fisher 2013). These interventions use play as therapy and as an outcome. In this type of treatment the goal is an improvement in play as an outcome of the intervention (Lynch et al. 2018). The numbers of interventions that meet these criteria are limited but include Learn to Play, Cognitive Orientation to Daily Occupational Performance (CO-OP), a play-based intervention for children with ADHD and the Cognitive-Functional (Cog-Fun) occupational therapy intervention.

■ **The Learn to Play programme** by Stagnitti (1998) is a specific play intervention that uses play as a therapeutic medium and as an outcome. This practical programme develops the imaginative play skills of children aged up to six years and is therapist facilitated but family-centred. Learn to Play addresses the area of play themes, sequences of play actions, object substitution, social interaction, role play and doll/teddy play and is suitable for use in a clinic or home setting. Following assessment using the Symbolic and Imaginative Play Developmental Checklist (Stagnitti 1998), the occupational therapist demonstrates developmentally appropriate play skill with the child and encourages the parent/carer to carry out the same. The play activities are supported with handouts and should be incorporated into the family play routine. The programme is regularly reviewed by the occupational therapist and the level of skill increased over a three- to six-month period (Stagnitti 1998). The Learn to Play programme can be used with children who have a range of difficulties including autistic spectrum disorders and attachment disorders.

- **CO-OP** is an intervention based on dynamic system or cognitive neuroscience approach in which there is an emphasis on the interaction between the person and the environment (Dawson et al. 2017). CO-OP can be applied to play but is not a play-specific intervention. The approach can be used with older age children in mental health settings with conditions such as autism spectrum disorders (Rodger, Ireland, et al. 2008; Rodger, Pham et al. 2008; Rodger and Brandenburg 2009). CO-OP is a client-centred, performance-based, problem-solving approach in which the therapist guides the child to discover and learn strategies to achieve their chosen goals. The occupational therapist establishes goals with the child, for example, to kick a ball in football and measures their current performance and satisfaction with the activity. The child is seen for 10 sessions in which the global strategy (goal, plan, do check) is used together with domain-specific strategies to improve performance of the activity itself (Dawson et al. 2017).

- **Play-based intervention for ADHD.** ADHD is a common condition seen in children and young people in mental health settings and is characterized by symptoms such as inattention and hyperactivity that impair everyday life (Barnes et al. 2017). Occupational therapists are specialists in understanding the impact of ADHD on daily occupations, including play. Recent studies have highlighted that children and young people with ADHD engage in less cooperative play and sharing, dominate play, lack interpersonal empathy, struggle with transitions between activities and are involved in more negative behaviours compared to typically developing peers (Leipold and Bundy 2000; Cordier et al. 2010, 2010a, 2010b). A play-based intervention delivered by therapists or parents has shown promising results (Barnes et al. 2017). The intervention has been systemically developed (Wilkes et al. 2011; Wilkes-Gillan et al. 2014) and includes five principles: (i) promoting the intrinsic motivation of children; (ii) teaching empathy; (iii) including a regular playmate; (iv) increasing parental involvement;

and (v) therapist modelling (Wilkes-Gillan 2016). The manualized intervention involves six 1-hour sessions, home activities and four parent-facilitated playdates. The long-term effectiveness of the intervention to improve play skills has begun to be established (Barnes et al. 2017).

- **Cog-Fun intervention for ADHD.** The Cog-Fun intervention is a manualized treatment approach that uses executive strategies and environmental adaptations (Hahn-Markowitz et al. 2016). Using a playful setting the therapist works with the child with ADHD to set meaningful goals, which could be in the area of play. Intervention strategies are delivered through games, such as Simon Says, that aim to compensate for difficulties commonly associated with ADHD. Parents are also involved in reinforcing strategies at home as well as using supporting strategies such as positive reinforcement, checklists and daily planners. This enables the child to transfer what they do in therapy to their natural contexts, such as playing board games with siblings or with friends on the school playground. The Cog-Fun has growing evidence of its long-term effectiveness (Maeir et al. 2014; Hahn-Markowitz et al. 2016) to improve the occupational performance of children in daily life, including during play activities.

SUMMARY

Play has always been an intrinsic part of occupational therapy practice. Occupational therapists have been influenced by the study of play in related areas such as psychology and sociology. This knowledge provides a foundation, but considering play as an occupation is unique to the occupational therapy domain of concern. Occupational therapists have developed an understanding of play as an interaction between the person, their environment and the occupation. Play occupations reflect societal and cultural roles, are influenced by the built and natural environment and transform through shared meaning. Play can therefore support healthy mental and physical development. Play deprivation has serious consequences for emotional development and behaviour. Mental health difficulties in children and young people can impact play and leisure occupations and therefore have further impact on health and well-being. Furthermore, parents with mental health issues can influence the child's development of a healthy range of play occupations. Occupational therapists working in this field have available an increasing range of play assessments and interventions that are occupation-focused. Research into play and occupational therapy is establishing the important role occupational therapists have in maintaining or establishing play occupations for children and young people with mental health difficulties.

QUESTIONS FOR CONSIDERATION

1. What do occupational therapists mean by the term 'play'?
2. Why does play deprivation have such a significant, negative affect on childhood development?
3. How could play be facilitated or encouraged when the child or family has limited resources?
4. Remembering your own experiences, what values can you identify that were learned or taught during play?
5. Research what might be considered play by people from another country or culture that is different to your own.
6. How might an occupational therapist observe each concept of Bundy's Playfulness Model while a child plays?
7. Design a table which outlines the strengths and differences between the model of processes transforming occupations (PTO) and the process for establishing children's occupations (PECO) that could aid an occupational therapist in their care plan approach. Consider age groups, purpose, assessment styles and drawbacks.
8. Write a brief summary of each of the following play-based interventions: Learn to Play, CO-OP, Cog-Fun and play-based intervention for children with ADHD.

REFERENCES

American Occupational Therapy Association (AOTA). (2017). Occupational therapy practice framework: Domain and process (3rd ed.). *American Journal of Occupational Therapy, 68*(Suppl. 1), S1–S48. https://doi.org/10.5014/ajot.2014.682006.

Barber, B. K. (2015). Political conflict and youth: A long–term view. In R. A. Scott, & M. C. Buchman (Eds.), *Emerging trends in the social and behavioral sciences: An interdisciplinary, searchable, and linkable resource.* London, UK: Wileyhttps://doi.org/10.1002/9781118900772.etrds0253.

Bardid, F., Rudd, J. R., Lenior, M., Polman, R., & Barnett, L. M. (2015). Cross-cultural comparison of motor competence in children from Australia and Belgium. *Frontiers in Psychology, 6,* Article 964.

Barnes, G., Wilkes-Gillan, S., Bundy, A., & Cordier, R. (2017). The social play, social skills and parent-child relationships of children with ADHD 12 months following a RCT of a play-based intervention. *Australian Occupational Therapy Journal, 64,* 457–465.

Bartie, M., Dunnell, A., Kaplan, J., et al. (2015). The play experiences of preschool children from a low-socio-economic rural community in Worcester, South Africa. *Occupational Therapy International, 23,* 91–102.

Berinstein, S., & Magalhaes, L. (2009). A study if the essence of play experience to children living in Zanzibar, Tanzania. *Occupational Therapy International, 15*(2), 89–106.

Bowlby, J. (1969). *Attachment.* New York: Basic Books.

Brackman, A. A., Rumugondo, E., Daniels, A., et al. (2017). Street play as occupation for pre-teens in Belhar, South Africa. *South African Journal of Occupational Therapy, 47*(2), 27–34.

Brown, F. (2018). Therapeutic play work: Theory and practice. In *Aspects of play work – play and culture studies* F. Brown, & B. Hughes (Eds.), (Vol. 14) (pp. 93–106). London: Rowman and Littlefield.

Brown, T., & McDonald, R. (2009). Play assessment: A psychometric overview. In K. Stagnitti, & R. Cooper (Eds.), *Play as therapy* (pp. 72–86). London: Kingsley.

Brown, F., & Patte, M. (2013). *Rethinking children's play.* London: Bloomsbury Academic.

Bundy, A. C. (1991). Play theory and sensory integration. In A. G. Fisher, E. A. Murray, & A. C. Bundy (Eds.), *Sensory integration: Theory and practice* (pp. 46–68). Philadelphia: FA Davis.

Bundy, A. C. (1999). *Test of Environmental Supportiveness (TOES).* Fort Collins, CO: Colorado State University.

Bundy, A. C. (2012). Children at play. In S. J. Lane, & A. C. Bundy (Eds.), *Kids can be kids: A childhood occupations approach* (pp. 28–43). Philadelphia: FA Davis.

Bundy, A. C., Nelson, L., Metzger, M., & Bingaman, K. (2001). Validity and reliability of a test of playfulness. *Occupational Therapy Journal of Research*, 21(4), 276–292.

Bundy, A. C., Waugh, K., & Brentnall, J. (2009). Developing assessments that account for the role of the environment: An example using the test of playfulness and test of environmental supportiveness. *Occupational Therapy Journal of Research*, 29(3), 135–143.

Case-Smith, J. (2015). Development of childhood occupations. In J. Case-Smith, & J. C. O'Brien (Eds.), *Occupational therapy for children and adolescents* (7th ed.) (pp. 65–101). St. Louis: Elsevier.

Cooper, R. (2009). Play focused therapy: Different settings, different approaches. In K. Stagnitti, & R. Cooper (Eds.), *Play as therapy* (pp. 218–233). London: Kingsley.

Cordier, R., & Bundy, A. (2009). Children and playfulness. In K. Stagnitti, & R. Cooper (Eds.), *Play as therapy* (pp. 45–58). London: Jessica Kingsley.

Cordier, R., Bundy, A., Hocking, C., & Einfield, S. (2010). Playing with a child with ADHD: A focus on the playmates. *Scandinavian Journal of Occupational Therapy*, 17(3), 191–199.

Cordier, R., Bundy, A., Hocking, C., & Einfield, S. (2010a). Comparison of the play of children with attention deficit hyperactivity disorder in subtypes. *Australian Occupational Therapy Journal*, 57, 137–145.

Cordier, R., Bundy, A., Hocking, C., & Einfield, S. (2010b). Empathy in play of children with attention deficit hyperactivity disorder. *Occupational Therapy Journal of Research*, 30(3), 122–132.

Costa, U. M., Brauchle, G., & Kennedy-Behr, A. (2017). Collaborative goal setting with and for children as part of therapeutic intervention. *Disability & Rehabilitation*, 39(16), 1589–1600.

Crepeau, E. B., Cohn, E. S., & Boyt Schell, B. A. (Eds.). (2009). *Willard and spackman's occupational therapy* (11th ed.). Philadelphia: Lippincott, Williams and Wilkins.

d'Entremont, L., Gregor, M., Kirou, E., et al. (2017). Developmental milestones for productivity occupations in children and youth: An integrative review. *Work*, 56, 75–89.

Darlington, Y., & Rodger, S. (2006). Families and children's occupational performance. In S. Rodger, & J. Ziviani (Eds.), *Occupational therapy with children* (pp. 22–40). Oxford: Blackwell.

Dawson, D. R., McEwen, S. E., & Polatajko, H. J. (Eds.). (2017). *Cognitive orientation to daily performance in occupational therapy*. Bethesda, MD: AOTA Press.

Desha, L. N., & Ziviani, J. M. (2007). Use of time in childhood and adolescence: A literature review on the nature of activity participation and depression. *Australian Occupational Therapy Journal*, 54, 4–10.

Drewes, A. A. (2009). Cultural considerations. In K. Stagnitti, & R. Cooper (Eds.), *Play as therapy* (pp. 159–173). London: Kingsley.

Fantuzzo, J., & Hampton, V. (2000). Penn interactive peer play scale: A parent and teacher rating scale for young children. In K. Gitlin-Weiner, A. Sandgrund, & C. Schaefer (Eds.), *Play diagnosis and assessment* (pp. 599–620). New York: John Wiley.

Felfe, C., Lechner, M., & Steinmayr, A. (2016). Sports and child development. *PLoS One*, 11(5), e0151729. https://doi.org/10.1371/journal.pone.0151729.

Fisher, A. (2013). Occupation-centred, occupation-based, occupation-focused: Same, same or different? *Scandinavian Journal of Occupational Therapy*, 20(3), 162–173.

Frech, A., & Kimbro, R. T. (2011). Maternal mental health, neighbourhood characteristics, and time invested in children. *Journal of Marriage and Family*, 73, 605–620.

Freud, S. (1961). *Beyond the pleasure principle*. New York: Norton.

Galvaan, R. (2015). The contextually situated nature of occupational choice: Marginalised young adolescents' experienced in South Africa. *Journal of Occupational Science*, 22(1), 39–53.

Gaskins, S. (2015). Yucatec Mayan children's play. In J. L. Roopnarine, M. M. Patte, J. E. Johnson, & D. Kuschner (Eds.), *International perspectives on children's play* (pp. 11–22). Maidenhead: Open University Press.

Gerlach, A., Browne, A., & Suto, M. (2014). A critical reframing of play in relation to indigenous children in Canada. *Journal of Occupational Science*, 21(3), 243–258.

Golchin, M. D., Mirakhani, N., Stagnitti, K., Golchin, M. D., & Rezaei, M. (2017). Psychometric properties of persian version of the "child-initiated pretend play assessment" for Iranian children. *Iranian Journal of Pediatrics*, 27(1), e7053.

Groos, K. (1901). *The play of man*. New York: Appleton.

Haga, M., Tortella, P., Asonitou, K., et al. (2018). *Cross-cultural aspects: Exploring motor competence among 7- to 8- year old children from Greece, Italy and Norway*. SAGE Open. April–June, 1–9.

Hahn-Markowitz, J., Berger, I., Manor, I., & Maeir, A. (2016). Efficacy of cognitive-functional (Cog-Fun) occupational therapy intervention among children with ADHD: An RCT. *Journal of Attention Disorders*, 1–12. https://doi.org/10.1177/1087054716666955.

Haight, W. L., Wang, X., Fung, H. H., Williams, K., & Mintz, J. (1999). Universal development and variable aspects of young children's play: A cross cultural comparison of pretending at home. *Child Development*, 70(6), 1477–1488.

Hall, G. S. (1920). *Youth*. New York: Appleton.

Hamm, E. M. (2006). Playfulness and the environmental support of play in children with and without developmental disabilities. *Occupational Therapy Journal of Research*, 26(3), 88–96.

Hammell, K. W. (2004). Dimensions of meaning in the occupations of daily life. *Canadian Journal of Occupational Therapy*, 71(5), 296–305.

Henry, A. D. (2000). *Paediatric interest profiles*. USA: Therapy Skill Builders.

Humphry, R. (2002). Young children's occupational behaviours: Explicating developmental processes. *American Journal of Occupational Therapy*, 56, 171–179.

Humphry, R. (2005). Model of processes transforming occupations: Exploring societal and social influences. *Journal of Occupational Science*, 12(1), 36–44.

Jaffe, L., & Cosper, S. (2015). Working with families. In J. Case-Smith, & J. C. O'Brien (Eds.), *Occupational therapy for children, seven* (pp. 129–151). St. Louis: Mosby Elsevier.

Johnson, J., Christie, J., & Yawley, T. (1999). *Play and early child development* (2nd ed.). New York: Longman.

Kemple, K. M., Oh, J., Kenney, E., & Smith-Bonahue, T. (2016). The power of outdoor play and play in natural environments. *Childhood Education, 92*(6), 446–454.

King, G., Law, M., King, S., et al. (2004). *Children's Assessment of Participation and Enjoyment (CAPE) and Preferences for Activities of children (PAC).* San Antonio: Harcourt Assessment.

Knox, S. (1997). Development and current use of the Knox preschool play scale. In D. Parham, & L. Fazio (Eds.), *Play in occupational therapy for children* (pp. 35–51). St. Louis: Mosby.

Knox, S. H. (2010). Play. In J. Case-Smith, & J. C. O'Brien (Eds.), *Occupational therapy for children* (6th ed.) (pp. 540–554). St. Louis: Mosby Elsevier.

Law, M. (2002). Participation in the occupations of everyday life. *American Journal of Occupational Therapy, 56*(6), 640–649.

Law, M., Cooper, B., Strong, S., Stewart, D., Rigby, P., & Letts, L. (1996). The person-environment-occupation model: A transactive approach to occupational performance. *Canadian Journal of Occupational Therapy, 65*(1), 9–23.

Leipold, E., & Bundy, A. C. (2000). Playfulness and children with ADHD. *Occupational Therapy Journal of Research, 20*(1), 61–79.

Lynch, H., & Moore, A. (2016). Play as an occupation in occupational therapy. *British Journal of Occupational Therapy, 79*(9), 519–520.

Lynch, H., Prellwitz, M., Schulze, C., & Moore, A. H. (2018). The state of play in children's occupational therapy: A comparison between Ireland, Sweden and Switzerland. *British Journal of Occupational Therapy, 81*(1), 42–50.

Maeir, A., Fisher, O., Bar-Ilan, R. T., et al. (2014). Effectiveness of cognitive-functional (Cog-Fun) occupational therapy intervention for young children with attention deficit hyperactivity disorder: A controlled study. *American Journal of Occupational Therapy, 68*(3), 260–267.

Manuel, P. M. (2003). Occupied with ponds: Exploring the meaning, bewaring the loss for kids and communities of nature's small spaces. *Journal of Occupational Science, 10*(1), 31–39.

Mathur, S. (2015). The ecology of play among young children of Mexican origin farmworkers. In J. L. Roopnarine, M. M. Patte, J. E. Johnson, & D. Kuschner (Eds.), *International perspectives on children's play* (pp. 49–61). Maidenhead: Open University Press.

Mead, G. H. (1934). *Mind, self, and society.* Chicago, IL: University of Chicago Press.

Moore, A., & Lynch, H. (2018). Understanding a child's conceptualisation of well-being through an exploration of happiness: The centrality of play, people and place. *Journal of Occupational Science, 25*(1), 124–141.

Njelesani, J., Sedgwick, A., Davis, J. A., & Polatajko, H. J. (2011). The influence of context: A naturalistic study of Ugandan children's doing in outdoor spaces. *Occupational Therapy International, 18*, 124–132.

Paley, V. G. (1986). *Boys and girls superheroes in the doll corner.* Chicago: University of Chicago Press.

Passmore, A. (1998). Does leisure have an association with creating cultural patterns of work? *Journal of Occupational Science, 5*(3), 61–165.

Passmore, A., & French, D. (2003). The nature of leisure in adolescence: A focus group study. *British Journal of Occupational Therapy, 66*(9), 419–426.

Pfeifer, L. I., Queiroz, M. A., Santos, J. L. F., & Stagnitti, K. E. (2011). Cross-cultural adaptation and reliability of the child-initiated pretend play assessment (ChIPPA). *Canadian Journal of Occupational Therapy, 78*(3), 187–195.

Piaget, J. (1936). *Origins of intelligence in the child.* London: Routledge.

Powrie, B., Kolehmainen, N., Turpin, M., et al. (2015). The meaning of leisure for children and young people with physical disabilities: A systematic evidence synthesis. *Developmental Medicine and Child Neurology, 57*, 993–1010.

Prellwitz, M., & Skär, L. (2016). Are playgrounds a case of occupational injustice? Experiences of parents of children with disabilities. *Children, Youth, and Environments, 26*(2), 28–42.

Ramugondo, E. L. (2012). Intergenerational play within family: The case for occupational consciousness. *Journal of Occupational Science, 19*(4), 326–340.

Ramugondo, E., F, A, Chung, D., & Cordier, R. (2018). A feasibility RCT evaluating a play-informed, caregiver-implemented, home-based intervention to improve the play of children who are HIV positive. *Occupational Therapy International*, Article ID 3652529. https://doi:10.1155/2018/3652529.

Rees, G. (2017). Children's activities and time use: Variations between and within 16 countries. *Children and Youth Services Review, 80*, 78–87.

Rigby, P., & Rodger, S. (2006). Developing as a player. In S. Rodger, & J. Ziviani (Eds.), *Occupational therapy with children: Understanding children's occupations and enabling participation* (pp. 177–195). Oxford: Blackwell.

Rodger, S., & Brandenburg, J. (2009). Cognitive orientation to (daily) occupational performance (CO-OP) with children with Asperger's syndrome who have motor-based occupational performance goals. *Australian Occupational Therapy Journal, 56*(1), 41–50.

Rodger, S., Ireland, S., & Vun, M. (2008). Can cognitive orientation to daily occupational performance (CO-OP) help children with Asperger's syndrome to master social and organisational goals? *British Journal of Occupational Therapy, 71*(1), 23–32.

Rodger, S., & Keen, D. (2017). Child and family-centred service provision. In S. Rodger, & A. Kennedy-Behr (Eds.), *Occupation-centred practice with children* (2nd ed.) (pp. 45–71). Oxford: Blackwell.

Rodger, S., Pham, C., & Mitchell, S. (2008a). Cognitive strategy use by children with Asperger's syndrome during intervention for motor-based goals. *Australian Occupational Therapy Journal, 57*(2), 103–111.

Roopnarine, J. L. (2015). Play as a culturally situated: Diverse perspectives on its meaning and significance. In J. L. Roopnarine, M. M. Patte, J. E. Johnson, & D. Kuschner (Eds.), *International perspectives on children's play* (pp. 1–8). Maidenhead: Open University Press.

Skaines, N., Rodger, S., & Bundy, A. (2006). Playfulness in children with autistic disorder and their typically developing peers. *British Journal of Occupational Therapy, 69*(11), 505–512.

Skard, G., & Bundy, A. C. (2008). Test of playfulness. In L. D. Parham, & L. S. Fazio (Eds.), *Play in occupational therapy for children* (2nd ed.) (pp. 71–93). St. Louis, MO: Mosby Elsevier.

Slagle, E. C. (1922). Training aides for mental patients. *Archives of Occupational Therapy, 1*, 11–17.

Smith, P. K. (2010). *Children and play*. Oxford: Wiley Blackwell.

Spencer, H. (Ed.). (1878). *The principles of psychology* (Vol. 2). New York: Appleton.

Stagnitti, K. (1998). *Learn to play*. West Brunswick: Co-ordinates.

Stagnitti, K. (2004). Understanding play: The implication for play assessment. *Australian Occupational Therapy Journal, 51*(1), 3–12.

Stagnitti, K. (2007). *Child initiated pretend play assessment kit*. West Brunswick: Co-ordinates.

Stagnitti, K. (2009). Pretend play assessment. In K. Stagnitti, & R. Cooper (Eds.), *Play as therapy* (pp. 87–101). London: Kingsley.

Stagnitti, K., & Unsworth, C. (2004). The test-retest reliability of the child initiated pretend play assessment. *American Journal of Occupational Therapy, 58*, 93–99.

Stagnitti, K., Unsworth, C., & Rodger, S. (2000). The development of an assessment to identify play behaviours that discrimi1nate between the play of typical pre-schoolers and pre-schoolers with suspected pre-academic problems. *Canadian Journal of Occupational Therapy, 97*(5), 291–303.

Stanton-Chapman, T. L., Toraman, S., Morrison, A., et al. (2018). An observational study of children's behaviors across two playgrounds: Similarities and differences. *Early Childhood Research Quarterly, 44*, 114–123.

Sutton-Smith, B., Rosenberg, B. G., & Morgan, E. F. (1963). Development of sex differences in play choices during pre-adolescence. *Child Development, 34*, 119–126.

Taylor, R. R. (Ed.). (2017). *Kielhofner's model of human occupation: Theory and application* (5th ed.). Philadelphia: Lippincott, Williams and Wilkins.

Thelen, E. (1995). Motor development. A new synthesis. *American Psychologist, 50*(2), 79–95.

Townsend, E.A., & Polatajko, H. J. (Eds.). (2013). *Enabling occupation II: Advancing an occupational therapy vision for health, well-being and justice through occupation.* (2nd ed.). Ottawa, ON: CAOT.

Uren, N., & Stagnitti, K. (2009). Pretend play, social competence and involvement in children aged 5-7 years: The concurrent validity of the child-initiated pretend play assessment. *Australian Occupational Therapy Journal, 56*, 33–40.

Vousden, B., Wilkes–Gillan, S., Cordier, R., & Froude, E. (2019). The play skills of children with high-functioning autism spectrum disorder in peer-to–peer interactions with their classmates: A multiple case study design. *Australian Occupational Therapy Journal, 66*(2), 183–192.

Vroman, K. (2015). Adolescent development: Transitioning from child to adult. In J. Case-Smith, & J. C. O'Brien (Eds.), *Occupational therapy for children and adolescents* (7th ed.) (pp. 102–121). St. Louis: Elsevier.

Wegner, L., & Flisher, A. J. (2009). Leisure boredom and adolescent risk behaviour: A systematic literature review. *Journal of Children and Young People's Mental Health, 21*(1), 1–28.

Whitcomb, D. A. (2012). Attachment, occupation and identity: considerations in infancy. *Journal of Occupational Science, 19*(3), 271–282.

Widmark, W., & Fristedt, S. (2018). Occupation according to adolescents: Daily occupations categorised based on adolescents' experiences. *Journal of Occupational Science.* https://doi:10.1080/14427591.2018.1546609.

Wilcock, A. A., & Hocking, C. (2015). *An occupational perspective of health* (3rd ed.). Thorofare, NJ: Slack.

Wilkes-Gillan, S., Bundy, A., Cordier, R., et al. (2014). Evaluation of a pilot parent-delivered play-based intervention for children with attention deficit hyperactivity disorder. *American Journal of Occupational Therapy, 68*(6), 700–709.

Wilkes-Gillan, S., Bundy, A., Cordier, R., et al. (2014a). Eighteen-month follow-up of a play-based intervention to improve the social skills of children with attention deficit hyperactivity disorder. *Australian Occupational Therapy Journal, 61*(5), 299–307.

Wilkes, S., Cordier, R., Bundy, A., et al. (2011). A play-based intervention for children with ADHD: A pilot study. *Australian Occupational Therapy Journal, 58*(4), 231–240.

Wiseman, J., Davis, J., & Polatajko, H. (2005). Occupational development: Towards an understanding of children's doing. *Journal of Occupational Science, 12*(1), 26–35.

World Federation of Occupational Therapists (WFOT). (2009). *WFOT statement on occupational therapy*. Available at: https://www.wfot.org/resources/statement-on-occupational-therapy.

Ziviani, J., & Rodger, S. (2006). Environmental Influences on children's participation. In S. Rodger, & J. Ziviani (Eds.), *Occupational therapy with children* (pp. 41–66). Oxford: Blackwell.

18 SELF-CARE

KEVIN CORDINGLEY ■ HANNAH SPREADBURY-TROY

CHAPTER OUTLINE

INTRODUCTION

Occupational therapists work with individuals with mental health problems to facilitate their recovery (see Chapter 2). For any occupational engagement and participation, biological health and physical safety needs (in other words, self-care) must be met (Matuska and Christiansen 2008). There are multiple forms of self-care required for recovery (Kelly et al. 2010). Occupational therapists have an important role in supporting service users' self-care (D'Amico et al. 2018). In this chapter we explore, define and describe self-care. We discuss wider social, cultural and economic impacts on self-care using a critical perspective. Also discussed are occupational therapists' assessments and interventions for self-care. The theory, practice and current research about self-care illustrates the discussion.

A BRIEF INTRODUCTION TO SELF-CARE

Self-care has been used to describe a range of activities of personal care that support other occupations and role performance. From a general societal perspective, self-care in Western societies has come to mean various activities ranging from having a bath, using fragrances and candles, to suggestions from Action for Happiness (2020) in their November calendar to use a new recipe or ingredient. These are suggestions to help increase happiness, for relaxation to help maintain mental health. They may be helpful, but they can also be de-contextualized from people who may lack resources and opportunities caused by factors outside of their control. This can contribute to restrictions in participating and engaging in occupations that can lead to forms of exclusion and marginalization. Furthermore, participation in self-care for a person with a formal diagnosis of a mental illness is a challenging experience.

Occupations related to self-care in the third edition of the Occupational Therapy Practice Framework (OTPF) (American Occupational Therapy Association (AOTA) 2014) include activities of daily living (ADLs) and instrumental activities of daily living (IADLs). The OTPF does not use self-care as a category but sees it as an obligatory occupation compared to leisure occupations (Parham and Fazio 1997 cited in AOTA 2014, p. 21). Nonetheless, in this chapter we use self-care as a category because of the importance of looking after oneself; we also use the OTPF's framework because the variety of I/ADLs in the latter is useful as a starting point for students and newly qualified therapists to develop their knowledge. There are, however, benefits and limitations with this choice, which will be discussed later. Now we provide key definitions and a table of the activities categorized in the OTPF (AOTA 2014).

Activities of Daily Living (ADL)

ADLs are basic or personal and are 'fundamental to living in a social world; they enable basic survival and well-being' (Christiansen and Hammecker 2001 cited in AOTA 2014, p. S19).

Instrumental Activities of Daily Living (IADL)

IADLs are 'activities to support daily life within the home and community that often require more complex interactions than in ADL' (AOTA 2014, p. S19). They are complex multistep activities requiring the integration of higher-level cognitive skills (McCreedy and Heisler 2004).

Table 18.1 helps identify various forms of self-care. The ADLs can be part of self-care, such as bathing/showering, and the IADLs include occupations for others, such as care of others/pets and child rearing. This highlights a challenge of using categories of occupation (Hammell 2009). When thinking about the occupation of self-care, consideration of context and environment is required; however, this cannot be incorporated into one table due to the vast array of characteristics and differences. Some aspects are discussed in the next few sections organized using a person, environment and occupation approach used by many occupational therapy models, such as the OTPF. We first consider influences on participation in the occupation of self-care.

TABLE 18.1	
Activities of Daily Living (ADL) and Instrumental Activities of Daily Living (IADL)	
Activities of Daily Living (ADL)	**Instrumental Activities of Daily Living (IADL)**
Bathing, showering	Care of others (including selecting and supervising caregivers)
Toileting and toilet hygiene	Care of pets
Dressing	Child rearing
Swallowing/eating	Communication management
Feeding	Driving and community mobility
Functional mobility	Financial management
Personal device care	Health management and maintenance
Personal hygiene and grooming	Home establishment and management
Sexual activity	Meal preparation and clean up
	Religious and spiritual activities and expression
	Safety and emergency maintenance
	Shopping

From AOTA 2014, p. S19–S20.

Factors that Influence Participation in Self-Care Activities

There are a variety of aspects that influence participation in any occupation, including self-care. Occupational participation and engagement in self-care involves doing tasks and activities that one may enjoy or has an obligation to do (Wilcock 1998, 2006). Various forms of self-care may be perceived in this way, depending on a variety of aspects and their interaction with a diagnosed mental illness that can impact participation (discussed later). A client-centered approach (Sumsion 1999) is required to understand the individual's perspective of self-care and his or her abilities, challenges and choices of self-care. These aspects must be balanced with the possibility of vulnerabilities such as self-neglect of I/ADLs that could harm peoples' health and well-being. Next, we discuss meaning in relation to participation and engagement in self-care.

Meaning and Value of Self-Care to the Service User

The interaction between the person and environment includes thinking about the meaning and value of occupation in relation to participation and engagement. Participation is the 'involvement in life situations through activity within a social context' (Creek 2010, p. 180). This definition emphasizes doing as performed and influenced by the norms and expectations of a given culture and social milieu (Creek 2010) impacting self-care, discussed later. Engagement is defined as 'a sense of involvement, choice, positive meaning and commitment while performing an occupation or activity' (Creek 2010, p. 166). These are linked to the person's experiences, thoughts and feelings when anticipating and performing occupations (Creek 2010; AOTA 2014; Lee and Kielhofner 2017). Therefore participation and engagement in occupations interact in a variety of ways.

The IADL of meal preparation and clean-up can show how participation and engagement interact. The OTPF definition is 'planning, preparing, and serving well-balanced, nutritious meals and cleaning up food and utensils after meals' (AOTA 2014, p. S20). These aspects can be experienced as pleasurable, creative, a symbol of caring for and sharing with others, as well as being fundamentally important for health and well-being. For some people, however, meal preparation and clean-up may be a mixture of pleasure and creativity in choosing, preparing and planning meals but can also be associated with the feeling that cleaning up is necessary but not pleasurable. Conversely, some people view meal preparation as a necessary but meaningless activity that they only perform to survive (Plastow et al. 2015).

Other influences on self-care that occupational therapists need to include are structural inequalities and intersections of disability, age, gender, ethnicity, class, culture, income, life chances and sexuality that combine to lead to oppression of people (Barker and Scheele 2016; Daley et al. 2019). Such intersections can restrict opportunities for occupational participation and engagement for effective self-care. We discuss some of these intersections below.

MENTAL ILLNESS AND IMPACT ON SELF-CARE

In general terms, mental illness impacts a person's capacity to participate and engage in occupations in various ways. It is important that the therapist checks the medical notes and records to know whether to assess for the impact of any combination of mental illness and physical illness, learning disability or difficulty and neuro diversity, along with other intersections.

It must not be assumed that all self-care challenges will be apparent for every diagnosis. Indeed, no relationship has been found between the diagnoses of schizophrenia and bipolar illnesses (mania or depression) and I/ADLs as measured by the Assessment of Motor and Process Skills (Moore et al. 2010). Some of the symptoms associated with various mental illnesses are similar and can impact I/ADLs. Table 18.2 shows the signs and symptoms related to the diagnoses of depression, anxiety, bipolar disorder, and schizophrenia from the International Classification of Diseases and Related Health Problems-11 (World Health Organization (WHO) 2019). The person is categorized with client factors in the OTPF (e.g., mental, sensory and neuromusculoskeletal body functions) (AOTA 2014) and their effects on self-care participation and engagement.

Difficulties with personal hygiene and grooming can be observed early in a person's acute admission to the hospital (see the description of 'A,' a person with psychosis described in Box 18.1). Also included in this example are challenges A has with clothing, which reflects the combination of I/ADL challenges that can be present.

Practice Example One shows how psychosis can impact a range of ADLs and IADLs at the same time. IADLs require a greater range of skills and abilities making participation in them multifaceted (AOTA 2014). Thus therapists need to understand the inter-relationship of different I/ADLs in self-care assessments and their limitations regardless of the model or framework that is used. There is a limitation with the IADL of financial management (AOTA 2014) in relation to A. The OTPF assumes that the person already has financial resources, which may not be the case (Aldrich et al. 2017). Thus it is

TABLE 18.2

Examples of I/ADLs, Diagnoses and Client Factors

I/ADLs (AOTA 2014)	Diagnosis Based on WHO (2018)	Signs & Symptoms (WHO 2018) and/ or Client Factors (AOTA 2014)	Examples and/or Supporting Literature
I/ADLs generally	Schizophrenia	Mental function of energy and drive (AOTA 2014).	A daily struggle and exhaustion (Urlic and Lentin 2010). Some I/ADL assistance is required at the acute stages of psychosis for some people (Hitch et al. 2013).
	Depression	Activity levels are reduced, with low energy/fatigue (anergia), changes in appetite (WHO 2018).	Not engaging in self-care to maintain nutritional and hydration needs. Self-neglect.
Personal hygiene and grooming – make-up, clothing	Hypomania (Bipolar type I & II disorders)	Euphoria, increased energy levels resulting in some social disinhibitions and acting out of character (WHO 2018).	Over-use of bright facial cosmetics, bright clothing.
Personal hygiene and grooming	Anxiety	Repetitive body-focused actions (WHO 2018). Autonomic signs of anxiety (WHO 2018).	Repeated hand washing causing chapped and painful hands. Biting nails and difficulties with nail care. Hair pulling leading to unkempt appearance and pain. Extreme grinding of the teeth causing jaw pain, affecting oral care (e.g., excessive teeth brushing, gum lesions) (Duncan and Prowse 2014). Excessive sweating leading to increased body odour (Duncan and Prowse 2014).
IADL - health management and maintenance - emotions	Schizophrenia, psychosis disorders	Specific mental function - emotional (AOTA 2014). Client factors and body functions - decreasing health risk behaviours for which energy and drive to control impulses and cravings (AOTA 2014).	Discomfort, anxiety and stress (Hitch et al. 2013). Self-monitoring and self-help activities linked to physical and mental health such as refraining from alcohol and drug use (Hitch et al. 2013).
IADL - health management and maintenance – weight gain	Schizophrenia, anxiety, major depressive, bi-polar and psychotic disorders	Client factors: body functions - Decreasing health risk behaviours for which energy and drive to control impulses and cravings (AOTA 2014).	Increased weight from anti-psychotic medications, sedentary lifestyles associated with depression and anxiety, diets low in fruit and fibre and high in saturated fats (Brown et al. 2018).
I/ADLs generally	Schizophrenia	Specific mental functions – higher level cognition and memory impaired (Green et al. 2000; AOTA 2014).	Cognitive difficulties with daily life task functioning (Rempfer et al. 2003). Awareness (insight) of problems (e.g., lack of knowledge or recognition of the deficits of the illness, leading to lack of initiation of activities and potentially limited success in rehabilitation) (Katz and Hartman-Maeir 2005). Executive function problems - initiating and performing tasks and solving new or conflicting problems in complex or unfamiliar situations (Green et al. 2000).

BOX 18.1

PRACTICE EXAMPLE ONE: OBSERVATIONS OF A SERVICE USER DURING ADMISSION TO AN ACUTE IN-PATIENT HOSPITAL

Service user 'A' has a possible untreated psychotic illness and requires a mental health act assessment at their home in the community. A is initially diagnosed with psychosis, pending further assessment and decision about their diagnosis and treatment during their admission.

INITIAL OBSERVATIONS AND ASSESSMENT

A has dirty, greasy and matted hair. A's fingernails are long and dirty and breath and body are malodorous. A's clothing is stained and does not fit well. A spends a lot of time in the bedroom, only leaving it to use the toilet and have meals in the ward dining area. A is quiet and responds minimally to questions from staff and service users. A does not provide many details to other staff about A's experience of psychosis.

ANALYSIS, PRACTICE/CLINICAL REASONING

The observations indicate that A is not engaging in ADLs (personal hygiene and grooming). Non-fitting clothing may indicate A is not engaging in other I/ADLs that may be affected by financial limitations such as shopping and cooking to maintain his nutrition and weight. The lack of participation and engagement may be associated with the diagnosed illness. This could include difficulty with higher-level cognitive function of insight and experience of self and time with lack of awareness of his body in relation to self-care (AOTA 2014). It is difficult to establish whether A believes they find his ADLs were found challenging as he does not communicate specific details. The therapist must explore A's lifestyle

choices unrelated to the diagnosed illness. A does not have a therapeutic relationship with any member of staff that may assist with discussing personal aspects of self-care.

ONGOING ASSESSMENT AND INFORMATION GATHERING FROM TEAM MEMBERS

Nurses assess the condition of covered areas of A's body (toenails, genitals, teeth, etc.), and they start to encourage A to engage in personal hygiene and grooming, providing supplies as required. The therapist and nurses discuss what ADLs A can do and how to do them, and he can discuss this with them if required.

Information to gather about A's home situation and IADLs.

INTERVENTIONS

The occupational therapist introduces himself or herself and his or her role to A and attempts to build a therapeutic rapport with A. The therapist has a brief discussion about the occupations A likes to do in the community. The occupational therapist establishes links between A's interests and the occupational therapy group programme and encourages A to engage with a group or groups if feeling ready. The occupational therapist also supports nurses as necessary to help A develop self-awareness of current personal hygiene and grooming and see how occupational therapy can help with motivating A and grading and adapting ADLs.

---

necessary to explore how a service user accesses finances to help clarify their context and whether other I/ADLs are affected. Combined ADLs and IADLs provide greater challenges for the person and need to incorporate environmental aspects, discussed next.

SELF-CARE AND THE ENVIRONMENT

Environment in the OTPF is formed of physical (natural and built) and social (people, groups and relationships) aspects (AOTA 2014). Context is related to environment but is less tangible and includes cultural (discussed later) and virtual contexts (AOTA 2014). All influence what occupations people do and why they do them and what may be restricting them (AOTA 2014). Therefore environments may offer or limit resources and opportunities for participating and engaging in occupations (Whiteford 2018).

The service user and therapist should discuss how far the person has control over environments and contexts. It can be that lack of resources such as personal, social, cultural, emotional, material, physical, spiritual and/ or assistive technology (Pereira 2017, p. 433) impacts their ability to perform I/ADLs. Therapists also need to consider opportunities such as the required circumstances or where therapists create and/or advocate for the service user (Pereira 2017) to find ways to perform I/ADLs. Thus therapists need to be attuned to where circumstances beyond the control of the individual impacts their mental illness and self-care. The home environment in Practice Example Two demonstrates some of these aspects.

It would be useful at this point to consider the IADL of shopping in more depth. The OTPF defines this as 'preparing shopping lists (grocery and other); selecting, purchasing, and transporting items; selecting method of payment;

BOX 18.2
PRACTICE EXAMPLE TWO: HOME ASSESSMENT OF A COUPLE (B AND C) LIVING TOGETHER

B and C each have a diagnosis of schizophrenia and substance misuse. They receive a home assessment and support from a community occupational therapist.

OBSERVATIONS AND DISCUSSION

B and C's accommodation was dirty, and waste food in the bin had maggots and flies in it. There was no fridge, and dirty dishes were over many of the kitchen surfaces. The couple has limited finances, and they cannot afford to buy meat and vegetables at the same time. They each shop for reduced priced foods on or past the best use-by date. They each, in turn, prepare the ingredients and add them to a saucepan of stock with meat and vegetables as they purchase them. They keep the pan on permanent low heat, 24 hours a day, 7 days a week. They eat this food for both lunch and the evening meal.

ANALYSIS, PRACTICE/CLINICAL REASONING

B and C are maintaining various IADLs to various degrees. IADL - meal preparation and clean-up are maintained in a way particular to the couple. IADL - financial management is on budget but utility costs may increase to keep the hob on permanently and low income impacts the quality of food they

can purchase in IADL - shopping. IADL - driving and community mobility appears intact. IADL - health management and maintenance may be challenging with possible nutritional deficiencies and/or physical health problems/at a potential risk to illnesses if the heat was not high enough and flies may get into the cooler sides of the saucepan that have dried food, thus bacteria may not be killed in the pot of food. IADL - home establishment and management may be compromised by potential fires with the hob being used permanently. They have no fridge to store fresh and cooked food, which may indicate why they keep adding ingredients to the pot and keep it warm.

INTERVENTIONS

The therapist is to discuss with B and C what is preventing the clean-up of surfaces, dishes and the bin and considers ways for B and C to complete these.

The therapist is to ask questions about B's and C's physical health and infections.

Consider other ways to balance provisioning healthy foods with cost-effectiveness using Beagan et al.'s (2018) findings linked to the OTPF IADLs in Table 18.3 in poverty and low-income section.

---

and completing money transactions; included are Internet shopping and related use of electronic devices such as computers, cell phones, and tablets' (AOTA 2014, p. S20).

Other aspects of shopping need to be explored with service users to ascertain what is relevant or not to their environments, cultures and context. The OTPF assumes that the person obtains food by shopping as the only method by which provisions can be sourced. Also suggested in shopping in the OTPF is that it is done in a mostly urban environment. It may be that people do not have opportunities to get to shops, have limited financial resources or live in more rural places with no, or limited, resources of shops and so will require alternatives to shopping.

Urban and rural environments may have resources such as access to a garden or land where individuals can grow some of their own produce rather than purchase them. If land is available, their main source of food can be growing their own. There may be bartering for provisions with others in the community. The gardening examples of course require the resources of land, tools/equipment and materials. These may, however, be borrowed, bartered for or purchased depending on the circumstances. The OTPF requires some critique and interpretation if used with people with limited finances, different cultures and geographical areas. We now consider some of those influences.

Culture

This section briefly introduces a diverse range of cultural differences in occupational participation and engagement of self-care. First, we consider the knowledge of the profession and culture.

Taking a critical perspective is helpful to question various aspects such as hidden assumptions, the purposes of competing theories, existing forms of practice and where they respond to situations of oppression and injustice, which can help create new possibilities for our service users (Ramugondo 2015; Farias and Laliberte Rudman 2016). The categorization of occupations, for instance, self-care, does not include survival occupations (Hammell 2009), which are contextually relevant and discussed later with poverty. Cultural values and beliefs, therefore, influence occupational patterns, choice of activity and perceptions of the value of occupations, all of which influence engagement (Chiang and Carlson 2003; Bonder et al. 2004).

Western concepts and ideas about occupation and their relationship with health reflect the individualistic religious, social and economic influences over their history and so are culturally laden (Kantartzis and Molineux 2011; Lee 2019). Indeed, the example about shopping from the OTPF created by American occupational therapists does not fit all cultures (Guajardo et al. 2015). Thus it is important to understand different cultures in relation to theories about occupation and occupational therapy.

Occupation and eastern cultures have been reviewed. Lee (2019) clarified how there needs to be more nuanced understanding of Asian cultures and occupation and highlighted that Asia includes regions (East Asia, South Asia, Southeast Asia and the Middle East) incorporating many different countries. Lee (2019) therefore questions how one country can be taken as representative of the diversity of Asia when broad descriptions of the binary categories of collectivist Asian countries and individualist western countries are used. His argument is that therapists need to understand how, why and in what ways and circumstances people engage in occupations that are part of Asian cultures (Lee 2019).

Participating and engaging in making tea has many approaches across the world. Making a hot drink, however, does not have a specific I/ADL in the OTPF, so the closest fit currently is to incorporate it into meal preparation and clean-up (AOTA 2014). This is not the most explicit categorization and therefore a limitation of the OTPF for an activity in self-care that is fundamental to maintaining hydration, whether that be through accessing water or other fluids.

Fair and Barnitt (1999) explored a range of different ways in which a cup of tea was made by 15 students and colleagues from South Asia, Africa, Europe and Australia. The ways of making tea, the meaning of doing this and the purpose for doing it varied between and as part of cultures and across generations. Also, gender influences are demonstrated in research on women's engagement in a traditional Japanese ceremony of making and drinking tea (Sakuae and Reid 2012). The interrelated principles of tea making associated with historical, social, aesthetic, environmental and traditional aspects, with personal experiences, learning and development are seen to impact the health and well-being of all involved (Sakuae and Reid 2012). Occupational therapists therefore need to be open to reviewing their existing and traditional practices of using hot drinks for assessment when working with service users from different cultures (Fair and Barnitt 1999).

Another western concept in occupational therapy is that of helping people to become independent in occupational participation. Research about service users' experience of self-care found some participants felt the focus on independence, and self-care was not culturally relevant (Notley et al. 2012). A study of 19 Hindu elders asking about four aspects of their self-care (i.e., dress, diet, bathing, and toileting) found issues relevant to occupational therapists (Gibbs and Barnitt 1999). Family members being expected to care for elders was valued, and the concept of independence, in that context, was not understood. Participants had an extended social group with the elder as part of it, indicating sensitivity must be shown to the familial group in assessment and treatment planning (Gibbs and Barnitt 1999). Therapists therefore need to consider a client-centred principle of respecting service users' strengths, experiences and knowledge (Law et al. 1995).

The examples above give an idea of some cultural aspects that need to be considered in relation to self-care. Therapists also need to be aware of their own cultural beliefs and actions and how those impact upon their understanding and sensitivity to others from a different background (Chiang and Carlson 2003). Even within a single society people have different backgrounds and therefore attach different meanings to the occupations they value (Darnell 2009; Lee 2019). Culture also has an emergent nature, so the therapist must recognize the cultural issues that are established and generate preliminary understandings that may need to be further explored with each client (Bonder et al. 2004). Another example of the potential impact of the environment related to poverty follows.

Poverty and Low Income

Social conditions of poverty and low income may affect people with mental illness who have no means of generating income or have a low-level financial support from government benefits. Existing literature about occupation and poverty is new and does not yet fully explore the relationship with mental illness, however, it is a relevant topic to present here. Sofo and Wicks (2017) provided an occupational perspective on the relationship between people living in poverty and the physical, social, cultural and political environments. They suggest that people in poverty need to spend a lot of time engaging in survival occupations, causing restrictions in other forms of occupational engagement (Sofo and Wicks 2017).

A survival occupation can be, for example, securing food. Research with a culturally mixed population of 31 low-income families without mental illness showed the effects on emotions and energy levels of providing food (Beagan et al. 2018). The IADL of health management and maintenance is relevant here because it includes awareness of nutrition, planning well-balanced nutritious meals in meal preparation and clean-up, shopping, driving and community mobility using public transport and financial management for cost effectiveness (AOTA 2014).

Shopping on a limited budget, with repeated denials to children of the things they want, can be exhausting, disenfranchising, stressful, unpleasant, and relentless (Power 2005 cited in Beagan et al. 2018, p. 108). The perceptions about the parents included others believing them to be lazy, uneducated and irresponsible in their role, plus showing intense judgement from the perception parents were not able to do familiar, mundane, and commonplace IADLs (Beagan et al. 2018). Consequently, they were stigmatized and marginalized (Beagan et al. 2018) and if this is combined with a mental illness it may exacerbate it. For a person diagnosed with a mental illness, who is also a parent with ongoing, long-term, food provisioning responsibilities, this may be challenging. Beagan et al.'s (2018) and Sofo and Wick's (2017) works can help to raise therapists' awareness and inform their questions and discussion with service users. There are suggestions in Beagan et al.'s work that can be applied to the IADLs in

the OTPF (see Table 18.3) to use for interventions, such as Practice Example Two.

So far, we have discussed some intersecting topics. We now turn to sexuality and self-care.

Sexuality

There is a gradually developing literature on sexuality and occupational therapy, but it is not often considered in practice. We introduce the topics here for two reasons. First, there is a client-centred principle of respecting service users' diversity (Sumsion and Law 2006; Hammell 2013). Second, the OTPF includes an ADL of sexual activity defined as 'engaging in activities that result in sexual satisfaction and/or meet relational or reproductive needs' (AOTA 2014, p. S19). There is also a related ADL of personal device care that incorporates caring for contraceptive and sexual devices (AOTA 2014). The OTPF therefore acknowledges the ADL of sexual activity as fundamental to survival, well-being and living in a social world (AOTA 2014). Therapists therefore need to be prepared to discuss sexuality in relation to occupational participation and engagement and their multifaceted nature.

The heterosexual and lesbian, gay, bisexual, transgender plus (LGBT+) identities may need discussion depending on the service user's needs. Sexuality is multifaceted, and for LGBT+ people, there are specific impacts to engagement in occupations related to familial, social, economic, political and spiritual perspectives. Due to the limited space to discuss this here, Barker and Scheele (2016) and other references are used to discuss a variety of aspects of LGBT+ experiences.

TABLE 18.3	
IADLs and Strategies Used by Low-Income Families	
IADLs (AOTA 2014)	**Strategies Used by Low-Income Families (Beagan et al. 2018)**
Financial management	Routinely using sales flyers, clipping coupons and comparing prices. Seeking sales, maximizing meals per dollar.
Driving and community mobility	Reducing transportation costs/time.
Health management and maintenance	Using less nutritional food.
Home establishment and management	Growing foods, minimizing waste.
Shopping	Creating shopping lists as a memory aid.
Meal preparation and clean-up	Using cheap convenience foods to go further, pouring non-branded products into brand name containers.

From Beagan et al. (2018).

Firstly, an introduction to terms and definitions is required. Sexuality, amongst other aspects, incorporates gender identities and roles, eroticism, pleasure, sexual orientation, intimacy, sex and reproduction (WHO 2006). WHO (2006) highlights that no international definition exists and current thinking has a contextual approach incorporating cultures, contexts, thinking and time periods to the understanding of and the practices of sexuality, gender and identity (Bergan-Gander and von Kurthy 2006; Sakellariou and Pollard 2009; Barker and Scheele 2016). The definitions used by the OTPF are less detailed than the WHO's, and the OTPF reduces sexuality to the physical act of sexual intercourse without relating it to the many other occupations through which sexuality can be expressed (McGrath and Sakellariou 2016). There is, however, an indication of the relationships involved in the ADL sexual activity in the OTPF, but that needs to be more nuanced and considered in relation to other parts of the OTPF such as leisure, work, education and social participation (AOTA 2014). Thus the range of facets of sexuality identified by WHO's and OTPF's definitions need to be combined.

There is a key need to discuss sexuality in both the literature and practice due to the impact of the majority of the world being heterosexual and LGBT+ people being minority groups. The discourse of that majority is therefore mostly heteronormative in which cultural assumptions that 'normal' or 'natural' forms of attraction and relationships are between one woman and one man that embodies conventional gender roles, norms and sex (Barker and Scheele 2016). If therapists only acknowledge a heteronormative discourse, this can limit the discussion, questioning and support of service users' mental health, sexuality and related occupations.

Therapists must be aware that the LGBT+ service user may find it difficult to discuss their sexuality. Therapists need to be sensitive and cannot assume that a LGBT+ service user has done this with anyone, including their closest family and friends. Essentially, when LGBT+ people meet any new person, they need to establish the context, sense of safety they feel, and the reasons for discussing sexuality, or not (Devine and Nolan 2007; Rose and Hughes 2018). It cannot be assumed that because a service user has discussed sexuality with others that they will always want to do so.

The choices, decisions and process of discussing sexuality can be a form of self-care and could be a part of the IADL of safety and emergency maintenance (AOTA

2014). The OTPF describes this as 'knowing and performing preventive procedures to maintain a safe environment' (AOTA 2014, S19). Indeed, safety awareness of monitoring others' actions and self-monitoring are a part of the social environment in relation to finding physical and architectural environments and people that accept LGBT+ people and are free from potential harm (Formby 2017), where they can engage in occupations. Furthermore, maintaining safety awareness by sourcing safe environments are especially important for LGBT+ people who may have experienced various physical, sexual, verbal or emotional trauma from others. All of these may form part of their experience of mental illness.

There are clearly implications for practice in which therapists need to be sensitive to LGBT+ service users. Some suggestions from research done in the physical setting are relevant to mental health. A therapist needs to be prepared to initiate discussion as it should not be the service user's responsibility to do so (Rose and Hughes 2018). They need to use nonjudgemental language and to clarify that it is okay to discuss feelings about sexuality (Rose and Hughes 2018).

In summary, occupational therapists' understanding about the structural inequalities and intersections noted above in relation to self-care helps the service user and decreases risks to their health and well-being. The occupational therapist and service user then decide the next steps in the occupational therapy process and self-care, discussed next.

Occupational Therapy Process and Self-Care

The following section looks at how occupational therapists assess and identify self-care abilities and challenges and establish interventions. The reader is directed to a useful resource of a case study employing research to inform practice that incorporates some aspects of self-care (Lannigan and Noyes 2019). First, we consider assessment of self-care.

Assessing Self-Care

There are various assessments (see Chapter 5) of I/ADLs. Some describe self-care through observations (such as the two examples above) and discussion or interviews. Others predict or evaluate change with standardized tools. Assessments are linked to a specific model of practice, or they are stand-alone, but in any event there should be a theoretical relationship to the assessments used. Assessment of self-care should be holistic, considering the person, environment and occupation.

Different forms of information gathering are required to gain an understanding of the person's history. Decisions can then be made about what form of discussion, interview and assessment is required. It is also important to know the purpose of using these various forms.

Therapists need to do activity analyses on various forms of self-care to establish the demands of participation for a healthy person to understand how they are done. Therapists then compare those analyses with various aspects: the service user's participation, their experience of mental illness and impact on body functions along with interactions with environments and individual preferences and abilities and challenges with self-care. It is possible to assess the simpler ADLs using this comparison. It becomes more intricate when there are combined I/ADL challenges, so activity analysis needs to be used in combination with other assessments.

Sensitivity and Assessing ADLs

The discussion, and particularly observational assessment of personal activities such as bathing, showering, bladder and bowel management and personal hygiene and grooming require empathy and observation. Initial observations of the person's mood are crucial as they may be anxious about being assessed. All attempts to prevent or minimize the service users' embarrassment should be made. Discussion would be better than a full observational assessment if service users' self-awareness is intact, but they may be unable to fully verbalize their abilities. Ultimately observation may be the only way to assess fully the specific difficulties.

Non-Standardized Assessment Observation Tools for I/ADLs

Assessment can take the form of a checklist of aspects of the activity that would be expected to be observed to perform it effectively. For example, the checklist might focus on making a cup of tea (see Table 18.4). Here a service user would be observed and a tick placed at the appropriate score and descriptor box, making additional comments as required.

The format in Table 18.4 may also be constructed for making a sandwich, the more multifaceted occupation of shopping for groceries, or the Practice Example Three below of a combined assessment and intervention with pre-prepared ingredients.

TABLE 18.4					
Making a Cup of Tea					
Making a Cup of Tea	1. Independent	2. Able with Verbal Prompts	3. Able with Physical and Verbal Assistance	4. Unable to Complete	Comments
Aware of use of equipment					
Organizes task in sequence					
Aware of safety factors					
Fills kettle appropriately					
Turns on gas/electricity switches					
Puts tea in pot/cup appropriately					
Pours boiled water in appropriately					
Uses sugar/milk appropriately					

Adapted from Finlay 2004.

BOX 18.3

PRACTICE EXAMPLE THREE: BASIC COOKERY. THIS EXAMPLE DEVELOPS FROM PRACTICE EXAMPLE ONE

OBSERVATION AND DISCUSSION/ INTERVIEWS

The occupational therapist has a concern that A was not eating healthily and may not know how to cook, which may relate to why they eat take away food.

A has a limited understanding of healthy eating and the impact of an inadequate diet on long-term physical health. A reports spending a lot of finances on take away meals and often being short of money. A agrees to participate in this individual cooking assessment.

INTERVENTION/ASSESSMENT

Start to plan the first session, considering a more basic healthy meal (e.g., eggs or beans on whole wheat toast) or something that will be successful and easily achievable with healthy pre-prepared ingredients. A says he can cook. A tells the therapist how he usually does the cooking task, but communication is minimal, and the therapist prompts as required:

1) What equipment is needed? (frying pan, baking sheet, saucepan)
2) What ingredients are required? (cook fish fillets in breadcrumbs, frozen oven chips and tinned baked beans)
3) What methods of ingredient preparation are required (minimal preparation, gathering ingredients, equipment, using hob and oven)?
4) What order do the ingredients need to be cooked in and for how long? (A is unclear about this.)

A's descriptions are minimal, but an activity analysis tells the therapist the answers to those questions and can judge the time required and can be prepared to help.

Encourage A to cook the ingredients as would ordinarily done; they can continue doing the cookery with minimal discussion.

ANALYSIS, PRACTICE/CLINICAL REASONING

The meal is not a fully healthy choice, suggesting A may not know how to make those choices. A's sequence indicates being unaware how to cook effectively, for example, the longest cooking time ingredient, oven chips, were put in the oven after the fish and beans in the saucepan had almost completed cooking. A put the food on a plate and waited for the chips to cook. By that time the other ingredients were cold. A returned the chips to the wire basket in the freezer but repeatedly pushed back as it would not slide into its place and could not close the freezer door. The therapist intervened to show A another bag of food had dropped through the basket, impeding correct positioning. Feedback from A indicated he did not believe there was a problem with any of the assessment. This indicated A did not identify the limitations and did not consider doing something different to try to correct the situation. A had the fullest opportunity to complete as much of the assessment as possible before the therapist intervened.

Practice Example Three shows assessment and intervention using observation and comparison with activity analysis. There are standardized assessments, considered next.

Assessing IADLs

There are a variety of assessments requiring observation, self-report or a combination that may or may not relate to a model.

There are assessments that can be used without training and are linked to models of occupation. The model of human occupation (MOHO; Taylor 2017) has the self-report Occupational Self Assessment (OSA) that is about the competence and values the person associates with various occupations and environmental impact (Kramer et al. 2017). OSA incorporates some self-care

including money management and taking care of oneself, others and one's home (Baron et al. 2002). The Canadian Occupational Performance Measure (COPM) (Law et al. 2005) is a semi-structured interview in which the service user identifies five of their most important occupational performance issues and their perceptions of change and satisfaction with performance. It incorporates self-care of personal care, functional mobility and community management. The COPM is theoretically linked to the Canadian model of occupational performance and engagement (Polatajko et al. 2007).

An observational assessment of I/ADLs is linked to MOHO and OTPF. The Assessment of Motor and Process Skills (AMPS; Fisher 2004) requires therapist training. AMPS incorporates a large variety of I/ADLs such as brushing teeth, ironing and vacuuming two rooms on different levels and some culturally relevant cooking including noodles cooked in a pot and fried green plantains (Fisher 2004).

There are also standalone, observational assessments. The Test of Grocery Shopping Skills (Hamera and Brown 2000; Rempfer et al. 2003) developed in America is used with people diagnosed with schizophrenia and schizoaffective disorder. This is not related to a model of practice.

Following the occupational therapy process of observation, assessment, interview and discussion, self-care intervention plans need to be established.

Interventions for Developing Self-Care

The intervention plan should be based upon the holistic and client-centred assessment of the specific and individual strengths and constraints of the service user and contextual limitations in resources and opportunities. Allied to this is the application of relevant research and practice knowledge from experience (Higgs et al. 2004; Cook and Wagenaar 2012) to inform the intervention plan. This means that the interventions and approaches will vary for each service user. There is, therefore, a range of methods that can be used for self-care interventions including basic requirements for self-care interventions, teaching and learning techniques and occupational therapy interventions.

Basic Requirements for Self-Care Interventions

The following aspects of planning and developing self-care interventions are fundamental preparations that aim to provide the optimal approach for each service user. It is at this stage that the assessment and other information gathered about the service user informs the therapist about how best to organize the environment, build on existing skills and abilities and provide the approach/es to promote learning skills.

Environment (Social and Place)

Social

At all stages of the therapeutic process the therapist must be aware of therapeutic approaches to self-care.

This includes the therapeutic use of self, client-centred practice and the use of core occupational therapy skills. Emotional and psychological support such as showing a genuine interest, a caring attitude, confidence and boundaries is required (Berkeland and Flinn 2005). This helps to build on the therapeutic relationship and develop the service user's trust in the therapist.

Places (Architectural, Natural)

The reader is referred to the initial observations about the environment that are also relevant in preparing and choosing an appropriate area to work with the service user. The interventions may start in a hospital or rehabilitation unit and develop into trips into the community working towards the service user's accommodation in the community. However, the service user's level of ability and self-care needs will dictate the location of intervention.

Teaching About Self-Care

Providing self-care interventions may require that some skills are taught to service users. There may be various reasons for this, which may include the service user never having developed the skills, they may have forgotten some aspects, mental illness may be impacting upon participating and learning self-care, or new or more effective ways of doing one's self-care are available. Learning to adapt to doing occupations in a different way or in a different social or physical (geographical, architectural) environment could also be required. In mental health service provision, occupational therapy uses teaching techniques and so practice is a blend of these therapeutic, teaching and learning approaches.

Occupational Therapy Core Skills and Self-Care

This section considers self-care interventions in occupational therapy in mental health settings.

A decision must be made about the overall approach to be followed, for example, a remedial or compensatory approach. Client factors in the OTPF such as the impact of attention limitations on self-care could indicate a remedial method that would try to improve attention through self-care (AOTA 2014). Compensatory approaches use occupational therapy core skills to adapt the activity or environment to enable effective self-care (AOTA 2014). For example, if a service user struggles with organizing his or her kitchen because it is difficult to find items in cupboards in the kitchen, the cupboards could be organized in a logical manner with hot drink–making dry ingredients in one place and tins of food (organized into vegetables, pulses, etc.) and pots and pans in other cupboards.

It needs to be determined how much self-care the service user would be able to effectively complete and what other types of occupational therapy core skills would be required to enable self-care development and performance, such as changes to the sequencing of tasks, grading the complexity of the activity and individual and group-based interventions. The example from Practice Example Four provides occupational therapy core skills for individual cookery with A.

BOX 18.4
PRACTICE EXAMPLE FOUR: FUTURE INDIVIDUAL COOKERY INTERVENTIONS

Establish A will agree to further cooking.

Grade cooking of a range of pre-prepared ingredients for basic meals to nutritional meals with fresh foods and healthy option, pre-prepared ingredients.

Adaptation of each meal with recipes with simpler instructions.

Provide education on healthy eating and the long-term impact of eating an inadequate diet.

Organize a food shopping trip with Mr B to help him plan the ingredients required and budget for them appropriately.

Research on the Effectiveness of Self-Care Interventions

It is a requirement for occupational therapists to incorporate critically evaluated research into their practice (College of Occupational Therapists 2015). Thus it would be helpful to readers to provide an overview of some of the existing research on self-care interventions.

First, we look at some disciplinary research about service users and their views about therapeutic approaches to self-care, which are from a western, United Kingdom, perspective. The practical focus to I/ADL development was valued by research participants (Di Bona 2004; Lim et al. 2007; Notley et al. 2012). Some studies used forms of group work (Brown et al. 2001) and individual approaches (Mairs and Bradshaw 2004) for interventions. Skills-based groups, particularly cookery, were positively experienced by participants (Di Bona 2004; Lim et al. 2007). Also, the opportunity to re-learn old skills (Di Bona 2004; Notley et al. 2012) and learn and practise new skills helped service users' participation in daily life, improving their confidence (Lim et al. 2007). Being offered choices, which were relevant to the participants' needs, were also valued (Notley 2012). Finally, service users in an acute setting valued the encouragement, support and choice offered by occupational therapists in a range of occupations (Bryant et al. 2016).

A systematic review of occupational therapy research supports I/ADL interventions. D'Amico et al. (2018) included a range of diagnoses of various mental illnesses, including the ones discussed in this chapter. In summary, they found the strongest support for I/ADL occupation interventions (along with cognitive-based therapy and psychoeducation) in community and residential settings when incorporating individualized client-centred goals (D'Amico et al. 2018). This is a useful summary, but therapists are guided to look at the research D'Amico et al. (2018) reviewed for the relevance to the service user's choices, identified I/ADL needs, goals and context of their practice.

SERVICE USER COMMENTARY

My perspective on self-care is that of someone whose main diagnosis is an eating disorder. My initial thought on the chapter was that it felt focused on a particular group of people who may experience mental illness and struggle with ADL tasks. Many people with mental illness may also be quite functional but require support with self-care for their recovery or to manage living with their mental health condition.

My personal view is that there is a disconnect within healthcare services and social care. My reflection on the chapter is how it may be necessary for occupational therapists to be able to signpost to other services to support people they are seeing. For example, if someone is in poverty, they may need support from an advice centre to access benefits/additional support or a referral for Adult Social Care to ensure their housing is suitable. They might also need personal assistant support from Adult Social Care to support them with their self-care.

My other reflection is how much medication may impact an individual's ability to self-care and how this may fluctuate in their treatment or support. Starting a new medication or withdrawing from a medication could completely impact someone's ability to engage in self-care activities, so the timing of activity or support is important.

I'm autistic and don't like to use showers for sensory reasons. On my first admission to the hospital, no-one told me there was a bath that I could use, so I didn't wash. When occupational therapists are seeing patients with additional needs, they may need to seek advice from specialist services about how to support someone with self-care. I find routine and structure really helpful, so when placed in an environment with no structure, I may completely withdraw or exhibit signs of distress. I may feel unable to self-care for this reason. When in the hospital it is helpful for an occupational therapist to support me with creating a visual timetable. Sensory difficulties may also make taking part in group activities difficult, particularly in a hospital setting. Understanding a patient's sensory needs may be helpful in finding out what barriers there might be to them engaging in support. For example, if there is loud music being played in a room, a patient may find it difficult to engage.

When it comes to my eating disorder professionals not familiar with eating disorders can completely miss the over exercise element of the disorder. In terms of self-care there may be some need around supporting someone to explore more sedentary tasks but that are still within their interests. Suggesting I take a walk when I am feeling depressed is ignoring that rest is a key part of recovery from my illness. I have found photography helpful for slowing myself down when outdoors or taking the focus away from the compulsions.

Self-care wise, it's important to understand the needs of the person you are working with. When transitioning from hospital to home, cooking from scratch has had the potential to take disordered short cuts in my eating disorder recovery. Helping someone to accept or understand that allowing someone else to cook for them or using ready meal options might be a necessary initial step in recovery.

Ruth Revell

SUMMARY

We have presented different ways of conceptualizing self-care and explanations about their relationship to categorizing occupations and challenges of doing this. The associations between I/ADLs (AOTA 2014) and self-care and the engagement and participation of service users in mental health settings have been discussed. Occupational therapy research about the impact of some diagnoses of mental illnesses on self-care and interventions have been provided. Examples from practice to illustrate how occupational therapists can work with self-care needs were also provided. The occupational therapy process has been highlighted with information on the observation and assessment of self-care and ways to work with service users that are relevant, client-centred, and sensitive to service users' diversity.

QUESTIONS FOR CONSIDERATION

1. Identify three self-care activities. Compare the meaning or value of these activities to you and to a service user you know well.

2. Consider the observations of 'A' in Practice Example One. Which ADLs might an occupational therapist initially try to build back into A's routine? What could be potential benefits or concerns to weigh up?

3. For someone who may not value self-care, how might you change their perspective or adapt a proposed ADL (such as making tea/eating) to suit their needs and ideas?

4. Consider difficulties affecting IADLs in low income families in rural areas versus urban areas. Do these need to be addressed in different ways?

5. Design your own observation checklist for an ADL or IADL (e.g., making sandwiches or grocery shopping) using Table 18.4 as an example.

6. Find two or three resources for self-care interventions or list two or three citations from this chapter to explore further.

REFERENCES

Action for Happiness. (2020). *New things November*. Available at: https://www.actionforhappiness.org/calendars.

Aldrich, R. M., Laliberte Rudman, D., & Dickie, V. A. (2017). Resource seeking as occupation: A critical and empirical exploration. *American Journal of Occupational Therapy, 71*(3), 7103260010p1–7103260010p9. https://doi.org/10.5014/ajot.2017.021782.

American Occupational Therapy Association (AOTA). (2014). Occupational therapy practice framework: Domain and process, third ed. *American Journal of Occupational Therapy, 68*(Suppl. 1), S1–S48. https://doi.org/10.5014/ajot.2014.682006.

Barker M-J., & Scheele J. (2016). *Queer: A Graphic History*. London: Icon Books Ltd.

Baron, K., Kielhofner, G., Iyenger, A., Goldhammer, V., & Wolenski, J. (2002). *The occupational self assessment (version 2.0)*. Illinois: University of Chicago.

Brenda L. Beagan, Gwen E. Chapman & Elaine Power. (2018). The visible and invisible occupations of food provisioning in low income families, *Journal of Occupational Science, 25*(1), 100–111, DOI: 10.1080/14427591.2017.1338192.

Bergan-Gander and von Kurthy 2006

Berkeland, R., & Flinn, N. (2005). Therapy as learning. In C. H. Christiansen, M. C. Baum, & J. Bass-Haugen (Eds.), *Occupational therapy: Performance, participation, and well-being* (3rd ed.) (pp. 421–442). Thorofare, NJ: Slack.

Bonder, B. R., Martin, L., & Miracle, A. W. (2004). Culture emergent in occupation. *American Journal of Occupational Therapy, 58*, 159–168.

Brown, F., Shiels, M., & Hall, C. (2001). A pilot community living skills group: An evaluation. *British Journal of Occupational Therapy, 64*(3), 144–150.

Brown, C., Geiszler, L. C., Lewis, K. J., & Arbesman, M. (2018). Effectiveness of interventions for weight loss for people with serious mental illness: A systematic review and meta-analysis.

American Journal of Occupational Therapy, 72, 7205190030p1–7205190030p1. https://doi.org/10.5014/ajot.2018.033415.

Bryant, W., Cordingley, K., Sims K., et al. (2016). Collaborative research exploring mental health service user perspectives on acute inpatient occupational therapy. *British Journal of Occupational Therapy*. https://doi.org/10.1177/0308022616650899.

Chiang, M., & Carlson, G. (2003). Occupational therapy in multicultural contexts: Issues and strategies. *British Journal of Occupational Therapy, 66*(12), 559–567.

Christiansen, C. H., & Hammecker, C. L. (2001). Self care. In Bonder, B.R., & Wagner, M.B. (Eds.), *Functional performance in older adults*. pp. 155–175. Philadelphia: F. A. Davis.

College of Occupational Therapists. (2015). Code of Ethics and Professional Conduct. London: College of Occupational Therapists.

Cook, S. D. N., & Wagenaar, H. (2012). *Navigating the Eternally Unfolding Present: Toward an Epistemology of Practice. The American Review of Public Administration, 42*(1), 3–38. https://doi.org/10.1177/0275074011407404

Creek, J. (2010). *The core concepts of occupational therapy*. London: Jessica Kingsley Publishers.

D'Amico, M. L., Jaffe, L. E., & Gardner, J. A. (2018). Evidence for interventions to improve and maintain occupational performance and participation for people with serious mental illness: A systematic review. *American Journal of Occupational Therapy, 72*(05), 1–11. https://doi.org/10.5014/ajot.2018.033332.

Daley, A., Costa, L., & Beresford, P. (2019). Introduction. In A. Daley, L. Costa, & P. Beresford (Eds.), *Madness, violence and power a critical collection* (pp. 20–35). Toronto: University of Toronto Press.

Darnell, R. (2009). Cross-cultural constructions of work, leisure and community responsibility: Some first nations reflections. *Journal of Occupational Science, 16*(1), 4–9.

Devine, R., & Nolan, C. (2007). Sexual Identity & Human Occupation: A Qualitative Exploration. *Journal of Occupational Science, 14*(3): 154–161.

Di Bona, L. (2004). What do they think of us? A satisfaction survey of users of occupational therapy services in an acute adult inpatient mental health unit. *Mental Health Occupational Therapy*, 9(3), 77–81.

Duncan, M., & Prowse, C. (2014). *Occupational Therapy for Anxiety, Somatic and Stressor-related Disorders*. In Crouch, R., & Alers, V. (Eds.). Occupational Therapy in Psychiatry and Mental Health (5th ed., pp.368–388. Chichester: Wiley.

Fair, A., & Barnitt, R. (1999). Making a cup of tea as part of a culturally sensitive service. *British Journal of Occupational Therapy*, 62(5), 199–205.

Farias, L., & Laliberte Rudman, D. (2016). A critical interpretive synthesis of the uptake of critical perspectives in occupational science. *Journal of Occupational Science*, 23(1), 33–50. https://doi.org/10.1080/14427591.2014.989893.

Finlay, L. (2004). *The practice of psychosocial occupational therapy* (3rd ed.). Cheltenham: Nelson Thomas Ltd.

Fisher, A. G. (2004). AMPS assessment of motor and process skills. *User Manual* (5th ed.) (Vol. 2). Fort Collins Colorado: Three Star Press Inc.

Formby, E. (2017). *Exploring LGBT spaces and communities*. Oxon: Routledge.

Gibbs, K. E., & Barnitt, R. (1999). Occupational therapy and the self-care needs of Hindu elders. *British Journal of Occupational Therapy*, 62(3), 100–106.

Green, M. F., Kern, R. S., Braff, D. L., et al. (2000). Neurocognitive deficits & functional outcome in schizophrenia: Are we measuring the "right stuff"? *Schizophrenia Bulletin*, 26(1), 119–136.

Guajardo, A., Kronenberg, F., & Ramugondo, E. L. (2015). Southern occupational therapies: Emerging identities, epistemologies and practices. *South African Journal of Occupational Therapy*, 45(1), 3–10.

Hamera, C., & Brown, C. E. (2000). Developing a context-based performance measure for persons with schizophrenia: The test of grocery shopping skills. *American Journal of Occupational Therapy*, 54(1), 20–25.

Hammell, K. W. (2009). Self-care, productivity, and leisure, or dimensions of occupational experience? Rethinking occupational "categories". *Canadian Journal of Occupational Therapy*, 76(2), 107–114.

Hammell, K. W. (2013). Client-centred occupational therapy in Canada: Refocusing on core values. *Canadian Journal of Occupational Therapy*, 80, 141–148.

Higgs, J., Richardson, B., & Abrandt Dahlgren, M. (Eds.). (2004). *Developing practice knowledge for health professionals*. Edinburgh: Butterworth Heinemann.

Hitch, D., Pepin, G., & Stagnitti, K. (2013). Engagement in activities and occupations by people who have experienced psychosis: A metasynthesis of lived experience. *British Journal of Occupational Therapy*, 76(2), 77–86. https://doi.org/10.4276/030802213X13603244419194.

Hoffmann, T. (2009). Educational skills for practice. In E. A. S. Duncan (Ed.), *Skills for practice in occupational therapy* (pp. 157–174). Edinburgh: Churchill Livingstone Elsevier.

Kantartzis, S., & Molineux, M. (2011). The influence of western society's construction of a healthy daily life on the conceptualisation of occupation. *Journal of Occupational Science*, 18(1), 62–80. https://doi.org/10.1080/14427591.2011.566917.

Katz, N., & Hartman-Maeir, A. (2005). Higher-level cognitive functions. In N. Katz (Ed.), *Cognition & occupation across the life span* (2nd ed.). Bethesda, MD: AOTA Press.

Kelly, M., Lamont, S., & Brunero, S. (2010). An occupational perspective of the recovery journey in mental health. *British Journal of Occupational Therapy*, 73(3), 129–135.

Kramer, J., Forsyth, K., Lavedure, P., et al. (2017). *Self-Reports: Eliciting Clients' Perspectives*. In Taylor, R.R. (Ed.), Model of Human Occupation. (5th ed.) (pp.248–274). Baltimore, MD: Lippincott, Williams and Wilkins.

Lannigan, E. G., & Noyes, S. (2019). Evidence connection — occupational therapy interventions for adults living with serious mental illness. *American Journal of Occupational Therapy*, 73(05), 1–5. https://doi.org/10.5014/ajot.2019.735001.

Law, M., Baptiste, S., & Mills, J. (1995). Client-centred practice: What does it mean and does it make a difference? *Canadian Journal of Occupational Therapy*, 62(5), 250–257.

Law, M., Baptiste, S., Carswell, A., McColl, M. A., Polatajko, H., & Pollock, N. (2005). *Canadian occupational performance measure manual* (4th ed.). Ottawa, ON: CAOT Publications.

Lee, S, W., & Kielhofner, G. (2017). Volition. In Taylor, R.R. (Ed.), *Model of Human Occupation* (5th ed.) (pp.38–56). Baltimore, MD: Lippincott, Williams and Wilkins.

Lee, B. D. (2019). Scoping review of Asian viewpoints on everyday doing: A critical turn for critical perspectives. *Journal of Occupational Science*, 26(4), 484–495. https://doi.org/10.1080/14427591.2019.1598475.

Lim, K. H., Morris, J., & Craik, C. (2007). Inpatients' perspectives of occupational therapy in acute mental health. *Australian Occupational Therapy Journal*, 54, 22–32.

Mairs, H., & Bradshaw, T. (2004). Self-care training in schizophrenia. *British Journal of Occupational Therapy*, 67(5), 217–218.

Matuska, K. M., & Christiansen, C. H. (2008). A proposed model of lifestyle balance. *Journal of Occupational Science*, 15(1), 9–19.

McCreedy, P., & Heisler, P. (2004). Occupation, purposeful activities, activities, the empowerment process, and client-motivated change. In J. Hinojosa, & M.-L. Blount (Eds.), *The texture of life purposeful activities in occupational therapy* (2nd ed.) (pp. 437–459). Bethesda, MD: AOTA Press.

Mc Grath, M., & Sakellariou, D. (2016). The Issue Is—Why has so little progress been made in the practice of occupational therapy in relation to sexuality? *American Journal of Occupational Therapy*, 70(1), 1–5. http://dx.doi.org/10.5014/ajot.2016.017707.

Moore, K., Merritt, B., & Doble, S. E. (2010). ADL skill profiles across three psychiatric diagnoses. *Scandinavian Journal of Occupational Therapy*, 17, 77–85.

Notley, J., Pell, H., Bryant, W., et al. (2012). 'I know how to look after myself a lot better now': Service user perspectives on mental health in-patient rehabilitation. *International Journal of Therapy and Rehabilitation*, 19(5), 288–298.

Parham, L. D., & Fazio, L. S. (Eds.). (1997). Play in occupational therapy for children. St. Louis, MO: Mosby. In American Occupational Therapy Association (AOTA). (2014).

Occupational therapy practice framework: Domain and process, third ed. *American Journal of Occupational Therapy* , 68(Suppl. 1), S1–S48. https://doi.org/10.5014/ajot.2014.682006.

Pereira, R. B. (2017). Towards inclusive occupational therapy: Introducing the CORE approach for inclusive and occupation-focused practice. *Australian Occupational Therapy Journal*, *64*, 429–435.

Polatajko, H.J., Townsend, E.A. & Craik, J. (2007). Canadian Model of Occupational Performance and Engagement (CMOP-E). In Townsend, E, A., & Polatajko, H, J. (Eds.), *Enabling Occupation II: Advancing an Occupational Therapy Vision of Health, Well-being, & Justice through Occupation.* (pp. 22–36), Ottawa, ON: CAOT Publications ACE.

Ramugondo, E. L. (2015). Occupational consciousness. *Journal of Occupational Science*, *22*(4), 488–501. https://doi.org/10.1080/14 427591.2015.1042516.

Rempfer, M. V., Hamera, E. K., Brown, C. E., et al. (2003). The relations between cognition and the independent living skill of shopping in people with schizophrenia. *Psychiatry Research*, *117*, 103–112.

Rose, N., & Hughes, C. (2018). Addressing sex in occupational therapy: A coconstructed autoethnography. *American Journal of Occupational Therapy*, *72*(3), 1–6. https://doi.org/10.5014/ajot.2018.026005.

Sakellariou, D., & Pollard, N. (2009). Three sites of conflict and cooperation: class, gender and sexuality. In Pollard, N., Sakellariou, D., & Kronenberg, F. (Eds), *A Political Practice of Occupational Therapy.* (pp69–89), Edinburgh: Churchill Livingstone Elsevier.

Sakuae, M., & Reid, D. (2012). Making tea in place: Experiences of women engaged in a Japanese tea ceremony. *Journal of Occupational Science*, *19*(3), 283–291. https://doi.org/10.1080/14 427591.2011.610775.

Sofo, F., & Wicks, A. (2017). An occupational perspective of poverty and poverty reduction. *Journal of Occupational Science*, *24*(2), 244–249. https://doi.org/10.1080/14427591.2017.1314223.

Sumsion, T. (Ed.). (1999). *Client-centred practice in occupational therapy* (2nd ed.). Edinburgh: Churchill Livingstone.

Sumsion, T., & Law, M. (2006). A review of evidence on the conceptual elements informing client-centred practice. *Canadian Journal of Occupational Therapy*, *73*(3), 153–162.

Taylor, R. R. (Ed.). (2017). *Kielhofner's model of human occupation: Theory and application* (5th ed.). Philadelphia: Wolters Kluwer.

Townsend, E. A., & Polatajko, H. J. (2007). *Enabling occupation II: Advancing an occupational therapy vision for health, well-being and Justice through occupation.* Ottawa, ON: CAOT Publications.

Ulric and Lentin 2010

Wilcock, A. A. (1998). Occupational for health. *British Journal of Occupational Therapy*, *61*(8), 340–345.

Wilcock, A. A. (2006). *An occupational perspective of health* (2nd ed.). Thorofare, NJ: Slack.

World Health Organization (WHO). (2006). *Defining sexual health: Report of a technical consultation on sexual health, 28–31 January 2002.* Geneva: WHO Press, Geneva. Available at https://www.who.int/reproductivehealth/publications/sexual_health/defining_sh/en/.

World Health Organization (WHO). (2019). *International statistical classification of diseases and related health problems 11th revision.* Version 4/2019. Available at: https://icd.who.int/browse11/l-m/en.

19

NATURE-BASED PRACTICE

JON FIELDHOUSE ■ JOE SEMPIK

INTRODUCTION

In the previous edition of this book this chapter was called 'Green Care and Occupational Therapy.' Whilst the term 'green care' is still widely used, the chapter's new title, 'Nature-Based Practice,' widens the scope to include both green care and aquatic blue care.

An awareness of nature-based practice care opens up many opportunities for occupational therapists to use the natural environment and its associated occupations in their practice. Many occupational therapists already use nature in their work, and many nature-based practitioners have an occupational therapy background. This chapter therefore aims to support nature-based practice by occupational therapists and others.

The chapter has four parts. Part 1 introduces nature-based interventions, Part 2 describes underpinning constructs and theories, Part 3 grounds the principles

333

of nature-based practice within an occupational therapy context to support therapists' professional reasoning and Part 4 highlights the growing evidence base for nature-based practice. Woven throughout the chapter are four illustrative case examples showing how nature-based practice operates in specific health and social care contexts; namely, an adult inpatient unit, a vocational rehabilitation service, a child and adolescent inpatient unit and a young people's counselling service.

Defining Nature-Based Practice

There are many types of nature-based practice (Fig. 19.1), but in all of them nature is an integral component of an active intervention. This distinguishes nature-based practice from passive encounters with nature (such as sitting in a garden) or people's self-directed engagement in nature-based occupations which feel beneficial or therapeutic, such as a woodland walk.

Whilst research-based evidence shows that experiencing the natural environment promotes physical health (Twohig-Bennet and Jones 2018) and psychological health and wellbeing (van den Berg et al. 2015),

such casual experiences are not designed as therapeutic interventions. So, the chapter adopts Sempik and Bragg's (2016) definition of nature-based practice as 'nature-based therapy or treatment interventions specifically designed, structured and facilitated for individuals with a defined need' (p. 100). Fig. 19.1 clarifies the distinction between the health benefits that people derive from their day-to-day nature connectedness and nature-based health or social care interventions.

In Fig. 19.1 Circle 3 (nature in everyday life) represents individuals' incorporation of nature-based occupations into their lifestyle. Circle 2 (nature-based health promotion) represents wider public health initiatives intended to encourage people to engage in nature-based occupations, which enhance wellbeing, by increasing physical activity, social contact or healthier eating, for example. In these outer circles the individual may or may not be vulnerable, and their engagement with nature is likely to be self-motivated or following the recommendation of a health worker, friend or family member. Circle 1 (nature-based practice) represents various intentional interventions designed to address specific health/social care needs and is the focus of this chapter.

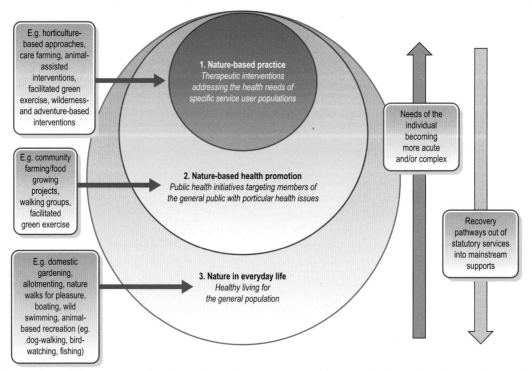

Fig. 19.1 ■ **Three different contexts in which an individual may engage with nature.** (Adapted from Bragg and Leck 2017.)

The two arrows on the right-hand side of Fig. 19.1 show how, as an individual's needs intensify, nature-based practice may be indicated. Conversely, because nature-based occupations are deeply embedded in society, individuals can progress out of statutory care services to less supported interventions as personal recovery journeys unfold. Alternatively, they may use such supports in a preventative way, such as through social prescribing.

Social prescribing is a means of connecting people who use primary care, including those with ongoing mental health problems, with a range of local, community-based, non-clinical services (see Chapter 6: Planning and Implementing Interventions). Social prescribers can link people with voluntary sector nature-based projects, an intervention often referred to as 'green social prescribing' (Leavell et al. 2019). Howarth et al. (2018) pointed to nature-based interventions being clinically valid in addressing mental health problems through social prescribing, noting a growing willingness of funders to support such projects. In 2020 the UK Government, spurred by the COVID-19 pandemic, which highlighted the positive impact of natural outdoor spaces on people's mental and physical health, funded seven test and learn sites in England to develop and evaluate green social prescribing. The activities included local walking for health schemes, community gardening and food-growing projects to address mental health problems and health inequalities (NHS England 2021).

Ethnocultural Issues

In a 2015/16 survey 41.9% of people in England said they had been to a natural setting in the previous seven days. White people were the most likely to have done so, and people with an Asian background were the least likely (UK Government 2020). Whilst over-generalizations about diverse Black, Asian and Minority Ethnic (BAME) groups' experiences should be avoided, an ethnocultural perspective of nature connection reveals health inequalities.

In the UK people of colour are more likely to be living in urban areas with less access to green spaces, defined in terms of travel time to green spaces and the quality and size of the space. However, other factors also make it less likely for them to visit natural settings for recreation (Natural England 2017). Collier's ethnographic UK study (2020) suggested that for people from some BAME groups, historical legacies of racism and colonialism generate this nature disconnect, both because being in nature is viewed as less socially acceptable than a more progressive urban materialism and also because of apprehensions about how they may be received in the countryside, including feeling unsafe and more exposed to racism (Collier 2020).

Inequalities of access to natural spaces were highlighted during the COVID-19 pandemic (UK Government 2021): 'In terms of nature it has illustrated that specific groups within society have less access to good quality natural spaces in proximity to where they live' (O'Brien and Forster 2020, p. 34). Inequality of access to health-promoting experiences is of particular concern given the mental health disparities that already exist regarding BAME populations in the UK, including poorer relations and engagement with services (Vahdadinia et al. 2020) and an increased risk of involuntary psychiatric detention (Bartlett et al. 2019) (see Chapter 12: Intersectionality).

PART 1: NATURE-BASED INTERVENTIONS

In this part of the chapter, nature-based interventions are introduced. Their effectiveness is based on a synergy between the person, the natural environment, and the occupation, whether it be gardening, birdwatching or surfing, for example. These interventions share a common set of core processes, which interact to determine the individual's performance. The intentional harnessing of these processes makes nature-based practice, like occupational therapy, a complex intervention (Sempik et al. 2010).

Horticulture-Based Interventions

Gardening and horticulture are the most widely used activities in nature-based practice and have the longest history as therapeutic media (Sempik et al. 2003). The term 'horticultural therapy' is more commonly applied in the United States of America, while the term 'social and therapeutic horticulture' (STH) is more common in the UK (Sempik and Spurgeon 2006). There is no protected job title, and accreditation or professionalization of STH has been the subject of debate (Fieldhouse and Sempik 2007). However, the existence of a horticulture-based practitioner profession would not take horticulture away from occupational therapists any more than the existence of art therapy or music therapy prevents occupational therapists using art or music as therapeutic media.

STH is probably the nature-based intervention which UK occupational therapists are most familiar with. The overall efficacy of STH interventions comprises restorative processes arising from the natural and social environments, highlighting STH's value as a route into the social capital of communities and as a focus for social prescribing (Howarth et al. 2018).

The largest service user groups accessing STH in the UK are people with mental health problems and with intellectual or learning disabilities (Sempik et al. 2005). Horticulture-based interventions have been used with people with a wide range of mental health problems, including schizophrenia (Oh et al. 2018), anxiety and depression (Gonzalez et al. 2009; Kim and Park 2018), dementia (Blake and Mitchell 2016), post-traumatic stress (Millman et al. 2017) and general mental health problems of war veterans (Wise 2015; Stowell et al. 2018). The case study of Amina, who engaged with nature-based interventions for her recovery, is presented in Box 19.1.

Care Farming

'Care farming is the therapeutic use of farming practices' (Social Farms and Gardens 2021 p. 2). Farming is fundamental to human life and, because the beginnings of civilization coincide with the development of agriculture (Shoemaker 1994), people's responses to the farm environment can be profound, eliciting behaviours and relationships (between people and farm animals, for example) that are transformative. Gorman (2019) noted that farm animals can serve as an experiential anchor solidly reinforced by the integration of sights, sounds and smells of animals. People experience themselves differently, and the farm becomes a place for biographical development and the (re-) construction of personal identity.

Diversity in the kinds of relationships possible is the key to engagement.

An individual may respond to 'something "cute" like lambs or, alternatively, "macho" thinking about the

---

BOX 19.1

HORTICULTURE-BASED PRACTICE IN AN INTENSIVE CARE UNIT

Amina was admitted to an adult psychiatric intensive care unit (PICU) following a psychotic episode. She had been violent towards her mother, with whom she lived, and then attempted to take her own life.

On the PICU Amina spent much of her time alone in her room. She was too agitated to engage in most PICU activities but occasionally walked in the garden, where she said she felt calmer. The occupational therapist noticed this and would join Amina briefly, pointing out colours in the garden, the weather or the feel of the breeze or picking salad leaves and herbs to taste and smell.

Following transfer to an acute ward, Amina found out about the gardening group, which had a small library of books about gardening and wildlife and a seating area, and provided hot drinks and snacks. The group encouraged participation by people of all levels of ability and/or motivation, and allowed Amina to drop in and out. Initially, she watched the people gardening from a distance, but, after seeing them planting seeds and potting-on seedlings, she asked to join. She was encouraged to make planting choices for the borders. Then, with other group members and the occupational therapist, she visited a garden centre to buy plants and seeds.

As Amina's commitment to the group increased, she offered to help clear up after a gardening activity, returning equipment to the therapies department. Within a few weeks, as her confidence grew, Amina attended an allotment group, also run by the therapist. Amina often remarked how she lost track of time while gardening and felt more able to deal with troubling thoughts. She talked to the occupational therapist about using this as a coping strategy.

Two months later Amina said she wanted to volunteer with a community gardening group after discharge. This informed her care plan, and she was referred to a weekly nature and wellbeing group in the community run by the local wildlife trust. This group combined horticultural and nature conservation activities with craft activities and discussions about wellbeing to build resilience and confidence. Amina attended for 6 months, first as a participant then as a buddy, supporting others; she wanted to give something back, she said.

Amina went on to volunteer on a placement at a local city farm that worked with a statutory vocational service supporting people with mental health difficulties into work. For the first time Amina felt that a job might be possible for her.

larger dairy animals and tropes of "cowboys", serves as a remedy to disinterested bravado' (Gorman 2019, p. 9). One care farmer noticed that a service user 'wouldn't even talk to someone when they started, and now, they're like, "oh yeah look at my rabbit, would you like to have a stroke"'

(Gorman 2019, p. 9).

Care farms serve the needs of people with a wide range of mental health problems, intellectual or learning disabilities, addictions and dementia (Bragg and Atkins 2016). They have also been used to address the problems of US war veterans (Greenleaf and Roessger 2017) and more general life-style problems, such as burnout. Care farms may assist in tackling depression and promoting social integration by providing 'a small-scale replica of normal socio-economic life' (Iancu et al. 2013, p. 318). Elsey et al. (2016) suggested they may also promote recovery through social connectedness and personal growth via the restorative effects of nature (see ART and SRT later). Different national healthcare contexts are reflected in different models of care farming internationally (Haubenhofer et al. 2010).

Animal-Assisted Interventions

Animal-assisted therapy is a therapist-directed intervention focused on specific goals (Berget and Braastad 2008), whilst animal-assisted interventions (AAIs), sometimes referred to as animal-assisted activities, are more generalized interventions using animals, such as care farming (Kruger and Serpell 2006; Sempik et al. 2010). The rationale for these interventions is that wellbeing and self-esteem develop through responding to an animal's needs and learning to communicate with them. Animals show affection in response to positive attention and are not judgemental (Katcher 2000).

Systematic reviews of AAI in dementia showed improved pro-social behaviour and quality of life in all studies reviewed, and reduced agitation and aggression in most (Yakimicki et al. 2018), and benefits for people living with depression and schizophrenia (in addition to those with dementia) have been shown by (Bert et al. (2016)). Benefits such as reduced anxiety and pain and improved mood and self-esteem were also reported for children who were hospital inpatients. Most studies

reviewed focused on vulnerable groups, such as children, psychiatric inpatients and elderly patients, possibly reflecting the most likely target groups for AAI.

Facilitated Green Exercise

Barton and Pretty (2010) described green exercise as 'activity in the presence of nature' (p. 3947), suggesting its efficacy arises from a synergy between physical activity and nature connection (Pretty et al. 2005). Green exercise has the potential to improve wellbeing in the general population, for example, through social prescribing, and can also be used as an intervention. Walking, cycling and running have all been used to address specific therapeutic goals (see Chapter 13: Physical Activity). Indeed, Mind (2007) has argued that GP referrals for facilitated green exercise sessions could be as effective as antidepressants for people with mild to moderate depression (Halliwell 2005; Richardson et al. 2005 as cited in Mind 2007).

A meta-analysis of 10 UK studies showed that green exercise improved mood and self-esteem, the latter being particularly evident in individuals with mental health problems (Barton and Pretty 2010). Patients with mild to moderate depression showed greater affective improvement after outdoor exercise compared to indoor exercise or a sedentary session (Frühauf et al. 2016). A review of literature on walking and mental health concluded that, although the evidence base was growing, more research was needed (Kelly et al. 2018).

Wilderness and Adventure-Based Interventions

Wilderness and adventure-based interventions use a variety of outdoor activities, such as canoeing, climbing and hiking, as the basis for experiential learning and self-reflection to address a range of emotional and mental health problems. Wilderness therapy combines the restorative qualities of remote, wild nature with individual and group-based therapy. It is a multi-disciplinary practice usually offered to adolescents with emotional, behavioural, psychological and/ or substance misuse difficulties (Bowen et al. 2016; Gabrielsen et al. 2018). The therapist-client relationship is experienced as being more natural and de-stigmatising than in clinic-based interventions

(Fernee et al. 2017). Wilderness therapy primarily operates in remote landscapes, whereas adventure therapy involves outdoor activities that can take place closer to home; however, the two terms have been used interchangeably in practice and in research (Fernee et al. 2017).

A group of adolescents participating in a wilderness adventure therapy programme was found to show significant improvements in emotional and mental wellbeing, which were evident at a three-month follow-up (Bowen et al. 2016). A meta-analysis of 197 studies of adventure therapy showed it was moderately effective at producing similar positive changes that were maintained in the longer term, while larger effects were reported in studies with older participants (Bowen and Neil 2013). This suggests that, whilst younger people are often offered wilderness/adventure programmes in the belief that their physical fitness will enable them to engage and benefit, such interventions may be helpful for people of all ages. A synthesis of seven qualitative primary wilderness therapy studies with 12 to 18 year olds highlighted therapeutic interactions between three factors (Fernee et al. 2017) (Table 19.1).

A brief overview of nature conservation volunteering and ecotherapy is now provided. Neither phenomenon is, strictly speaking, a type of intervention, but both are often written about within nature-based practice.

Nature-Conservation Volunteering

The nature conservation sector aims to preserve and restore the natural environment (including various habitats and species), promote biodiversity and raise awareness of environmental issues. Nature conservation volunteering promotes social relationships between generations, genders and people of different backgrounds (Sloane and Pröbstl-Haider 2019) and can help to develop people's social and vocational skills (O'Brien et al. 2008). Bragg and Atkins (2016) identified 22 studies reporting improved mental wellbeing, self-esteem and social contact/inclusion and reduced stress. Similarly, an evaluation of conservation projects provided by the UK Wildlife Trusts showed significantly increased scores of mental wellbeing, feelings of positivity, nature relatedness and pro-environmental behaviour (Rogerson et al. 2017).

Ecotherapy

Ecotherapy is not so much an intervention as an approach to any/all nature-based practice (Sempik and Bragg 2013). Personal health is viewed as being directly related to the health of the natural world, or ecosystem, of which humans are a part (Chaudhury and Banerjee 2020). Ecotherapy integrates health promotion activities that simultaneously serve individual, community and global goals (Burls 2007). For example, horticulture, in addition to benefitting individuals, ' ... helps the community, too, particularly when

TABLE 19.1	
Therapeutic Factors Associated with Wilderness Therapy	
Therapeutic Factor	**Features**
Wilderness	The 'semi-unpredictable wilderness environment' (p. 115) provided an initial shock but ultimately evoked self-confidence and promoted reflection and peacefulness, with the wilderness acting as a metaphor for healing and peace.
Physical self	The presence of challenges (such as long hikes and rock-climbing) and lack of customary comfort (due to outdoor living and physical effort) elicited resilience, physical strength and feelings of accomplishment; self-efficacy and enhanced awareness of self, others and the environment (such as finding peace in the woods after having experienced turmoil and loss in their personal lives).
Psychosocial self	Separation from habitual supports, challenges to habitual relational patterns of behaviour, surfacing of personal issues (and reflection on these), recognition of personal priorities, activation of attachments (through sincere self-expression), individuation, reliance on peers, cooperative activities and pro-social processes all fostered self-reliance and trust, although it is frequently conceptualized as an individual journey (e.g., using rites of passage practices). Treatment resistance and stigma decreased also.

From Fernee et al. 2017.

it involves growing fruit and vegetables locally, thus decreasing dependency on chemically treated food products seized from exhausted, nitrate-singed soils and trucked or flown in from thousands of miles away' (Chalquist 2009, p. 68).

Ecotherapy overlaps with green politics and the sustainability agenda (see later). For example, a therapeutic horticulture project is likely to use organic methods that serve to protect the environment (Sempik et al. 2005).

Blue Care

Britton et al. (2018) defined 'blue care' as 'pre-designed activities or programmes (typically physical) in a natural water setting, targeting individuals to manage illness, promote or restore health and/or wellbeing for that group' (p. 2). The 'blue space' where this happens is 'all visible, outdoor, natural surface waters with potential for the promotion of human health and wellbeing' (p. 2), which excludes swimming pools and garden ponds, for example.

The human association of water with healing is centuries old; for example, sacred springs, holy wells, spas, medicinal sea-bathing and holidays and leisure activities promoting restoration and renewal at the coast (Bell et al. 2015). The capacity of seascapes to draw an individual's thoughts outwards, countering rumination, is captured in this personal experience: 'If I'm kind of upset about anything or if I just need to get away for a bit, I find that being by water and just staring at the waves crashing in kind of washes your emotions away … you can get lost in that' (Bell et al. 2015, p. 59).

A systematic review of 33 blue care studies showed many positive effects for psycho-social wellbeing but relatively few for physical health (Britton et al. 2018) (Table 19.2). It is 'blue space', rather than 'blue care' that is most often associated with wellbeing, reflecting the relative importance of access to blue spaces as part of a healthy lifestyle (Gascon et al. 2017) and health promotion interventions. For instance, proximity to the coast is an indicator of better general and mental health, but a propensity to take coastal walks is the key factor (Elliott et al. 2018). Access to the coast may reduce activity inequalities, since coastal walking, engages a more diverse population than woodland walking; being more likely to attract females, older people and those from lower socioeconomic groups (Elliott et al. 2018).

The boundaries between green and blue elements in a totality of experience are often diffuse (Britton et al. 2018). For example, walking along a river locates a traditional green care–related activity in a blue space (Marselle et al. 2013) and wilderness/adventure-based interventions often include water-based activities. However, blue care has some additional properties, for example, the lower gravity in saltwater improves mobility and

---

TABLE 19.2
Summary of Britton et al.'s (2018) Review of 33 Blue Care Studies

Area of Need Addressed/ Outcomes Measured (n = No. of Studies)	Blue Space Location	Features of the Activity	Outcomes Shown
Mental health n = 5 Physical disability n = 4 Addiction n = 1 Post-traumatic stress disorder n = 5 Behavioural (young people) n = 2 Breast cancer n = 7 Learning disability and physiological needs n = 1 Psychosocial benefits (resilience, confidence) n = 8	Marine/coastal n = 19 Freshwater n = 14 [One study used a mix of green and blue space, and one used a wetland or nearshore marsh location]	Activities are typically classified as action sports or requiring learned skills. A tendency exists to emphasize the immersive and experiential qualities of these activities in blue space. Little mention of more accessible activities (e.g. swimming) which require minimal resources or funding. Passive and conservation-based activities and approaches are somewhat lacking in blue care, unlike in green care.	Positive changes in self-esteem, self-efficacy, social confidence, anxiety level, mood, social interactions/ relationships, pro-social behaviours, sense of belonging Positive outcomes for health and wellbeing, especially mental health and psychosocial wellbeing in the short-term

cardio-respiratory function, boosting opportunities for muscular workout as a contribution to overall wellbeing (Hignett et al. 2017).

The range of interventions described in Part 1 highlights the diversity of nature-based interventions whilst focusing on their common ingredient, the natural environment. Part 2 gives an overview of how the human relationship with nature is theorized and how these theories can inform practitioners' professional reasoning.

PART 2: CONSTRUCTS AND THEORIES

The theoretical underpinnings of nature-based practice are approached here from a psycho-evolutionary perspective and by exploring phenomena and constructs used to understand the human relationship with the natural world.

Psycho-Evolutionary Perspective

From this perspective, humans find natural environments restorative because we have not evolved effective responses to the stressors of modern, urban life (Ulrich 1983). Human disconnection from our natural surroundings is a characteristic of the Anthropocene age, the current geological age in which human activity is the dominant influence on climate and the environment (Levin and Poe 2017), and more than 50% of the global population are city-dwellers (Engemann et al. 2019). Indeed, in industrialized nations, people spend between 1% and 5% of their time outdoors; the lowest amount of time at any point in human history (Chalquist 2009).

> *If we compress human evolution into 24 hours, then for around 23 hours and 58 minutes – more than 99% of our time as the human species – we lived and worked in the great outdoors. In this wild and wonderful but mostly challenging environment, despite the lack of medicines, technology, far-ranging communications, and our relative weakness and vulnerability to many predators, homo sapiens became the planet's dominant species.*
>
> *Lister 2018, pp. 38–39*

Two theoretical frameworks have been proposed to explain nature's restorative effects: stress reduction theory (SRT) (Ulrich 1983; Ulrich et al. 1991) and attention restoration theory (ART) (Kaplan and Kaplan 1989; Kaplan 1995). Both frameworks are based on the human affinity towards nature (biophilia) being a still-active remnant from our species' evolutionary past.

Biophilia

The biophilia hypothesis suggests that humans have an innate desire to connect with nature (MacKerron and Mourato 2013), which is strongly determined by survival instincts established early in our species' evolution (Wilson 1984; Kellert and Wilson 1993). This desire is hard-wired and adaptive, being integral to people's physical, psychological and social development. Nature is seen to stimulate certain values and behaviours that positively influence human development (Box 19.2). For example, a utilitarian value generates the human ethic of conservation and care for nature and bio-diversity and is at the core of an ecological perspective of life (see earlier).

The biophilia hypothesis theorizes that humans attune to the condition of nearby animals and plants as a way of deriving information about their shared environment. An animal at rest signals wellbeing and safety, and this impression is transmitted to the person (see AAI). Similarly, healthy plants convey a relaxed feeling of

---

BOX 19.2

VALUES AND FEATURES OF HUMAN DEVELOPMENT ASSOCIATED WITH BIOPHILIA

- **An aesthetic value** – The beauty of nature attracts human curiosity, exploration and adaptability.
- **A humanistic value** – A shared emotional attachment promotes trust, cooperation and sociability.
- **A moralistic value** – An appreciation of the wholeness and integrity of the natural world generates feelings of harmony with it and belonging to it.
- **A negativistic (or resisting, questioning) value** – A healthy respect for the power of nature and the sense of wonder it fosters promotes positive attitudes to risk-taking and self-management.
- **A symbolic value** – The figurative and metaphorical significance of natural objects, processes and rhythms encourages greater understanding of one's own life and mortality.
- **A utilitarian value** – One's dependence on nature's finite material resources (e.g., food) is appreciated.

From Burls 2007.

being in a bountiful natural setting that will also benefit humans (Melson 2000 as cited in Sempik et al. 2010).

Stress Reduction Theory

SRT draws on evolutionary psychology. Ancestral humans adapted to live in natural, vegetation-rich environments, which held the potential for food, water and shelter. Modern humans are therefore predisposed to experience a reduction in psycho-physiological stress in natural settings (Tooby and Cosmides 1992).

The health implications of this theory are wide-ranging. Modern cultural values and norms often detach people from the natural world that shaped our evolutionary path, making modern life less orientated to exercising the older bio-psychosocial capacities necessary for maintaining health (Wilcock and Hocking 2015). Modern living bombards people with sensory over-stimulation that may lead to damaging levels of psychological and physiological arousal, whereas natural environments contain visual patterns that reduce stress levels (Ulrich et al. 1991; Pretty et al. 2005).

Attention Restoration Theory

ART focuses on an individual's ability to concentrate attention on something while blocking out unwanted, distracting stimulation (Kaplan and Kaplan 1989; Kaplan 1995). There are two types of attention:

- **directed attention**, which is the volitional, effortful control of attention that depletes over time, causing mental fatigue, and
- **involuntary or effortless attention**, which is experienced as an instinctive attraction. Effortless attention needs no conscious control, allowing directed attention to rest and replenish itself, and is often referred to as 'fascination.'

ART suggests that fascination is one of four essential features of a restorative environment (Box 19.3). Fatigue is eased and information-processing is enhanced by a restorative environment, so concentration improves and capacity for reflection and planning increases. Kaplan and Kaplan (2011) used the term 'reasonableness' to describe the kind of wellbeing experienced in restorative environments, contrasting this with the irritability, impulsiveness, impatience, distractibility and error-prone performance associated with attentional fatigue.

BOX 19.3

FOUR QUALITIES OF A RESTORATIVE ENVIRONMENT

1) **Fascination** – the ability to maintain attention effortlessly so that directed attention can be rested and attentional fatigue eased
2) **Being away** – the subjective sense of having escaped or feeling removed (physically or conceptually) from habitual stressors
3) **Extent** – a sense that the environment is 'rich enough and coherent enough so that it constitutes a whole other world' (Kaplan 1995, p. 173) which the individual can become immersed in.
4) **Compatibility** – the individual's personal inclinations to becoming active are matched by the opportunities for action, which the environment affords. In other words, an individual may feel inclined to pull a weed off a plant, pick a ripe apple or swim in the sea.

From Kaplan 1995.

People have been shown to prefer environments where they expect to function effectively, responding unconsciously to environmental cues. These cues include the feeling of coherence (the sense that the environment is knowable with a degree of predictability) and the sense of complexity (that there is more to be learned, arousing curiosity) (Kaplan and Kaplan 2011).

Basu et al. (2019) explored 400 participants' experience of four occupations: walking in nature, watching television, hanging out at home and using a smartphone. They found that *soft* fascination stimuli associated with nature walks, 'such as wind blowing through leaves or ripples of water travelling across a pond' (p. 1057), were the most restorative because they exert only a modest attentional hold. By contrast, *hard* fascination stimuli, associated with film, television and computers, 'forcefully grab one's attention and are difficult to resist ... they tend to fill the mind, leaving little room for peripheral mental activity or reflection' (p. 1057). In other words, 'walking in nature can engage the mind [effortlessly] without filling it' (p.1059), leaving 'head space', or processing capacity, known as *mental bandwidth*, to deal with the thoughts running around in one's head (p. 1059). Restoring bandwidth resolves internal noise and allows recovery from mental fatigue. For example, a service user said gardening

'... puts you in a state where it's just enough to stop you from having thoughts about this, that or the other and you're focused' (Howarth et al. 2018, p. 485). Similarly, Bell et al. (2015) studied coastal restorative experiences using ART to understand how views of the oceanic horizon helped participants to clear the head and create internal spaciousness.

ART can therefore inform practitioners' professional reasoning regarding people's occupational balance and the occupations most supportive of recovery.

'Although many people turn to television as a way to relax, the low available bandwidth raises doubts about the restorative benefits of this activity.'
Basu et al. 2019, pp. 1061–1062

The Human Relationship with the Natural World

In this section phenomena and constructs that recur in the nature-based practice literature are explored, each drawn from close observation and inquiry into people's experiences as they engage with the natural world. Such experiences may be considered as here and now manifestations of the psycho-evolutionary viewpoints presented earlier.

The health benefits arising from exposure to nature, as summarized by Lord and Coffey (2019), are presented in Box 19.4, and Chalquist's (2009) overview of the evidence for the impacts of nature-based interventions is shown in Box 19.5.

To encourage thinking about how nature-based occupations can be adapted as occupational therapy interventions, the effects listed in Boxes 19.4 and 19.5 can be explored using concepts and phenomena such as sensory processing and sensory integration, temporality, personal narratives, spirituality, flow, productivity, work and social inclusion and certain qualities of human relationships with plants and/or animals.

Sensory Processing and Sensory Integration

Sensory processing refers to the way the body receives, analyses and responds to information from its environment; sensory integration is the neurological process that organizes these sensations, plus those from one's own body, to enable effective functioning (Dunn 2009; Beyer et al. 2019).

BOX 19.4

HEALTH BENEFITS ARISING FROM EXPOSURE TO NATURE

- Stress reduction
- Attention restoration
- Improved mood
- Slowing of cognitive aging
- Increased frequency of exercise
- Increased life satisfaction
- Social connection
- Better sleep hygiene
- Improved immune function

From Lord and Coffey 2019.

BOX 19.5

IMPACT OF NATURE-BASED INTERVENTIONS

- Reduce anxiety
- Alleviate frustration
- Relieve depression
- Increase subjective health
- Enhance self-esteem
- Develop self-relatedness
- Increase social connectedness
- Promote joy

From Chalquist 2009.

As described previously, natural environments allow individuals to easily extract the information they need to function effectively (Kaplan and Kaplan 2011). Furthermore, there is an abundance of multisensory input during nature-based occupations, both from the activity (for example, the crunch of the spade into soil when digging or the whole-body rhythmical sensation of riding a horse) and from the natural environment (such as the shape, colour and scent of plants or the sound of birdsong). These sensory experiences are authentic, uncontrived and naturally integrated during occupation, supporting optimal cognitive functioning that occurs when external cues (sensory input from the environment) correspond with internal proprioceptive, vestibular and somatosensory cues arising from the act of doing (Dunn 2009).

Although some sensory integrative interventions may require post-registration training, sensory-based approaches are within the scope of occupational therapy and are particularly relevant in mental health. For example, the social functioning of people living with schizophrenia may be affected by sensory processing difficulties with motion, decoding facial information or in recognizing and conveying emotion in the voice (Champagne and Frederick 2011). Sensory processing difficulties have also been associated with social anxiety and agoraphobia (Champagne and Frederick 2011) and with the difficulties in self-awareness and agency associated with schizophrenia (Harrison et al. 2019).

Temporality

Nature-based occupations can give individuals a strong sense of being located within a particular temporal framework, known as 'temporality' (Clark 1997). They may heighten the individual's awareness of a growing season, perhaps of daily rhythms, such as milking cows or ocean tides.

The rapid pace of modern life can dislocate the temporality of occupations resulting in 'doing without being' (Clark 1997, p. 86). Nature-based occupations can help restore the sense of being in the world in relation to past, present and future events, with an awareness of the passage of time and a commitment to the present (Larson 2004). This then orientates behaviour towards the formulation of goals and a re-connection with, or re-construction of, personal narratives.

Personal Narrative

Constructing a personal narrative, or life story, is a fundamental human sense-making process. Narratives enable people to develop identities and understand their experiences in terms of an ongoing story that is being lived. Individuals instinctively seek to behave within the story they create for themselves, therefore developing a positive identity is conducive to recovery (Robertson et al. 2020).

Certain nature-related experiences can help positive personal narratives emerge. ART theorizes that, after an initial phase of clearing the head, an individual will reflect on personal issues and goals (Kaplan 1995). In nature-based occupations this reflective process can imbue a person's narrative with affirming metaphors of nurturing and growth drawn from the natural environment. This attitude allows a narrative to be simultaneously reviewed, adapted, and unfolded forwards into the future.

Nature-based practice may be regarded as a positive metaphor made real, one which meshes with the individual's own life through their engagement with the world;

'The garden is a metaphor for the process of recovery. During the winter months we must work hard although we do not see the results, in the hope that they will arrive in the spring.'

Simo 2011, p. 358

Spirituality

The term 'spirituality' refers not only to a connection with something transcendent, or outside the self, but also to an affirmation of one's sense of self (Koenig 2010; see Chapter 2: The Grounds for Occupational Therapy). Spiritual beliefs have been found to correlate with better mental health, particularly regarding anxiety, depression and substance misuse (Koenig 2010). In nature-based practice individuals often express their spirituality in their connection with nature and their sense of purpose within it (Sempik et al. 2005). Spirituality could therefore be described as a secular experience of finding meaning through moments of absorbed doing (Egan and Delaat 1994; Urbanowski and Vargo 1994; Howard and Howard 1997; Humbert 2016).

For some people, especially those with life-limiting illness or otherwise confronting their own mortality, gardens have been found to have a religious significance (Unruh 2004); a resonance with creation and, ultimately, a creator. Spirituality is often associated with an appreciation of place as a facet of identity and finding oneself, the natural setting being a focal point for feelings of belonging, kinship, stories, image and metaphor (Chalquist 2009).

Flow

Flow is a subjective, psychological state arising when an individual becomes totally absorbed in the act of doing as they navigate the cusp between feeling skilful and feeling challenged (Reid 2011). Flow is characterized by feelings of enjoyment, self-motivation, self-worth and competence (Czikszentmihalyi 1992; Emerson 1998) and such absorbed engagement that the individual may forget their embodied being-in-the-world altogether (Reid 2011). Flow is thus both an absorbed engagement in the now and an encounter with 'possibilities of being' (Reid 2011, p. 52), echoing Wilcock's

(2007) notion that occupation (doing) involves an awareness not only of being, but also of becoming or transforming (see Chapter 2 and later).

Reflecting on flow, Wright (2004) noted that an occupation is likely to be most therapeutic when:

- it has the full attention of the individual;
- it provides clear, immediate, unambiguous feedback;
- it takes place in an uncontrived, real-life environment; and
- it occurs when the individual feels relaxed.

Nature-based occupations have the potential to meet all these requirements. The individual's focused attention on their own challenge-skill balance, combined with flow's capacity to exclude competing negative thoughts, leads to the restorative experiences described earlier.

Productivity, Work and Social Inclusion

Growing produce is integral to many nature-based occupations and this productivity has many therapeutic applications. Growing fruit and vegetables can appeal at a basic nutritional/survival level, as well as offering an aesthetic appeal or soft fascination (Cziksentmihalyi and Rochberg-Halton 1981). Taking home fresh food to share reinforces a provider role for individuals who may otherwise primarily feel cared for and enables people to explore topics such as healthy eating, cooking, numeracy and literacy. Harvesting produce collectively can become a symbolic means for a group to reinforce its own identity. For example, one service user recounted, 'I had those runner beans that me and you planted ... and they were nice' (Fieldhouse 2003, p. 293).

Nature-based occupations may be experienced as therapy, leisure, a hobby, education, training, voluntary work and employment, depending on the context. With planned adaptations, occupational therapists can present an occupation such as horticulture as a continuous recovery pathway from occupational therapy into occupation as in the case studies in Boxes 19.1 and 19.6 (see also Fig. 19.1). Occupations related to food production can have many characteristics of work, providing opportunities to be productive, develop skills and status, make friends, structure time and sometimes transfer to paid employment. Staff at horticultural projects are frequently drawn from former service users (Box 19.6).

Productivity can promote social inclusion through volunteering or employment (see Boxes 19.1 and 19.6 and Chapter 20: Work). Nature-based projects aim to

---

BOX 19.6

NATURE-BASED PRACTICE IN A VOCATIONAL SERVICE

Liz is the manager of New Blooms, a UK social enterprise providing a supportive work environment for people referred by local community mental health and learning (intellectual) disabilities teams. The project has 30 places, and trainees attend for 1–3 days per week for vocational training to increase self-esteem and social contact and as a pathway into open employment, education and training. Staff include horticulturalists, florists and support workers, all of whom instruct in and accredit City and Guilds qualifications, which are recognized by land-based industry employers throughout England, Wales and Northern Ireland.

With the increasing awareness of air miles associated with cultivated flowers, New Blooms devotes its 9-acre rural site to the cultivation of organically grown English cottage flowers which are sold via their website and through a weddings and events service. Production is based on a range of commercial tasks performed by trainees including seed sowing, planting, watering and packing plants for dispatch. The large volumes of plants and flowers means the work involves much repetition, so skills and confidence grow quickly and trainees are engaged in full working days.

The project has become a focus for local community cohesion. In the growing season Liz is overwhelmed with offers from local people who want to help pick flowers, weed the beds or just be part of something they feel is authentic and positive. The financial viability of the business has enabled New Blooms to recruit eight of its staff from former trainees, modelling inclusive employment to other local businesses.

Hamzah left his job as contracts manager in a construction business following severe depression, which left him anxious, isolated, housebound and feeling despondent. His community mental health team referred him to New Blooms and he quickly felt safe there. After a busy summer in the flower nursery he responded to its supportive social milieu and strong work ethic by embarking on a National Vocational Qualification (Level 2) in Amenity Horticulture. This involved work placements in local parks and gardens, which his support worker arranged with the local government authority (council). Hamzah later gained employment as a Horticultural Support Worker with New Blooms and now draws on his own experience to foster trainees' hopes and aspirations about gaining employable skills.

---

enable participants to be productive according to their abilities, promoting inclusion without applying undue pressure. Democracy and service user involvement are common in many nature-based projects, shifting the power dynamic of the service provider/service user relationship in positive, enabling ways (Sempik et al. 2010; Fieldhouse et al. 2014; Howarth et al. 2018).

The Human Relationship with Plants and/or Animals

In many nature-based occupations the direct and obvious response of plants and animals to care or neglect provides immediate reinforcement of an individual's sense of agency;

> 'In nature there are neither rewards nor punishments. There are consequences'
> **Ingersoll as cited in Jiler 2006, p. 91**

The notion of caring in a person-animal relationship has many interpretations from care farming to Harkness's (2019) account of how mindful bird-watching was instrumental in his own self-management of anxiety and obsessive-compulsive behaviour and in his ultimate recovery. Such caring relationships offer non-discriminatory, non-threatening, positive returns for the carer without imposing the emotional burden of an interpersonal relationship that they may not want or not yet feel ready for (Fieldhouse 2003).

PART 3: GROUNDING NATURE-BASED PRACTICE WITHIN OCCUPATIONAL THERAPY

Nature-based practice and occupational therapy are interwoven in many ways; there is much common history, a shared interest in occupational science and practice grounded in person-environment-occupation models. Joint work frequently occurs between practitioners, including shared professional reasoning using certain frames of reference as well as skills, such as group work. Each of these connection points will now be examined in turn.

A Shared History

Occupational therapy has always had a strong connection with nature-based practice. Observing the improved outcomes for patients who worked in the market gardens and farms of the old psychiatric asylums was a formative influence on the emerging occupational therapy profession in the UK (Paterson 2014). These horticultural and agricultural resources were lost in the move from institutional to community care (Leff 2001). However, arguably, as a response to the shortcomings of community care, they have reappeared as an intervention option for the same service user groups as before (Mind 2007).

Nature-Based Practice, Occupational Science and Sustainability

Occupational scientists have signalled the health risks arising from being disconnected from natural environments from where humans evolved and where their capacities flourished (Wilcock 1995, 1998). There are negative impacts from patterns of living shaped wholly by sociocultural and socioeconomic contexts:

> In today's deskbound workplaces and with our homes crammed with labour-saving devices, we have little need to exert ourselves. Whereas until quite recently our diet varied with the seasons and was produced without chemicals, the transport industries, agri-business and Big Food have changed all that ... Evidently, we have a symbiotic relationship with the natural world, and it's one we break at our own, and its, peril.
> **Lister 2018, p. 39**

The psycho-evolutionary perspectives described earlier emphasize how change at a human genetic level is much slower than the transformation of society and lifestyle, meaning we have outstripped our biology (Wilcock 1995). Early humans, endowed with an enlarged occupational brain (Wilcock 1995) and faced with environments that could sustain or threaten survival developed the capacity to analyse situations and make decisions about the prospect of food, water and shelter (Lewis 1994). As described earlier, people still show strong preferences for natural environments, such as a 'brightly lit area that is partially obscured by foreground vegetation' (Kaplan and Kaplan 2011, p. 311) and the presence of water and/or trees.

The mechanisms presented earlier (sensory integration, temporality, narrative, spirituality and flow) can be interpreted using Wilcock's (2007) doing-being-becoming-belonging theoretical framework (see also Chapter 2), where d = doing, b^3 = being, becoming and belonging, and sh = survival and health. Applying this framework to the evolutionary and ecological dimensions of nature-based occupations highlights how they can anchor and reinforce an individual's sense of being, which is the necessary starting point for any therapeutic change. In other words, 'doing', when it involves a strong sense of 'being' in a real world of passing time and physical space, can foster an individual's sense of their own capacity for self-transformation, or 'becoming'. They are then connected with their sense of self, their community and their culture, promoting feelings of 'belonging'. These connections permit individuals to do more than merely survive, but to thrive and enjoy good health.

From an ecological perspective, common ground also exists between nature-based practice and the World Federation of Occupational Therapists' (WFOT) guiding principles for sustainability. Practitioners are urged to educate themselves about ecosystem sustainability and use their professional skills to guide individuals and communities in making occupational choices that lead to healthy, sustainable lifestyles (WFOT 2018).

Using Occupational Therapy Models of Practice

Nature-based practice offers an experience that integrates a wide range of physiological, psychological and social processes, woven together in natural, uncontrived ways. A service user's lived experience is likely to incorporate all of these processes at the same time, so it would be arbitrary to highlight any single process. Appreciating this synergy leads the practitioner to consider that the positive impacts of nature-based practice may be due to the totality of experience created; one that envelops people completely.

Understanding the Totality of Experience

Occupational therapists see individuals as separate and linked complex, dynamic systems in continuous interaction with their environment (see Chapters 2, 3 and 4). This supports our understanding of a totality of experience during nature-based occupations (and how to harness this as occupational *therapy*) because activity analysis can be used to identify elements of the person, the natural environment and the occupation which synergize as a single, coherent experience.

The connection between nature-based practice and occupational therapy is therefore not just a practical one but also a conceptual one. For example, in 2010 an occupational therapy model of practice, the Person-Environment-Occupation-Performance (PEOP) model (Baum and Christiansen 2005), was adopted by an international group of nature-based practitioners as a basis for developing a European conceptual framework for green care (Sempik et al. 2010).

The PEOP model was adopted because of its conception of the dynamic relationship between the person, the natural environment and the activity or occupation determining the individual's performance. In Fig. 19.2 these domains of the nature-based practitioner's professional reasoning are shown, with performance at the point of convergence and in which the totality of experience occurs through the act of doing. Intervention can be targeted at any one or all of the PEO areas because change in one area will stimulate change in the others, as with any complex system. Therefore there

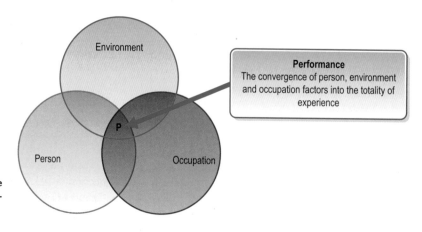

Fig. 19.2 ■ **The domains of the nature-based practitioner's professional reasoning.**

are multiple starting points for intervention when working with individuals who have multiple/complex needs or those who appear hard to engage.

The emergence of PEOP and related models indicated a conceptual shift within occupational therapy away from a focus on mastery of the environment (via occupation) towards a more ecological appreciation of occupation as a means of participation within it (Turpin and Iwama 2011). This shift develops our conception of the service user beyond the individual to include families, groups, communities and populations and widens our gaze from a biopsychosocial perspective of health to a socioecological one (Cracknell et al. 2019). Interventions that benefit the individual can also enhance communities and nature itself.

This ecological perspective forges links with a wider sphere of practice partners beyond the traditional confines of health and social care, such as farmers, gardeners, conservationists, landscape designers, human geographers, architects, town-planners and public health agencies, with the potential to integrate services. The importance of interdisciplinary and inter-agency work has long been highlighted within occupational science (Wilcock and Hocking, 2015; WFOT, 2018) and is increasingly widely recognized within nature-based practice (Nesshöver et al. 2017).

Frames of Reference

People in prolonged contact with mental health services do not often have access to psychological therapies (Roy-Chowdhury 2010). However, nature-based practice may be a medium for challenging this convention and applying a range of therapeutic approaches in natural environments, beyond traditional clinical settings (Grut 2003; Chalquist 2009; Haubenhofer 2010; see case studies in Boxes 19.7 and 19.8). Nature may be used in relationship building, as a metaphor in narrative therapy and in role play or modelling (Cooley et al. 2020).

Frames of reference are used to link theory to practice (see Chapter 2, 3 and 4), so an overview of some widely-used therapeutic frames of reference may assist practitioners in understanding better how nature-based practice works. In Boxes 19.7 and 19.8 case studies offer examples in practice.

BOX 19.7
NATURE-BASED PRACTICE IN A YOUTH COUNSELLING SERVICE

YouthVoice is a city-centre mental health charity serving 11- to 25-year-old youth who experience low mood, depression, anxiety, self-harm, eating disorders and suicidal ideation. Referrals come from Child and Adolescent Mental Health Services, community child health agencies, schools, pastoral services within local universities and self-referral.

As well as psychological therapies, YouthVoice runs the Natureways project, which offers a weekly drop-in, residential camps and counselling in natural, outdoor settings. The drop-in accommodates 5 to 10 young people after the school/work day (4 to 7 pm) in a local community garden, using horticulture, cooking, food-sharing and simple nature connection practices, such as sensory grounding, to encourage group and individual reflection and peer support.

Camps are held two or three times a year primarily for 11- to 14-year-old children and accommodate up to 12 people. Each camp has four staff members, two volunteers and a therapist (present 9 to 5 pm only) and lasts 3 days (2 nights), offering an immersive social and nature-based experience. The camping party travels together by minibus to a conservation site managed by a local city farm. The young people do not use phones or devices during the camp, there is minimal artificial light and cooking is mostly done on open fires. Consequently, young people's rhythms become more attuned to those of the natural world and of each other. Experiences such as this in early adolescence can promote lasting behavioural change and support successful life-stage transitions.

Outdoor counselling is offered as a stand-alone option within YouthVoice but also features in the drop-ins and camps, offering opportunities to recognize and work with the thoughts and feelings that emerge from young people when in nature. It takes place on an allotment and in public woodland all year round and in all weathers. The outdoor settings help redress the therapist-client power imbalance associated with clinic-based settings and optimizes the sensory-integrative experience, enabling clients to feel wholly present. The therapeutic process combines a young person's deepening understanding of their inner world, their connection to the wellbeing–promoting qualities of nature and recognition of the supportiveness of community resources.

Cognitive-Behavioural Frame of Reference

A cognitive-behavioural frame of reference harnesses an individual's ability to acknowledge the automatic connection between their thoughts and behaviour, to modify the relationship between these, and thus bring about changes

BOX 19.8
NATURE-BASED PRACTICE IN A CHILD AND ADOLESCENT MENTAL HEALTH SERVICE

The Families in Nature (FIN) Project runs each spring and summer within a Child and Adolescent Mental Health Service. It was set up by Anne (an occupational therapist) and Sara (a family therapist) for people aged 13 to 18 years old who are inpatients and day patients at The Oaks adolescent unit. The young people have one or more mental health diagnoses and face challenges related to self-harm and suicidal thoughts/attempts, often arising in the context of family issues.

Anne and Sara developed FIN with a local community interest company Iruko (which takes city-dwelling young people into rural settings for self-development) and with a local city farm. Iruko provides equipment for cooking, music and craft activities, and FIN staff (Anne, Sara and nursing staff from The Oaks) oversee the therapeutic input and risk management.

Family relationships need rebuilding alongside the care of the young person, and this normally happens through parent groups and family therapy at The Oaks. FIN complements these interventions through the enhanced relationship-building that occurs when families do creative, exploratory and fun things together during a weekend event in a natural green space; a setting which many family members say feels more authentic than a therapy room. All parents/carers and siblings of the young people are invited to attend the event over two consecutive days. There is no sleepover, and families make their own way to the site each day.

The therapists use nature-based activities to prepare parents/carers to take over the full care of their young people when discharged. This may include dealing positively with challenging behaviour or adopting a positive risk management approach, such as by allowing a young person who self-harms to whittle wood.

Family members value the collective peer support between families, the relaxed relationships with staff (around a campfire, for example) and building skills for life. As the mother of a young person with anorexia put it, 'What a lovely environment to eat together for the first time in over a month and not focus on just the food.'

On the second FIN day, each family is supported by a staff member to hold a family pow-wow involving time for reflection in a favourite natural space, for example, a cob roundhouse, a willow wigwam, or a secluded woodland bench. The family write a postcard to themselves, pledging what they will do differently as a result of the FIN experience. Anne posts these out to families after a month to consolidate new learning.

in performance (Lee and West 2014). As described earlier, nature-based interventions can enhance the individual's capacity for reflection and their sense of agency. They can enable an individual to experience themselves differently and unlearn unhelpful patterns of thinking and doing.

Humanistic Frame of Reference

A humanistic frame of reference focuses on each individual's sense of self and agency. By reflecting on the experience of being that individual, greater congruence can be achieved between the actual self (how one is) and the ideal self (how one would like to be) (Finlay 2004). This perspective is implicitly about self-creation, as people search for meaning in life, and relates closely to aspects of personal narrative, spirituality and flow, as described earlier.

Psychodynamic Frame of Reference

People often describe the emergence of strong feelings while immersed in nature. Natural settings can prompt contemplation of accumulated thoughts and feelings while also stimulating a capacity to process them (Basu et al. 2019). In nature-based practice these thoughts and feelings can be woven into an occupation that is an expression of care for living things. This experience can connect individuals with the fact of life, with growth and with issues of oneness with a natural order and a life/death cycle.

Psychodynamic processes flourish in natural settings and generate positive intrapersonal change (Linden and Grut 2002). The safe, dependable relationship that people develop with the natural world can foster projection and transference. Projective identification, when infused with positive natural metaphors and social coherence, can link individuals' inner and outer worlds, leading to the strengthening of identity, attachment and social inclusion. Grut (2003) highlighted the strong connection between horticulture, personal narrative and spirituality;

Nature provides a metaphor to help integrate all aspects of life. The psyche is reflected in nature... This means we are in connection with a reality that reflects our inner landscape. We can see there, before us, what is happening inside us and when we realize this we become part of the vastness of nature and of the universe.

Grut 2003, p. 188

Nature-Based Group Work

Many of the occupations associated with nature-based practice, such as horticulture, conservation volunteering and wilderness pursuits, take the form of group-based activities, where practitioners use group work principles to amplify therapeutic potential. The therapeutic processes associated with nature-based practice are widely acknowledged to promote social functioning and group cohesiveness. Gonzalez et al. (2011) showed that, for a group of adults with depression, the efficacy of a horticulture group was related to group cohesiveness arising from horticultural as well as group psychotherapeutic factors. The sense of shared experience across group members, termed 'universality' by Yalom and Leszcz (2005), is an important therapeutic factor in group psychotherapy (see Chapter 15: Client-Centred Groups). This experience has much in common with the humanistic implications of biophilia described earlier, whereby a shared emotional attachment to the natural world can promote norms of trust, cooperation and sociability among those who work together within it, with the net result that 'group cohesiveness serves beneficial change' (Gonzales et al. 2011, p. 126). In other words, the gardening group has a therapeutic effect because of both the gardening experience and the group experience. There is a synergy, echoing the notion of a totality of experience described earlier.

PART 4: THE GROWING EVIDENCE BASE

Nature-based practice embraces many different interventions, each of which comprises a variety of activities and all of which are conducted with a range of service user groups. This variation presents any researcher with a challenge: a heterogeneous group of participants and no standardized intervention. Hence, it is difficult to conduct randomized controlled trials and no large-scale trials of effectiveness have been carried out in this area to date. Additionally, the variety of terms used to refer to nature-based interventions can make it difficult to compare research studies or synthesize the findings to strengthen the evidence for effectiveness. Nonetheless, the research output has increased substantially since a review of STH by Sempik et al. (2003), concluded that it was effective but there was a lack of hard evidence.

Different methods have been used to examine particular aspects of nature-based practice. Sempik et al. (2014) used a quantitative methodology to show that STH can increase social interaction among participants with learning difficulties and mental health problems; Harris' (2017) focus group exploration of STH showed that the key facilitator of engagement was the social element.

Some researchers have pooled information in the form of narrative and systematic reviews. Annerstedt and Währborg (2011) conducted a systematic review of controlled and observational studies. They concluded that the evidence base was small but reliable with indications of significant improvements for people with diverse diagnoses, so it was important to consider 'nature as an important resource ... and the value of putting further efforts into research' (p. 385). A systematic review of four randomized controlled trials in horticultural therapy by Kamioka et al. (2014) indicated some effectiveness for a range of mental health problems. However, the authors acknowledged that the poor quality of methodology and reporting prevented definitive conclusions within the criteria of systematic reviews. In a review of the effectiveness of three nature-based mental health interventions (nature conservation, STH and care farming), Bragg and Atkins (2016) analysed 69 primary research studies, noting a range of benefits for mental health and quality of life.

Nature-based practice 'is not a collection of disparate interventions but a coherent philosophy and strategy that uses nature (and the interdependency of humans and nature) in a deliberate way to promote health and wellbeing' (Sempik and Bragg 2013, p. 25). Many of the observations relating to specific nature-based interventions apply equally to others; for example, research has highlighted the similarities between nature-based practice and therapeutic communities (Sempik 2008; Sempik et al. 2010). Both create cohesive communities with a common purpose that provide support and therapy through their group identity and shared activities (Hickey 2008).

Capturing a Totality of Experience in Research

As described in this chapter, the evidence for nature-based practice in mental healthcare is growing, and interventions are becoming more widely understood and used. Nevertheless, there are challenges to capturing the interplay between intrapersonal, interpersonal and non-human environmental factors. Diverse research methods and wider perspectives on what constitutes evidence in nature-based practice are required. However, this diversity is sometimes threatened by pressure to fit interventions into an evidence-based healthcare culture that demands quantitative measurement to satisfy existing systems and policy frameworks (Nesshover et al. 2017; Lord and Coffey 2019).

An efficiency culture that reduces nature to a resource for human use will set it 'on the way to becoming indistinguishable from a box of tablets on a pharmacy shelf' (Lord and Coffey 2019, p. 9). This concern 'seems particularly pertinent in the failure of solely medical approaches to provide a meaningful response to the complexities of people's experiences of mental illness' (Lord and Coffey 2019, p. 12). This technological drift is implicit in medicalized language such as 'dose' (Cox et al. 2017) and 'prescription' (Ulmer et al. 2016) and in new pseudo-technical terms like 'nature deficit disorder' (Dickinson 2013).

Britton et al. (2018) observed that the anecdotal experience of people benefitting from nature-based interventions often drives their growth rather than the initiatives of the research establishment. Without formal researcher involvement, there are risks of increased difficulty with accurate evaluations of the processes driven by contributions from 'settings, activity, role of participant and researcher' (p. 16). However, the research establishment favours linear research methods which are not sensitive to the 'dynamics and complexities of nature-based messy or ill-structured problems' (p. 16). Nesshöver et al. (2017) advocated participatory and codevelopment approaches to complement quantitative methods, suggesting that the inclusion of contextual information about the human experience may be more relevant for politicians and decision-makers. These approaches can support initiatives and prompt change within health care systems because of their emancipatory basis (Lord and Coffey 2019).

For occupational therapy researchers, these issues underline the value of occupational science's interdisciplinarity as a resource for understanding nature-based practice (as distinct from traditional medical sciences). The experiences of people engaged with nature-based interventions can be captured with new paradigm post-positivist, qualitative and participatory approaches (Kinsella 2012).

CONCLUSION

The natural environment can be an integral component of therapy with many benefits. Nature-based practice is a recovery-orientated phenomenon comprising a range of accessible, adaptable and increasingly evidence-based interventions that occupational therapists can use either directly or in collaboration with others. Cross-pollination between occupational therapists and nature-based practitioners can be mutually beneficial.

Nature-based practice will not appeal to all service users. The notion of compatibility, the personal inclination to engage with a natural environment, helps us to understand the impacts of nature-based interventions. From another perspective, it may also be regarded as a kind of selection bias; those individuals who participate have chosen to do so. Not all service users will find nature-based occupations attractive: some may not enjoy being outdoors, getting cold and wet, getting their hands dirty, dealing with the emotional impact of farm animals being sent to slaughter or plants dying. However, some individuals who are reluctant to engage with nature in the first instance may subsequently find it enjoyable and beneficial. The occupational therapist, as always, explores the views and preferences of the service user and guides them towards nature-based interventions if it is appropriate for them.

Nature-based practice can be regarded as an emerging phenomenon with ancient roots. A psycho-evolutionary perspective suggests humans are hard-wired to respond positively to the natural world. However, nature-based interventions are still comparatively marginal within statutory health and social care services. It is hoped that this chapter will encourage occupational therapists to discover, use and evaluate nature-based interventions and to work closely with other practitioners. The benefits of nature-based practice can reach more people when learning, evaluations and research about these interventions and the joint work is shared.

Acknowledgments

The authors would like to thank the following people whose expertise informed this chapter: Rosie Backhouse, Rachel Bragg, Sian Brewer, Rob Dixon, Tim George, Roy Kareem, Sarah Rideout, Nicki Townsend, Patrick Tumilty, Jo Wright and Olivia Woodhouse.

QUESTIONS FOR CONSIDERATION

1. What are the common health benefits of nature connectedness in day-to-day life and what impacts can they have for people with mental health problems?

2. Are there initiatives locally to you for increasing access to natural spaces for people in urban areas? If so, how might they contribute to addressing health inequalities in society?

3. How might an occupational therapist measure/evaluate the outcomes of the nature-based interventions discussed?

4. Research into nature-based interventions show largely positive results but what risks are possible/unavoidable in nature-based practice?

5. Regarding the ethical standpoint of animal rights in person-animal relationships, how might this work where the service user is in a position of primary responsibility for an animal's care and wellbeing?

SERVICE USER COMMENTARY

I'm an older woman and mental health researcher, diagnosed with bipolar. I've benefitted from different forms of nature-based therapy in different contexts as an inpatient within third-sector projects and by my own volition.

During my first hospital stay we visited a dogs' home where we each took a dog for a walk. I chose an energetic lurcher. Walking or being dragged by him was invigorating and unsettled my depressed lethargy! Being pulled and shocked may sometimes help, though it may just seem traumatic and difficult.

Another activity was making hanging-baskets for the ward. I wasn't keen and didn't like my basket. However, I later visited the ward and noticed how beautiful the baskets looked once they had grown and flowered. I learned that growing things was an investment in 'hope,' one of the five dimensions of recovery in CHIME, namely connectedness, hope, identity, meaning and empowerment (Leamy et al. 2011).

Now I motivate myself to sow vegetable seeds in my garden every spring, knowing that seeing them grow will feed my hope. The short sowing and growing seasons remind me to seize the day; to be guided by Earth's natural rhythms and anchor myself in the current season – or temporal framework, as described in the chapter. Tending to plants or nurturing things in nature enables me to nurture myself better. Being in the garden helps me feel more rooted and grounded, that I have a place in the world, counteracting feelings of weightlessness associated with a bipolar high.

Recently I joined a well-being course with my local Wildlife Trust, which focused on one aspect of the Five Ways to Wellbeing model (Aked et al. 2008) each week, as all these Five Elements of Well-being can be experienced through nature. I particularly recall an exercise in Taking Notice. We were asked to find and collect as many different shades of green as possible. About ten! Counting the number of flowers in my garden or on a walk helps me learn by observation.

I have swum in pools with occupational therapists, but I prefer wild-swimming – the total body sensation shifts my mind from everything else, especially in rough seas. The chapter describes well how nature-based therapies provide multi-sensory experiences, but for me being forced to focus on one sensation (temperature) can suddenly change my mood. During cold-water swimming my body struggles to adapt to the initial temperature shock, especially in winter; I can think of nothing else for a short time. The beauty of the water and scenery around me, level with ducklings and damselflies, helps me escape my worries and ruminations for a while. I'm more aware that I'm part of nature, of being in the world. Embodied rather than disassociated. I get a sense of achievement with wild-swimming: overcoming my trepidation and the fear that limits my life during depressions. After swimming for several days I can feel unusually relaxed.

I've learned how to be quieter, slower, more observant and meditative in nature. Looking mindfully and deeply at a plant, flower or leaf can lift me out of deep depression into a more restful space.

Ruth Sayers

REFERENCES

Aked J, Marks N, Cordon C, Thompson S: *Five Ways to Wellbeing*, London: 2008, New Economics Foundation. Available at: https://neweconomics.org/uploads/files/five-ways-to-wellbeing-1.pdf.

Annerstedt, M., & Wahrborg, P. (2011). Nature-assisted therapy: Systematic review of controlled and observational studies. *Scandinavian Journal of Public Health, 39*, 371–388.

Bartlett, P., Mackay, E., Matthews, H., et al. (2019). Ethnic variations in compulsory detention under the mental health act: A systematic review and meta-analysis of international data. *The Lancet Psychiatry, 6*, 305–317.

Barton, J., & Pretty, J. (2010). What is the best dose of nature and green exercise for improving mental health? A multi-study analysis. *Environmental Science & Technology, 44*(10), 3947–3955.

Basu, A., Duvall, J., & Kaplan, R. (2019). Attention restoration theory: Exploring the role of soft fascination and mental bandwidth. *Environment and Behavior, 51*(9–10), 1055–108̶1. https://doi.org/10.1177/0013916518774400.

Baum, C., & Christiansen, C. (2005). Person-environment-occupation-performance: An occupation-based framework for practice. In C. H. Christiansen, C. M. Baum, & J. Bass-Haugen (Eds.), *Occupational therapy: Performance, participation, and well-being* (3rd ed.), 243–259. Thorofare NJ: Slack.

Bell, S. L., Phoenix, C., Lovell, R., & Wheeler, B. W. (2015). Seeking everyday wellbeing: The coast as a therapeutic landscape. *Social Science & Medicine, 142*, 56–67.

Berget, B., & Braastad, B. O. (2008). Theoretical framework for animal-assisted interventions – implications for practice. *Theoretical Communities, 29*(3), 323–337.

Bert, F., Gualano, M. R., Camussi, E., Pieve, G., Voglino, G., & Siliquini, R. (2016). Animal assisted intervention: A systematic review of benefits and risks. *European Journal of Integrative Medicine, 8*, 695–706.

Beyer, O., Butler, S., Murphy, B., et al. (2019). Sensory integration and sensory processing... What's in a name? *Journal of Occupational Therapy, Schools, & Early Intervention, 12*(1), 1–37. https://doi.org/10.1080/19411243.2019.1589702.

Blake, M., & Mitchell, G. (2016). Horticultural therapy in dementia care: A literature review. *Nursing Standard, 30*(21), 41–47.

Bowen, D. J., & Neill, J. T. (2013). A meta-analysis of adventure therapy outcomes and moderators. *The Open Psychology Journal, 6*, 28–53.

Bowen, D. J., Neill, J. T., & Crisp, S. J. R. (2016). Wilderness adventure therapy effects on the mental health of youth participants. *Evaluation and Program Planning., 58*, 49–59.

Bragg, R., & Atkins, G. (2016). *A review of nature-based interventions for mental health care*. Natural England Commissioned Reports. Number 204.

Britton, E., Kindermann, G., Domegan, C., & Carlin, C. (2018). Blue care: A systematic review of blue space interventions for health and wellbeing. *Health Promotion International, 35*(1), 50–69. https://doi.org/10.1093/heapro/day103.

Burls, A. (2007). People and green spaces: Promoting public health and mental well-being through ecotherapy. *Journal of Public Mental Health, 6*(3), 24–39.

Chalquist, C. (2009). A look at the ecotherapy research evidence. *Ecopsychology, 1*(2), 64–74.

Champagne, T., & Frederick, D. (2011). Sensory processing research advances in mental health: Implications for occupational therapy. *Occupational Therapy Practice*, 7–12, June 6th.

Chaudhury, P., & Banerjee, D. (2020). Recovering with nature": A review of ecotherapy and implications for the COVID-19 pandemic. *Frontiers in Public Health, 8*. https://doi.org/10.3389/fpubh.2020.604440.

Clark, F. (1997). Reflections on the human as an occupational being: Biological need, tempo and temporality. *Journal of Occupational Science, 4*(3), 86–92.

Collier, B. (2020). *The Race factor in access to green space. Runnymede trust*. Available at: https://www.runnymedetrust.org/blog/the-race-factor-in-access-to-green-space.

Cooley, S. J., Jones, C. R., Kurtz, A., & Robertson, N. (2020). 'Into the wild': A meta-synthesis of talking therapy in natural outdoor spaces. *Clinical Psychology Review, 77*, 101841. https://doi.org/10.1016/j.cpr.2020.101841.

Cox, D. T., Shanahan, D. F., Hudson, H. L., et al. (2017). Doses of nearby nature simultaneously associated with multiple Health benefits. *International Journal of Environmental Research and Public Health, 14*(2). Available at: https://pubmed.ncbi.nlm.nih.gov/28208789/.

Cracknell, D., Lovell, R., Wheeler, B., & White, M. (2019). *Valuing nature paper VNP19: Demystifying health metrics*. Available at: https://valuing-nature.net/sites/default/files/images/VNP19-DemystifyingHealthMetrics-A4-36pp-200dpi_0.pdf.

Czikszentmihalyi, M. (1992). *Flow: The psychology of happiness*. London: Rider.

Czikszentmihalyi, M., & Rochberg-Halton, E. (1981). *The meaning of things – Domestic symbols and the self*. Cambridge: Cambridge University Press.

Dickinson, E. (2013). The misdiagnosis: Rethinking "nature deficit disorder". *Environmental Communication, 7*(3), 315–335.

Dunn, W. (2009). Sensation and sensory processing. In E. B. Crepeau, E. S. Cohn, & B. A. Boyt Schell (Eds.), *Willard and Spackman's occupational therapy* (11th ed.) (pp. 777–791). Philadelphia: Lippincott Williams & Wilkins.

Egan, M., & Delaat, M. D. (1994). Considering spirituality in occupational therapy practice. *Canadian Journal of Occupational Therapy, 61*(2), 95–101.

Elliott, L. R., White, M., Grellier, J., Rees, S., Waters, R., & Fleming, L. (2018). Recreational visits to marine and coastal environments in England: Where, what, who, why, and when? *Marine Policy, 9*, 305–314.

Elsey, H., Murray, J., & Bragg, R. (2016). Green fingers and clear minds: Prescribing "care farming" for mental illness. *British Journal of General Practice, 66*(643), 99–100. https://doi.org/10.3399/bjgp16X683749.

Emerson, H. (1998). Flow and occupation: A review of the literature. *Canadian Journal of Occupational Therapy, 65*(1), 37–44.

Engemann, K., Pedersenc, C., Arge, L., Tsirogiannis, C., Mortensen, P., & Svenning, J. (2019). Residential green space in childhood is associated with lower risk of psychiatric disorders from adolescence into adulthood. *Proceedings of the National Academy of Sciences of the United States of America, 116*(11), 5188–5193. https://doi.org/10.1073/pnas.1807504116.

Fernee, C. R., Gabrielsen, L. E., Andersen, A. J. W., & Mesel, T. (2017). Unpacking the black box of wilderness therapy: A realist synthesis. *Qualitative Health Research, 27*(1), 114–129.

Fieldhouse, J. (2003). The impact of an allotment group on mental health clients' health, wellbeing and social Networking. *British Journal of Occupational Therapy, 66*(7), 286–296.

Fieldhouse, J., Parmenter, V., & Hortop, A. (2014). Vocational rehabilitation in mental health services: Evaluating the work of social and therapeutic horticulture community interest company. *Mental Health and Social Inclusion*, *8*(3), 155–163. https://doi.org/10.1108/MHSI-01-2014-0002.

Fieldhouse, J., & Sempik, J. (2007). 'Gardening without borders': Reflections on the results of a survey of practitioners of an 'unstructured' profession. *British Journal of Occupational Therapy*, *70*(10), 449–453.

Finlay, L. (2004). *The practice of psychosocial occupational therapy* (3rd ed.). Cheltenham: Nelson Thornes.

Frühauf, A., Niedermeier, M., Elliott, L. R., Ledochowski, L., Marksteiner, J., & Kopp, M. (2016). Acute effects of outdoor physical activity on affect and psychological well-being in depressed patients – a preliminary study. *Mental Health and Physical Activity*, *10*, 4–9.

Gabrielsen, L. E., & Harper, N. J. (2018). The role of wilderness therapy for adolescents in the face of global trends of urbanization and technification. *International Journal of Adolescence and Youth*, *23*(4), 409–421.

Gascon, M., Zijlema, W., Vert, C., White, M. P., & Nieuwenhuijsen, M. J. (2017). Outdoor blue spaces, human health and well-being: A systematic review of quantitative studies. *International Journal of Hygiene and Environmental Health*, *220*, 1207–1221.

Gonzalez, M. T., Hartig, T., Patil, G. G., Martinsen, E. W., & Kirkevold, M. (2009). Therapeutic horticulture in clinical depression: A prospective study. *Research and Theory for Nursing Practice*, *23*, 312–328.

Gonzalez, M. T., Hartig, T., Patil, G. G., Martinsen, E. W., & Kirkevold, M. (2011). A prospective study of group cohesiveness. *International Journal of Mental Health Nursing*, *20*, 119–129.

Gorman, R. (2019). Thinking critically about health and human-animal relations: Therapeutic affect within spaces of care farming. *Social Science & Medicine*, *231*, 6–12.

Greenleaf, A. T., & Roessger, K. M. (2017). Effectiveness of care farming on veterans' life satisfaction. *Journal of Humanistic Counseling*, *56*(2), 86–110.

Grut, J. (2003). Horticulture and psychotherapy: The healing fields. *Therapist Communities*, *24*(3), 187–191.

Harkness, J. (2019). *Bird therapy*. London: Unbound.

Harris, H. (2017). The social dimensions of therapeutic horticulture. *Health and Social Care in the Community*, *25*(4), 1328–1336.

Harrison, L. A., Kats, A., Williams, M. E., & Aziz-Zadeh, L. (2019). The importance of sensory processing in mental health: A proposed addition to the research domain criteria (RDoC) and suggestions for RDoC 2.0. *Frontiers in Psychology*, *10*, 103. Available at: https://www.frontiersin.org/articles/10.3389/fpsyg.2019.00103/full.

Haubenhofer, D. K., Elings, M., Hassink, J., & Hine, R. E. (2010). The development of green care in Western European countries. *Explore*, *6*(2), 106–111.

Hickey, B. (2008). Lothrorien community: A holistic approach to recovery from mental health problems. *Therapist Communities*, *29*(3), 261–272.

Hignett, A., White, M. P., Pahl, S., Jenkin, R., & Froy, M. L. (2017). Evaluation of a surfing programme designed to increase personal well-being and connectedness to the natural environment among at risk young people. *Journal of Adventure Education and Outdoor Learning*, *18*, 53–69.

Howard, B. S., & Howard, J. R. (1997). Occupation as spiritual activity. *American Journal of Occupational Therapy*, *51*(3), 181–185.

Howarth, M., Rogers, M., Withnell, N., & McQuarrie, C. (2018). Growing spaces: An evaluation of the mental health recovery programme using mixed methods. *Journal of Nursing Research*, *23*(6), 476–489.

Humbert, T. K. (2016). *Spirituality and occupational therapy: A model for practice and research*. American Occupational Therapy Association Press.

Iancu, S. C., Bunders, J. F. G., & van Balkom, A. J. L. M. (2013). Bridging the gap: Using farms to enhance social inclusion of people with chronic mental disorders. *Acta Psychiatrica Scandinavica*, *128*, 318–319.

Jiler, J. (2006). *Doing time in the garden: Life lessons through prison horticulture*. Oakland, CA: New Village Press.

Kamioka, H., Tsutani, K., Yamada, M., et al. (2014). Effectiveness of horticultural therapy: A systematic review of randomized controlled trials. Complement. *Therapeutic Medicine*, *22*, 930–943 (2014).

Kaplan, S. (1995). The restorative benefits of nature: Toward an integrative framework. *Journal of Environmental Psychology*, *15*, 169–182.

Kaplan, R., & Kaplan, S. (1989). *The experience of nature: A psychological perspective*. New York: Cambridge Press.

Kaplan, R., & Kaplan, S. (2011). Well-being, reasonableness, and the natural environment. *Applied Psychology: Health and Well-Being*, *3*(3), 304–321.

Katcher, A. H. (2000). The future of education and research on the animal-human bond and animal-assisted therapy. Part B: Animal-assisted therapy and the study of human-animal relationships: Discipline or bondage? Context or transitional object? In A. H. Fine (Ed.), *Handbook on animal-assisted therapy* (pp. 461–473). New York: Academic Press.

Kellert, S. R., & Wilson, E. O. (Eds.). (1993). *The biophilia hypothesis*. Washington, DC: Island Press.

Kelly, P., Williamson, C., Niven, A. G., Hunter, R., Mutrie, N., & Richards, J. (2018). Walking on sunshine: Scoping review of the evidence for walking and mental health. *British Journal of Sports Medicine*, *52*, 800–806. https://doi.org/10.1136/bjsports-2017-098827.

Kim, K.-H., & Park, S.-A. (2018). Horticultural therapy program for middle-aged women's depression, anxiety, and self-identify. *Complementary Therapies in Medicine*, *39*, 154–159.

Kinsella, E. A. (2012). Knowledge paradigms in occupational science: Pluralistic perspectives. In G. E. Whiteford, & C. Hocking (Eds.), *Occupational science: Society, inclusion, participation* (pp. 69–85). Chichester: Wiley-Blackwell.

Koenig, H. G. (2010). Spirituality and mental health. *International Journal of Applied Psychoanalytic Studies*, *7*(2), 116–122.

Kruger, K. A., & Serpell, A. (2006). Animal-assisted interventions in mental health. In A. H. Fine (Ed.), *Handbook on animal-assisted therapy* (2nd ed.), 21–38. San Diego: Academic Press. Theoretical Foundations and Guidelines for Practice.

Larson, E. A. (2004). The time of our lives: The experience of temporality in occupations. *Canadian Journal of Occupational Therapy*, *71*(1), 24–35.

Leamy, M., Bird, V., Le Boutillier, C., Williams, J., & Slade, M. (2011). A conceptual framework for personal recovery in mental health: Systematic review and narrative synthesis. *British Journal of Psychiatry*, *199*, 445–452.

Leavell, M. A., Leiferman, J. A., Gascon, M., Braddick, F., Gonzalez, J. C., & Litt, J. S. (2019). Nature-based social prescribing in urban settings to improve social connectedness and mental well-being: A review. *Current Environmental Health Reports*, *6*, 297–308. https://doi.org/10.1007/s40572-019-00251-7.

Lee, S., & West, R. (2014). Cognition approaches to intervention. In W. Bryant, J. Fieldhouse, & K. Bannigan (Eds.), *Creek's occupational therapy and mental health* (5th ed.) (pp. 224–240). Edinburgh: Churchill Livingstone.

Leff, J. (2001). Why is care in the community perceived as failure? *British Journal of Psychiatry*, *179*, 381–383.

Levin, P. S., & Poe, M. R. (2017). *Conservation for the Anthropocene ocean: Interdisciplinary science in support of nature and people*. Academic Press.

Lewis, C. A. (1994). The evolutionary importance of people-plant relationships. In J. Flagler, & R. P. Poincelot (Eds.), *People-plant relationships: Setting research Priorities* (pp. 239–254). New York: Food Products/Haworth Press.

Lister, C. (2018). Rediscovering human-nature connectedness through social prescribing. *Journal of Holistic Healthcare*, *15*(3), 38–40.

Lord, E., & Coffey, M. (2019). Identifying and resisting the technological drift: Green space, blue space and ecotherapy. *Social Theory & Health*. https://doi.org/10.1057/s41285-019-00099-9.

MacKerron, G., & Mourato, S. (2013). Happiness is greater in natural environments. *Global Environmental Change*, *23*, 992–1000.

Marselle, M. R., Irvine, K. N., & Warber, S. L. (2013). Walking for well-being: Are group walks in certain types of natural environments better for well-being than group walks in urban environments? *International Journal of Environmental Research and Public Health*, *10*, 5603–5628.

Millman, C., McAnuff, A., & Sempik, J. (2017). *Blossoms at larne lough horticultural therapy pilot "wellbeing with nature" evaluation final report*. Belfast: Public Health Agency.

Mind. (2007). *Ecotherapy: The green agenda for mental health*. London: Mind. Available at: https://festinalente.ie/wp-content/uploads/2019/01/Ecotherapy_The_green_agenda_for_mental_health.pdf.

Natural England. (2017). *Monitor of engagement with the natural environment*. Available at: https://assets.publishing.service.gov.uk/government/uploads/system/uploads/attachment_data/file/612705/mene-technical-report-2015-16.pdf.

Nesshöver, C., Assmuthe, T., Irvine, K. N., et al. (2017). The science, policy and practice of nature-based solutions: An interdisciplinary perspective. *The Science of the Total Environment*, *579*, 1215–1227.

NHS England. (2021). *Green social prescribing*. Available at: https://www.england.nhs.uk/personalisedcare/social-prescribing/green-social-prescribing/.

O'Brien, L., & Forster, J. (2020). *Engagement with nature and COVID-19 restrictions: Quantitative analysis 2020*. Available at https://www.forestresearch.gov.uk/research/engagement-nature-and-covid-19-restrictions/.

O'Brien, L., Townsend, M., & Ebden, M. (2008). *Environmental volunteering: Motivations, barriers and benefits*. Forest Research: Report to the Scottish Forestry Trust and Forestry Commission.

Oh, Y.-A., Park, S.-A., & Ahn, B.-E. (2018). Assessment of the psychopathological effects of a horticultural therapy program in patients with schizophrenia. *Complementary Therapies in Clinical Practice*, *36*, 54–58.

Paterson, C. F. (2014). A short history of occupational therapy in mental health. In W. Bryant, J. Fieldhouse, & K. Bannigan (Eds.), *Creek's occupational therapy and mental health* (5th ed.) (pp. 2–13). Edinburgh: Churchill Livingstone/Elsevier.

Pretty, J., Peacock, J., Sellens, M., & Griffin, M. (2005). The mental and physical health outcomes of green exercise. *International Journal of Environmental Health Research*, *15*(5), 319–337.

Reid, D. (2011). Mindfulness and flow in occupational engagement: Presence in doing. *Canadian Journal of Occupational Therapy*, *78*(1), 50–56.

Robertson, S., Carpenter, D., Donovan-Hall, M., & Bartlett, R. (2020). Using lived experience to develop a personal narrative workshop programme in order to aid mental health recovery. *Journal of Mental Health*, *29*(4), 483–491. Available at: https://doi-org.ezproxy.uwe.ac.uk/10.1080/09638237.2019.1677877.

Rogerson, M., Barton, J. ,, Bragg, R., & Pretty, J. (2017). *The health and wellbeing impacts of volunteering with the wildlife trusts*. Colchester: University of Essex.

Roy-Chowdhury, S. (2010). IAPT and the death of idealism. *Clinical Psychology Forum*, 25–29.

Sempik, J. (2008). Green care: A natural resource for therapeutic communities? *Therapeutic Communities*, *29*(3), 221–227.

Sempik, J., Aldridge, J., & Becker, S. (2003). *Social and therapeutic horticulture: Evidence and messages from research*. CCFR, Reading, Thrive and Loughborough.

Sempik, J., Aldridge, J., & Becker, S. (2005). *Health, well-being and social inclusion: Therapeutic horticulture in the UK*. Bristol: The Policy Press.

Sempik, J., Beeston, A., & Rickhuss, C. (2014). The effects of social and therapeutic horticulture on aspects of social behaviour. *British Journal of Occupational Therapy*, *77*(6), 313–319.

Sempik, J., & Bragg, R. (2013). Green care: Origins and activities. In C. Gallis (Ed.), *Green care: For human therapy, social Innovation, rural Economy, and education*, 11–31. Hauppauge, NY: Nova Science Publishers.

Sempik, J., & Bragg, R. (2016). Green care: Nature-based interventions for vulnerable people. In J. L. Barton, R. Bragg, C. Wood, & J. N. Pretty (Eds.), *Green exercise linking nature, health and well-being*, 100–113. London: Routledge.

Green care: A conceptual framework. In J. Sempik, R. Hine, & D. Wilcox (Eds.), (2010). *A report on the working group on the health benefits of green care*. Loughborough: Loughborough University.

Sempik, J., & Spurgeon, T. (2006). Lessons learnt – evidence from practice: The use of plants and horticulture in promoting health and well-being. In *Proceedings of the 6th international congress on education in botanic gardens*. Richmond/Oxford: Botanic Gardens Conservation International in association with University of Oxford Botanic Garden.

Shoemaker, C. A. (1994). Plants and human culture. In J. Flagler, & R. P. Poincelot (Eds.), *People-plant relationships: Setting research priorities* (pp. 3–7). New York: Food Products/Haworth Press.

Simo, S. (2011). Universities and the global change: Inclusive communities, gardening, and citizenship. In F. Kronenberg, N. Pollard, & D. Sakellariou (Eds.), *Occupational therapies without borders Towards an Ecology of occupation-based practices: Vol. 2*. (pp. 357–365). Edinburgh: Churchill Livingstone.

Sloane, G., M-T., & Pröbstl-Haider, U. (2019). Motivation for environmental volunteering: A comparison between Austria and great Britain. *The Journal of Outdoor Recreation and Tourism, 25*, 158–168.

Social Farms and Gardens. (2021). *Growing care farming leaflet*. Social Farms and Gardens/Thrive. Available at: https://www.farmgarden.org.uk/sites/farmgarden.org.uk/files/sfg_growing_care_farming_leaflet_final.pdf.

Stowell, D. R., Owens, G. P., & Burnett, A. (2018). A pilot horticultural therapy program serving veterans with mental health issues: Feasibility and outcomes. *Complementary Therapies in Clinical Practice, 32*, 74–78.

Tooby, J., & Cosmides, L. (1992). The psychological foundations of culture. In J. H. Barkow, L. Cosmides, & J. Tooby (Eds.), *The adapted mind. Evolutionary psychology and the generation of culture* (pp. 19–136). New York: Oxford University Press.

Turpin, M., & Iwama, M. K. (2010). *Using occupational therapy models in practice*. Edinburgh: Elsevier.

Twohig-Bennett, C., & Jones, A. (2018). The health benefits of the great outdoors: A systematic review and metaanalysis of greenspace exposure and health outcomes. *Environmental Research, 166*, 628–637.

UK Government. (2020). *Ethnicity facts and figures: Visits to the natural environment*. Available at: https://www.ethnicity-facts-figures.service.gov.uk/culture-and-community/culture-and-heritage/visits-to-the-natural-environment/latest.

Ulmer, J. M., Wolf, K., Backman, D., et al. (2016). Multiple health benefits of urban tree canopy: The mounting evidence for a green prescription. *Health & Place, 42*, 54–63.

Ulrich, R. S. (1983). Aesthetic and affective response to natural environment. In I. Altman, & J. Wohlwill (Eds.), *Human behavior and environment* (Vol. 6) (pp. 85–125). New York: Plenum Press.

Ulrich, R. S., Simons, R. F., Losito, B. D., Fiorito, E., Miles, M. A., & Zelson, M. (1991). Stress recovery during exposure to natural and urban environments. *Journal of Environmental Psychology, 11*, 201–230.

Unruh, A. M. (2004). The meaning of gardens and gardening in daily life: A comparison between gardeners with serious health problems and healthy participants. *Acta Hortic, 639*, 67–73.

Urbanowski, R., & Vargo, J. (1994). Spirituality, daily practice, and the occupational performance model. *Canadian Journal of Occupational Therapy, 61*(2), 88–94.

Vahdaninia, M., Simkhada, B., van Teijlingen, E., Blunt, H., & Mercel-Sanca, A. (2020). Mental health services designed for black, asian and minority ethnics (BAME) in the UK: A scoping review of case studies. *Mental Health and Social Inclusion, 24*(2), 81–95. Available at: https://www.emerald.com/insight/content/doi/10.1108/MHSI-10-2019-0031/full/html.

van den Berg, M., Wendel-Vos, W., van Poppel, M., Kemper, H., van Mechelen, W., & Maas, J. (2015). Health benefits of green spaces in the living environment: A systematic review of epidemiological studies. *Urban Forestry and Urban Greening, 14*, 806–816.

Wilcock, A. A. (1995). The occupational brain: A theory of human nature. *Journal of Occupational Science, 2*(1), 68–73.

Wilcock, A. A. (1998). Occupation for health. *British Journal of Occupational Therapy, 61*(8), 340–345.

Wilcock, A. A. (2007). Occupation and health: Are they one and the same? *Journal of Occupational Science, 14*(1), 3–8.

Wilcock, A. A., & Hocking, C. (2015). *An occupational perspective of health* (3rd ed.). Thorofare, NJ: Slack Inc.

Wilson, E. O. (1984). *Biophilia: The human bond with other species*. Cambridge: Harvard University Press.

Wise, J. (2015). *Digging for victory: Horticultural therapy with veterans for post-traumatic growth*. Karnac Books.

World Federation of Occupational Therapists (WFOT). (2018). *Sustainability Matters: Guiding principles for sustainability in occupational therapy practice, education and Scholarship, WFOT*. Available at: https://www.wfot.org/resources/wfot-sustainability-guiding-principles.

Wright, J. (2004). Occupation and flow. In M. Molineux (Ed.), *Occupation for occupational therapists* (pp. 66–77). Oxford: Blackwell.

Yalom, I., & Leszcz, M. (2005). *The theory and practice of group psychotherapy* (5th ed.). New York: Basic Books.

Yakimicki, M. L., Edwards, N. E., Richards, E., & Beck, A. M. (2018). Animal-assisted intervention and dementia: A systematic review. *Clinical Nursing Research, 28*(1), 9–29. https://doi.org/10.1177/1054773818756987.

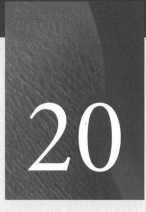

20 WORK

ELLIE FOSSEY ■ SALLY BRAMLEY

INTRODUCTION

Work is a defining feature of everyday life for people around the world, although only a small portion of it is paid work (Gammarano 2019). The right to work is enshrined in the Universal Declaration of Human Rights (United Nations (UN) General Assembly 1948). All people have a right to work, productive employment, fair working conditions and protection against unemployment. This includes access to vocational training and policies to realize the right to work (UN General Assembly 1966). Since the declaration was published, all people with disabilities have gained the right to work on an equal basis with others in freely chosen work and open, accessible and inclusive workplaces (UN General Assembly 2006).

Many people worldwide do not yet have access to equitable and safe forms of work. International labour standards provide an important means of promoting decent and productive work, with fair pay and working conditions for men and women worldwide. The International Labour Organization calls for the elimination of forced or compulsory labour, unsafe labour practices and discrimination in employment for people in all countries, regardless of the level of economic development (International Labour Organisation 1998).

Work is a major occupational role of adulthood that individuals and their families depend on for many aspects of their personal, social and material well-being (Waddell and Burton 2006). Consequently, work powerfully shapes people's lives socially and economically, as well as their sense of productivity, dignity and identity within society.

> *'What do you do?' Having an answer to that question gives us immediate entrée to the normal flow of life ... Work gives us the opportunity to develop relationships in which we can feel good about ourselves. ... We know deeply that we are being taken seriously and respectfully by someone who is depending on us to complete a job.*
>
> **Vorspan 1992, p. 52**

This quote emphasizes the significance of work for mental health and well-being. Not surprisingly, illness-related disruptions to people's working lives, prolonged unemployment and exclusion from work are profoundly felt by individuals, families and communities. People with mental ill-health experience wide-ranging work-related challenges and barriers to employment, yet there are many effective ways to support them to access employment and pursue work-related goals.

This chapter addresses:

- what is meant by work, productivity and vocation;
- how and why people with mental health issues face restrictions and barriers to work;
- how to support people with mental health issues so that they can pursue their goals and access jobs and careers;
- how occupational therapists can bring a vocational focus to their practice.

OCCUPATION, WORK, PRODUCTIVITY AND VOCATION

Occupation is often understood as a person's work, vocation or employment, and paid occupations are most readily recognized and categorised as work. Work is such a commonplace idea that its meaning may be taken for granted; yet defining the concept of work is not straightforward (Jarman 2010). Frequently, the terms 'work' 'jobs' and 'employment' are used interchangeably. In comparison, people undertaking child-rearing, caring and domestic activities are not necessarily paid, but they may still regard these occupations as work.

In considering what is meant by work and productive occupations, Ross (2007) suggested distinctions between paid, unpaid, hidden and substitute work.

Paid work is any form of paid employment or job, including self-employment. It typically takes place with an agreement, where a person's labour is exchanged for a specified payment. This includes formal contracted employment and non-regulated arrangements between employers and employees, the latter being more common working conditions in many developing countries (Chopra 2009). Paid work imposes a structure on a person's time and is typically more highly socially valued than unpaid work; however, the types of paid work that people do, their working conditions and experiences of working vary widely. Precarious employment situations in which work is time-limited or dependent on the needs of the employing organization, can provide useful supplemental income. However, these situations offer limited opportunity to control working hours or work activities, which can be detrimental to workers' mental health (Kirsh and Gewurtz 2012).

Unpaid work is labour that contributes to sustaining and enriching society but does not attract pay, such as unpaid domestic work, caring and volunteering (Ross 2007). Often not highly visible, and therefore undervalued, the economic contribution of unpaid work to society is substantial if there is consideration of financial cost of the paid work necessary to replace it. Much unpaid housework and caring work is informal, carried out within the home or family roles. In comparison, volunteering usually occurs within a community group or organization where particular interests or concerns are pursued and social connections and relevant skills are developed. Some people choose volunteering as a meaningful occupation in its own right; others volunteer for personal development or to gain skills and experiences relevant to employment (Fegan and Cook 2014). Like volunteering, education and training are unpaid and offer people opportunities for personal and vocational development. Education and training are also similar to paid work in some ways because they impose structure on a person's time.

Hidden work includes work in which services are exchanged for cash, goods, or other services that are not formally counted as income, such as child-minding or house-sitting for extended family (Ross 2007). Some hidden work involves illegal activities, such as trading illicit drugs or exploitation through forced labour for little or no money and without safe and decent working conditions.

Substitute work is a segregated form of work, also referred to as sheltered work (Ross 2007). Traditionally, this was organized to provide daily structure and work-like activity for disabled people as a substitute for employment but without access to the same rights, pay, and working conditions as the mainstream workforce. It was seen as prevocational training, but this type of work often created segregated substitutes for employment rather than pathways into jobs that afford the social and economic benefits of community life (Schneider 2005). Given the lack of pay and conditions comparable to those in the mainstream labour market this form of work has been recognized as discriminatory in the context of the rights of disabled workers (UN General Assembly 2006).

These four forms of work (paid, unpaid, hidden and substitute) signal the importance of exploring what people mean when talking about work (Ross 2007). Work is not easily distinguished from other forms of human activity and effort merely based on whether or not it is paid. How we understand that the concept of work is shaped by meanings and values ascribed to different kinds of occupation by individuals, communities and cultures over time (Ross 2007). To illustrate, sociological, psychological and occupational perspectives offer overlapping and somewhat different views (Ross 2007; Jarman 2010).

Perspectives of the Concept of Work

Work is often described as labour by sociologists. The division of labour offers a way to understand work and productivity from a sociological perspective. Originating from French sociologist Emile Durkheim, the division of labour points to the relative value and status in society of different types of work; the differing class, race and gender composition of occupations and how these relate to broad patterns of social inequality and disadvantage (Jarman 2010). Sociologists consider the structural factors in societies that explain why some people are more likely to be excluded from paid work than others. Changes in the economy and labour market shape social responses so that, in times of economic hardship, people with mental health issues are more likely to be excluded from paid work (Warner 2004). In comparison, social psychologists have identified benefits of employment for health. These benefits include a time structure and demand for activity, regular shared experiences, individual goals being linked to collective purposes, access to social networks and defining one's identity (e.g., Jahoda 1981). This perspective highlights the potential benefits that people can gain from securing decent and productive employment.

An occupational perspective on work includes paid employment, study, volunteering and unpaid domestic, parenting and caring work. These are ways of being productive and contributing to families, communities and the economy. The Canadian model of occupational performance and engagement (Townsend and Polatajko 2007) describes three major categories of occupations: self-care, productivity and leisure. Productivity refers to those occupations where people make economic and social contributions or economically sustain themselves. For occupational therapists, productive occupations are also understood in terms of their meaning, temporal, contextual and performance dimensions (Christiansen and Townsend 2010). Put another way, this perspective leads us to ask questions about:

■ why people choose to engage in particular occupations;
■ what meanings these occupations hold;
■ how these occupations are integrated into regular patterns and routines of daily life;
■ and where these occupations are undertaken and how.

An occupational perspective on work therefore also involves consideration of a person's vocational interests or pursuits. A person's vocation is described as a calling or a strong feeling about a particular job or profession (Collins English Dictionary 2020) and reflects a preferred job, career or occupation to which the person is strongly attracted and wishes to invest most time. Traditionally, vocational rehabilitation was focused on training people in the skills and knowledge needed to do their preferred work (Lloyd 2010). Vocational specialists take a broader focus, as explored later in this chapter.

An occupational perspective of work also focuses on dynamic relationships and the fit between persons, their occupations and their environments

(Christiansen and Townsend 2010). In a process called job matching, occupational therapists explore a person's interests, preferences, skills and experiences to identify matches with suitable potential employment options (Bond et al. 2008). If a person is already employed, their job is evaluated to assess the fit between the person, the demands of their job and their workplace environment. This can lead to identifying necessary work adjustments to improve this fit. Occupational therapists also attend to how patterns related to work and other occupations in daily life affect health, well-being and social inclusion (Backman 2010; Eklund et al. 2010; Wagman et al. 2012). This is often described as occupational balance.

MENTAL ILL-HEALTH AND EMPLOYMENT

There are many economic, social and health-related reasons for being concerned about employment and mental health. In high-income countries the Organisation for Economic Cooperation and Development (OECD 2012) indicates that the majority of people with common mental health problems are employed (around 60%–70%). In comparison, around half of people with severe disorders are employed. Mental ill-health is also a leading cause of both sickness absence from the workforce and long-term work incapacity (Dewa and McDaid 2011; OECD 2012). This means that many people who experience mental health issues are employed but are likely to be struggling in their jobs (Dewa et al. 2012; OECD 2012). Mental ill-health may also account for a substantial proportion of disability payments, being the reason for between one-third and one-half of all new disability benefit claims and higher among young adults in high-income countries (OECD 2012). In lower income countries the absence of a welfare system means the financial impact is more likely to be borne by working family members (Benach et al. 2007). So, for individuals, families and communities, there are significant economic costs associated with inadequate support for people to retain and return to their jobs following sickness absence. It is, therefore, important not to ignore the vocational issues of unemployed people with ongoing mental health issues.

The relationships between employment and mental health are complex and not fully understood. Paid employment is beneficial for health and well-being when jobs provide opportunities for control, using skills, pursuing goals, variety, physical security, money, social contact and a valued social position (Waddell and Burton 2006; Ross 2007). This means that the nature, quality and social context of work are important for mental health and well-being. Conversely, poor working conditions, such as job insecurity, high job demands and role ambiguity, can be detrimental for mental health (Butterworth et al. 2011; Kirsh and Gewurtz 2012).

Unemployment has many adverse effects for people who experience job loss and lack of work, including loss of income, purpose, structure, identity and social status, as well as poorer physical and mental health (Waddell and Burton 2006). For unemployed people with enduring mental ill-health, these losses are likely to worsen their circumstances, highlighting the inextricable links between profound employment challenges and social inequalities (Warner 2004; Grove et al. 2005). Low levels of workforce participation do not imply that people with enduring mental health problems are incapable of or do not want to work, especially since the majority report that they want meaningful and productive work. With the right support people with enduring mental ill-health can and do engage in education, employment and other productive occupations (Fossey and Harvey 2010).

Benefits of Employment for Mental Health and Well-Being

Several benefits of employment are central to the process of recovery: meaningful opportunities to be productive and contribute to community life; a decent standard of living; and inclusive relationships (Krupa 2004; van Niekerk 2009). People with mental health issues have reported that gaining employment creates a sense of wellness, improved relationships, more positive self-appraisals and greater optimism (Fossey and Harvey 2010). Other benefits of being employed are shared with other employed people: more structured time use; greater autonomy; status and acceptance within society; a sense of purpose; feeling productive and useful to others; affirmation of ability; and opportunities for social contact and personal development (Fossey and Harvey 2010). However, people with mental health issues face many challenging systemic, employer and job-related barriers to finding and maintaining meaningful employment, in addition to personal and illness-related factors.

Barriers to Employment

The availability of jobs influences the likelihood of being employed. People who are at risk of job loss and instability include the young and inexperienced, those with fewest vocation-related skills and qualifications, older workers, those in poor health and disabled people (Ross 2007). Employment barriers vary in individuals' different circumstances, requiring personalized vocational interventions and support (Rinaldi et al. 2010; Krupa 2011; OECD 2011; Vorhies et al. 2012; Roy et al. 2017).Young people whose ill-health starts in adolescence or early adulthood are at risk of disruption to their education or their transition from school to work, potentially limiting their vocational development and career choices. For better educational outcomes and school to work transitions, they could require support to access mental health interventions at school, along with supported education and employment programs.

Employees with mental health issues whose mental ill-heath fluctuates have an increased risk of job loss. The situation can be worse with poor access to mental health services, workplace supports, flexibility and reasonable work adjustments. To address the situation, workplace-based interventions are required to put in place workplace support and reasonable adjustments along with mental health interventions. Policy changes can promote and develop mentally healthy workplaces. Employees on sick leave face barriers caused by inadequate assistance and support for returning to work. These increase the risk of job loss, curtailed career prospects and economic insecurity. Workplace-based interventions may overcome these barriers by providing information and support for return to work. Policy changes can promote better coordination with healthcare.

Unemployed people with a lack of recent work experience or relevant work skills are least likely to obtain work and are at greatest risk of long-term economic marginalization and exclusion. Support for education, volunteering and employment should strengthen their vocational options and pathways along with initiatives to create new, accessible employment options.

There are barriers to participation which occur in education and employment settings, affecting all groups.

- **Prejudice and discrimination** for young people at school or college and people in work-training sessions. Stigma can be expressed by how language is used, performance expectations, social interactions and performance management.
- **Inflexibility** in working practices and educational course structures limits paid work and study choices, particularly for people with fluctuating or episodic conditions.
- **Limited knowledge** among employers about how to accommodate people with mental health issues in the workplace can result in reluctance to hire them.
- **Low expectations** or limited knowledge among mental health staff about the opportunities for people with mental health issues to study and work. As a result, mental health services either do not attend to vocational issues or convey pessimism about study and work prospects.
- **Views** can be held by mental health staff and/or carers that work or study is too stressful or harmful, especially when it is identified as a trigger factor for a person's ill-health. As a consequence, return to study or work can be discouraged.
- **Inadequate support** is another barrier to participation within the workplace or educational setting.
- **Dilemmas about illness disclosure** can be ongoing because of possible adverse consequences in job-seeking, returning to study or work following sick leave and during education or employment.
- **Limited income and resources** to enable job-seeking or study, such as transport, clothing and equipment.
- **Homelessness and insecure housing** disrupt the ability to access and register for services, seek jobs or create a stable routine.
- **Medication side-effects** or illness-related factors impact on managing study and work demands. This may cause fears about not performing well enough and the consequences of becoming unwell.

■ **Employment disincentives,** which mean that by getting a new job, people lose entitlement to welfare benefits. If they then lose the job, it is difficult to regain the welfare benefits.

■ **Complex systems** are barriers to access education, job-seeking assistance and financial entitlements.

Vocational services, career advice and financial counselling are variable in effectiveness to address these issues (Blitz and Mechanic 2006; Ringeisen et al. 2007; Time to Change 2012; Harris et al. 2014; Ennals et al. 2015; Hielscher and Waghorn 2015; Gmitroski et al. 2018).

FINDING AND KEEPING WORK

Substitute work has a long history in psychiatry, associated with the 18th century moral treatment methods of William and Samuel Tuke at The Retreat in York, England, and Philippe Pinel at Bicêtre and La Salpêtrière in Paris, France. People worked in kitchens, laundries, gardens and workshops in mental institutions in which, as part of their treatment, their often unpaid labour actively contributed to running these institutions (Wilcock 2001, see Chapter 1). Later, industrial therapy workshops provided substitute work in protected environments for those preparing to leave the institutions. However, the restrictive working conditions provided few opportunities for vocational development and little access to mainstream employment. These workshops lost favour because they were inconsistent with recognized workers' rights (Schneider 2005; UN General Assembly 2006).

Over the past three decades services have shifted towards supporting people to find and sustain employment of their own choosing. This is more in keeping with recovery-oriented practice and fosters self-determination (Slade 2009). It also places emphasis directly on addressing working conditions and practices that perpetuate disadvantage or exclusion, which is consistent with a social model of disability (Burchardt 2004). There has also been greater attention paid to mental health in the workplace (Dewa et al. 2012; OECD 2012). Addressing employment barriers at individual, workplace and societal levels is essential to include and support people within and outside the workforce (Kirsh et al. 2009; Krupa 2011; Kirsh and Gewurtz 2012).

Employment Support

The primary goal of supported employment is to secure a job in a mainstream workplace on an equivalent wage, following a competitive process. The support includes rapid job search, job placement and on-the-job support without lengthy pre-vocational assessment or training. The job search and placement process is tailored to match jobs to people's vocational preferences; then follow-along support is provided to retain employment (Bond et al. 2008). Vocational specialists are integrated into mental health teams, enabling them to regularly meet and interact, formally and informally. These elements of employment support originally defined the Individual Placement and Support (IPS) approach and are now seen as general principles for evidence based supported employment at international level (Bond et al. 2012; Modini 2016; Munoz-Murillo et al. 2018; Latimer et al. 2019; Waghorn et al. 2019).

There is strong evidence of the effectiveness of supported employment for assisting young people with psychoses and adults with persistent mental illness to obtain employment (Bond et al. 2008; Modini 2016; Dewa 2018; Munoz-Murillo et al. 2018; Latimer et al. 2019; Waghorn et al. 2019). Originally developed in the United States, it is effective in other countries provided the IPS principles are maintained (Bond et al. 2012). Outcomes are also influenced by national policy factors (Waghorn et al. 2007; Boyce et al. 2008; Bond et al. 2012).

Success in securing a job does not necessarily translate into long-term employment for many reasons. A range of strategies are recommended to improve the rate of success of occupational therapists and others in assisting people to keep their jobs (Bond et al. 2008; Modini 2016; Williams et al. 2016; Dewa 2018; Waghorn et al. 2019). These strategies involve more thorough job-matching processes, offering support for problem solving and attending to work adjustments, workplace supports and employer education. Service users have reported that the ongoing support is helpful in many ways (Johnston et al. 2009; Fossey and Harvey 2010; Blank et al. 2011; Williams et al. 2016):

■ To develop personalized strategies for maintaining their job and well-being;

■ To see disclosure as an ongoing process at work;

■ To access financial and career advice;

■ To weigh up the benefits and drawbacks of vocational options to make informed choices.

To improve career options and vocational success, there needs to be more involvement of people with lived experience of mental ill-health in developing solutions and strategies that address their work challenges (Boeltzig et al. 2008; Shaw and Sumsion 2009).

Education Support

The onset of mental ill-health can disrupt the successful completion of schooling and qualifications in adolescence or early adulthood, making it more challenging to obtain employment or develop a career (Waghorn et al. 2011). The goal of supported education is to improve career options. It is an individualized approach focused on supporting people to access and successfully participate in their chosen educational courses within mainstream settings (Ringeisen et al. 2017).

Supported education operates in a number of ways. With personalized support, students are enabled to attend mainstream classes and to use on-campus learning support available to all. Alternatively, separate classes can be offered to accommodate the specific learning needs of students with mental health issues (Rudnick and Gover 2009). Supported education can also be integrated with supported employment to enhance vocational outcomes (Murphy et al. 2005; Killackey et al. 2017). Supported education improves employment options and outcomes for people with mental health issues, including young people and homeless adults (Rudnick and Gover 2009; Ferguson et al. 2011; Killackey et al. 2017; Ringeisen et al. 2017).

Creating New Employment Options

An alternative approach to improving the available job options is to create new workplaces with embedded support. One approach involves actively developing new employment options within communities, where the working conditions that disadvantage people are eliminated (Krupa et al. 2003; Roy et al. 2014). These include social enterprises and affirmative businesses that adopt an economic development approach to create new employment options (Krupa et al. 1998; Mandiberg 2012). These workplaces are designed with built-in adjustments to make employment accessible and sustainable for those who struggle whilst offering equitable working conditions for all workers (Svanberg et al. 2010; Williams et al. 2010). Occupational therapy

is evident in a range of social enterprise initiatives, including a café in Singapore, a catering company in Canada, a cleaning company in Australia and an enterprise providing organic produce in the United Kingdom (Stickley and Hall 2017).

Another possibility is employment within mental health services as a lived experience practitioner or peer support worker. This offers a unique work context where lived experience of mental health issues is a positive quality for work, rather than an experience to be hidden for fear of discrimination. People may choose this option to give something back, support others in simiilar situations to themselves and make a difference to services (Joint Commissioning Panel for Mental Health 2016). However, safe, sustainable and equitable employment depends on addressing the culture and practices of human resources departments and organizations (Wolf et al. 2010; Bennetts et al. 2013).

Self-employment is not often considered as an option, but it can provide flexible and self-managed work (Hamlet Trust et al. 2007). Many self-employed people run small businesses part-time and choose self-employment for the freedom, flexibility and work–life balance (Ostrow et al. 2019). They use their creative, artistic or other talents to develop their own businesses. Others choose to provide expertise as advocates, educators and researchers within the mental health sector on a consultancy basis (Gammon et al. 2014). For those interested in self-employment, development of effective peer supports, alternative learning opportunities and resources is needed (Ostrow et al. 2018).

Volunteering

Opportunities for volunteering in communities are diverse. Some offer scope to pursue interests and personal development, involving activities such as art or animal care. Others focus on contributing to community life, involving provision of care or other services. Volunteering is valued as an altruistic and meaningful occupation that benefits others. It can also be pursued as an addition to or substitute for paid work (Fegan and Cook 2014). The benefits of volunteering with community groups or organizations include better mental health and well-being, more social connections and valued role participation (Fegan and Cook 2014; Pérez-Corrales et al. 2019). Volunteering can enable people with severe mental health issues to regain confidence, a sense of competence and accomplishment and rebuild their self-identity. All these benefits support recovery (Fegan and Cook 2014; Blank et al. 2015; Pérez-Corrales et al. 2019). However, the effectiveness of volunteering as a route to paid employment is less clear. Volunteering can be a less financially risky initial step towards re-engaging with employment (Fegan and Cook 2014), but this depends on welfare policies and income support arrangements, which are internationally variable. Volunteering can also provide a setting for practising employment-related skills and strategies for managing mental health at work, but it does not directly redress economic disadvantage (Farrell and Bryant 2009; Fegan and Cook 2014).

Supported volunteering offers people access to voluntary roles, assisted by resources from health services and the wider community. For supported volunteering to offer meaningful occupation and real opportunities for vocational development, it is essential to match the role to the person's interests, preferences and capabilities (Fegan and Cook 2014). The principles of a supported volunteering service developed in the United Kingdom by Fegan and Cook (2014) are:

1. A dedicated coordinator, preferably an expert by experience as leader;
2. Volunteering is part of the individual's vocational goal;
3. Standard employment processes are used (e.g., for applications and appraisals);
4. A dedicated mentor is in the workplace with time for supervision;
5. An honorary agreement is drawn up that outlines expectations of the volunteer role, conduct, confidentiality, sickness absence and handling grievances as for any paid worker;
6. There is access to appropriate training relevant to the role and a standard induction into the organization;
7. Regular review and appraisal is performed with the volunteer to ensure progress.

Peer support initiatives have also generated opportunities for volunteering and paid positions in service user–led, mental health and community services. These include the development of recovery colleges in the United Kingdom, North America, Western Europe, Australia, Hong Kong and Japan. These colleges draw on the expertise of both people with mental health issues and practitioners to coproduce and codeliver courses (Perkins et al. 2018). The development of these roles, as voluntary or paid positions, varies across different service settings and countries. Although some people prefer to volunteer as peers, this situation could also be viewed as exploiting and devaluing their expertise (Bennetts et al. 2013; Perkins et al. 2018).

BRINGING A VOCATIONAL FOCUS TO MENTAL HEALTH PRACTICE

To bring a vocational focus to their practice in mental health services, occupational therapists draw on occupational perspectives and frameworks. Using this knowledge they investigate and appreciate how health, disability and other life circumstances impact on participation in occupation. Kielhofner's model of human occupation (MOHO) (Taylor 2017) provides one framework for appreciating how occupations shape and sustain our sense of who we are (occupational identity); what we are capable of (occupational competence) and how personal and environmental factors contribute to disruptions or problems in work and other occupations:

- A person's values, interests and sense of abilities that shape choosing work and sustaining participation in it (volition);
- A person's daily routines, roles and habits for organizing work (habituation);
- The particular job demands and required performance;
- The physical and social workplace characteristics and relationships which either support working or create barriers (environment).

Occupational therapists understand and address occupational issues related to work and productivity. They can also ensure that these issues are routinely considered in mental health services (NHS Scotland 2011; Noyes et al. 2018). By regularly asking questions about work and productivity from initial assessment through all phases of service contact and in discharge-planning, occupational therapists can refocus on mental health services. This refocusing can challenge myths that equate working and productivity with wellness, and mental ill-health with worklessness being unproductive or incapable of work. This avoids leaving service users with the belief that they are not capable of work because of what they are experiencing.

People's capabilities and drives to be active, occupied and productive are encouraged in occupational therapy, extending interest in people beyond their symptoms. Their vocational aspirations are a means of facilitating recovery, because exploring these aspirations can instill hope and create opportunities to address self-efficacy, self-determination and citizenship. Within occupational therapy, opportunities can be created for effective and meaningful working alliances, based on a common experience as people who want to do, achieve and be seen as working, contributing and productive members of local communities.

Occupational therapists initiate and continue conversations with service users about their concerns regarding working, supporting them to weigh up options and develop strategies for dealing with issues such as jobseeking, disclosure, negotiating work adjustments and financial implications. Many people experience significant pressure to be economically productive, so talking about work means these concerns are not silenced, support can be offered and strategies agreed.

This means that occupational therapists can support people to pursue vocational goals of their own choosing, including gain and sustain employment. Within mental health services they can implement IPS approaches and provide leadership on these issues (Hitch et al. 2017; Noyes et al. 2018).

BEING A VOCATIONAL SPECIALIST

Some occupational therapists work specifically as vocational specialists, while others have a vocational leadership element within a broader occupational therapy role within a team, service or organization (Perkins et al. 2009; NHS Scotland 2011). Being a vocational specialist involves using a flexible, practical, capability-focused and often creative approach, acting like a navigator to create a working alliance (College of Occupational Therapists/National Social Inclusion Programme 2007). Trusting relationships are developed to enable cooperation and collaboration. A shared vision about possible vocational options and the variety of routes to reach them is developed. To know how to navigate the service systems, the potential obstacles

and who else knows the way, the vocational specialist builds networks and uses curiosity to acquire information and provide practical support. As a navigator or guide they must also have the courage to acknowledge when they need to ask others for directions, since the pathway will vary for each service user.

There are five key elements of a productive working alliance:

1. creating relationships with individuals,
2. sustaining partnerships with other mental health workers and supporters,
3. collaborating with other agencies and services,
4. developing relationships with employers and workplaces, and
5. supporting mental health and well-being.

Using these elements the vocational specialist develops mutual respect and lays the foundations to enable vocational success. Next, these elements are briefly described.

Working with Individuals

Trust, collaboration, reassurance, hope, flexibility and a capability focus are crucial to the development of an effective, trusting relationship and shared vision between the vocational specialist and service users (Johnson et al. 2009). Initially, individuals may need significant encouragement to believe they can have aspirations. They may need reassurance about their ability to succeed and support to contemplate change. It is important to take an approach that recognizes and validates each individual. Consideration of their choices, preferences, interests and prior experiences is important. There will be variations in motivation, self-efficacy, confidence, responses to change and the complexity of individual situations (McQueen et al. 2012; RCOT 2017).

Employment is often an anxiety-provoking prospect to consider, so gaining an understanding of what work means to the person is an important way to begin to understand their motivations and vocational aspirations (Bertram et al. 2015). For this purpose, The WORKS framework (Bramley and Mayne 2010) and resource manual is useful (Fig. 20.1)

The WORKS framework (Bramley and Mayne 2010) was developed with active mental health service

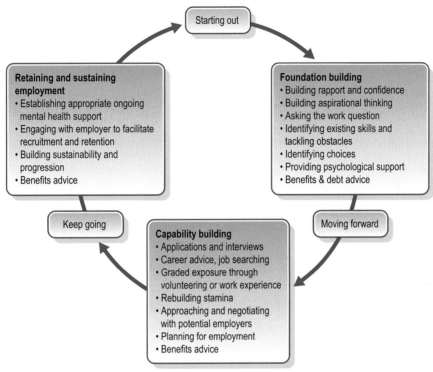

Fig. 20.1 ■ **The WORKS framework.** (©Sally Bramley.)

users' and workers' collaboration in Sheffield, England. People generally start from any of these three points in the framework.

Starting out - Some people do not believe they can ever achieve employment because of the barriers they face. They feel that they do not have any skills and abilities and experience poor self-esteem and low confidence. They may have adopted the attitude that people with mental health issues should not work or are unable to be employed, a form of internalized stigma. To progress from here the vocational specialist collaborates with the person to build a strong foundation.

Moving forward - People may have some experience of employment and/or vocational preferences. They want to explore their options but lack confidence in their skills and abilities and information about the next step. They may want to try some things out in a graded way to ease the transition. To move forward the person builds their

capability, guided and supported by the vocational specialist.

3. **Keep going and growing** - People want to identify how to meet their on-going support needs so that they continue to develop. This stage is focused on retaining and sustaining employment.

To understand what work means to the person and where they are in the framework, resources in The WORKS manual may be useful (Bramley and Mayne 2010). 'My Vocational Profile' (Box 20.1) could support discussion about the person's perceptions of themselves and their role or potential vocational role. There is scope in The WORKS framework for individuals to share details of their unique skills, experiences and preferences and to address the different opportunities and challenges that individuals face in identifying and achieving their vocational aspirations.

For example, Cassinello and Bramley (2012) described how The WORKS resources can be used

---

BOX 20.1
MY VOCATIONAL PROFILE

The person identifies every relevant aspect of:
- What work means to me
- My current vocational status
- My current obstacles/challenges
- My strengths
- My vocational support networks
- My current financial situation
- Any other relevant information

This information is then used to create an action plan. From Sheffield Health and Social Care NHS Foundation Trust 2012. For full details see

Fossey and Bramley 2014, pp. 339–340 © Sally Bramley.

BOX 20.2
WORKER ROLE INTERVIEW

The Worker Role Interview (WRI) comprises a semi-structured interview and a rating scale (Braveman et al. 2005; Lohss et al. 2012). The interview guide can assist a therapist to talk with a person about their past, present and future employment situation in an individualized, conversational manner, and may be used to explore employment readiness, return to work following injury, or work ability following long-term sick leave (Ekbladh and Sandqvist 2015; Lee and Kielhofner 2010). Informed by key MOHO concepts of volition, roles, habits and environment, the interview questions address the following areas: the person's views of their own abilities and expectations of success in work; their work-related values and goals; work interests and enjoyment; work role identity and expectations; habits and routines related to working; and the person's views of their workplace and supports. The WRI rating scale allows the therapist to document the extent to which each of these areas supports or interferes with the person working.

---

to support self-directed re-engagement with volunteering and working. Using The WORKS framework Cassinello explored her capabilities and aspirations for returning to work initially as a volunteer and later in a paid position as a peer worker (Cassinello and Bramley 2012). An Australian community mental health service used The WORKS to bridge gaps between local mental health and employment support service systems (Robertson 2015; Hitch et al. 2017). To reconnect people experiencing longstanding mental health issues, a series of workshops based on the 'Starting out' phase of The WORKS were cofacilitated by occupational therapists and peer workers. Participants appreciated meaningful ways to talk about working, aspirations and concerns while the involvement of peer facilitators fostered sharing of experiences in a respectful and supportive environment. People identified transferable skills, reconnected with vocational goals and redefined themselves as employable (Hitch et al. 2017).

The role of the occupational therapist as vocational specialist involves guiding people to identify the obstacles and challenges to their vocational aspirations. This requires time, sensitivity and patience. Establishing a shared understanding of the obstacles and challenges is essential to develop strategies to tackle the challenges and manage the pace of change. Identifying strengths and supports can widen possible strategies and solutions. 'My Vocational Profile' (Box 20.1) could be useful in starting conversations about potential obstacles or challenges, as well as strengths and supports.

Two useful work-specific interview tools are the Worker Role Interview (WRI) (Braveman et al. 2005; Lohss et al. 2012) and Work Environment Impact Scale (WEIS) (Moore-Corner et al. 1989; Williams et al. 2010) (Boxes 20.2 and 20.3). Informed by MOHO (Taylor 2017), both tools explore return-to-work issues and the impact of the workplace on a person's participation. Other interview and self-report tools are also helpful, especially those designed to consider role participation, investigate time use and activity patterns and explore activity-related interests and values (see Taylor 2017 for further examples).

Partnerships with Supporters and Mental Health Workers

Working in partnership with supporters and mental health workers is an important part of addressing employment barriers. Supporters can be motivating and supportive but sometimes can also be disempowering, thwarting the person's efforts to find and keep work. This depends on their views of the person in relation to mental health issues, capabilities and work prospects. Negative views usually arise from concerns to keep people safe and well. This can be useful for keeping the person and the vocational specialist focused on aiming

BOX 20.3
THE WORK ENVIRONMENT IMPACT SCALE

The Work Environment Impact Scale (WEIS) (Moore-Corner et al. 1989) focuses on how workplace characteristics impact a worker. The WEIS interview is designed to support a person in talking about a particular job environment, and to identify workplace characteristics or supports that may enhance employment success (Lee and Kielhofner 2010; Williams et al. 2010).

The WEIS questions are semi-structured and cover workplace characteristics, including: time and task related demands; the appeal of work tasks; work schedule; interactions with colleagues, managers or supervisors; work role; rewards; sensory qualities, physical arrangement and social atmosphere of the workplace; physical objects/equipment and amenities, and the meaning of work. The WEIS rating scale documents the level of support or interference of specific workplace characteristics for the person in or returning to work.

The WEIS is suitable for interviewing workers who are experiencing difficulties in their current job or for interviewing people who anticipate returning to a specific job or type of work. Its use may help to identify and plan strategies with individuals to overcome work-related difficulties or negotiate work adjustments when needed (Lexén et al. 2013), as well as to identify organisational changes that could be made to create more inclusive workplaces (Williams et al. 2010).

for the right opportunities at a pace that is likely to be successful and fosters recovery (Blank et al. 2011).

Collaborating with other workers and supporters about a person's vocational plans means important information can be included about existing coping strategies; prevention and support plans; ways of recognizing triggers and signs of relapse. While the person manages transitions and change, active involvement of others sustains a sense of safety and continuity. Working together can enhance the knowledge of other workers about vocational issues, as well as broadening their understanding of a particular individual's capabilities, strengths and aspirations. Occupational therapists can suggest possible outcomes and issues based on their knowledge of mental health issues and vocational rehabilitation. The person and their supporters will usually feel safer with access to this knowledge and expertise, enabling them to consider risks that are necessary to move forward.

Collaboration with Other Agencies and Services

Effective collaboration with other agencies and services is often required of a vocational specialist. All the information required to enable a person to follow their vocational aspirations is very unlikely to be held by one person or agency. Welfare and return-to-work services are often complex in structure and organization and change frequently depending on the social, economic and political context. Therefore good working alliances with employment agencies and providers (such as Jobcentre Plus in the United Kingdom) are crucial.

Having established good working alliances the vocational specialist can learn of possible opportunities and identify their relevance to individuals. They can also share their working knowledge of the practices and provisions of other services and agencies. This makes it easier to decide what would be helpful and then to navigate through the service systems and processes. In the United Kingdom a direct link to personal advisers at Jobcentre Plus helps with providing accurate financial information to calculate the impact of employment on benefits. This is essential for people to fully understand their financial situation. It can remove perceived barriers to employment associated with loss of welfare entitlements (NHS Scotland 2011).

Developing Relationships with Employers and Workplaces

It is not possible to support individuals in work or into work without developing relationships with employers and line managers (Sainsbury Centre for Mental Health 2009). This requires the vocational specialist to understand the world of work, the employer's priorities and responsibilities, as well as individual employee rights. It also requires awareness, tact and mutual respect.

The vocational specialist plays a significant and useful role by signposting useful sources of employer support and information (Mental Health Foundation 2016), developing employers' understanding of how to work with employees with mental health issues. With the person's and employer's agreement the vocational specialist can:

▪ negotiate return-to-work plans; suggest temporary or on-going reasonable work adjustments and support an employee to discuss the potential impact of a health condition with his or her employer.

Alternatively, the vocational specialist may have no direct contact with an employer with whom an individual is seeking work through an employment agency or other intermediary. In both situations, a thorough understanding of the culture and functioning of workplaces and their demands is essential so that the vocational specialist can work for the best fit between a person, the employer and the workplace.

Supporting Mental Health and Wellness

To sustain engagement in education or employment, people require strategies. Drawing on their internal and external resources, they can manage work and their mental health and maintain wellness (Ennals et al. 2015; Williams et al. 2016). Developing health management strategies helps the person keep in touch with employers through situations such as crises, episodes of acute mental ill-health, substance misuse and in times of financial or housing instability (Harris et al. 2014). Unexpected life events may require working jointly with other services and supporters to manage issues and adjust vocational planning to take account of circumstances.

When an individual's mental health fluctuates or deteriorates, ongoing collaboration with them will be needed to review the potential impact on vocational plans and study or work transitions. The vocational specialist reinforces the person's established and effective strategies for maintaining wellness. The Wellness Recovery Action Plan is a useful tool (Cook et al. 2010). Smartphone apps, a form of mobile technology, can be used to enhance cognitive skills and coping strategies. For example, the Working Well smartphone app was designed for self-management and recovery support to enable people to keep working (Nicholson et al. 2017).

Regular review is crucial for recognizing achievements and maintaining momentum, focus and direction. Using a mobile app could enable the person to identify and chart their own skills acquisition and progress. Keeping track of agreed areas will maintain a recovery perspective during periods of fluctuating health by offering a clear record of achievements. There is much scope for collaboration with service users to create innovative approaches and strategies for supporting mental health, employment and other vocational aspirations.

Promoting Mentally Healthy and Safe Workplaces

Mental health promotion in the workplace is important to reduce work-related stress, the prevalence of mental ill-health among staff and work-related disability of people who experience mental health issues (Dewa et al. 2012). Individual, team and organizational level strategies are needed (Kirsh and Gewurtz 2012). Settings for occupational therapy with such opportunities include return-to-work programs, Employee Assistance Programs, workplace health and safety teams and health and community care organizations. Occupational therapy theoretical frameworks can be used to understand the fit between workers, work and workplaces. An occupational therapist could analyse specific job requirements from psychosocial and physical safety perspectives. This analysis could be used to educate employers and employees about reasonable work adjustments to support return-to-work and job retention. At an organizational level, an occupational therapist could contribute to inclusive policies and practices that support staff to balance the demands of their work and personal lives.

SUMMARY

Work is a major role of adulthood. Therefore occupational therapists working with adults and young people address productivity, employment and vocational issues. These issues are significant for economic and social inclusion and supporting recovery. There is extensive evidence that people experiencing mental health issues can pursue their chosen vocational goals with the right support. Vocational specialism involves supporting mental health service users for those in employment making the best arrangements and supports to sustain it; and for those without work exploring and pursuing vocational goals. Occupational therapists, as vocational specialists, can provide leadership within mental health services and local communities on these issues.

QUESTIONS FOR CONSIDERATION

1. What benefits and challenges may be experienced by service users in employment?
2. List factors that contribute to poor working conditions for everyone's mental health and consider how they could be addressed.
3. Using the list of barriers to work participation, reflect on the different ways young people, employees and unemployed people might experience each barrier.
4. What are three reasons for why substitute work difficult to align with a recovery-oriented approach?
5. What are the primary principles for individualised support to enable service users to secure employment?
6. Reflect on what you know about supported education in schools, colleges and universities. What makes this kind of support helpful for young people with mental health issues?
7. Which local or national initiatives are you aware of that offer embedded workplace support for people with mental health issues?
8. Compared to an occupational therapist in an inpatient mental health service, who might an occupational therapist working as a vocational specialist liaise with and why?

SERVICE USER COMMENTARY

'So, Mark, what is it that you do?' That one question I always dread which never fails to cause my stomach to churn and stinging beads of sweat to trickle down my lower back...

As someone who has lived with Obsessive Compulsive Disorder throughout his adult life, I know all too well that having something meaningful to do each day can and does bring huge benefits, particularly in relation to my mental health. Unfortunately, I have also experienced the difficult position of being in the opposite situation, often for long periods, resulting in damaging and unwanted consequences. To have the opportunity to work, together with the potential of enjoying a healthy and all-round fulfilling existence are two fundamental privileges which are inextricably connected and must be viewed as such. On a personal level it has come as no surprise to me that my better times have nearly always coincided with a suitably stimulating occupation, which has been both structured and consistent.

A significant factor in the improvement of my well-being over the past 2 years has undoubtedly been the vocational focus adopted by my former occupational therapist; she quickly realized that my needs and expectations associated with work had to be both challenging and rewarding. Her therapeutic approach began by identifying my strengths and capabilities, which lead on to the development of practical and realistic strategies fit for future implementation. I began to not only better understand my difficulties, but also to take positive and tangible steps towards enjoying and re-identifying with the many benefits that having structured work can bring.

I particularly resonated with the section that dealt with the perspectives relating to the concepts of work, in particular the notion that occupation not only defines one's inner self worth, but also influences and categorises society's perceptions in the outside world. Clinicians and employers alike must meaningfully embrace an individual's personal and specific set of needs; it simply cannot be and must not be a 'one size fits all' approach!

I have always been mindful about the relative value and status of any previous work, which I have been well enough to undertake. Time and experience have taught me how to better manage the obstacles I face, as well as to come to terms with the inevitability of their reoccurrence. I have also become acutely aware of my own capabilities, what I see myself doing, as well as how I am considered by my peers and those around me. I strive to be valued in the work I undertake, realize my potential and not accept external definitions derived either from my difficulties or my diagnosis. On too many occasions I have encountered clinicians who not only appear to prioritize my limitations, but, frustratingly, seem to place little worth on the importance of my own perception of what I am able to do and how I want others to define me. The importance of creating open and transparent environments, in line with an acceptance of honest and candid dialogue, are two ways to alleviate this most unhelpful practice in terms of both initial engagement and the long-term.

Mark Weightman

REFERENCES

Backman, C. (2010). Occupational balance and well-being. In C. H. Christiansen, & E. A. Townsend (Eds.), *Introduction to occupation: The art and science of living* (2nd ed.) (pp. 231–249). Upper Saddle River, New Jersey: Prentice Hall.

Benach, J., Muntaner, C., & Santana, V. (2007). *Employment conditions and health inequalities: Final report to the WHO Commission on Social Determinants of Health (CSDH).* Barcelona.

Bennetts, W., Pinches, A., Paluch, T., & Fossey, E. (2013). Real lives, real jobs: Sustaining consumer perspective work in the mental health sector. *Advanced Mental Health, 11*(3), 308–320.

Bertram, M., & McDonald, S. (2015). From surviving to thriving: How does that happen. *The Journal of Mental Health Training, Education and Practice, 10*(5), 337–348.

Blank, A., Harries, P., & Reynolds, F. (2011). Mental health service users' perspectives of work: A review of the literature. *British Journal of Occupational Therapy, 74*(4), 191–199.

Blank, A. A., Harries, P., & Reynolds, F. (2015). 'Without occupation you don't exist': Occupational engagement and mental illness. *Journal of Occupational Science, 22,* 197–209.

Blitz, C. L., & Mechanic, D. (2006). Facilitators and barriers to employment among individuals with psychiatric disabilities: A job coach perspective. *Work, 26*(4), 407–419.

Boeltzig, H., Timmons, J. C., & Marrone, J. (2008). Maximising potential: Innovative collaborative strategies between one-stops and mental health systems of care. *Work, 31*(2), 181–193.

Bond, G., Drake, R. E., & Becker, D. R. (2008). An update on randomized controlled trials of evidence-based supported employment. *Psychiatric Rehabilitation Journal, 31*(4), 280–290.

Bond, G. R., Drake, R. E., & Becker, D. R. (2012). Generalizability of the individual placement and support (IPS) model of supported employment outside the US. *World Psychiatry, 11,* 32–39.

Bramley, S., & Mayne, N. (2010). *The WORKS a resource to support you in achieving your employment ambitions.* Sheffield: Sheffield health and social care NHS Foundation Trust.

Braveman, B., Robson, M., Velozo, C., et al. (2005). *The Worker Role Interview (WRI) (version 10.0) model of human occupation clearinghouse.* Chicago: University of Illinois at Chicago.

Burchardt, T. (2004). Capabilities and disability: The capabilities framework and the social model of disability. *Disability & Society, 19*(7), 57–102.

Butterworth, P., Leach, L. S., Strazdins, L., Olesen, S. C., Rodgers, B., & Broom, D. H. (2011). The psychosocial quality of work determines whether employment has benefits for mental health: Results from a longitudinal national household panel survey. *Occupational and Environmental Medicine, 68*(11), 806–812.

Cassinello, K., & Bramley, S. (2012). Keeley's journey: From service user to service provider. *Work, 43*(1), 91–97.

Chopra, P. (2009). Mental health and the workplace: Issues for developing countries. *International Journal of Mental Health Systems, 3,* 4. doi.org/10.1186/1752-4458-3-4.

Christiansen, C., & Townsend, E. (2010). Introduction to occupation. In C. H. Christiansen & E. A. Townsend (Eds.), *Introduction to occupation: The art and science of living* (2nd ed.) (pp. 1–340). Upper Saddle River, New Jersey: Prentice Hall.

College of Occupational Therapists/ National Social Inclusion Programme. (2007). *Work matters: Vocational navigation for occupational therapy staff. College of occupational therapists, national social inclusion programme and department of health.* London.

Collins English Dictionary. (2020). Available at: https://www.collinsdictionary.com/dictionary/english/vocation. Accessed 23/02/20.

Cook, J. A., Copeland, M. E., Corey, L., et al. (2010). Developing the evidence base for peer-led services: Changes among participants following Wellness Recovery Action Planning (WRAP) education in two statewide initiatives. *Psychiatric Rehabilitation Journal, 34*(2), 113–120.

Dewa, C. S., & McDaid, D. (2011). Investing in the mental health of the labor force: Epidemiological and economic impact of mental health disabilities in the workplace. In I. Z. Schultz, & E. S. Rogers (Eds.), *Work accommodation and retention in mental health* (pp. 33–51). Springer.

Dewa, C. S., Corbiere, M., Durand, M., & Hensel, J. (2012). Challenges related to mental health in the workplace. In R. J. Gatchel, & I. Z. Schultz (Eds.), *Handbook of occupational health and wellness* (pp. 105–129). Springer.

Dewa, C. S. (2018). The effectiveness of augmented versus standard individual placement and support programs in terms of employment: A systemic literature review. *Journal of Mental Health, 27*(2), 174–183.

Ekbladh, E. & Sandqvist. J. (2015). Psychosocial factors' influence on work ability of people experiencing sick leave resulting from common mental disorders. *Occupational Therapy in Mental Health, 31*(3), 283–297, DOI: 10.1080/0164212X.2015.1055530.

Eklund, M., Erlandsson, L. K., & Leufstadius, C. (2010). Time use in relation to valued and satisfying occupations among people with persistent mental illness: Exploring occupational balance. *Journal of Occupational Science, 17*(4), 231–238.

Ennals, P., Fossey, E., & Howie, L. (2015). Postsecondary study and mental ill-health: A meta-synthesis of qualitative research exploring students' lived experiences. *Journal of Mental Health, 24*(2), 111–119. https://doi.org/10.3109/09638237.2015.1019052.

Farrell, C., & Bryant, W. (2009). Voluntary work for adults with mental health problems: A route to inclusion? A review of the literature. *British Journal of Occupational Therapy, 72*(4), 163–173.

Fegan, C., & Cook, S. (2014). The therapeutic power of volunteering. *Advances in Psychiatric Treatment, 20,* 217–224. https://doi.org/10.1192/apt.bp.113.011890.

Ferguson, K. M., Xie, B., & Glynn, S. (2011). Adapting the individual placement and support model with homeless young adults. *Child and Youth Care Forum, 41*(3), 277–294.

Fossey, E., & Harvey, C. A. (2010). Finding and sustaining mainstream employment: A qualitative meta-synthesis of mental health consumer views. *Canadian Journal of Occupational Therapy, 77*(5), 303–314.

Fossey, E., & Bramley, S. (2014). Work and vocational pursuits. In W. Bryant, J. Fieldhouse, K. Bannigan, (Eds.), *Creek's occupational therapy and mental health* (pp. 328–344). Edinburgh: Elsevier.

Gammarano, R. (2019). *Work and employment are not synonyms.* Available at: https://ilostat.ilo.org/work-and-employment-are-not-synonyms/.

Gammon, D., Strand, M., & Eng, L. S. (2014). Service users' perspectives in the design of an online tool for assisted self-help in mental health: A case study of implications. *International Journal of Mental Health Systems*, 8, 2. Available at: https://bmjopen.bmj.com/content/8/12/e024487.

Gmitroski, T., Bradley, C., Heinemann, L., et al. (2018). Barriers and facilitators to employment for young adults with mental illness: A scoping review. *British Medical Journal Open 8*, e024487. https://doi.org/10.1136/bmjopen-2018-024487.

Grove, B., Secker, J., & Seebohm, P. (2005). Introduction: Rethinking employment and mental health. In B. Grove, J. Secker, & P. Seebohm (Eds.), *New thinking about mental health and employment* (pp. xiii–xxii). Abingdon: Radcliffe Publishing Ltd.

Hamlet Trust, Project North East, and College Research & Training Unit (Royal College of Psychiatrists). (2007). Business minds: Mainstreaming business support for mental health. *Research findings from the newcastle demonstration project*. Available at: http://www.socialfirmsuk.co.uk.

Harris, L. M., Matthews, L. R., Penrose-Wall, J., Alam, A., & Jaworski, A. (2014). Perspectives on barriers to employment for job seekers with mental illness and additional substance-use problems. *Health & Social Care in the Community*, 22(1), 67–77.

Hielscher, E., & Waghorn, G. (2015). Managing disclosure of personal information: An opportunity to enhance supported employment. *Psychiatric Rehabilitation Journal*, 38(4), 306–313.

Hitch, D., Robertson, J., Ochteco, H., et al. (2017). An evaluation of a vocational group for people with mental health problems based on the WORKS framework. *British Journal of Occupational Therapy*, 80(12), 717–725.

International Labour Organisation (1998). ILO Declaration on Fundamental Principles and Rights at Work. ILO: Geneva, Switzerland https://www.ilo.org/declaration/lang--en/index.htm.

Jahoda, M. (1981). Work, employment and unemployment: Values, theories and approaches in social research. *American Psychologist*, 36(2), 184–191.

Jarman, J. (2010). What is occupation? Interdisciplinary perspectives on defining and classifying human activity. In C. H. Christiansen, & E. A. Townsend (Eds.), *Introduction to occupation: The art and science of living* (2nd ed.) (pp. 81–99). Upper Saddle River, New Jersey: Prentice Hall.

Johnson, R., Floyd, M., Pilling, D., et al. (2009). Service users' perceptions of the effective ingredients in supported employment. *Journal of Mental Health*, 18(2), 121–128.

Joint Commissioning Panel for Mental Health. (2016). *Guidance for commissioners of rehabilitation services for people with complex mental health needs*. London: Royal College of Psychiatrists.

Kirsh, B., & Gewurtz, R. (2012). Promoting mental health within workplaces. In R. J. Gatchel, & I. Z. Schultz (Eds.), *Handbook of occupational health and wellness* (pp. 243–265). Springer.

Kirsh, B., Stergiou-Kita, M., Gewurtz, R., Didredre, D., Krupa, T., & Shaw, L. (2009). From margins to mainstream: What do we know about work integration for persons with brain injury, mental illness and intellectual disability? *Work*, 32(4), 391–405.

Krupa, T. (2004). Employment, recovery, and schizophrenia: Integrating health and disorder at work. *Psychiatric Rehabilitation Journal*, 28(1), 8–15.

Krupa, T. (2011). Employment and serious mental health disabilities. In Schultz, I.Z (Ed.), *Work accommodation and retention in mental health* (pp. 91–101). Rogers, E.S: Springer.

Krupa, T., Lagarde, M., & Carmichael, K. (2003). Transforming sheltered workshops into affirmative businesses: An outcome evaluation. *Psychiatric Rehabilitation Journal*, 26(4), 359–367.

Krupa, T., Lagarde, M., Carmichael, K., Hougham, B., & Stewart, H. (1998). Stress, coping and the job search process: The experience of people with psychiatric disabilities in supported employment. *Work*, 11(2), 155–162.

Latimer, E., Bordeleau, F., Methot, C., et al. (2019). Implementation of supported employment in the context of a national Canadian program: Facilitators, barriers and strategies. *Psychiatric Rehabilitation Journal*. https://doi.org/10.1037/prj0000355. [Epub].

Lee, J., & Kielhofner, G. (2010). Vocational intervention based on the model of human occupation: A review of evidence. *Scandinavian Journal of Occupational Therapy*, 17(3), 177–190.

Lexén, A., Hofgren, C., & Bejerholm, U. (2013). Reclaiming the worker role: perceptions of people with mental illness participating in IPS. *Scandinavian journal of occupational therapy*, 20(1), 54–63. https://doi.org/10.3109/11038128.2012.693946.

Lloyd, C. (2010). Evidence-based supported employment. In C. Lloyd (Ed.), *Vocational rehabilitation andmental health* (pp. 19–32). Chichester: Wiley-Blackwell.

Lohss, I., Forsyth, K., & Kottorp, A. (2012). Psychometric properties of the worker role interview (version 10.0) in mental health. *British Journal of Occupational Therapy*, 75(4), 171–179.

Mandiberg, J. M. (2012). The failure of social inclusion: An alternative approach through community development. *Psychiatric Services*, 63(5), 458–460.

McQueen, J. M., & Turner, J. (2012). Exploring forensic mental health service users' views on work: An interpretative phenomenological analysis. *British Journal of Forensic Practice*, 14(3), 168–179.

Mental Health Foundation. (2016). *Added value. Mental health as a workplace asset*. Available at: https://www.mentalhealth.org.uk/publications/added-value-mental-health-workplace-asset.

Modini, M. (2016). Supported employment for people with severe mental illness: Systematic review and meta-analysis of the international evidence. *British Journal of Psychiatry*, 209(1), 14–22.

Moore-Corner, R., Kielhofner, G., & Olsen, L. (1989). *A user's guide to Work Environment Impact Scale (WEIS) version 2.0. Model of human occupation clearinghouse, department of occupational therapy, college of applied health sciences*. Chicago: University of Illinois at Chicago.

Munoz-Murillo, A., Esteban, E., Avila, C. C., et al. (2018). Furthering the evidence of the effectiveness of employment strategies for people with mental disorders in europe: A systematic review. *International Journal of Environmental Research and Public Health*, 15, 838.

Murphy, A. A., Mullen, M. G., & Spagnolo, A. B. (2005). Enhancing individual placement and support: Promoting job tenure by integrating natural supports and supported education. *American Journal of Psychiatric Rehabilitation, 8*(1), 37–61.

Nicholson, J., Carpenter-Song, E. A., MacPherson, L. H., et al. (2017). Developing the workingwell mobile app to promote job tenure for individuals with serious mental illnesses. *Psychiatric Rehabilitation Journal, 40*(3), 276–282.

Noyes, S., Sokolow, H., & Arbesman, M. (2018). Evidence for occupational therapy intervention with employment and education for adults with serious mental illness: A systematic review. *American Journal of Occupational Therapy, 72,* 7205190010. https://doi.org/10.5014/ajot.2018.033068.

Organisation for Economic Co-operation and Development (OECD). (2012). Sick on the Job? Myths and Realities about Mental Health and Work, OECD Publishing, Paris, https://doi.org/10.1787/9789264124523-en.

Ostrow, L., Nemec, P., & Smith, C. (2018). Self-employment for people with psychiatric disabilities: Advantages and strategies. *Journal of Behavioral Health Services & Research.* https://doi.org/10.1007/s11414-018-9625-8.

Ostrow, L., Smith, C., Penney, D., & Shumway, M. (2019). "It suits my needs": Self –employed individuals with psychiatric disabilities and small businesses. *Psychiatric Rehabilitation Journal, 42*(2), 121–131.

Perkins, R., Farmer, P., & Litchfield, P. (2009). *Realising ambitions: Better employment support for people with a mental health condition. A review to government. Department of work and pensions.* London.

Perkins, R., Meddings, S., Williams, S., & Repper, J. (2018). *Recovery colleges 10 Years on.* Nottingham: ImROC.

Ringeisen, H., Langer Ellison, M., Ryder-Burge, A., Biebel, K., Alikhan, S., & Jones, E. (2017). Supported education for individuals with psychiatric disabilities: State of the practice and policy implications. *Psychiatric Rehabilitation Journal, 40*(2), 197.

Ross, M. (2007). *Vocational rehabilitation and occupational therapy.* Chichester, West Sussex: Wiley & Sons Ltd.

Royal College of Occupational Therapists (RCOT). (2017). *Professional standards for occupational therapy practice.* London: College of Occupational Therapists.

Roy, L., Vallee, C., Kirsh, B., Marshall, C., Marval, R., Low, A., 2017. Occupation-based practices and homelessness: A scoping review. *Canadian Journal of Occupational Therapy, 84*(2), 98–110. http://journals.sagepub.com/doi/full/10.1177/0008417416688709.

Roy, M. J., Donaldson, C., Baker, R., & Kerr, S. (2014). The potential of social enterprise to enhance health and well-being: A model and systematic review. *Social Science & Medicine.* https://doi.org/10.1016/j.socscimed.2014.07.031.

Rudnick, A., & Gover, M. (2009). Frontline report: Combining supported education with supported employment. *Psychiatric Services, 60*(12), 1690.

Sainsbury Centre for Mental Health. (2009). *Delivering job retention services. A knowledge and skills set for employment advisory services located in primary care settings. Sainsbury Centre for Mental Health.* London.

Schneider, J. (2005). Getting back to work: What do we know about what works? In B. Grove, J. Secker, & P. Seebohm (Eds.), *New thinking about mental health and employment. Radcliffe publishing ltd* (pp. 37–49) Abingdon.

Scotland, N. H. S. (2011). *Realizing potential. An action plan for allied health professionals in mental health.* Edinburgh: Scottish Government.

Shaw, L., & Sumsion, T. (2009). There is so much more to do: Strategies and research needs to support work transitions for persons with chronic mental health conditions. *Work, 33*(4), 377–379.

Slade, M. (2009). *Personal recovery and mental illness: A guide for mental health professionals.* Cambridge: Cambridge University Press.

Stickley, A., & Hall, K. (2017). Social enterprise: A model of recovery and social inclusion for occupational therapy practice in the UK. *Mental Health and Social Inclusion, 21*(2), 91–101.

Svanberg, J., Gumley, A., & Wilson, A. (2010). How do social firms contribute to recovery from mental illness? A qualitative study. *Clinical Psychology & Psychotherapy, 17*(6), 482–496.

Taylor, R. R. (Ed.). (2017). *Kielhofner's model of human occupation: Theory and application* (5th ed.) Philadelphia: Wolters Kluwer Health.

Time to Change. (2012). Children & young peoples programme development. *Summary of Research and Insights London.* Available at: www.time-to-change.org.uk.

Townsend, E. A., & Polatajko, H. J. (2007). *Enabling occupation II: Advancing an occupational therapy vision for health, well-being, and justice through occupation.* Ottawa: CAOT Publications ACE.

United Nations (UN) General Assembly. (1948). *Universal declaration of human rights.* Available at: https://www.un.org/en/universal-declaration-human-rights/.

United Nations (UN) General Assembly. (1966). *International covenant on economic, social and cultural rights, 16 December 1966. United Nations: Treaty Series. 3,* 993. Available at: https://www.refworld.org.

United Nations (UN) General Assembly. (2006). *Convention on the Rights of Persons with Disabilities (CRPD).* Available at: https://www.un.org/development/desa/disabilities/convention-on-the-rights-of-persons-with-disabilities.html.

Van Niekerk, L. (2009). Participation in work: A source of wellness for people with psychiatric disability. *Work, 32*(4), 455–465.

Vorhies, V., Davis, K. E., Frounfelker, R. L., & Kaiser, S. M. (2012). Applying social and cultural capital frameworks: Understanding employment perspectives of transition age youth with serious mental health conditions. *The Journal of Behavioral Health Services & Research, 39*(3), 257–270.

Vorspan, R. (1992). Why work works. *Psychosocial Rehabilitation Journal, 16*(2), 49–54.

Waddell, G., & Burton, K. (2006). *Is work good for your health and wellbeing?* London: Her Majesty's Stationery Office.

Waghorn, G., Chant, D., Lloyd, C., & Harris, M. (2011). Earning and learning among australian community residents with psychiatric disorders. *Psychiatry Research, 186*(1), 109–116.

Waghorn, G. R., Collister, L., & Killackey, E. (2007). Challenges to implementing evidence-based supported employment in Australia. *Journal of Vocational Rehabilitation, 27,* 29–37.

Waghorn, G., Killackey, E., Dickson, P., Brock, L., & Skate, C. (2020). Evidence-based supported employment for people with psychiatric disabilities in Australia: Progress in the past 15 years. *Psychiatric Rehabilitation Journal, 43*(1), 32–39. https://doi.org/10.1037/prj0000370.

Wagman, P., Hakansson, C., & Bjorklund, A. (2012). Occupational balance as used in occupational therapy: A concept analysis. *Scandinavian Journal of Occupational Therapy, 19*(4), 322–327.

Warner, R. (2004). *Recovery from schizophrenia: Psychiatry and political economy* (3rd ed.). London: Routledge.

Wilcock, A. A. (2001). *A journey from prescription to self health. Occupation for health.* (Vol. 2). London: College of Occupational Therapists.

Williams, A. E., Fossey, E., Corbiere, M., Paluch, T., & Harvey, C. (2016). Work participation for people with severe mental illnesses: An integrative review of factors impacting job tenure. *Australian Occupational Therapy Journal, 63,* 65–85.

Williams, A. E., Fossey, E., & Harvey, C. (2010). Sustaining employment in a social firm: Use of the work environment impact scale v.2.0 to explore views of employees with psychiatric disabilities. *British Journal of Occupational Therapy, 73*(11), 531–539.

Wolf, J., Lawrence, L. H., Ryan, P. M., & Hoge, M. A. (2010). Emerging practices in employment of persons in recovery in the mental health workforce. *American Journal of Psychiatric Rehabilitation, 13*(3), 189–207.

Section 5

PEOPLE AND SETTINGS

21

THE ACUTE SETTING

KATHERINE L. SIMS

INTRODUCTION

In many places people with mental health problems are supported at home when their mental state deteriorates. However, there will always be some who are admitted to a unit in a hospital for a period of inpatient treatment. In this chapter the word 'treatment' is used to refer to the hospital setting, where the focus is on acute symptoms and difficulties addressed by a multidisciplinary team (MDT). Within this setting there is a clear role for occupational therapy and the use of occupation for assessment and intervention. Focusing on an individual's strengths to support their return to occupational function is an important component of recovery from an acute episode.

This chapter starts with some essential information about the acute setting, followed by an analysis of how services are changing in response to the continued development of community mental health services. The staff and others working in acute units are described, followed by brief explanations of relevant legislation, which may impact their work. Specific considerations for occupational therapy are then discussed in terms of the occupational therapy process, indicating the importance of building rapport and assessment. Working with groups and individuals prevents relapse and promotes recovery and social inclusion. Following this, the occupational therapy role in the psychiatric intensive care unit (PICU) is briefly explored. Finally two case examples are used to illustrate and summarize occupational therapy in the acute setting.

An Acute Episode

An acute episode of mental ill-health is characterized by symptoms that may affect a person's cognitive processes, beliefs, perceptions and behaviour. There may be a sudden onset of symptoms or a gradual deterioration leading to admission. There is increasing recognition of the role that trauma has in contributing to mental ill-health. This may be just one event or a series of events that reduces a person's ability to cope (Sweeney et al. 2016). Within any acute unit there will be a diverse population with many different diagnoses, including severe depression, bipolar affective disorder, psychosis, drug-induced psychosis, schizophrenia and personality disorders. It is important to remember that this is often a very distressing time for the service user and their family and friends. Any member of staff working in an acute setting will have a responsibility to support all involved and offer reassurance.

The Environment

An acute mental health unit serves the local population and largely reflects the ethnicities and cultures in the community. The unit has gender-specific wards or areas within a ward. A modern purpose-built unit may have individual rooms and ensuite faculties to maintain dignity and privacy. Some have an occupational therapy department with facilities such as group rooms, kitchen, computer access, art room and a gym (Birkin and Bryant 2019). There may be designated areas on the ward for activity. Wards are staffed by registered mental health nurses who work with support staff. The built environment is important as a therapeutic space that is clean and welcoming. All staff is responsible for ensuring that environmental standards are maintained and problems are reported. Acute units are smoke-free, meaning smoking is not allowed anywhere on site. Local policies determine how people on the unit can safely access places where smoking is permitted. Support is given in the form of nicotine replacement therapy and smoking cessation sessions. This approach supports the physical health of service users acknowledges the high rate of smoking in people with mental health issues and meets the current guidance by the National Institute for Health and Care Excellence (NICE) (NICE 2021).

Maintaining Dignity and Privacy

When someone is admitted to an acute unit, they may behave in a way that is unusual for them. They may be verbally abusive or aggressive, sexually disinhibited or emotionally labile, lacking control of their emotions. It is therefore important that both the environment and staff support an individual in maintaining their dignity and privacy and help them to keep safe. This may be as simple as knocking on a bedroom door before entering, supporting someone in being appropriately dressed and listening to someone's concerns (Chambers et al. 2014).

THE CHANGING NATURE OF ACUTE SERVICES

Prolonged inpatient admissions of months or years are now avoided for many people. As mental health services have evolved and community services have developed and diversified (see Chapters 22), acute settings have become more focused on minimizing the duration of a person's stay.

More Acuity

People on an acute unit will be very unwell with treatment aimed at stabilizing them for discharge to community services for longer-term work (NHS England 2016). The emphasis is on admission as a last resort when all other options are no longer considered appropriate, effective or safe. Admission to an acute unit may be legally enforced, for example in England and Wales under the Mental Health Act (2007), when people are deemed to be a risk to themselves or others and do not agree to be admitted to the hospital voluntarily. If they are admitted under the Mental Health Act, they are said to be 'under' or 'on section' referring to the different sections of the act (see below).

Substance Misuse

Another change in the population profile is the increase in dual diagnosis. This is where a mental health service user also uses illicit drugs and/or alcohol. Due to their vulnerability people with mental health problems can be at increased risk of substance misuse. This may be a way of managing their symptoms, coping with social isolation or due to being targeted by those who perceive and exploit their vulnerability. Occupational therapists in an acute setting will need to know about substance misuse and the impact on mental health and recovery. They will also need to have an awareness of the local substance misuse services and seek advice and training accordingly.

Austerity

Austerity measures implemented as a result of the global financial crisis and also recent changes to the benefits system in the United Kingdom may have contributed to increased impacts on mental health and well-being (Stuckler et al. 2017). This may be due to unemployment, financial hardships, loss of social support and/or homelessness. Occupational therapists working with people in acute crisis may therefore find multiple factors contributing to the situation. With complex situations, agreeing priorities for occupational therapy will be important.

Shorter Admissions/Community Support

In acute care the aim is for admission to be as short as possible, with early discharge being made easier with community support. The development of crisis teams and similar services has supported shorter admissions (NHS England 2016), which limits the time available

for occupational therapists on acute units to provide a service. This means having a flexible working attitude as well as being able to work under pressure. There may be a requirement for working out of regular office hours, in the evenings and at weekends. These attitudes and approaches enhance the response of occupational therapy services to the changing needs of service users and the unit as a whole. Assessments need to be completed quickly. However, the focus needs also to be on good-quality care, maintaining the person-centred philosophy of occupational therapy. A good knowledge of the local community and its resources is also required to ensure appropriate provision of information and onward referral.

THE BROADER CONTEXT FOR ACUTE SERVICES

Occupational therapists consider the broader context for acute services partly to provide information and onward referral to other services. The broader context also shapes the focus of occupational therapy depending on the person's situation and needs, reflecting the resources available. Current organizational and multidisciplinary approaches to service delivery and care pathways also form part of the broader context.

Bed Management

The reduction of inpatient beds in mental health units in the United Kingdom has meant that there is an ongoing need to manage bed use as effectively as possible (NHS England 2016). This ongoing need is due to both the cost of inpatient services and the understanding that hospital is not always the best place for people to receive treatment. The management of beds is often led by a bed manager specifically employed for this purpose. Occupational therapists, as a part of the MDT, need to be involved in this daily task. This may include attending meetings, contributing to care plans, undertaking home visits, actively supporting discharge plans and assisting people to be aware of, and gain access to, community resources. Decisions are often made quickly, and the occupational therapy team has to be responsive whilst supporting safe discharge. Clear and effective communication is vital including to the service user and any carers or family. Links with statutory and voluntary organizations and charities ensure robust community support. There may also be practical issues that need addressing with the service user and their families to support safe and effective discharge.

Sensory Integration

While an inpatient, people may find it difficult being in a restricted environment with other people who are very unwell. One way of addressing this difficulty is to consider individual sensory needs. This is recognized as a focus for occupational therapy in many fields using sensory integration (Scanlan and Novak 2015). This approach starts with an assessment of how a person processes sensory input, which is then developed or inhibited using a variety of techniques. Sensory integration is an area in acute mental health that is increasingly being led by occupational therapists. It can be provided in a graded way depending on resources and the environment. One format is the provision of individual sensory boxes that people can use in times of distress. Some wards may have sensory rooms which provide a safe space for people to de-escalate. These rooms support them in managing emotions of anger or thoughts of self-harm.

Preparing for Discharge

Early discharge is encouraged once a person has recovered from an acute phase and is no longer a risk to themselves or others. Occupational therapy supports preparation for discharge in many ways, for example with functional assessments, home assessments, linking with community services, and employment advice. Due to the limited time available for inpatient occupational therapy, work may be completed in the community after discharge as part of an outreach service. This is not always possible, but the advantage is that the person continues to work with a familiar member of staff and is supported through the vulnerable stage of transition.

Community Services

Admission to a unit, while sometimes necessary, can be a disempowering and frightening experience for people. Treatment in a home environment, if possible and appropriate, is preferred. There are cost implications of acute inpatient care so alternatives to admission within the community are favoured (NHS England 2016). These community services are described in detail in Chapter 22 and it is important for occupational therapists in acute settings to know what they offer. Many people are supported by community mental health team. Crisis and home treatment teams aim to prevent admission in acute phases. These teams may work in partnership with community mental health teams for enhanced support in the short term. People experiencing psychosis for the first time may receive services from an early intervention team. If admission is required, some mental health services operate a triage ward. Triage is an intensive process aiming to assess, stabilize, and determine the best course of action for a person in an emergency or crisis situation. Triage wards are highly staffed, with very regular team reviews to clarify the need for admission and promote early discharge.

Self-Management

People with severe and enduring mental health problems will be encouraged by all the MDT to learn about self-management, which has been described by Lean et al. (2019) as:

> *the provision of information and education on a condition and its treatment, collaboratively creating an individualized treatment plan, developing skills for self-monitoring symptoms and strategies to support adherence to treatment including medication, psychological techniques, lifestyle and social support.*
>
> *Lean et al. 2019, p. 260*

Many aspects of occupational therapy in an acute setting will support self-management in individual and group work.

Well-Being and Resilience

Supporting well-being and building resilience is an essential part of recovery and contributes to maintaining good mental health. Well-being can be seen as an outcome of engagement in occupation (Wilcock 2006), so people can experience a sense of well-being by participating in occupational therapy. Ayed et al. (2018) suggest that resilience is understood in two ways in mental health research and practice. First, resilience can be seen as a characteristic shaped by personal and social resources. People who are acutely unwell may use their resilience to support their recovery if they are well resourced personally and socially. Second, resilience can be seen as a process. People lacking resilience in acute settings may not have much capacity to endure difficult circumstances. However, by engaging in occupational therapy they will have an opportunity to overcome their difficulties by building their resilience or capacity to cope (Ayed et al. 2018). This can be achieved with the support of a variety of approaches (See Chapters 4 and 6).

The Use of Apps and Websites

Increasingly, people are choosing to access online resources as a way of seeking information and supporting recovery. There is a wide variety of such resources including websites, specialist organizations and support groups, blogs, chat rooms and apps. Whilst many people have access to smartphones, this is not always the case, and occupational therapists have a role to play in supporting access and providing instruction if required. Guidance can be provided as to which online resources are considered the most helpful and useful for an individual, keeping this information up to date. Accessing online resources encourages self-management and provides people with help that they can access at any time. Choosing and trying online resources can empower people to take more control of their own recovery. Online resources can also be a useful addition in groups, individual work and information leaflets.

Issues can arise when people do not have access to these resources either through lack of Information Technology knowledge or access to equipment. Supporting people to access training and be made aware of local internet cafes or libraries is helpful. It is always important to remember that not all the material accessed online is helpful and supportive. Enabling and guiding people to access the most useful information and chat rooms will prevent difficulties arising.

Carers

Carers are defined as anyone who supports a service user. Some services use the word 'supporter' rather than 'carer.' This may not be a family member but a close friend, work colleague or neighbour. An occupational therapist may have contact when carers visit the ward, at a home visit or when gathering information to inform a intervention plan. Carers have specific needs and concerns that require consideration. The period leading up to admission may have been very stressful and distressing for a carer. Awareness of the impact of this period can enable occupational therapists to signpost carers to local assessments, groups and other sources of support, to prepare for discharge.

People may not want their carers to be involved in their admission or discharge planning, which requires a sensitive approach from all staff. It is important to remember that it is still possible to listen to a carer's point of view and experience without breaching confidentiality. This can be done by listening but not providing any information if permission from the service user has not been given (see also Chapter 9). If a person gives permission for staff to contact their carer, then a systematic approach to planning should be undertaken, particularly at the stage of discharge. This approach considers those involved in an individual's life as part of a complete system so that changes in one area will affect everyone in different ways, with many implications for future plans. Occupational therapists may also be involved in the education and support of carers by providing information, by promoting carer assessments and sometimes by facilitating support groups for carers.

Service User and Carer Involvement

Collaborative work with service users and their carers is valued by mental health services and has many forms, such as the formal care programme approach (CPA) (See Chapter 22). Other forms of collaborative work include risk assessment, service user evaluations, audit and research and relapse prevention (Bryant et al. 2016). Collaboration can often take place in meetings between the MDT, service users and carers. Even when someone appears very unwell, person-centred practice is an approach used at all stages of the occupational therapy process (see chapter 4). Providing choice, considering needs and planning collaborative care are essential (Department of Health (DH) 2009).

Coproduction

Coproduction is another way of involving service users, based on the belief that users, staff and others involved can work together on an equal basis to improve and design the services provided (Momori and Richards 2017) (see also Chapter 12). This may be undertaken while someone is currently on the unit, but also by inviting recently discharged people to take part and use their recent experiences. True coproduction takes longer, but the results are often more productive. This may include coproducing welcome packs and information leaflets and reviewing reception areas and notice boards on a regular basis. Service users are often involved in coproducing recovery and well-being colleges.

Recovery and Well-Being Colleges

In the United Kingdom recovery and well-being colleges offer an educational approach to providing information, guidance and self-help to a range of people. The resources for these colleges are coproduced in a collaborative process. This means that people with mental health problems contribute their lived experience as a resource, by leading sessions or influencing how the college develops (Meddings et al. 2014). This approach can be adapted for the inpatient setting with courses being made shorter and more 'bite-sized' whilst losing none of their principles of coproduction and codelivery. Courses can introduce people to the principles of recovery while inpatients can offer hope at a challenging time and can provide them with a useful resource once they are discharged.

Star Wards

Involving service users can have benefits beyond the individual. For example, the Star Wards UK initiative is a service user–led movement started by Marion Janner in 2006 to support the development of best practice and care on inpatient mental health wards (Star Wards 2006). The aim is to improve both the inpatient experience and outcomes. The information provided ranges from practical advice and suggestions through to publications and newsletters. Good practice and ideas are shared by staff and people on a website. There are many references to activities and occupation, and the website is a valuable resource and information tool for those working in acute setting (Star Wards Impact Review 2013).

Care Pathways

In the United Kingdom an acute service has a care pathway, which outlines the care through admission, treatment and discharge (Leading Change, Adding Value Team 2019). It gives an indication of what will happen, when and by whom. This is multidisciplinary but each profession, including occupational therapy, may have its own parallel care pathway. Current guidelines and evidence are used to write care pathways to promote the most appropriate and effective interventions (Fig. 21.1).

STAFFING

In an acute unit the MDT can consist of medical staff, nurses, occupational therapists, pharmacists, psychologists, social workers, arts psychotherapists, support staff and community staff (NHS England 2017). Good teamwork is essential, often indicated by effective communication in team meetings and informally. Some units have psychiatrists (medical consultants) who work across inpatients and the community in specific areas, treating the same people, regardless of whether they are an inpatient or not. However, in some units there is a functional split with inpatient consultants and community consultants.

Therapy Services

Therapy services in acute settings are provided by a team which could include support staff, peer support workers, activity coordinators, other therapy staff and teachers, technicians and volunteers. Each team varies in its skills mix and level of staffing, depending on the size of the unit, needs of the people and funding provided (NHS England 2017).

Support staff assist occupational therapists in delivering occupational therapy. This may be by cofacilitating groups or by undertaking specific individual work under guidance. Peer support workers use their own experience of mental health issues and services to share hope and communicate that recovery is possible. This experience is known as 'lived experience' in many services. Activity coordinators provide activities for groups or individuals, often in the evenings or at weekends in the ward settings. Other therapy staff include arts therapists, such as art psychotherapists, drama therapists, music therapists and dance and movement

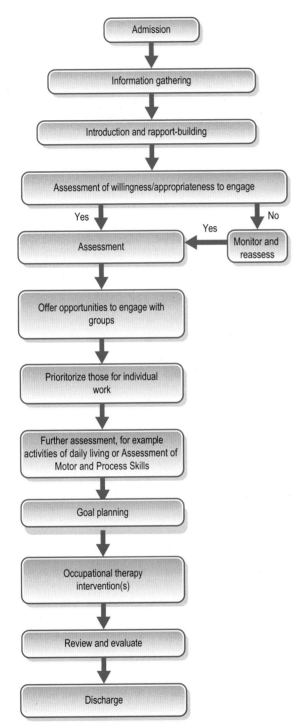

Fig. 21.1 ■ **Care pathway.**

therapists. They contribute their own specific skills to the service and work alongside occupational therapists to enhance the therapeutic milieu. Other teachers and technicians may be present, particularly on a sessional basis, providing a specific resource to the service (for example, yoga teachers, T'ai Chi instructors and sports technicians). Coordinating therapy services for an individual and liaising about their progress with other members of the team is an important aspect of occupational therapy in this setting.

Support and Supervision

It is generally acknowledged that those working in acute care face particular stresses (Scanlan and Still 2013) not only due to the fast pace of work and high turnover of service users, but also because mental health problems can be presented in a very distressing way. Presentation refers to how people appear, behave and communicate: they may be behaving unusually, responding to voices, self-harming and/or be suicidal. Some people have distressing histories with sexual abuse or neglect. It is particularly important that staff or students who are new to the acute setting have opportunities to discuss their emotional response to their work. All staff should have access to informal support and formal supervision. This is usually provided on an individual basis with a named supervisor but may also be part of the team's processes. Some teams have access to group supervision with an external supervisor. This enables the staff to discuss challenges and issues within their working practice and problem-solve together (Ashby and Ryan 2012).

Volunteers, Peer Support Workers and Advocates

Volunteers can have many roles, including providing activities and organising visits. Those who have experienced mental health problems themselves can provide specific insights into the user experience and offer support and hope to others. For staff development, volunteers can provide insight into direct experiences of mental health issues and services. Others may use their own personal or direct experience to inform their role as an employed peer support worker. They work as part of the staff group and facilitate groups or undertake individual work under the direction and supervision of qualified staff. They may be based on a ward or in an occupational therapy department. (Peer support is also discussed in Chapters 10 and 12.)

Every setting has access to advocacy services for comments and complaints. Awareness of how these services work enables occupational therapists to provide appropriate support and guidance to service users and carers, particularly, as many individuals may have been admitted involuntarily. Advocacy services include patient advice and liaison services, independent mental health advocates and independent mental health capacity advocates.

LEGISLATION

Many people are compulsorily admitted to an acute unit because they are seriously unwell, although they may not have insight into the severity of their problems. The power to detain people for treatment for mental health problems is subject to legal constraints to prevent human rights abuses. Sharing the outcomes of occupational therapy is essential for informing decisions about a person's legal status on an acute unit. In the United Kingdom relevant legislation is concerned with mental health, mental capacity and safeguarding; and English laws are discussed here briefly. The Department of Health and Social Care (2018, 2021) is consulting on reform of the Mental Health Act (2007), following an independent review.

The Mental Health Act 2007

The Mental Health Act 2007 is used to detain (or 'section') a person in a place of safety if they are considered to be a danger to themselves or others. This may be for an assessment period or for assessment and treatment, depending on which section of the act is used to justify their detention (Rethink Mental Illness 2011). For example, Section 4 allows detention for up to 72 hours for assessment, whereas Section 3 allows detention for up to six months for treatment. It is usual for an acute unit to care for people under a section of the Mental Health Act while others are there on a voluntary or 'informal' basis. Those people 'on section' will have limitations placed on their movements, particularly with regard to leaving the unit, which has implications for participation in occupational therapy. They may be able to leave the unit if they have Section 17 leave, which has to be signed for by their consultant psychiatrist. This enables someone to leave the unit either with or without a staff member for a specified amount of time. It is therefore essential that the occupational therapist is aware if someone is on a section and what the relevant restrictions are. Sections can be lifted or imposed at any time, so close liaison is required with ward staff.

Mental Capacity Act 2005

The Mental Capacity Act 2005 prevents decisions being taken on behalf of people without justification. Everyone is assumed to have mental capacity to consent unless it is established by the MDT that the individual lacks such capacity. In acute settings lack of capacity is usually a temporary state during the acute phase of illness. A person may lack capacity to make some decisions but have capacity to make others. Any staff working within an acute unit may at times have to make decisions on behalf of a person when they are very unwell, but wherever possible the person must be supported to make their own decisions.

Under the Mental Capacity Act 2005, Deprivation of Liberty Safeguards were introduced to protect people in care homes and hospitals from being inappropriately deprived of their liberty. However, they do not apply if someone is detained under the Mental Health Act but would for informal or voluntary patients.

Safeguarding Vulnerable Groups Act 2006

To protect vulnerable people, legislation was introduced to enforce vetting of employees for previous criminal activity and require staff to raise any concerns they might have about the safety of others. Safeguarding seeks to ensure that no vulnerable adult or child is exploited or harmed by others. This includes physical, sexual, financial and emotional abuse. All staff, whether qualified or otherwise, have a duty of care to the vulnerable adults they work with. Mental health services have a safeguarding lead and staff need to inform them if they have a safeguarding concern. This includes any safeguarding concerns regarding children that may be in the family.

OCCUPATIONAL THERAPY PROCESS

The process of providing occupational therapy follows a pattern (see Chapter 4) to ensure that the service provided is based on the best available information and adapted to meet individual needs and goals. In the acute setting this process may be completed within a very short time period. Due to rapid changes in presentation of a person, any assessment process will often be completed quickly. Deciding in advance which people have priority because of their needs will enable an occupational therapist to provide interventions effectively. These priorities are usually defined in an occupational therapy care pathway.

Referral and Information Gathering

Occupational therapists often have a blanket referral system in acute settings, which means that all the people admitted to the unit have access to an occupational therapist. This system has the advantage that the occupational therapist makes the decision as to who is appropriate to receive services. Collaborative work with the MDT is required to ensure that colleagues understand the occupational therapy role and that occupational therapy is aligned with other interventions.

All assessments follow a process of information gathering from records held by the unit and others such as care coordinators, nurses and carers. Information can also be obtained by an occupational therapist introducing themselves to the service user to build rapport. However, the person may be too unwell for the assessment process to be taken further at this stage. In this situation the occupational therapist would monitor their progress on a regular basis, judging when it would be best to resume the assessment process.

Rapport Building

Rapport building could continue as part of this monitoring stage and could involve the occupational therapist simply making short daily interactions with the person so that they become familiar with them. Sitting and chatting to a person may appear casual, but the occupational therapist will be observing and assessing their mental state, concentration, motivation, orientation and communications skills. All this will inform the occupational therapist when to move onto a more formal assessment process and introduce activity. Services users newly admitted to a ward may be frightened, disorientated, confused and withdrawn. It is vital for the occupational therapist to become a familiar and reassuring presence to build a collaborative therapeutic relationship with a person (Lim et al. 2007).

Risk Assessment

A robust risk assessment is always a priority for people admitted to an acute unit, because of their vulnerability (see also Chapter 5). There is an MDT risk assessment with different levels of observations for each person. Some may be on close observation, which means they are at risk and within sight of a staff member at all times. However, service user presentations change rapidly and someone who was on close observation due to risk one day might be significantly improved the next day and able to engage with the occupational therapist. Similarly, someone who is engaging well might deteriorate quickly and then be unable to leave the ward. Effective communication between team members is essential to maintain safe practice.

To keep themselves and others safe, the occupational therapist follows safeguarding procedures to be aware of risks from forensic history, substance misuse or history of violence. Staff may be required to wear personal alarms. Judging whether or not someone can leave the ward environment or go into the community is usually an MDT decision. Certain activities that involve sharp implements or other potentially self-harming equipment, such as kitchen knives, may need to be restricted. There are local procedures regarding sharps and hazardous equipment which should be followed, such as locking up procedures to ensure safety and minimize risk.

Positive risk management is often a part of discussions within the MDT, with the carers and the person themself. This is to ensure that, while risk is minimized as much as possible, the person is supported to take responsibility for their own safety whenever possible (see also Chapter 22).

Assessment

The occupational therapist has a significant contribution to make within the overall MDT assessment of a person. This includes having an occupational focus that identifies strengths as well as areas needing development. Occupational therapists can contribute a unique perspective on a person's occupational performance, function and engagement (see chapter 2). Most importantly, this will also include the person's own views on their strengths and areas needing development and support. Assessment takes place through both individual and group work and may also be focused on activities of daily living (ADL). The occupational therapist also considers a person's physical health needs and addresses these as appropriate.

Assessment is discussed in detail in Chapter 5. One example of a standardized occupational therapy assessment that may be used within an acute unit is the model of human occupation screening tool (MOHOST). This is an observational tool that assesses motivation of occupation, pattern of occupation, communication and interaction skills, process skills, motor skills and the environment (Taylor 2017). Assessment enables collaborative planning of intervention goals and outcomes. Case formulation, following assessment, directs the therapist's aims for an intervention. Assessments can be re-administered and used as an outcome measure (See Chapters 4-6).

Function

Occupational therapists may often be required to assess a person's function or ability to do specific activities or tasks, for example, their ability to organize washing their own clothes. This functional assessment may take place in the unit or the person's home to inform decisions about their capacity for returning home or the need for a care package or alternative placement. Their previous accommodation could be unsuitable, unavailable, unsafe or not meeting their needs. The occupational therapy assessment of function will be essential in contributing to the decision made. It could involve assessment of self-care and domestic functioning, mobility, safety and risk, as well as the home environment itself.

Physical Health

Enduring mental ill-health is associated with increased vulnerability to other health problems, including being physically frail due to age, neglect or substance misuse. Assessing and meeting the physical health needs of service users is now a requirement of services. People with long-term and severe mental health problems have a reduced life expectancy, because they are more likely to have other health problems, for example, related to smoking. Historically, mental health services have not addressed these problems effectively, and other health services have not adapted to meet the specific needs of people with multiple health problems. Occupational therapy knowledge and skills can be used to assess physical health needs in an acute mental health service, reflecting a holistic approach to care. Occupational therapists may need to assess for assistive equipment items and order, fit and instruct in their use. It is therefore essential that occupational therapists maintain and develop their knowledge and skills to address functional problems arising from physical impairments. Occupational therapists also provide assessment and interventions to promote and support people's physical health and well-being (see chapter 14). This might be through the process of 'making every contact count' (Public Health England 2016) and looking at exercise, diet, sleep, alcohol and drug use, smoking and general well-being. The assessment process, groups or 1:1 interventions should meet this need.

Communication

Good communication is the key to building rapport and forming positive therapeutic relationships. Within an acute unit people may be disorientated, confused and frightened. Their admission may have been traumatic and they find themselves in an unfamiliar environment. When service users are very unwell, they may not be able to retain information or comprehend what is being said to them. They may not share a common language to communicate verbally with occupational therapists.

In this setting, occupational therapists are creative and communicate through a variety of media. This may include written information, information boards, leaflets, pictures, community meetings, individual verbal reminders and using interpreters (Parkinson 1999). They may have to repeat information many times and spend time orientating people to their surroundings and unit routines. Reassurance, support and maintaining hope are key within this process. It is important to remember that, even though very unwell, people often have a memory of interactions with staff when they recover, even if they do not appear at the time to comprehend what is said to them. Staff and students reflect on how it must feel to be very unwell in an unfamiliar setting and remember it is vital to treat someone with dignity and respect at all times (NICE 2021).

Goal Planning And Intervention

Occupational therapy in the acute setting often focuses on specific skills in individual and/or group sessions, aiming to prepare for discharge, prevent relapse and promote recovery and social inclusion. Sometimes the assessment and intervention will merge as a person progresses quickly. In contrast, following assessment, careful goal planning may be required for an intervention, such as confidence building within a cooking skills group.

Occupation

The main medium used for both assessment and intervention is occupation (Wimpenny et al. 2014). The overall aim is to enable a person to identify their occupational goals and maintain skills, regaining those lost and returning to a level of occupational functioning for a safe discharge (see chapter 6). They may also learn new skills to sustain their recovery. Because of the limited time available, the occupational therapist needs to establish strong working links with community services to refer the person on for continued work, if appropriate (see Chapter 23).

Occupational therapy sessions are individual, group or a combination of both, taking into consideration individual skills and interest. Motivation may be an issue, requiring the occupational therapist to spend time encouraging and supporting a person to engage with occupational therapy. Group sessions include those that develop skills and support function (see Chapter 15), with a protocol that explains the function and aims as well as the process and evidence. Social and recreational groups are often provided by support workers, activity coordinators and volunteers, taking place in evenings and at weekends as well as during weekdays.

In an acute unit groups have to be flexible to accommodate those who are unwell. It is inappropriate to have very rigid boundaries, as any group has a fluctuating population and attendance from day to day. This requires great flexibility so that occupational therapists can facilitate and adapt the group according to the needs of the participants in the room. People who

are acutely unwell may have difficulties understanding and retaining information, so repetition is important.

The consideration of individual cultural and religious needs influence groups and individual work. Some people are unable or unwilling to participate in a group. There are also needs that can be addressed only through individual work. These can be identified through building rapport, assessment and identifying specific goals for intervention. Individual work might focus on confidence building, skills building, relapse prevention, seeking or returning to employment, structuring the day, re-engagement with community activities and identification of roles.

Relapse Prevention

For people with severe and enduring mental health problems, relapse prevention focuses on the reasons for the acute episode or triggers. These may be environmental, physical, circumstantial or emotional. Relapse prevention involves exploring what led up to the admission and what behaviours were associated with this time. The aim is to put support in place to prevent another acute episode. This process is led by the person themselves to produce a personal relapse prevention plan. The plan encourages recognition of relapse signatures (i.e., what a person recognizes as the behaviours and thoughts that indicate that they are becoming unwell) as well as what to do in a crisis, with important contact details for help and support.

It is important to explore relapse prevention to support people in their discharge and reduce or prevent future admissions. The acute setting can be a safe place to discuss what triggers led up to their current admission and what could be done differently next time to support them. Triggers could be times or situations such as an anniversary of a bereavement, forgetting medication or becoming physically unwell. Behaviours could be poor sleep patterns, withdrawal from family and friends or a decrease in self-care. Information about these triggers and behaviours might emerge during occupational therapy, where they are explored with the individual and then shared with the MDT as avoiding relapse is an important component of recovery.

Building resilience is also an important component of relapse prevention and supports people to build skills that will enable them to manage challenges and stresses in their lives (Echezarraga et al. 2019). Adverse life events are a part of life, and research suggests that, rather than avoiding events, it is more realistic to support people to build the skills to cope with them (Seery 2011). Occupational therapists can support this approach by confidence building through occupational engagement, social engagement to reduce isolation and specific skills building (e.g., relaxation and mindfulness skills training).

Recovery

Recovery does not necessarily mean a clinical recovery from illness itself. In mental health services it means recovery of a meaningful life, which will include occupation. This may be in the form of roles such as paid employment or parenting or activities (Perkins and Repper 2015). The focus is on instilling and sustaining hope, not on symptoms and limitations (see Chapters 4, 10 and 12). Service users going through an acute episode may experience a sense of hopelessness and low self-esteem and confidence. Supporting them to rebuild their sense of worth is a key role for occupational therapy. The person-centred approach of occupational therapy enables recovery principles to be practised within an acute unit. This may involve enabling choices to be made within a group, recognizing skills and roles, involving individuals in goal-setting and enabling them to participate in activities that promote and develop their interests (Kelly et al. 2010).

Community engagement is an important component of recovery. This is the process by which people engage with their community and services, including those that are mainstream services and available for everyone in the community (see Chapters 23 and 29). Using and getting involved with local community facilities and networks takes time but enables people to focus on their strengths and capacities. This may include employment and education, as well as attending religious services, using the local gym or going to adult education classes. All occupational therapists in the acute setting will develop a working knowledge of what is available within the community, so they can discuss this information with people and carers. This in turn will support the reduction of stigma of mental health.

Evaluation

Evaluation has two aspects: one is concerned with the person being treated by the occupational therapist and the other aspect is concerned with the quality of the service provided. Regarding the former, the occupational therapist refers back to the original assessment and evaluates whether the occupational goals have been achieved. The latter involves service evaluation, which is an essential part of any service delivery, as well as an opportunity to contribute to individual continuing professional development and the evidence base of the profession (Royal College of Occupational Therapists 2019) (see Chapters 7). Evaluation can take many forms, including audit, research and service user feedback. It is essential that occupational therapists take part in evaluation to meet both professional and service requirements. For commissioning purposes and at times of reorganization and redesign, the need for occupational therapy within acute care needs to be evidenced. This would also be of use when external evaluation of a service, for example by independent bodies such as the Care Quality Commission is undertaken.

PSYCHIATRIC INTENSIVE CARE UNIT

A PICU is commonly found within an adult acute unit and is a locked ward with a higher level of security and staffing. The people may be on court orders, from detention centres or unable to be safely managed on an adult acute ward. PICUs are often gender-specific, that is, either male or female.

Assessment and interventions with an occupational focus are similar in acute units and PICUs. The main difference is that the unit may be gender-specific, which needs to be considered for activity provision. The increased risk issues will inhibit what tools and equipment can be used, posing restrictions similar to those experienced by occupational therapists in forensic settings (see Chapter 27). The occupational therapist often works within the ward environment, and there are significant limitations on people being able to leave, with some being confined to the ward. Provision of a programme of varied activities is essential, requiring liaison with the ward and therapy teams.

CASE STUDIES

Case Studies 21.1 and 21.2 illustrate how a significant amount of recovery can be achieved in a limited time and the importance of awareness of risk.

CASE STUDY 21.1

Amir

Amir was a 22-year old man admitted on Section 2 of the Mental Health Act following an episode of psychosis. He was already known to mental health services, had been engaged with the Early Intervention service community mental health team for 2 years and had a diagnosis of drug-induced psychosis. Amir had been struggling to cope in his flat for some time. He was known to take his prescribed medication but also used cannabis on a regular basis. Amir was socially isolated in the community but did have contact with his sister and her family. On admission, on a Section 2, Amir presented as dishevelled and was responding actively to auditory hallucinations. He appeared frightened at times and spent a lot of time in his room.

The occupational therapist began to engage with Amir from the start of his admission. An increase in his medication enabled his psychotic symptoms to become less evident, which meant he was then able to engage in activities on the ward and attend the groups in the occupational therapy department. A need for increased support for Amir at home was quickly identified and acknowledged so, together with his care coordinator, the occupational therapist completed an activity of daily living assessment on a home visit. This was specifically to look at the home environment and Amir's ability to live independently.

There was a possibility that he required more supported accommodation. However, following the visit and in discussion with Amir and his care coordinator, returning home to his flat was the preferred option. Further discussion with Amir and his sister identified areas at home that he found more challenging, which included shopping, maintaining an adequate diet and keeping his environment clean. A request of a short-term care package was made following the occupational therapist recommendations.

Amir had engaged in the more physical based activities on the unit, and the occupational therapist provided him with information on local walking groups and a football group that he was keen to become involved in. There were discussions with his care coordinator as to how he could be supported to engage in these activities on discharge. His care coordinator had been working with him to possibly engage in further education courses at the local college, and these discussions continued with the occupational therapist. Amir expressed a desire to the occupational therapist to reduce his cannabis use, which was discussed together with the multidisciplinary team and his care coordinator. Partnership working with the local addictions services was supported.

Amir was discharged home after 4 weeks.

CASE STUDY 21.2

Lucy

Lucy was a 64-year old woman admitted to the unit following a suicide attempt. She had been diagnosed with bipolar disorder in her 20s but had been stable for many years and had been under the care of her GP only. Lucy had recently experienced several life events, the major one being the sudden death of her husband who had been a significant support to her over the years. She described this loss as 'devastating' and, together with the continuing decline of her elderly mother with a diagnosis of dementia, Lucy

had become very depressed. Her suicide attempt had led to her initially being admitted to the general hospital for medical supervision and assessment, but she had then been transferred to the mental health unit. Treatment at home under the Home Treatment Team had been considered, but the risks were deemed too high.

Lucy presented as severely depressed with poor self-care and very limited appetite. She was monitored by nursing staff on close observation initially

Lucy (Continued)

who had a fluid and food intake chart for her. Medication was restarted as Lucy had stopped this due to her bereaved state.

Occupational therapists initially had daily contact with Lucy, building rapport and gathering information. The activity coordinator was asked to take her some activities that she could complete on her own (self-occupying) and to involve her in the ward smoothie-making group if possible. Over time Lucy was increasingly able to engage in ward activities and then attend the groups in the occupational therapy department. A model of human occupation screening tool assessment identified Lucy's main issues as motivation, with some deficits in motor and process skills. The occupational therapist had identified that Lucy was a very passionate gardener and this was the main activity used initially to engage her and then to support her in regaining her confidence. Tasks were graded to ensure that she was successful, and this helped her self-esteem. (See chapter 6). She was encouraged to be involved in the unit's gardening group and was eventually able to advise and help with the planning. Contacts with local gardening groups and societies were explored.

Lucy's husband had been the main cook and Lucy felt underconfident in this task, which added to her sense of not being able to cope with practicalities on discharge. Together with the occupational therapist, Lucy identified small, easy meals she could prepare and practised these in the occupational therapy groups and 1:1 sessions with the support worker. Practical support also included learning how to do shopping for food online.

Lucy had reduced mobility following a car accident many years earlier in which she had broken her femur and pelvis. She walked with a stick and now had increasing pain, and her GP had recently referred her for an orthopaedic review. Assistive equipment items for both the home and use in the garden were assessed for and provided, Lucy was made aware of other equipment she could purchase. Orders were placed for rails in her home to enable her to use steps safely and to prevent falls. Major adaptations and equipment were not required for safe discharge, but Lucy was made aware of equipment and resources she may require in the future. An occupational therapy report was completed, and occupational therapists in the community mental health teams were informed.

Together with the occupational therapist Lucy explored social activities in the community. She expressed an interest in volunteering but did not feel ready for this yet. She was provided with community contacts and agencies that would be helpful for her in the future, but in the meantime she focused on planning to join a local peer-led support group which was of interest to her following her discharge.

Time was given for Lucy to express her feelings of loss following her husband's death, and bereavement counselling was explored for her to engage in following discharge. She was also provided with information on the local Alzheimer's Society carers' support groups so she could feel better supported in meeting her mother's needs.

SUMMARY

This chapter has highlighted the importance of occupational therapy as part of the MDT provision in an acute setting. The various challenges and the need for close MDT working and communication have been identified. The occupational therapy process has been discussed and the unique contribution of occupation in the recovery process in the acute setting has been highlighted. The case examples have indicated the value of collaborative, person-centred work for everyone involved and the importance of an occupational focus in determining and achieving occupational and recovery goals.

QUESTIONS FOR CONSIDERATION

1. What contributes to stigma around inpatient treatment?
2. Why is minimizing a person's inpatient admission preferable?
3. How can the experience of trauma in a person's life contribute to a mental health crisis?
4. How else could inpatient staff be supported in their own mental health?
5. What could an occupational therapist do to build rapport with service users in an acute setting?
6. How can occupational therapists assess the service user's level of comfort with a session as well as their progression?
7. What possible societal expectations or pressures could have affected Amir as a 22-year-old (Case Study 21.1) man? What could have contributed to the psychosis he was experiencing?
8. Given Lucy's history and multiple issues (Case study 21.2), how can occupational therapists in acute settings work with her and community services to enable her recovery in the long term?

SERVICE USER COMMENTARY

If you were with occupational therapy cookery, you'd be collected and escorted to the occupational therapy suite. This exotic excursion could last all afternoon. We first decided on a recipe, bought the corresponding ingredients from a supermarket, followed the recipe and the results were served to all the patients.

It took a while for me to understand that occupational therapy wasn't a therapy aimed at a paid occupation following discharge. I thought occupational therapy cookery, if you showed competency, meant you'd get a job cooking somewhere after discharge. Without ever getting any job offers, the real purpose of occupational therapy cookery came as some relief.

Post-discharge support from an occupational therapist would've been great, but this never happened. Of all the different types of staff, occupational therapists usually were more positive and practical in implementing new, meaningful habits.

I thought the mental health service was Mafia-run. Why else would these kind professionals want to help me individually unless preparing us for murders? The cannabis I was using often prevented realistic thought.

It sometimes felt good to be on a multidisciplinary team (MDT) ward round with so many professionals. I'd leave some of those meetings slightly lightheaded with all the attention. On occasion, I'd even mishear news of any leave increases.

Many small, happy interactions with somebody normal (the occupational therapist) are often far better than occasional gestures of goodwill and heaps better than none at all. Outside of these chats, the patient might not meaningfully speak with anybody else. Small talk, even if just attempted, can really improve the mood.

Motivation when ill was a big problem. On one admission, it took weeks to get into the occupational therapy gym group. After I'd been greenlighted in ward round, I was raring to go. Sadly, the occupational therapist came round at about 9 am in the morning. This was terrible planning – everyone was still asleep!

Repetition regarding important information can be crucial. I might have seemed attentive on the outside, but inside, I'd be distracted. I'd often forget that my behaviour in a ward round could decide further leave during the coming week. Getting the balance right between repetition and condescension is a delicate thing, especially in a group setting. Here, stronger service users can seize on this as a weakness to be exploited.

An occupational therapist aware of the social opportunities presented by the local community (for the patient after discharge) is worth their weight in gold. Sadly for me, I got the impression that the occupational therapists for our ward lived miles away and so were quite detached. I'm not really sure they thought it their role to give such advice.

If, say, my occupational therapist put me in touch with a local football team, I'd naturally try to conceal my illness. I'd then be worried about being in big groups buying beer or shots of tequila or smoking weed afterwards at someone's house if we won a contest. It takes a lot of strength to define your own social boundaries, and this might need extra input and coping strategies to make workable.

Ad Gridley

REFERENCES

Ashby, S. E., & Ryan, S. (2012). Factors that influence the professional resilience of occupational therapists in mental health practice. *Australian Occupational Therapy Journal, 60*(2), 110–119.

Ayed N, Toner S, Priebe S. (2019) Conceptualizing resilience in adult mental health literature: A systematic review and narrative synthesis. *Psychol Psychother.* Sep;92(3):299–341. doi: 10.1111/papt.12185.

Birken, M., & Bryant, W. (2019). A photovoice study of user experiences of an occupational therapy department within an acute inpatient mental health setting. *British Journal of Occupational Therapy. 82*(9), 532–543. https://doi.org/10.1177/0308022619836954.

Bryant, W., Cordingley, K., Sims, K., et al. (2016). Collaborative research exploring mental health service users perspectives on acute inpatient occupational therapy. *British Journal of Occupational Therapy, 79*(10), 607–613.

Chambers, M., Gallagher, A., Borschmann, R., et al. (2014). The experiences of detained mental health service users: issues of dignity in care. *BMC Medical Ethics,* 15(50). Available at: https://www.ncbi.nlm.nih.gov/pmc/articles/PMC4114162/.

Department of Health (DH). (2002). *Mental health policy implementation guide: Adult acute inpatient care provision.* London: Department of Health.

Department of Health (DH). (2009). *New horizon: A shared vision for mental Health.* London: Department of Health.

Department of Health (DH). (2018). *Modernising the mental health act.* London: Department of Health and Social Care.

Department of Health and Social Care. (2021). Reforming the Mental Health Act. https://www.gov.uk/government/consultations/reforming-the-mental-health-act/reforming-the-mental-health-act#contents.

Echezarraga, A., Las Hayas, C., Lopez de Arroyabe, E., et al. (2019). Resilience and recovery in the context of psychological disorders. *Journal of Humanistic Psychology.* 1–24. Available at: https://journals.sagepub.com/doi/pdf/10.1177/0022167819851623.

Fitzpatrick, N. K., Thompson, C. J., Hemingway, H., et al. (2003). Acute mental health admissions in inner London: Changes in patient characteristics and clinical admission thresholds between 1988 and 1998. *Psychiatric Bulletin, 27*(1), 7–11.

Glover, G., Arts, G., & Babu, K. S. (2006). Crisis resolution/home treatment teams and psychiatric admission rates in England. *The British Journal of Psychiatry, 189*(5), 441–445.

Hummelvoll, J. K., & Severinsson, E. (2001). Coping with everyday reality: Mental health professionals' reflections on the care provided in an acute psychiatric ward. *Australian and New Zealand Journal of Mental Health Nursing, 10*(3), 156–166.

Kelly, M., Lamont, S., & Brunero, S. (2010). An occupational perspective of the recovery journey in mental health. *British Journal of Occupational Therapy, 73*(3), 129–135.

Leading Change, Adding Value Team. (2019). The Atlas of Shared Learning. Case Study. https://www.england.nhs.uk/atlas_case_study/improving-care-in-mental-health-services-an-acute-care-pathway/.

Lean, M., Fornells-Ambrojo, M., Milton, A., et al. (2019). Self-management interventions for people with severe mental illness: Systematic review and meta-analysis. *British Journal of Psychiatry, 214*(5), 260–268.

Lim, K. H., Morris, J., & Craik, C. (2007). Inpatients' perspective of occupational therapy in acute mental health. *Australian Occupational Therapy Journal, 54*(1), 22–32.

Meddings, S., Byrne, D., Barnicoat, S., et al. (2014). Co-delivered and co-produced: Creating a recovery college in partnership. *Journal of Mental Health Training, Education and Practice, 9*(1), 16–25.

MIND, & Ward Watch. (2004). *MIND campaign to improve hospital conditions for mental Health patients.* London: MIND.

Momori, N., & Richards, G. (2017). Service user and carer involvement: Co-production. In C. Long, J. Cronin-Davis, & D. Cotterill (Eds.), *Occupational therapy evidence in practice for mental Health.* Chichester: John Wiley and Sons Ltd.

National Institute for Health and Care Excellence (NICE). (2011). *Service user experience in adult mental health: Improving the experience of care for people using adult NHS mental health services.* NICE Clinical Guideline 136. Available at: http://www.nice.org.uk/nicemedia/live/13629/57534/57534.pdf.

National Institute for Health and Care Excellence (NICE). 2021 Tobacco: preventing uptake, promoting, quitting and treating dependence. NICE guideline [NC209]. https://www.nice.org.uk/guidance/ng209/chapter/recommendations-on-treating-tobacco-dependence#behavioural-support-in-acute-and-mental-health-services.

National Institute for Mental Health in England (NIMHE). (2007). *New ways of working for everyone.* London: NIHME Workforce Development Programme.

NHS England. (2016). *Implementing the five year forward view for mental health.* London: NHS England.

NHS England. (2017). *Stepping Forward to 20/21.* London: The Mental Health Workforce Plan for England.

Parkinson, S. (1999). Audit of a group programme for inpatients in an acute mental health setting. *British Journal of Occupational Therapy, 62*(6), 252–256.

Perkins, R., & Repper, J. (2015). Recovery is possible for everyone? *Society and Mental Health Inclusion, 19*(2) doi.org/10.1108/MHSI-03-2015-0006.

Public Health England (PHE). (2016). *Making every contact count.* London: PHE.

Rethink Mental Illness. (2011). *Detention under the mental health act factsheet.* London: Rethink Mental Illness. Available at: http://www.rethink.org.

Royal College of Occupational Therapists (RCOT). (2019). *Royal college of occupational therapists research and development strategy.* London.

Scanlan, J. N., & Novak, T. (2015). Sensory approaches in mental health: A scoping review. *Australian Occupational Therapy Journal, 62*(5), 277–285.

Scanlan, J. N., & Still, M. (2013). Job satisfaction, burnout and turnover intention in occupational therapists working in mental health. *Australian Occupational Therapy Journal, 60*(5), 310–318.

Seery, M. (2011). Resilience: A silver lining to experiencing adverse life events. *Current Directions in Psychological Science, 20*(6), 390–394.

Simpson, A., Bowers, L., Alexander, J., et al. (2005). Occupational therapy and multidisciplinary working on acute psychiatric wards: The tompkins acute ward study. *British Journal of Occupational Therapy, 68*(12), 545–551.

Star Ward Impact Review. (2013). *Star Wards. Bright, London.* Available at: https://www.starwards.org.uk/download/impact-review-report-2013-with-tangible-results-appendix-1-docx/.

Star Wards. (2006). *Star Wards. Bright, London.* Available at: http://www.starwards.org.uk/.

Stuckler, D., Reeves, A., Loopstra, R., et al. (2017). Austerity and health: The impact in the UK and Europe. *European Journal of Public Health, 27*(4), 18–21.

Sweeney, A., Clememnt, S., Filson, B., et al. (2016). Trauma-informed mental healthcare in the UK: What is it and how can we further its development. *Mental Health Review Journal, 21*(3), 174–192.

Taylor, R. (2017). *Kielfhofner's model of human occupation: Theory and application* (5th ed.). Baltimore, MD: Lippincott Williams and Wilkins.

Wilcock, A. (2006). *An occupational perspective on health* (2nd ed.). Thorofare, NJ: Slack.

Wimpenny, K., Savin-Baden, M., & Cook, C. (2014). A qualitative research synthesis examining the effectiveness of interventions used by occupational therapists in mental health. *British Journal of Occupational Therapy, 77*(6), 276–288.

22

COMMUNITY PRACTICE

HAZEL PARKER ■ SIMON HUGHES

INTRODUCTION

This chapter introduces the community as a context for work with people with severe and enduring mental health problems, identifying how ill-health is defined and exploring the drivers that shape community mental health services. The approaches used by these services are explained as a basis for understanding teamwork. There is a section on medication, which is important for many people with severe and enduring mental health problems, followed by an overview of the different services in the community mental health setting in the United Kingdom.

From a global perspective challenges for people with mental health problems are primarily concerned with access to services and reduced life expectancy often associated with stigma within and beyond health services. The majority of people receive no treatment. This is reported as 75% of people in low-income countries (World Health Organization (WHO) 2018). In the United Kingdom, despite improvements in care, only 60% of people with common mental health problems were in receipt of care in a survey in 2014 (McManus et al. 2016), with 19% of individuals identified with a diagnosis of a psychosis. Life expectancy is reduced by up to 20 years for men and 15 years for women in the United Kingdom (McManus et al. 2016). Factors contributing to this include alcohol and drug use as well as suicides and accidents, producing higher rates of unnatural deaths. However, early deaths from heart disease, diabetes, and cancer present significant challenges to service providers in ensuring that physical healthcare needs are also considered. Smoking and use of other substances contribute to physical health problems which reduce life expectancy (Wahlbeck et al. 2011). WHO (2013) has agreed a Mental Health Action Plan, with the overall goal:

'to promote mental well-being, prevent mental disorders, provide care, enhance recovery, promote human rights and reduce the mortality, morbidity and disability for persons with mental disorders.'

Details of how to achieve this goal was developed further by Patel et al. (2013), exploring how to address the need for empowerment, a diverse workforce, collaborative team working, the use of technology, early intervention and prevention of premature death. All of these aspects are relevant to occupational therapists working with people with severe and enduring mental health problems.

Severe and Enduring Mental Health Problems

Diagnosis is often a requirement for treatment within mental health services. The two main frameworks that are used to define and identify mental health problems are WHO's International Classification of Diseases, 11th Revision (ICD-11), and the American Psychiatric Association's Diagnostic and Statistical Manual of Mental Disorders, 5th Edition (DSM-5). There are similarities between the two systems, which focus on symptoms to aid diagnostic reasoning and categorization. Common diagnose within community mental health teams include schizophrenia, psychotic disorders, bipolar disorder, anxiety, and depression. An individual may have more than one diagnosis, and diagnoses may change over time. Many people find a

diagnosis beneficial. However, there is greater recognition that a biomedical perspective of mental health has limitations and does not fully consider an individual's life experiences and beliefs (Mind 2017). Most Western countries agree on a similar set of clinical diagnoses and treatments for mental health problems. However, cultures in which there are other traditions or beliefs may not use these terms. For example, in Syria mental illness may be called dementia, which can cause confusion when working with Syrian families, especially as there may not be a direct translation for some diagnoses (Hassan et al. 2015).

Mind (2017) has identified a range of factors that adversely impact on mental health including:

- physical, sexual or emotional abuse in either childhood or adulthood;
- stress that may be linked with poverty, unemployment and poor housing;
- social isolation or loss of people close or stigma;
- long-term physical health conditions and drug and alcohol misuse.

Factors such as employment, diet and exercise play a part in managing mental health, but severe and enduring mental health problems are usually associated with multiple factors. For example, a participatory research study by Sayer et al. (2019) revealed the many social determinants for poor diet and obesity collaborating with African-American people with direct experience of severe mental health problems. Social determinants are discussed further in Chapter 12.

When the impact on an individual's level of functioning is severe, people often require ongoing contact with services. There may also be a significant level of risk to self or others or risks from others due to vulnerabilities. Enabling people to overcome difficulties in coping with daily living occupations such as work, household chores and maintaining safe housing is important, recognizing a person's potential for recovery and self-management.

Occupational therapy offers a valuable means for people to address these difficulties, working on occupations, activities, skills and tasks. Therapeutic occupation is used to address thinking skills, practical activities and self-management (See Chapter 6). Thinking skills include problem-solving, instilling hope, improving motivation, developing meaning and building confidence. Whenever possible specific practical activities are negotiated collaboratively with the individual. Examples include budgeting, shopping, cooking, getting out and about, using public transport and using community facilities. Organizational skills, such as balancing different activities, structuring the day, establishing routines and making good use of time can also be promoted. These different areas of practice are supported by different policies which drive the direction and shape of community mental health services.

Drivers

Community mental health services are driven by local, national and international policies. The WHO Mental Health Action Plan (WHO 2013) highlights essential conditions to enhance healthy living. These conditions include income security, an appropriate and fair level of social protection, decent living conditions, good social and human capital, decent work and employment conditions and good-quality and accessible health services. The emphasis is on creating societies that reduce the social determinants of ill-health and effectively intervene when people need help and support.

In the United Kingdom the Five Year Forward View is a strategic vision for transforming mental healthcare (Department of Health (DH) 2016). The key objective for adult community mental health services is to provide timely access to evidence-based, person-centred care which is focused on recovery and integrated with primary and social care and other sectors. The strategy also emphasizes the need to reduce premature mortality because of physical health causes as well as lowering the suicide rate nationally. The Five Year Forward View was developed following the publication of the Health and Social Care Act (2012) which outlined its aim of enabling users of mental health services to have parity of esteem. In comparison with other NHS services this means:

> 'equal access to effective care and treatment, equal efforts to improve the quality of care, equal status within healthcare education and practice, equally high aspirations for service users and equal status in the measurement of health outcomes'
>
> *Gilburt 2018, online*

Key aspects in the delivery of this vision include the ability of the NHS to recruit and retain the workforce as well as the need for a greater emphasis on prevention rather than treatment. This presents opportunities and challenges for occupational therapists to develop practice beyond addressing existing health problems and disability, for example, by working in a more proactive way within primary care services and particularly non-statutory services.

The NHS (DH 2019) People Plan highlights the role of allied health professionals in leading the transformation of care. Essential features of this process involve the delivery of person-centred and evidence-based care, breadth of skills and the ability to work across different aspects of people's lives and across current boundaries between health and social care settings. The expertise of allied health professionals is key in this shift from an over reliance on expensive hospital-based care as sustainable services are developed. The occupational needs of individuals and communities can be championed by occupational therapists that are aware of this changing landscape and involved in shaping services.

Regardless of the actual composition of services, priorities for delivery have to be agreed upon. Priorities which drive the shape and direction of services include ensuring that value for money is achieved with effective interventions. This has fostered processes for regulation and accountability at multiple levels, from individual professional accountability to an organizational and sector provider level (see Chapter 8).

Another driver is concerned with involving service users and carers in service development and evaluation to give voice to their experiences and expectations. This trend aims for more personalized services with an emphasis on continued well-being and recovery. Accessible services require increasing use of digital media to communicate, assess, intervene and evaluate. Innovative practice involves developing entrepreneurship and understanding change management (see Chapter 7). Therefore many contextual factors for community practice are considered when deciding how to deliver occupational therapy.

SUPPORTING MODELS AND APPROACHES

The community setting offers many opportunities to demonstrate the importance and effectiveness of occupational therapy for people with severe and enduring mental health problems. Core principles can be aligned with specific supporting models and approaches (see chapter 4), such as recovery-oriented practice, a strength-based approach, cycles of change, the stress vulnerability model and a trauma-informed approach.

Recovery-Oriented Practice

Recovery is a central theme in mental health and is covered more broadly elsewhere in this book (see Chapters 4, 10 and 12). Clinical recovery is viewed in the United Kingdom as a state of being symptom free. Recovery-oriented practice introduces the idea of personal recovery, where a person's life goals are considered (Slade 2009). The focus of this chapter is on issues relevant to people with severe and enduring mental health problems.

In the United Kingdom the shift to recovery-oriented practice was initially signalled in 2001 through a policy emphasizing that services would be as focused on recovery as they had been on symptoms and illness (DH 2001a). Community mental health services could support people in settings of their own choosing, prompting access to community resources including housing, education, work and friendships or whatever the individual felt would be critical to their own recovery (DH 2001a, p. 24). The idea of promoting social inclusion supported this alongside breaking down the stigma of mental ill-health as one of the typical barriers to an individual's recovery. Occupational therapy involvement and leadership of recovery-oriented services have enabled the shift to this more holistic kind of service provision (Nugent et al. 2017).

Although recovery is identified as a unique and individual experience, interventions have been focused on agreed areas. For example, Leamy et al (2011) developed a recovery framework called CHIME, using findings from a systematic review. CHIME stands for five areas of recovery:

- connectedness
- hope and optimism for the future
- identity
- meaning in life
- empowerment.

From an occupational perspective this is consistent with developing meaning and purpose from occupation in real-world settings while seeing oneself as more than just a diagnosis. In the long term a stance of hope and optimism is necessary for an individual. People may not have this stance of hope at points of their journey through services. At these times the hope of the occupational therapist or those around them can help sustain them (Nugent et al. 2017).

The management of symptoms with medication has been consistently ranked as an important priority for service users and carers, alongside the desire to see the development of new innovative drug treatments. Turton et al. (2010) highlighted the importance of medication in supporting recovery. In addition, there has also been an emphasis on focusing on strengths and the value of structure and routine.

Strengths-Based Approach

Statutory services have typically tended to be focused on providing care based on solving problems. A person is asked to identify their deficits. Time is then spent with the person trying to improve such areas. To focus on deficits can act as a regular reminder of the problems or difficulties that are experienced. In contrast, the strengths-based approach encourages a focus on a person's strengths:

- What is the person good at?
- What have they achieved in their lifetime?
- What does the person get most out of in their life?
- What do they want most in their life right now?

The principles of the strengths-based approach have been documented by Ryan and Morgan (2004), who view the service user as the director of the process. They place strong emphasis on the use of community and neighbourhood services as resources for integration, rather than focusing solely on mental health resources, making this approach compatible with recovery-oriented practice and promoting social inclusion.

Cycle of Change

An understanding of the cycle of change can support collaboration, informed by models such as the transtheoretical model of behavioural change (Prochaska and DiClemente 1986). This model uses a behavioural frame of reference to describe stages of change, starting with the present. Appropriate approaches and interventions towards the maintenance of healthier behaviour are identified. People may progress incrementally through the stages or move backwards (relapse) or forwards (recovery), including jumping between the six stages.

Pre-contemplation

At this stage the person is not ready to change. Their lack of readiness to change is validated by the therapist, who feeds back to the individual their understanding of the situation and their wishes to remain in the current situation. An evaluation of the individual's current behaviour is encouraged while clarifying that any decision to change is theirs. An educational approach may be used to explore and personalize the risks and benefits of current behaviour.

Contemplation

The person is getting ready to change. Exploration of the pros and cons of behavioural change is encouraged, and it is recognized that ambivalence regarding change can delay action. The individual's current perspective continues to be validated while reinforcing that the choice to change is theirs.

Preparation

The person is ready to change. A graded approach is used to define appropriate challenges. Potential obstacles are identified and a problem-solving approach used to explore possible solutions. Social support networks are involved when possible to support and encourage the planned behaviour change. Skill acquisition may be necessary at this stage to enable the individual to change previous behaviours.

Action

The person has started to make changes to their behaviour. Newly acquired skills may be consolidated into habits and routines. Consistency and persistence are encouraged and minor setbacks dealt with. Feelings of loss for previous lifestyle or friendship groups may be present, therefore the long-term benefits and rewards for current behaviour need to be reinforced.

Maintenance

The person has continued with the planned behavioural change. Progression to greater self-efficacy is emphasized. Dealing with stressful situations and potential relapse is explored to reinforce coping strategies and identify support mechanisms, including emergency or crisis contacts.

Relapse

The person may return to previous behaviours. This may occur at any point. The setback needs to be validated while recognizing that change can still occur with the potential for new learning from the experience. The triggers for relapse can be explored while reassessing the stage of readiness to progress again. Coping strategies and support networks can be revisited and strengthened when necessary.

The cycle of change is particularly relevant for community practice, and its use can support the delivery of person-centred occupational therapy. Jointly agreed interventions can engender change and develop understanding of the individual's situation. This understanding can be used from the perspective of stress and vulnerability, as discussed in the following section.

Stress Vulnerability

The stress vulnerability model was originally described by Zubin and Spring (1977), who saw individuals as having a predisposition or vulnerability to developing psychotic disorders. Individual exposure to stress can trigger psychotic experiences. This simple model shows that more vulnerable people may need fewer stressors to develop a psychotic reaction. In contrast, less vulnerable people may need more stressors to develop psychosis. Vulnerability is explained by a range of factors, for example, genetic predisposition to illness, childhood trauma or loss of a caregiver in early life or poor social circumstances. The model describes psychosis as being on a continuum, challenging stigma by suggesting that anyone could develop schizophrenia or psychosis given enough stressors in relation to their own vulnerability.

The stress vulnerability bucket (Brabban and Turkington 2002) is a useful tool in understanding the role of helpful and unhelpful occupations, indicating where effective adaptations can be made. Box 22.1 describes how this tool is used.

Trauma-Informed Approach

Knowledge of how personal trauma events can impact a person has become far more widely recognized in

BOX 22.1
STRESS VULNERABILITY BUCKET

Imagine each individual has a bucket. The size of the bucket will vary according to the individual's vulnerabilities. Those with higher vulnerability will have a smaller bucket.

Stressors are held in the bucket, like a bucket holding water. For example, work stress, financial difficulties, housing problems, difficulty in relationships, physical health worries, poor diet, lack of exercise and poor sleep are stressors in the bucket.

Imagine then as the stressors are building up, they will reach a point where no more can be held. This is like the bucket is being filled with more and more water so it overflows. The water that overflows is seen as representing symptoms of mental or physical ill-health.

There are different ways to control the overflow, or reduce the stress. Most importantly, support can be offered to identify activities which effectively relieve stress for the person, acting like taps or holes in the bucket to release some of the water. These activities, or taps or holes, will be uniquely placed and combined for each person.

It is important in recovery-oriented practice to ensure that stressors are not simply avoided but that appropriate management strategies are identified. If the focus is on minimizing or avoiding stress, it may lead to risk-averse practice, fostering low expectations of what individuals can achieve and undermining recovery-oriented practice and positive risk management (see also Chapter 10).

Vulnerability can therefore be reduced by developing problem-solving skills, coping skills, social skills and support networks. Working with the person on activities that are found to be relaxing and absorbing can reduce personal levels of stress. Environmental stressors such as housing issues may be addressed directly through changes to that environment or indirectly by relocating to more supportive and less demanding environments (see chapter 19). The stress vulnerability model incorporates biological as well as psychological and social elements by considering the effects of stress on body functions and structures. As a biopsychosocial approach (Zubin and Spring 1977), it is relevant to all health professionals, enabling them to work together in teams. This also allows profession-specific interventions, for example, occupational therapists focusing specifically on occupation.

---

relation to mental ill-health to help make sense of a person's experiences. To develop a trauma-informed approach, Dillon et al. (2012) suggest that services need to shift focus to a person's story and their experiences of trauma. Any harmful or life-threatening events that have lasting impacts on a persons' mental or physical well-being can be identified as trauma. They can occur at any time in a person's life and can be a single event or multiple events over time (Machtinger et al. 2019). Links between trauma and severe and enduring mental health conditions have become more evident. A body of knowledge is developing to suggest that trauma-informed approaches and trauma-informed services need to be taken seriously (Sweeney et al. 2016).

Mental health services have been responsible for retraumatizing people through practices involving control and power over individuals. For example, the use of the Mental Health Act takes away many aspects of a person's choice and control for the period of time they are detained (see chapter 21). This also then allows some treatments to be given against the will of the individual, such as rapid tranquillization injections to calm and settle a distressed patient (Sweeney et al. 2016). The experience of being coerced can often lead to flashbacks to past traumas, a further sense of loss of control over one's life and a fear or mistrust of those professionals whose main aim is to care and support.

Occupational therapists, as with all health and social care staff, are required to have a good understanding of the impact trauma can play in a person's mental health. When possible it is important to be able to understand the nature of a person's past trauma as this may directly impact the ability to complete occupations or to work with occupational therapists on certain occupations. For example, a woman identifies she is struggling with food preparation activities because of poor concentration and would like to be more independent in this area. However, she also avoids sessions in the kitchen in her own home. Part of her trauma history is that she was physically abused by her ex-partner, always in the kitchen. Therefore the idea of being in the kitchen with an occupational therapist is causing her increased distress, despite the wish to develop skills. Without this knowledge of the background history, the occupational therapist might see her as unwilling to engage and consider discharging her from the service if the reasons for non-engagement are not explored. Support to develop coping skills may need to be offered before beginning sessions in the kitchen. Awareness of trauma is therefore vital in all areas of occupational therapy practice, as trauma can often shape the way in which people develop their own understanding of events or interpret information. This can lead to individuals being unable to access and receive the appropriate support (Machtinger et al. 2019).

TEAM WORKING AND COORDINATED CARE

Team working is essential for providing a comprehensive and coordinated approach to the provision of mental health services. In the United Kingdom the care programme approach (CPA) (DH 2008) has been developed to ensure services are coordinated effectively.

The Care Programme Approach

The CPA (DH 2008) was introduced in England in 1991 and reviewed in 2008 by the Department of Health. The CPA continues to be used in organizing the delivery of care to people who access secondary mental health services. Health and social care services work together, coordinating their approach for individuals, agreeing care packages, and seeking to provide the best care available.

The aim of the CPA is to put the person at the centre of the care planning process and empower them to take ownership of this process by considering all aspects of their lives. It is for people with complex needs who require services from a number of agencies and/or professionals, because of the greater risks associated with their mental health problems. It is based on a whole systems approach led by a care coordinator (DH 2008). The CPA includes:

- comprehensive assessment of needs;
- consideration and planning of all available resources to meet these needs;
- regular assessment and review of risk issues and management plans.

It should also include people who have a caring role, so that their needs can also be assessed and met when possible. This helps clarify expectations about roles and responsibilities, setting boundaries for individuals and agencies involved. Occupational therapists are included in the range of professionals that may be involved and are often care coordinators.

The Care Coordinator

The CPA requires that all individuals have a care coordinator who is a named professional who aims for a strong, sustainable and hope-inspiring professional relationship with the service user (Repper and Perkins 2003). To empower the service user to draw on their valuable expertise, it is important that the care coordinator focuses on strengths and needs and is not distracted by the agendas and priorities of others involved. The agreed care plan should be specific to the individual.

For anyone with severe and enduring mental health problems, it is important that regular reviews take place. Within the CPA the care coordinator is responsible for ensuring that an individual's care plan is reviewed on a regular basis and that goals are specific, measurable, achievable, realistic and timely (SMART). Care plans are altered accordingly by the coordinator following agreement at each review. The care coordinator is not necessarily responsible for providing care but monitors that others are providing appropriate and timely care as agreed.

The role of the care coordinator is clearly defined by the CPA policy (DH 2008) and is not profession specific. The process for identifying care coordinators for service users varies across teams, considering:

- the needs of the service user;
- caseload sizes;
- complexity of the case;
- staff skills.

Care coordination should not take away from each individual profession's ability to provide more specific intervention plans but raises issues about the tension between generic and profession-specific working.

Care coordination involves considering problems with symptoms, medication, housing, legal issues and risks. Discussing these issues could be negative if a good therapeutic relationship has not been formed. Occupational therapists can establish a good therapeutic relationship based on appreciating the person's strengths as part of an occupational journey to recovery (Kelly et al. 2010). However, often there are barriers to recovery due to lack of resources such as funding, opportunities, education and peer support. Overcoming these barriers requires creative thinking, using occupational therapy specialist skills to support people effectively.

In the UK, NHS mental health services are required to follow CPA, which has remained largely unchanged since its introduction in 1991. The idea of recovery, however, has been a moving and shifting focus for services (see chapter 4). A user experience study of the

CPA alongside recovery-oriented practice found there was a risk that administrative processes pushed service users away from the centre of a therapeutic approach (Gould 2012). Services are often under pressure to demonstrate effectiveness by completing reviews and care plans within set timescales. This risks the process of review becoming primarily administrative, losing focus on recovery and what the individual needs to live the life they choose. Occupational therapists can consider different ways in which service users can be empowered to take ownership within the CPA process. Recovery-oriented practice, which ensures specific and realistic goals are identified, can inform the timing and focus of reviews.

Generic Versus Specialist Working

There has been much debate around generic and specialist ways of working over the past two decades (Scanlan et al. 2019). Community mental health teams are formed from various health professionals and support staff, who share the work that anyone can do (generic) and take responsibility for work that is their professional speciality. Time taken with generic work can overshadow specialist work and cause tension, especially as mental health services are frequently reconfigured, requiring new ways of working. In the United Kingdom services such as assertive outreach or early intervention in psychosis teams use the skills that occupational therapists have but advertise for any person with nursing, social work or occupational therapy registration. Where occupational therapists take up these posts, they can use their creativity and leadership to ensure that their professional knowledge and skills are used effectively. Some occupational therapists take on leadership and management for multidisciplinary teams, using their skills, for example, in activity analysis and adaptation, which can inform understanding of a team's functioning or enable an absent member to return to work after a period of sickness.

To provide specialist occupational therapy services, occupational therapists must spend the majority of their time using assessments and interventions that are occupation-centred (College of Occupational Therapists 2006; see Chapter 4). In contrast, care coordination is often identified as generic work. However, as already identified, being a care coordinator does not mean providing services to a person but coordinating their delivery. Profession-specific assessments and interventions

are provided alongside other elements of care. When working in teams and identifying appropriate care coordinators, people with greater occupational needs can be allocated to an occupational therapist. This may enhance many aspects of care. For example, obtaining appropriate housing may be viewed as a generic task for care coordination, as housing often needs addressing as a priority to promote stability. The occupational therapist as care coordinator can support and enable people to use the skills required. Practically, the occupational therapist could work jointly on completing forms, for example, enabling the person to share ownership of the process at each stage. Meeting a basic need such as safe and long-term accommodation can ultimately promote a sense of belonging.

Partnership Working

Working in community mental health as an occupational therapist involves forming and sustaining working relationships with users of mental health services, families, carers, colleagues and other services. Tait and Shah (2007) also highlight the benefits of non-statutory organizations being involved in partnership working. These organizations enhance statutory services through advocacy and campaigning roles. They focus on practical help with housing, welfare and financial advice. Social exclusion can be addressed with local services providing opportunities for work, training, leisure and social contact. Non-statutory services are sometimes more able to engage with people who distrust statutory services, being responsive to their needs but not associated with compulsory detention and treatment, especially in black and ethnic minority communities (Vahdaninia et al. 2020).

For effective partnership working, there needs to be a clear understanding of what different services provide, where there is an overlap of provision and what the unique aspects of a service are. Services need to be coordinated with timely signposting so that people can make informed decisions to meet their needs and navigate their way around multiple agencies. The Kings Fund (2010) identified elements of successful partnership working, which included having bespoke solutions to meet local needs, having a focus on the desired outcomes and clarifying responsibilities. One example is social prescribing in which people with long-term health issues are directed to community activities by primary care staff. Working in partnership with local primary care teams gives community mental health occupational therapists valuable knowledge and insight into local provision (Thew et al. 2017).

Risk

Public perceptions mean people with severe mental health problems are likely to be seen as potentially violent whereas, in reality, they are more likely to be victims of violent crime (Time to Change 2020). This means that assessment and management of risks in a community setting can be broadly concerned with the impact of crime on service users and the likelihood of future problems. The influence of coexisting alcohol or substance abuse may also be important to understanding historical risk and the context of that risk.

Risk has implications for all areas of community practice. The level of risk is dynamic and often cannot be eliminated. Empowering people to make their own choices and decisions requires thorough consideration of risks, minimizing incidents through assessment and management. All practitioners must ensure decisions are defensible through gathering as much information as possible and making clear, reasoned action plans.

There are formal processes for clinical risk assessment and for people working alone. The community setting involves working in varied venues, requiring ongoing risk assessment, but there should always be positive risk management to balance avoidance with opportunities. There are specific considerations of risk in relation to mental capacity (Jones 2020), and shared decision-making is applicable in all settings (Reed and Jaxson 2019) (see also Chapter 9).

Clinical Risk Assessment

All members of multidisciplinary teams are responsible for contributing to clinical risk assessment, which takes place throughout a person's journey within mental health services. Workplaces have local policies and training for team members regarding risk, and these must always be consulted for guidance when completing documents. In the United Kingdom the CPA (DH 2008) requires that detailed risk assessments are carried out regularly. Depending on the setting, occupational therapists may be involved in assessing and addressing safeguarding concerns to protect the person from possible abuse and neglect (Mind 2018). A multiagency risk assessment conference is a

risk management meeting during which information is shared on high-risk cases of domestic violence and abuse and a risk management plan is put in place (Eley 2018). Multi-agency public protection arrangements meetings are where the assessment of risks posed by sexual and/or violent offenders takes place and a management strategy is devised.

Lone Working

Community working often means lone working. All employers and organizations should provide a lone working policy. While visiting people in their own homes, a number of safety issues should be considered including:

- Does the person live alone or are there others in the house?
- How well is the person known to the service?
- Do any members of the household pose any known risks to others?
- Is the surrounding area safe, or is there potential risk posed by others?

If any of the above is a concern, action must be taken accordingly and in line with any relevant organizational policies.

Considerations might include:

- A visit with two staff present;
- Ensure a system is in place at base for notifying others of whereabouts and expected time of return;
- Use mobile phones to inform others at base of time of arrival and of leaving property;
- Use other agencies, such as police, for support;
- Identify an alternative safe place to see the person.
- Are there animals in the household, and is the owner able to keep them under control for the duration of the visit?
- Do people smoke within the household, and are they able to abstain during the duration of the visit?

Sometimes if staff are concerned about visiting a particular household, they will try to get in and out of the house as quickly as possible. This does not provide the person with the optimum level of service and places staff at risk; therefore if there is such a concern, it is suggested that alternative arrangements are made.

Working in Varied Environments

Risk assessments must also be considered when arranging to meet at alternative venues. Other venues and considerations may include:

- Community mental health resource centres or the team office base: consideration must be given to using personal attack alarms and ensuring other staff are aware of any response required if alarm is sounded;
- Alternative health and social care buildings such as GP surgeries: consideration must be given to any safety procedures including fire alarms, personal alarm systems and how to notify resident staff when entering and leaving the building;
- Community leisure facilities such as libraries or sports centres: consideration must be given particularly to confidentiality.

Positive Risk-Taking

Positive risk-taking is deciding to do something in which the positive outcome is worth taking a risk for (Morgan 2020). It can be an important part of a care plan. To avoid taking risks is to limit opportunities to learn and develop, as everybody takes risks in their lives (Ryan and Morgan 2004, p. 230). However, pressures on mental health services to minimize risk and negative publicity have an impact on willingness to take risks. This in turn can jeopardize recovery as opportunities are missed. A collaborative and positive approach to managing risk empowers individuals, promoting a sense of responsibility while considering the impact of identified problems. The aim is to enable people to make their own decisions and choices with appropriate support. For example, graded activity could be used to minimize risk, informed by the stress vulnerability model.

When working with people with dementia and others with cognitive impairments, positive risk-taking may need to be carefully discussed with carers (Bamford et al. 2019). The challenges to positive risk management are not just about avoiding adverse events, as there are other pressures to minimize or avoid risk. These pressures are indicated by an over-emphasis on treating symptoms, judging effectiveness of services by avoiding admission, staff assuming a role as the expert and overriding service users. Services have to find balance between measuring risks and being the experts, favouring practices that are evidence-based and empowering the person as the expert of their own experiences and choices (Bonney and Stickley 2008). Positive risk-taking can pose ethical dilemmas within practice, as services have a responsibility to protect the public yet also to protect the service user. A narrative approach to risk is proposed by Stickley and Felton (2018) who suggest that greater understanding can be gained through exploring events with the individual. This helps to contextualize events and offers opportunities to explore strengths, resilience and coping rather than focusing on possible negative outcomes. Positive risk-taking should conform to relevant local guidelines, be based on the best information available and be clearly documented, and the relevant people should be informed.

The term 'therapeutic risk-taking' is also used as an alternative to positive risk-taking. Felton et al. (2017) discuss it with particular reference to challenges in mental health services, focusing on organizational influences, the need to listen to service users to understand what they think is risky and the importance of ethical decision-making. One common risk for service users is taking medication, risking adverse side effects in the hope of improvements to their symptoms (Felton et al. 2017).

MEDICATION

Medication has a large part to play in the management of mental health problems. It could be argued that it does not fit within the remit of occupational therapists, who are primarily concerned with occupational performance issues. However, if occupational therapists are to provide comprehensive interventions, then medication has to be a consideration because of its impact on occupational performance. For example, Conn et al. (2019) identified that obesity was a significant side effect of many medications for people with severe and enduring mental health problems, proposing a tailored intervention. Two aspects of medication are considered within this section. The first is medication management as an activity. The second regards the effects of medication and implications for occupational performance.

Medications can be categorized into four major groups:

- Antipsychotics: used for the treatment of psychosis, for example, to lessen hallucinations or delusions and reduce agitation;

- Antidepressants: primarily used for the treatment of depression although may also be licensed for some anxiety disorders;
- Mood stabilizers: used primarily in bipolar disorder to control episodes of mania;
- Minor tranquillizers: includes sleeping tablets and benzodiazepines used for short-term sleeping problems and as sedatives for severe anxiety or distress; can be prescribed for short-term use only due to their addictive properties.

Medication Management

Medication is an important factor in a person's wellbeing when severe and enduring mental health problems exist. Often, people will be expected to take medications for indefinite periods of time, complying with instructions and sticking to the recommended regimen for taking medication, known as 'adherence' (WHO 2003). Medication management requires that appropriate community mental health team members are able to communicate effectively with a person to gain a clear agreement to adherence (Mitchell and Selmes 2007). There is a significant rate of non-adherence with medication for many mental health problems. The reasons for this can be varied but include the following:

- Cognitive difficulties: forgetfulness, confusion, memory, disorientation;
- Belief: faith, insight, hope;
- Knowledge: understanding of effects and side-effects, experience of undesirable side-effects, such as tiredness or increased appetite;
- Barriers to accessing services: chaotic lifestyles, difficulties with community travel, financial costs for attending appointments/paying for prescriptions.

Medication management must therefore be considered as much an occupation as brushing teeth. Occupational therapists provide advice and education that is within their professional scope of practice (Royal College of Occupational Therapists (RCOT) 2019). When there are problems, as with any other occupation, it is important that the therapist aims to identify the reasons for non-adherence with medication. If there are poor routines or forgetfulness, then specific prompts and reminders could be suggested, such as

setting mobile phone alerts or placing a note on the fridge door. Some medications (e.g., clozapine and lithium) require regular attendance for blood tests and health checks. If a person does not keep an appointment, it is possible that some medications cannot be provided until the necessary health checks have been carried out. The occupational therapist could address issues, such as accessing public transport to attend regular health checks.

Medication and Occupational Performance

While medication is used effectively by many people to reduce psychotic symptoms or improve mood, some may experience side-effects. These can include over-tiredness, difficulty getting up or increased appetite. It is important that occupational therapists are aware of medications and their possible effects on people. This information can be used in the assessment of an individual's occupational performance. However, the occupational therapist should always be careful to liaise with medical and nursing colleagues to ensure it is appropriate to use interventions such as altering routines, adding exercise into daily activities and menu planning to ensure a regular, healthy diet.

There may be some community settings where it is essential to have a greater understanding of medication, for example, a crisis resolution team (see later section in this chapter). Medication may also be crucial at particular times to achieve the best outcome. The occupational therapist should know when to engage other team members. This decision should be informed with knowledge of commonly used medications, including:

- Names of commonly used drugs;
- Common side-effects of each drug;
- Major contra indications;
- Form of drug – oral tablet, liquid or injection;
- Length of time for medication to take effect and expected outcome;
- Details of any blood monitoring and other health checks required and frequency;
- Action required if medications are not taken.

SERVICE SETTINGS

Community mental health services aim to address the diverse needs associated with mental health problems from resolving acute crises to long-term care. In the United Kingdom occupational therapists work across these NHS services: crisis resolution and home treatment, early intervention in psychosis, community mental health teams, assertive outreach services, trauma-informed services, veterans' services and liaison psychiatry services. Each of these services is briefly outlined below.

Occupational therapists are also employed by non-statutory organizations, including charities, not-for-profit companies and commercial businesses. These are often developing areas that present challenges and opportunities for occupational therapists, requiring the development of entrepreneurial skills (see Chapters 7, 10 and 29). Regardless of the service provider or setting, the mental health and well-being of the community can be addressed by occupational therapy (NHS England 2019; NHS Collaborating Centre for Mental Health 2019). Occupational therapists may be employed in these settings specifically to deliver occupational therapy, as general mental health workers or in a combined role. It is important for the individual therapist to be clear when they are delivering the governed therapy of occupational therapy as laid out by the Health and Care Professions Council and when they are delivering services as a mental health worker.

Crisis Resolution and Home Treatment Teams

In the United Kingdom NHS crisis resolution and home treatment teams are required to provide a 24/7 service for anybody experiencing an acute mental health crisis. These teams were established to reduce demand for inpatient care, quickly resolving crises when possible and following up with intensive contact at home (see Chapter 21) (DH 2000; Stulz et al. 2020). Policy guidance defined the structure of teams and best practice (DH 2001b), and many aspects have been found to be helpful to people supported by them, including occupational therapy (Morant et al. 2017). These specialist multidisciplinary teams offer a service to people in the following groups, who are experiencing an acute crisis which would otherwise require hospital admission:

- adults with a severe and enduring mental health diagnosis;
- adults with a personality disorder;

- adults with a coexisting mental health diagnosis and learning disability;

The teams aim to:

- provide comprehensive assessment of mental state and associated risk;
- act as gatekeepers for hospital admissions;
- provide a service to promote and facilitate early discharge from the hospital;
- provide a care plan for intensive home treatment that is a suitable option;
- continue with intensive home treatment until the individual is stabilized and referral to or transfer back to an alternative team can be made.

The teams are set up to provide high ratios of staff to service users to allow for up to two to three visits per day. The range of interventions carried out by the teams is varied and includes brief solution-focused interventions, practical problem-solving, medication management and support with daily activities (Morant et al. 2017). Interventions are brief as once the crisis is resolved, the process of discharge or transfer to another service will begin. Based on short-term goal-setting, interventions can include practical problem-solving, identifying and building on occupational strengths. People may be enabled to engage in self-care and leisure activities. It is important for occupational therapists within these teams to use a recovery-oriented approach, not allowing problems to become the prominent factor. Engaging in meaningful occupation can enable the person to rediscover their own strengths and coping strategies (National Institute for Mental Health in England 2004).

Early Intervention in Psychosis

The rationale of early intervention is that intensive support at an early stage for people experiencing psychosis will reduce future need. Norman and Malla (2001) explored the duration of untreated psychosis and found that the earlier treatment can be started, the greater chance that symptoms can be reduced. Specialised early-intervention teams have been developed in several countries, and evidence is still emerging of the effectiveness of the approach. Interventions focused on employment and family therapy have been found to be beneficial (Marshall and Rathbone 2011).

Early intervention services have two main objectives. The first is one of early detection, identifying and working with people with prodromal symptoms, which indicate there is a risk of developing psychosis. The second objective is to provide effective interventions for those who are newly experiencing psychotic phenomena, maintaining existing support mechanisms and social roles (Neale and Kinnair 2017). This might involve promoting independence and recovery, emphasizing education and work-related outcomes. Many of the approaches and interventions are occupation-focused and supportive to the maintenance and development of life roles, requiring occupational therapy involvement.

Community Mental Health Teams

Where there is identified need following on from involvement with early intervention services, it is likely a person will be transferred to a community mental health team. These teams address complex needs, coordinating care through a multidisciplinary approach (National Collaborating Centre for Mental Health (NCCMH) 2019). Within the United Kingdom these teams may often be providing integrated NHS and social care services. They can include community psychiatric nurses, psychiatrists, social workers, occupational therapists, psychologists, pharmacists, art therapists, cognitive behavioural therapists and support staff. They may also access additional resources, such as dietetics or physiotherapy, as necessary. Some teams have been divided to provide specialist mental healthcare according to diagnosis or need. For example, affective disorder teams alongside psychosis teams, or recovery and rehabilitation teams (NCCMH 2019).

Based on collaborative working, the focus is on recovery and hope while promoting quality of life. Teams aim for the person to manage their life better by enabling them to identify a sense of purpose and meaning to their occupations and form stronger relationships. Using a strengths-based approach, the person is enabled to improve their chances of finding work, gaining education and maintaining suitable accommodation (DH 2011). In this setting, occupational therapists aim to enable and empower individuals to become the makers and directors of getting their own lives back on track. This involves focusing on participation and quality of life to improve mental health and well-being (RCOT 2018).

Assertive Outreach

Assertive outreach teams aim to engage people who struggle to access services often because they have limited insight into their mental health problems. Alternatively, they may have had compulsory inpatient treatment and struggle to trust mental health professionals (see Chapter 25). Assertive outreach teams also work with people who are unable to easily access services due to chaotic lifestyles. Most people have severe and enduring mental health problems, usually a psychotic disorder. They would be vulnerable or would present with high levels of risk if not engaged and appropriate interventions provided with an assertive approach.

Assertive outreach teams were first developed in the United States in the 1980s to reduce hospital readmission rates following the closure of many of the old institutions (Stein and Santos 1998). They use a flexible and creative approach to engaging and establishing therapeutic relations.

Occupational therapists within assertive outreach teams can focus on occupation for effective work with service users, identifying what is important to a person and where their strengths lie. Focusing on everyday life can provide a welcome break from focusing on symptoms and medication. This everyday life focus can include self-care and domestic tasks, social and recreational opportunities and work and education. Practical problem solving can build hope for the future, which is essential in a person's recovery (Slade 2009).

Housing

Housing problems and homelessness can be associated with severe and enduring mental health problems for many reasons but often occur because of fluctuating support needs over a long period of time. The issue of housing is historically linked to deinstitutionalization, with the closure of large hospitals and the shift of resources from inpatient to community settings. Razzouk (2019) investigated the costs and complexities of meeting the needs of long-term service users who often struggle to engage with local communities and facilities. As the stability of housing increases, rates of serious mental health problems decrease. For people with a severe and enduring mental health problem, the sense of being at home where they live can be helpful for managing their lives (Fossey et al. 2020).

Supported housing offers different levels of support according to need, often with an expectation that people will progress through services from levels of high support to levels of low support (Fossey et al. 2020). For people with severe and enduring mental health problems, this assumption may not reflect their ongoing needs and has led to instability in housing. Rees (2009) suggests that more positive outcomes are achieved by close working between housing, substance misuse and mental health services with assertive approaches. The role of the occupational therapist involves working with the individual to identify the most suitable accommodation to meet the individual's needs. There will also be work to develop skills to support their security of tenancy and progression to less supported environments.

Homelessness

People with severe and enduring mental health problems have a much higher risk of becoming homeless than the general population (O'Donovan et al. 2019). Being homeless includes living in any insecure accommodation, such as staying with friends, sleeping on the sofa as an alternative to living on the streets. Boland and Cunningham (2019) explored homelessness from an occupational perspective, identifying macro, meso and micro aspects. At a macro level, homelessness is a global issue caused by poverty, poor housing supply, unemployment and welfare priorities. At a meso level, homelessness support services are often provided by charities, with expectations of users about how they will engage with the service, which can be challenging for many. At a micro level, individuals vary in how they engage with occupation: some are focused on time use, avoiding boredom; some engage in non-sanctioned occupations, such as drinking alcohol; and others resist structured occupations (Boland and Cunningham 2019).

Occupational therapists can be involved with providing activity sessions for homeless people to promote and develop occupational engagement (Silva et al. 2018). For homeless people making the transition to supported accommodation, occupational therapy staff in one service offered a range of interventions including developing knowledge of a new place, accessing community resources, teaching life skills and fostering a sense of belonging. Being responsive to the needs of people with severe and enduring mental health problems was central to this approach (O'Donovan et al. 2019).

Personality Disorder Services

Borderline personality disorder is characterized by instability in interpersonal relationships and impairment of social, psychological and occupational functioning (National Institute for Health and Care Excellence 2009). This combination of difficulties raises challenges for community mental health services, and so specialist services have been established in some areas. The global prevalence of personality disorders has been estimated at 7.8%, being higher in high-income countries (9.6%) and lower in low-income countries (4.3%) (Winsper et al. 2020). Diagnosis of borderline personality disorder varies globally for unknown reasons, although Winsper et al. (2020) suggest increased wealth and inequality could be a factor. Harding (2020), an occupational therapist, has highlighted the stigma associated with the diagnosis for many people.

Key interventions are similar to other approaches to working with people with enduring mental health problems. Identifying long-term goals, including those relating to employment and occupation, are carried out in collaboration with the individual. These goals are then linked to realistic and achievable short-term objectives. Psychological approaches that support people to live with a diagnosis of borderline personality disorder include dialectical behaviour therapy and systems training for emotional predictability and problem solving (Federici and McMain 2009). Psychological approaches may inform occupational therapy for those in generic roles, such as psychoeducational groups (Leppanen et al. 2016).

Military Personnel and Veteran Mental Health Services

Reactions to and experiences of traumatic events such as armed conflict can lead to a range of mental health problems. The welfare and mental well-being of military personnel and veterans has renewed prominence due to prolonged conflicts throughout the world (Murphy et al. 2016). Occupational therapists have promoted their role in the treatment and management of post-traumatic stress disorder (Baum and Michael 2008). They argue that, in addition to medication and talking, therapies that focus on functioning through social and other therapeutic activities are critical to recovery. Kashiwa et al. (2017) highlight the role of occupational therapy and suicide prevention for veterans, engaging in suicide prevention training, fostering coping strategies and addressing occupational performance issues.

Liaison Psychiatry

Liaison psychiatry teams provide the interface between mental health and physical health services (Walker et al. 2018), carrying out specialist mental health assessments with people in general hospitals. These teams assess people who are experiencing difficulty in adjusting to physical health problems or who have diagnosed mental health problems. They also attend to people who have self-harmed and carry out a comprehensive mental health and risk assessment. A person may then be transferred on to one of the other community mental health services. Where there are felt to be occupational needs, occupational therapists are often accessed through other teams either within the general hospital or via the other community mental health teams according to need.

CONCLUSION

The different community settings outlined offer many opportunities and challenges for working with people with severe and enduring mental health problems. Using supporting models and approaches can enhance practice and the experience of the person receiving services. Awareness of historical and current issues, as well as being alert to emergent themes, can aid appropriately responsive collaborative care. Multidisciplinary teams may exert pressure for the therapist to work generically, while professional groups have an expectation that a specialist role is retained. The reality is that occupational therapists undertake a dual role and are competent mental health practitioners. Care coordination and recovery-oriented practice recognize and support the skilled use of occupation as a therapeutic medium. There is also the need to work flexibly to best meet people's needs. Responding to current demands and expectations requires a clear focus on how to make the most effective and efficient contribution within diverse community mental health teams and services.

QUESTIONS FOR CONSIDERATION

1. What do occupational therapists mean by 'community' in relation to mental health service provision?
2. Consider the steps in the Cycle of Change framework. Have you experienced behaviour change that relates to these steps? Has someone else you know experienced this?
3. What aspects of care coordination make it possible for occupational therapists to take on the role?
4. What does a narrative approach to positive risk-taking involve?
5. Why might there be a problem with non-adherence to prescribed medication?
6. What are the two main objectives for early intervention for psychosis services?
7. How do occupational therapists work in assertive outreach teams?
8. There are many reasons that mental health is challenged by homelessness or housing difficulties. What are some of the most significant reasons, and how could an occupational therapist respond?

SERVICE USER COMMENTARY

During the early phase of a severe mental illness, a patient may be having experiences that they cannot put a name to. So, it is true that 'many people find a diagnosis beneficial,' because they realize that they are ill.

'Parity of esteem' is very important as the stigma attached to being diagnosed can mean that patients feel that they are being treated like second-class citizens, particularly when accessing mainstream health services. Also, in some places, the idea that there is now a 'greater emphasis on prevention rather treatment' is not uniformly true. Some workers do still focus on symptoms and illness despite the fact that recovery is now the priority.

The 'cycle of change' gives a name to something that I have experienced for myself without realizing what it was. It is relevant and I know of a few people who have been moving forwards and backwards between various stages for years.

The reality of the situation is that mental health services do retraumatise people, and this is not limited to 'rapid tranquilisation injections.' The long-term treatment of certain people is at best shabby, with patients being ignored for months by the people that are supposed to be caring for them.

Stress is a factor in mental illness that some people do not pay as much attention to as they should, and I believe that 'childhood trauma' was a major factor in the development of my long-term illness. That said, I find that the 'stress vulnerability bucket' is an over-simplification of the many ways in which stress can affect a person's life experiences.

I would like to take issue with the statement that 'the aim of the CPA is to put the person at the centre of the planning process and empower them.' That certainly didn't happen with me; once the plan had been written, that was it and I never saw it again. It wasn't referred to either.

I would like to note that, while the chapter is almost free of jargon, there are a few phrases that need to be highlighted. Patients are supposed 'to take ownership within the CPA process'; 'A narrative approach to risk is proposed.' What do these statements actually mean? And what does the word 'biopsychosocial' mean?

Later on, it is stated that 'positive risk-taking is deciding to do something for which the positive outcome is worth taking a risk for.' In my experience some therapists try to eliminate any risk-taking behaviour on the basis that the patient has a history of alcohol and or substance abuse and so should avoid risk completely. In effect, they wrap the patient up in cotton wool.

People take medication because they are told to; they trust the mental health workers that work with them. Side-effects are a big problem because patients are already dealing with the symptoms of their illness, and then the medication makes them over-tired as well. Medication needs to be managed because sometimes patients don't want to move on: despite the severity of their symptoms, it is what they have become used to.

Christopher Wood

REFERENCES

Anthony, W. A. (1993). Recovery from mental illness: The guiding vision of the mental health service system in the 1990s. *Psychosocial Rehabilitation Journal, 16*(4), 11–23.

Bamford, C., Wheatley, A., Shaw, C., & Allan, L. M. (2019). Equipping staff with the skills to maximise recovery of people with dementia after an injurious fall. *Aging & Mental Health, 23*(11), 1524–1532. https://doi.org/10.1080/13607863.2018.1501664.

Baum, C., & Michael, E. (2008). *Statement of the american occupational therapy association presented to the United States house of representatives committee veterans' affairs subcommittee on health.* Bethesda, MD: AOTA.

Boland, L., & Cunningham, M. (2019). Homelessness: Critical reflections and observations from an occupational perspective. *Journal of Occupational Science, 26*(2), 308–315. https://doi.org/10.1080/14427591.2018.1512006.

Bonney, S., & Stickley, T. (2008). Recovery and mental health: A review of the literature. *Journal of Psychiatric and Mental Health Nursing, 15*(2), 140–153.

Brabban, A., & Turkington, D. (2002). The search for meaning detecting congruence between life events, underlying schema and psychotic symptoms. In A. P. Morrison (Ed.), *A casebook of cognitive therapy for psychosis* (pp. 59–75). New York: Brunner-Routledge.

Coid, J., Yang, M., Tyrer, P., et al. (2006). Prevalence and correlates of personality disorder in Great Britain. *British Journal of Psychiatry, 188*, 423–431.

College of Occupational Therapists. (2006). *Recovering ordinary lives: The strategy for occupational therapy in mental health services 2007–2017.* London: Royal College of Occupational Therapists.

Conn, A., Bourke, N., James, C., & Haracz, K. (2019). Occupational therapy intervention addressing weight gain and obesity in people with severe mental illness: A scoping review. *Australian Occupational Therapy Journal, 66*(4), 446–457. Available at: https://pubmed.ncbi.nlm.nih.gov/30972772/.

Department of Health (DH). (2000). *The NHS plan: A plan for investment, a plan for reform.* London: HMSO.

Department of Health (DH). (2001a). *The journey to recovery – the government's vision for mental health Care.* London: HMSO.

Department of Health (DH). (2001b). *The mental health policy implementation guide.* London: HMSO.

Department of Health (DH). (2008). *Refocussing the Care programme approach: Policy and positive practice guidance.* London: HMSO.

Dillon, J., Johnstone, L., & Longden, E. (2012). Trauma, dissociation, attachment and neuroscience: A new paradigm for understanding severe mental distress. In E. Speed, J. Moncrief, & M. Rapley (Eds.), *De-medicalising misery II* (pp. 226–234). London: Palgrave Macmillan.

Eley, A. (2018). *The role of the mental health representative at marac.* Available at: https://safelives.org.uk/practice_blog/role-mental-health-representative-marac.

Federici, A., & McMain, S. (2009). Recent advances in psychosocial treatments for borderline personality disorder. *Medical representatives, 1,* 51.

Felton, A., Wright, N., & Stacey, G. (2017). Therapeutic risk-taking: A justifiable choice. *BJPsych Advances, 23*(2), 81–88. https://doi.org/10.1192/apt.bp.115.015701.

Fossey, E., Harvey, C., & McDermott, F. (2020). Housing and support narratives of people experiencing mental health issues: Making my place, my home. *Frontiers in Psychiatry, 10,* 939. https://doi.org/10.3389/fpsyt.2019.00939.

Gilburt, H. (2018). *Funding and staffing of NHS mental health providers: Still waiting for parity.* The Kings Fund. Available at: https://www.kingsfund.org.uk/publications/funding-staffing-mental-health-providers.

Gould, D. (2012). *Service users experience of recovery under the 2008 Care programme approach – a research study.* Available at: https://www.mentalhealth.org.uk/sites/default/files/CPA_research_study.pdf.

Harding, K. (2020). Words matter: The royal College of psychiatrists' position statement on personality disorder. *The Lancet Psychiatry, 7,* e25.

Hassan G, Kirmayer LJ, Mekki Berrada A, et al. *Culture, Context and the Mental Health and Psychosocial Wellbeing of Syrians: A Review for Mental Health and Psychosocial Support staff working with Syrians Affected by Armed Conflict.* ;16–17. Geneva: UNHCR; 2015.

Jones, S. (2020). A functional perspective to information gathering, risk assessment and insight-building. In A. Janice, K. Mackenzie, & E. Wilkinson (Eds.), *Assessing mental capacity: A handbook to guide professionals from basic to advanced practice.* Routledge. ISBN 9781315103440.

Kashiwa, A., Sweetman, M. M., & Helgeson, L. (2017). Centennial topics—occupational therapy and veteran suicide: A call to action. *American Journal of Occupational Therapy, 71,* 7105100010. https://doi.org/10.5014/ajot.2017.023358.

Kelly, M., Lamont, S., & Brunero, S. (2010). An occupational perspective of the recovery journey in mental health. *British Journal of Occupational Therapy, 73*(3), 129–135.

Leamy, M., Bird, V., Le Boutilier, C., Williams, J., & Slade, M. (2011). A conceptual framework for personal recovery in mental health: Systematic review and narrative synthesis. *British Journal of Psychiatry, 199*(6), 445–452.

Leppänen, V., Hakko, H., Sintonen, H., & Lindeman, S. (2016). Comparing effectiveness of treatments for borderline personality disorder in communal mental health care: The oulu BPD study. *Community Mental Health Journal, 52*(2), 216–227.

Machtinger, E. L., Davis, K. B., Kimberg, L. S., et al. (2019). From treatment to healing: Inquiry and response to recent and past trauma in adult health care. *Women's Health Issues, 29*(2), 97–102. Available at: https://www.whijournal.com/article/S1049-3867(18)30550-4/fulltext.

Marshall, M., & Rathbone, J. (2011). Early intervention for psychosis. *Cochrane Database of Systematic Reviews, 6,* CD004718.

Mind. (2017). *Mental health problems: An introduction.* Available at: https://www.mind.org.uk/information-support/types-of-mental-health-problems/mental-health-problems-introduction/causes/.

Mind. (2018). *Health and social care rights: What is safeguarding in social Care?* Available at: https://www.mind.org.uk/information-support/legal-rights/health-and-social-care-rights/safeguarding-in-social-care/#:~:text=Safeguarding%20means%20protecting%20your%20right,are%20at%20risk%20of%20either).

Mitchell, A. J., & Selmes, T. (2007). Why don't patients take their medicine? Reasons and solutions in psychiatry. *Advances in Psychiatric Treatment, 13*(5), 336–346.

Morant, N., Lloyd-Evans, B., & Lamb, D. (2017). Crisis resolution and home treatment: Stakeholders' views on critical ingredients and implementation in England. *BMC Psychiatry, 17*(254).

Morgan, S. (2020). *Why positive risk-taking is so misunderstood.* Available at: https://strengthsrevolution.net/category/positive-risk-taking/.

Murphy, D., SpencerHarper, L., Carson, C., et al. Long-term responses to treatment in UK veterans with military-related PTSD: An observational study. *British Medical Journal Open, 6,* e011667. https://doi.org/10.1136/bmjopen-2016-011667.

National Collaborating Centre for Mental Health (NCCMH). (2019). *The community mental health framework for adults and older adults.* Available at: https://www.england.nhs.uk/wp-content/uploads/2019/09/community-mental-health-framework-for-adults-and-older-adults.pdf.

National Institute for Health and Care Excellence (NICE). (2009). *NICE clinical guideline 78 – Borderline personality disorder.* London: NICE.

Neale, A., & Kinnair, D. (2017). Early intervention in psychosis services. *British Journal of General Practice, 67*(661), 370–371. https://doi.org/10.3399/bjgp17X692069.

NHS England. (2019). *NHS mental health implementation plan 2019/20 – 2023/24.* Available at: https://www.longtermplan.nhs.uk/wp-content/uploads/2019/07/nhs-mental-health-implementation-plan-2019-20-2023-24.pdf.

National Institute for Mental Health England. (2004). *Crisis resolution and home treatment.* UCE Birmingham: NIMHE.

Norman, R., & Malla, A. K. (2001). Duration of untreated psychosis: A critical examination of the concept and its importance. *Psychological Medicine, 31*(3), 381–400.

Nosowska, G. (2010). OT: Are we ready to put people first? *Occupational Therapy International, 6,* 50.

Nugent, A., Hancock, N., & Honey, A. (2017). Developing and sustaining recovery-orientation in mental health practice: Experiences of occupational therapists. *Occupational Therapy International.* https://doi.org/10.1155/2017/5190901.

O'Donovan, J., Russell, K., Kuipers, P., Siskind, D., & Elphinston, R. A. (2019). A place to call home: Hearing the perspectives of people living with homelessness and mental illness through service evaluation. *Community Mental Health Journal, 55,* 1218–1225.

Patel, V., Saxena, S., De Silva, M., & Samele, C. (2013). *Transforming lives, enhancing communities: Innovations in mental health.* Available at: https://www.imperial.ac.uk/media/imperial-college/institute-of-global-health-innovation/public/WISH_Mental_Health_Report.pdf.

Prochaska, J., & DiClemente, C. (1986). Toward a comprehensive model of change. In W. Miller, & N. Heather (Eds.), *Treating addictive behaviours: Processes of Change.* New York: Plenum Press.

Rapp, C. A. (1998). *The strengths model: Case management with people suffering from severe and persistent mental Illness.* New York: Oxford University Press.

Razzouk D. Accommodation and Health Costs of Deinstitutionalized People with Mental Illness Living in Residential Services in Brazil. *Pharmacoecon Open.* 2019;3(1):31–42. https://doi.org/10.1007/s41669-018-0078-z.

Reed, K., & Jaxson, L. (2019). Shared decision making: Exploring the experience of mental health practitioners. *New Zealand Journal of Occupational Therapy, 66*(3), 5–10.

Rees, S. (2009). *Mental ill health in the adult single homeless population. A review of the literature.* London: Crisis.

Repper, J., & Perkins, R. (2003). *Social inclusion and recovery: A model for mental health practice.* London: Bailliere Tindall.

Royal College of Occupational Therapists (RCOT). (2019). *Medicines management and administration Responsibilities.* London: Royal College of Occupational Therapists.

Ryan, P., & Morgan, S. (2004). *Assertive outreach: A strengths approach to policy and practice.* London: Churchill Livingstone.

Sayer, J., Paniagua, D., Ballentine, S., et al. (2019). Perspectives on diet and physical activity among urban African Americans with serious mental illness. *Social Work in Health Care, 58*(5), 509–525. https://doi.org/10.1080/00981389.2019.1587662.

Scanlan, L. M., Devine, S. G., & Watkins, D. L. (2019). Job satisfaction of mental healthcare workers in multidisciplinary teams. *Journal of Mental Health, 30*(1), 80–87. https://doi.org/10.1080/09638237.2019.1644489.

Silva, C. R., Silvestrini, M. S., Poellnitz, J. C. V., Prado, A. C. S. A., & Leite Junior, J. D. (2018). Creative strategies and homeless people: Occupational therapy, art, culture and sensitive displacement. *Cadernos Brasileiros de Terapia Ocupacional, 26*(2), 489–500.

Slade, M. (2009). *The handbook of recovery.* Cambridge: Cambridge University Press.

Stein, L. I., & Santos, A. B. (1998). *Assertive community treatment of persons with severe mental illness.* London: Norton.

Stickley, T., & Felton, A. (2006). Promoting recovery through therapeutic risk taking. *Mental Health Practice, 9*(8), 26–30.

Stulz, N., Wyder, L., Maeck, L., et al. (2020). Home treatment for acute mental healthcare: Randomised controlled trial. *British Journal of Psychiatry, 216*(6), 323–330. https://doi.org/10.1192/bjp.2019.31.

Sweeney, A., Clement, S., Filson, B., & Kennedy, A. (2016). Trauma informed mental health care in the UK: What is it and how can we further its development? *Mental Health Review Journal, 21*(3), 174–192.

Tait, L., & Shah, S. (2007). Partnership working: A policy with promise for mental healthcare. *Advances in Psychiatric Treatment, 13,* 261–271.

The National Archives, 1959. Available at: www.legislation.gov.uk/ukpga/Eliz2/7-8/72/enacted.

Thew, M., Bell, F., & Flanagan, E. (2017). Social prescribing: An emerging area for occupational therapy. *British Journal of Occupational Therapy, 80*(9), 523–524.

Time to Change. (2020). *Violence & mental health.* Available at: https://www.time-to-change.org.uk/media-centre/responsible-reporting/violence-mental-health-problems.

Turton, P., Wright, C., White, S., et al. (2010). Promoting recovery in long-term institutional mental health care: An international delphi study. *Psychiatric Services, 61*(3), 293–299.

United Nations. (2006). *Convention on the rights of persons with disabilities.* New York: United Nations.

Vahdaninia, M., Simkhada, B., van Teijlingen, E., et al. (2020). Mental health services designed for black, asian and minority ethnics (BAME) in the UK: A scoping review. *Mental Health and Social Inclusion, 24*(2), 81–95.

Wahlbeck, K., Westman, J., Nordentoft, M., et al. (2011). Outcomes of nordic mental health systems: Life expectancy of patients with mental disorders. *British Journal of Psychiatry, 199*(6), 453–458.

Walker, A., Barrett, J. R., Lee, W., et al. (2018). Organisation and delivery of liaison psychiatry services in general hospitals in England: Results of a national survey. *British Medical Journal Open, 8,* e023091. doi: 10.1136/bmjopen-2018-023091.

Winsper, C., Bilgin, A., Thompson, A., et al. (2020). The prevalence of personality disorders in the community: A global systematic review and meta-analysis. *British Journal of Psychiatry, 216*(2), 69–78.

World Health Organization (WHO). (2003). *Adherence: Setting the scene.* Available at: https://www.who.int/chp/knowledge/publications/adherence_Section1.pdf?ua=1.

World Health Organization (WHO). (2013). *mhGAP: Mental health gap action programme: Scaling up care for mental, neurological and substance use disorders.* Geneva: WHO.

Zubin, J., & Spring, B. (1977). Vulnerability: A new view on schizophrenia. *Journal of Abnormal Psychology, 86*(2), 103–126.

23 OLDER PEOPLE

JENNIFER WENBORN

CHAPTER OUTLINE

INTRODUCTION

Globally, the number of older people is growing, albeit with geographical differences, including those surviving into very old age, due to advances in medicine and management of disease, lower rates of fertility and infant mortality, and improved public health awareness. Compared to 962 million people aged 60 and over in 2017, the number is expected to more than double to 2.1 billion by 2050 with the proportion of people aged 80 and above also rising from 137 million in 2017 to 425 million in 2050 (United Nations, Department of Economic and Social Affairs Population Division 2017). Older people are often supported and cared for by family and friends, many of whom are older themselves. Hence, there is a huge financial and social cost of caring for older people, especially those with dementia.

The practice examples and terminology used in this chapter are primarily from the United Kingdom, where older people are the biggest users of health and social care services. Occupational therapists, therefore, work with older people in many settings, including specialist older adults' mental health and dementia services, as well as psychiatric liaison, emergency departments, medical and surgical wards in general hospitals and local authority social services. Specialist mental health services are provided to older adults in inpatient wards and increasingly via a range of community-based services such as community mental health teams, home treatment teams, dementia crisis teams, and memory services. Occupational therapists increasingly provide services within care homes, often on an in-reach basis. Many of these services are provided in other countries albeit referred to by different titles.

Services are provided within the context of ever-changing health and social care policy, but primarily focused on a number of consistent themes. These include raising awareness of mental health issues and dementia; early diagnosis and timely access to services to support older people and their families; the need for all staff in contact with older people to be aware of, and appropriately trained to meet, their needs; and specialist staff being available in consultative, advisory, and educational roles. There is an emphasis on enabling older people to remain as independent as possible for as long as possible within their own homes with dignity, respect, and choice at the heart of service provision. There is also a key health promotion agenda focused on encouraging people to age healthily and actively, both mentally and physically.

Older people can experience a combination of physical, psychological, sensory and cognitive challenges as they age. Many older people also experience the impact of losses that often occur in later life, such as loneliness, social isolation, loss of independence and roles, and bereavement. However, it is important to remember that depression and dementia are not inevitable features of the ageing process. Therefore occupational therapists need to be able to differentiate between changes caused by 'normal' ageing and the impact of other physical or mental health conditions that are not an inevitable consequence of getting older.

Each older person is unique but 'older people' are often depicted as a homogeneous group by the media using negative stereotypes. Older people can experience ageism and discrimination in terms of service provision, with health and social care professionals making prejudicial assumptions about the validity of interventions (Age UK 2016; Royal College of Psychiatrists (RCOT) 2018).

Occupational therapists usually work as members of a multidisciplinary team, often linking with other statutory and voluntary agencies. Within older adults' mental health services, it is common for occupational therapists to cover a combination of generic mental health and specialist occupational therapy roles and activities. While this offers the opportunity to develop more generic skills in managing risks and crises, service demands may reduce the capacity to deliver occupation-focused interventions (Swinson et al. 2016). A range of interventions are used by occupational therapists working with older people, both on a one-to-one and a group basis (see Chapter 16 on the therapeutic use of groups). There is growing evidence to support the effectiveness of these as well as of occupational therapy specific programmes.

The first half of this chapter describes the importance of occupation in maintaining health and well-being in older age, highlighting health-promoting occupation-based interventions. The causes and impact of later life depression and the potential occupational therapy role are summarized. The causes, prevalence and diagnosis of dementia are outlined along with a description of person-centred care and the range of evidence-based non-pharmacological interventions that are commonly used by occupational therapists within their practice. The second section describes the occupational therapy assessment of older people and the most commonly used assessment tools. The role of community occupational therapy in dementia and occupational therapy provision to care homes is illustrated through examples of the profession's developing evidence base. Finally, practice issues such as mental capacity, assessing and managing risk, and working with carers are discussed.

OCCUPATION FOR MENTAL HEALTH AND WELL-BEING IN LATER LIFE

The urge to engage in purposeful and meaningful activity is a basic human drive that is essential for physical and mental health and well-being regardless of age. Our individual personality, life story, interests, values and beliefs influence our choice of activity and what we do partly defines who we are. It has long been recognized that participation in meaningful activity has a positive effect on the health, self-esteem, happiness and life satisfaction of older people (Gregory 1983; Bowling et al. 1997). It also reduces mortality (Glass et al. 1999) and is a key contributor to quality of life (Age Concern and Mental Health Foundation 2006). Older people are advised to 'use it or lose it' (Gilhooly et al. 2003) as physical activities can postpone cognitive decline (van Gelder et al. 2004) and frequent cognitively stimulating activity can reduce the risk of dementia (Verghese et al. 2003).

The Well Elderly Study

Conducted in southern California the 'Well Elderly Study' (Clark et al. 1997; Jackson et al. 1998) recruited 361 people aged 60 or over who lived independently in the community. Participants were randomly assigned to either the preventative occupational therapy 'Lifestyle Redesign®' programme; a social activity group; or a control group. Results showed significant benefit for people attending the occupational therapy group in terms of general health, physical and social functioning, mood and well-being. The social activity programme was no more effective in promoting health and well-being than receiving no intervention.

Lifestyle Redesign®

Lifestyle Redesign® is an occupation-based approach to healthy ageing. It aims to empower older people to examine and analyse their own occupations to enable participation in meaningful activity, thus maximizing independence and function, and potentially preventing or reducing a negative spiral of ill-health and disability. The programme is facilitated by occupational therapists and runs for nine months. Participants attend a weekly, two-hour group session and also have a monthly hour-long one-to-one meeting with a facilitator to focus on achieving their individual goals. Sessions include didactic teaching alongside activity engagement, with participants rating the impact of each activity on their own health and well-being. The social activity intervention was a programme of the same duration run by non-professional staff providing activities to promote social interaction. The control group did not receive any intervention.

Lifestyle Matters

Inspired by Lifestyle Redesign®, a similar, occupation-based health promotion intervention tailored for the UK population 'Lifestyle Matters' was developed through consultation with older people (Craig and Mountain 2007). The intervention aims to enable community living older people to make positive lifestyle choices and participate in new or neglected activities through increasing self-efficacy. It consists of weekly group meetings in addition to some one-to-one sessions and runs over four months. A feasibility study measured impact on cognition, mood, functional dependency and quality of life, and indicated an upward trend in quality of life; whilst a qualitative analysis indicated that participants experienced benefits such as improved self-efficacy (Mountain et al. 2008). The efficacy and cost-effectiveness of Lifestyle Matters was subsequently evaluated through a randomized controlled trial (RCT; Mountain et al. 2017). In that study 288 independently living people aged 65 and above were recruited and randomly allocated to either participate in the intervention or to continue with their usual schedule. The primary outcome was mental well-being at 26 weeks post-randomization as measured by the mental health dimension of the SF-36, but the intention to treat analysis showed no evidence of clinical effectiveness. A purposeful sample of 13 participants allocated to the intervention were interviewed at 24 months post-randomization to explore whether it had any impact on their lifestyle choices, participation in meaningful activities and well-being (Chatters et al. 2017). The majority reported minor benefits and increases in self-efficacy, but there were significant and lasting benefits for two of the participants, who reported having also experienced a significant life-changing event preceding the study. The findings raise the question as to how to most effectively target the delivery of preventative interventions such as this to reach those who are at greatest risk of decline. Further analysis of this qualitative data suggests that the intervention could have a positive effect, but only if it is targeted at older adults at most risk of age-related decline and if the intervention is delivered as planned (Mountain et al. 2020). The subsequent development of this intervention for use with people in the early stages of dementia, namely 'Journeying through Dementia,' is discussed later in this chapter.

Based on the earlier evidence, occupational therapy interventions such as Lifestyle Matters were recommended within the UK National Institute for Health and Care Excellence (NICE) public health guidance regarding 'Mental wellbeing in over 65s: occupational therapy and physical activity interventions' (NICE 2008). Occupational therapy input to train health and social care staff to effectively enable older people to participate in activities that help maintain or improve health and well-being was also recommended. The later NICE guideline 'Older People; independence and mental wellbeing' (NICE 2015) recommends interventions such as group activities, one-to-one activities and volunteering to maintain and improve the mental well-being and independence of people aged 65 and above. It states that certain life events or circumstances are more likely to increase the risk of decline, for example, an older person whose partner has died in the last two years. Practitioners need to be aware that the people who are at most risk of decline are also those who: are carers; live alone and have little opportunity to socialise; have recently separated or divorced; have recently retired (particularly if involuntary); were unemployed in later life; have a low income; have recently experienced or developed a health problem (whether or not it led to hospital admission); have had to give up driving; have an age-related disability; and are aged 80 or older. Both guidance documents were reviewed in 2018 following which the earlier document is currently being updated in the light of new evidence to support the effectiveness of occupational therapy interventions, and physical activity interventions such as yoga, Pilates, and tai chi. The most recent NICE pathway for mental well-being and independence in older people (NICE 2020) recommends the types of information older people need to maintain or improve their well-being, as well as recommendations for individual interventions and group activities. Volunteering, walking schemes, and exercise programs are other recommended interventions that occupational therapists can support older people to access.

DEPRESSION IN LATER LIFE

Depression is a mood disorder, characterized by continued low mood and/or loss of interest and pleasure in nearly all activities for most of each day for the preceding two weeks accompanied by one or more of the following symptoms: marked weight loss or gain, or increased/decreased appetite; disturbed sleep pattern; psychomotor agitation or retardation; feelings of fatigue or loss of energy; guilt or worthlessness; poor concentration or indecisiveness; recurrent thoughts of death or suicide or a suicide attempt or specific plan (Diagnostic and Statistical Manual of Mental Disorders (DSM-5) criteria; American Psychiatric Association 2013). Its severity can range from experiencing low mood and depressive symptoms to a major depressive episode.

Prevalence

The percentage of people with depression is higher in the older age group than any other age group and it is the most common mental health disorder in older people, estimated to affect 22% of men and 28% of women aged 65 and above (RCOT 2018; Age UK 2019). An estimated 4.6-9.3% of adults aged 75 and over have a major depressive disorder, with up to 37.4% experiencing subthreshold depressive symptoms (Frost et al. 2019). It is estimated that approximately 25% of older people living in the community have some degree of depressive symptoms requiring intervention, with the prevalence trebling for those residing in care homes (RCOT 2018).

Risk and Protective Factors

This higher percentage occurs in old age as people become more vulnerable to risk factors such as being widowed or divorced, experiencing physical ill-health or disability, lacking family support, being lonely or socially isolated, being retired or unemployed and having a history of depression. Older people may also develop depression due to genetic susceptibility (which increases with age), neurobiological changes associated with ageing or medication prescribed for other conditions. Major life events such as bereavement, separation, acute illness, moving into institutional care, major financial crisis, negative interactions with family, loss of a 'significant other' (including a pet) or caring for a family member (Rodda et al. 2011) can also trigger depression. Depression in older adults is associated with poorer quality of life, increased risk of death, cognitive and functional decline and suicide; proportionately more people aged 65 and above commit suicide, mostly due to major depression (Rodda et al. 2011; Frost et al. 2019).

Presentation

Depression is diagnosed using the same criteria as for younger adults. However, the presentation in older people often differs and is therefore not always recognized or treated. Older people are more likely to present somatic symptoms such as loss of appetite or fatigue that may be falsely attributed to a coexisting medical condition or just put down to 'old age.' Older people may minimize any feelings of sadness they have, being a generation not used to 'bothering' their doctor about how they feel. If left untreated, a person's behaviour can resemble that of someone with dementia. This is sometimes referred to as 'pseudodementia.' It is vital to differentiate between depression and dementia to offer the appropriate care. The onset of depression can usually be pinpointed to a specific date, whereas the onset of dementia is more insidious. Depression and dementia can also coexist.

Alcohol and Substance Misuse in Later Life

The body's tolerance to alcohol diminishes with age, thus leading to an increased risk of intoxication. Approximately one in five older men and one in ten older women drink alcohol at a potentially harmful level; and one in three of those aged 65 and over who misuse alcohol developed this problem later in life (Drink Wise Age Well 2019). Alcohol misuse can be precipitated by many of the same risk factors as for depression, namely, bereavement, loss and loneliness, physical ill-health, disability, pain and increasing dependence; and is more likely to go undetected among older people. Likewise, substance misuse is also increasing in the older age group, with 8% of those admitted to hospital due to poisoning by illicit drugs in 2016–2017 being aged 65 and over, compared with 6% in 2010–2011 (RCOT 2018). Older people are also at high risk of misusing prescription drugs such as benzodiazepines and opioids (RCOT 2018).

Diagnosis

To understand what is affecting a person, a detailed history is obtained from the person and family and should cover major adverse life events, previous coping strategies and personality traits and drug and alcohol usage. Blood tests are taken to identify physical conditions that may resemble depression such as hypothyroidism or any deficiencies that commonly occur in people who are depressed, such as folate levels, which may fall due to malnutrition caused by appetite loss. A screening assessment tool will also be used. Those commonly used with working age adults do not necessarily have validity and reliability for use with older people, so the most frequently used tools with this age group are:

- Patient Health Questionnaire (PHQ-9) (Kroenke et al. 2001). This is self-rated with 9 questions that score each of the DSM criteria from 0 (not at all) to 3 (nearly every day). Scores indicate the following levels of depression: 0–4 none, 5–9 mild, 10–14 moderate, 15–19 moderately severe, 20–27 severe. This tool is available in over 50 languages, making it useful in range of different contexts.
- The Geriatric Depression Scale (GDS-15) (Yesavage et al. 1983). This is self-rated with 15 questions requiring a yes or no answer. Scores above 5 indicate depression.
- Hospital Anxiety and Depression Scale (HADS) (Zigmond and Snaith 1983). This is self-rated using two subscales that measure anxiety and depressive symptoms over the preceding week. Scores above 8 indicate depression.
- Cornell Scale for Depression in Dementia (Alexopoulos et al. 1988). This is specifically designed for use with people who have dementia and is completed through an interview with the person themselves and/or a relative or carer, depending on the severity of dementia. Scores above 8 indicate depression.

Intervention

Later-life depression is often managed in primary care with 87.1% of patients being prescribed antidepressant medication (Frost et al. 2019) despite increased age being associated with reduced efficacy and more side-effects. Psychological therapies such as cognitive behavioural therapy have been shown to be equally effective in older and younger adults with depression (Cuijpers et al. 2009a) but are not always offered (Rodda et al. 2011; Frost et al. 2019). A combination of pharmacological and psychological therapies has been shown to be more effective than psychological therapy alone for older people (Cuijpers et al. 2009b).

Impact on Occupational Performance

Depression can affect people's motivation and ability to initiate or carry out activity. Someone who is depressed may lack concentration and confidence in their abilities and find it difficult to make choices. Lack of appetite and changed sleep patterns can result in low energy, slowness and generalized aches and pains. People may become uninterested in or neglect their appearance. Feelings of anxiety can lead to agitation, wandering and behaviour that family and carers can find difficult to cope with. It is difficult to say categorically whether it is a lack of activity that leads to depression or if being depressed reduces participation. It is probably a combination of both. When an older person experiences lowered mood precipitated by other risk factors, such as poor physical health or bereavement, this is likely to lead to reduced opportunities to participate in personally meaningful activities. The risk of depression can be reduced by taking regular exercise, planning for major life transitions such as retirement or moving to a care home, seeking support when bereaved, maintaining activities and social involvement.

Occupational Therapy

Bearing in mind the link between participation in activities and maintaining mental well-being, occupational therapists have an important role in the detection and management of later life depression. The primary aim of occupational therapy intervention is to enable the older person to engage in valued daily occupations and roles. Occupational therapists use many of the interventions outlined previously, delivered with an occupational emphasis and incorporating the following principles:

- Encouraging an individual to attempt activity;
- Using familiar activities to increase self-confidence;

- Using personally meaningful activities to increase motivation and self-confidence;
- Limiting the number of choices to be made;
- Enhancing self-confidence through self-care activities, such as hairdressing or manicures;
- Providing reassurance and opportunities to wander safely to reduce agitation;
- Encouraging people who are fatigued to do 'little and often';
- Setting short term, realistically achievable goals;
- Using activities that quickly provide a successful end result for positive reinforcement;
- Providing opportunities for social interaction for those who have withdrawn or become isolated due to anxiety or bereavement;
- Supporting people to utilize community resources, such as day clubs and transport schemes;
- Supporting people to manage their mental and physical health conditions.

DEMENTIA

The diagnostic criteria now categorize dementia as a neurocognitive disorder (NCD) reflecting that the major symptom is cognitive decline due to physical changes within the brain (DSM-5 criteria, American Psychiatric Association 2013). NCD is then divided into two categories: mild and major, with the former having modest impact on cognitive performance and unlikely to affect day-to-day living other than the most complex tasks; whilst the latter has substantial impact on cognitive performance and interferes with basic activities of daily living (ADLs). For simplicity the term 'dementia' is used within this text.

'Dementia is an umbrella term for several diseases that are mostly progressive, affecting memory, other cognitive abilities and behaviour, and that interfere significantly with a person's ability to maintain the activities of daily living' (World Health Organization 2017, p. 2). Early onset dementia refers to an onset before the age of 65 and late onset applies to an onset at 65 years or older. The presentation and progression of dementia varies from individual to individual, partly due to the underlying pathology, but is also influenced by the person's own personality and their unique combination of practical and emotional support networks. What is common is its progressive nature.

Causes

There are many causes of dementia with the most common type being Alzheimer's disease, which changes the chemistry and structure of the brain and accounts for approximately 60% to 70% of cases globally. Other types include: vascular dementia, which results from poor oxygen supply to the brain; mixed dementia (Alzheimer's and vascular combined); dementia with Lewy bodies, which is caused by protein being deposited within nerve cells, and shares features of Parkinson's disease, such as slowness of movement; plus rarer causes of dementia including frontotemporal dementia, human immunodeficiency virus/acquired immunodeficiency syndrome, Huntington's disease, Creutzfeldt-Jakob disease, Korsakoff syndrome and Pick's disease.

Prevalence

Whilst dementia is not specifically a condition of old age, prevalence does increase exponentially with age so the number of people living with dementia is due to increase in tandem with the increasing ageing population (Livingston et al. 2020). Globally, the number of people living with dementia was 50 million in 2018, of whom 66% lived in low- and middle-income countries. This figure is due to rise to 152 million in 2050, of whom 72% will live in low- and middle-income countries, which equates to someone being diagnosed with dementia every 3.2 seconds (Patterson 2018). However, the incidence has recently decreased in some areas, primarily due to the improved management of modifiable risk factors, such as treating hypertension in middle to later life (Livingston et al. 2020), thus emphasizing the importance of promoting preventative strategies. It is estimated that 40% of dementia worldwide could be prevented or delayed by addressing 12 modifiable risk factors: less education, hypertension, hearing impairment, smoking, obesity, depression, physical inactivity, diabetes, low social contact, excessive alcohol consumption, traumatic brain injury and air pollution (Livingston et al. 2020).

Impact on Occupational Performance

A person with dementia can find it increasingly difficult to remember things, know where they are, recognize other people, keep track of time, organize themselves, understand what is being said to them,

communicate with other people, make decisions and learn new things. As a result, the person will experience increasing difficulty in carrying out everyday tasks. The need to engage in activity is intrinsic to all human beings and people with dementia are no exception, but they increasingly need the help of caregivers, be they family and friends (informal, unpaid) or health and social care staff (formal, paid), to do this (Kitwood 1997). As the person with dementia loses their skills, abilities and former roles, their family often experience a feeling of increased burden and stress, which can impact on their own occupational opportunities and performance.

Neuropsychiatric or behavioural and psychological symptoms of dementia, such as disturbed perception, thought content, or mood; or challenging behaviour, such as physical or verbal aggression, occur in approximately one-third of people with mild dementia, and in two-thirds of those with more severe impairment. These problems are known to contribute to increased caregiver burden, institutionalisation and decreased quality of life for the person themselves and their carers (Livingston et al. 2017). The prevalence of depression in people with dementia is estimated to be at least 20%; this can reduce quality of life, exacerbate cognitive and functional impairment; and is associated with increased mortality and carer stress and depression (Livingston et al. 2017). In addition, there is moderate evidence to suggest that antidepressant treatment does not improve symptoms (Livingston et al. 2020).

Diagnosis

Many countries have policies in place that emphasize the need for early diagnosis by a specialist service, to enable people with dementia and their family to access support and make informed choices to plan accordingly for their future. Within the United Kingdom, for example, the establishment of dedicated Memory Services within community mental health services enables early diagnosis by specialist multidisciplinary teams that often include occupational therapists.

The diagnosis process includes obtaining a history, physical examination, review of medication, blood tests and use of a structured cognitive assessment. The Mini Mental State Examination (MMSE) (Folstein et al. 1975) is a well known screening tool that has long been in frequent clinical and research use. It has the advantage of being quick and easy to administer but concerns about its validity with people with visual or language impairment, those with low intellectual ability or poor literacy skills, or non-English speakers have been raised. More recently, due to copyright issues and the cost of purchasing the necessary licence, other tools are increasingly used, such as the Addenbrooke's Cognitive Examination-III (ACE-III) (NeuRA 2012) which is available in several languages; the Montreal Cognitive Assessment (MoCA) (Nasreddine et al. 2005) which is particularly sensitive when used for people with Parkinson's disease or dementia with Lewy bodies; and the Rowland Universal Dementia Assessment Scale (RUDAS) (Storey et al. 2014) which is suitable for use with those whose first language is not English or whose literacy is poor.

Impact on function and ADLs will also be screened, possibly using a validated scale, such as the Bristol Activities of Daily Living Scale (BADLS) (Bucks et al. 1996), which was developed specifically for use with community dwelling people with dementia and has been shown to be sensitive to change over time (Byrne et al. 2000). It is a carer rated scale comprising 20 personal care and instrumental daily living activities. An overall score of 0 indicates independence in all areas, while higher scores, up to a maximum of 60, indicate higher dependency.

Person-Centred Care

Kitwood (1997) first described the concept of person-centred care for people with dementia. Person-centred care is described as 'V + I + P + S,' where 'V' refers to *valuing* people with dementia, 'I' refers to treating them as *individuals*, 'P' refers to trying to understand their *personal perspective*, and 'S' refers to supportive *social* psychology. VIPS also stands for 'very important persons,' which – as a portrayal of the endpoint service user – is perhaps a simpler way of understanding the essence of person-centred care (Brooker 2007). Kitwood's enriched model of dementia described the experience of living with dementia as a combination of five factors, represented by the mnemonic 'D = NI + H + B + P + SP'; where D = dementia, NI = neurological impairment, H = health and physical fitness, B = biography/life history, P = personality and SP = social psychology (Brooker 2007). Personality and biography cannot be changed – what has happened in the past cannot be altered – but greater knowledge about these factors informs assessment and planning. The nature of neurological impairment varies from individual to individual, depending on the type and rate of progression of the underlying disease, and there is ongoing debate about the degree to which this damage can be reversed. Carers therefore need to enhance well-being through promoting and maintaining physical health and improving the social and psychological context within which the person lives.

Dementia care mapping (DCM) evaluates the quality of person-centred care. A 'mapper' observes six people simultaneously over a six-hour period. The nature of activity being engaged in and their perceived degree of well-being is noted every five minutes. Well-being scores are produced for each individual, plus examples of positive ('uplifts') and negative ('putdowns') interactions between staff and service users. These data are used to inform and train staff to recognize and understand peoples' behaviour and thereby improve care planning and provision. There is mixed evidence of the success of DCM in improving dementia care (Surr et al. 2018; Surr et al. 2020). Nevertheless, there is the potential for occupational therapists to take leadership in the full implementation of cycles of observation, planning and action to improve person-centred care.

Interventions

Currently there is no cure for dementia. Cholinesterase inhibitor medication has been shown to have some clinical benefit for cognitive symptoms in those with Alzheimer's disease, dementia with Lewy bodies or Parkinson's disease dementia. Alongside this, a range of non-pharmacological interventions have been developed and found to have varying levels of clinical or cost benefit for people with dementia and their carers (be that family and friends or paid health and social care staff), with the most effective type: having a number of related components, being tailored to the individual, and including training for carers to maximize their communication skills and coping strategies (Clarkson et al. 2017; Livingston et al. 2017; Nickel et al. 2018; McDermott et al. 2019; Oyebode and Parveen 2019; Livingston et al. 2020). Occupational therapists often incorporate these interventions within their practice, usually presenting them with an increased focus on occupational engagement.

OCCUPATIONAL THERAPY AND OLDER PEOPLE

This section of the chapter describes occupational therapy assessment of older people and the most commonly used assessment tools. It illustrates the potential role of occupational therapy in community-based dementia care and in care homes, drawing on the profession's developing evidence base in these areas. It also discusses issues such as mental capacity, assessing and managing risk and working with carers.

Occupational Therapy Assessment of Older People

Assessment has to be timely; not whilst the person is psychologically unstable, but in sufficient time to allow for future planning. Assessment should be carried out at a realistic time of day, related to the person's normal routine. For example, carrying out personal care tasks in the morning if that is when the person usually washes and dresses. Performance can fluctuate at certain times of the day, possibly due to the condition itself or caused by medication.

Peoples' homes are the most realistic venue for assessment and intervention. They provide a fuller picture and the occupational therapist may identify significant factors that have previously gone unnoticed by the individual, for example, potential fall hazards. Equipment can be installed, demonstrated and practised *in situ* and with the carer if needed. Most importantly, older people, including those with dementia, perform instrumental ADLs significantly better in their own home (Park et al. 1994; Tullis and Nicol 1999).

The aspects most commonly considered when assessing an older person include:

- Communication: what is the person's preferred form of address? What is their first language? What verbal and non-verbal methods of communication are used? Are there any speech or language impairments?
- Sensory issues: this includes smell, movement, touch, vision, hearing and taste. Does the client usually wear a hearing aid and/or glasses? Are these available for use at the time of assessment?

- Orientation to time, place and person: does the person know the time of day, the day and date, where they are and who they and others are?
- Cognition: areas to consider here include short- and long-term memory, concentration, visual-spatial awareness, sequencing and problem-solving abilities;
- Mood: does the person currently enjoy well-being or not? Are they happy, relaxed, cheerful and realistic or sad, anxious and fearful?
- Mobility: can the person mobilize indoors and outside? Can they use stairs? Do they need to use mobility aids?
- Transfers: can the person transfer from their bed/chair/toilet/bath/shower? It is also important to note the height, type and layout of furniture;
- Personal care tasks: does the person have any problems with eating/drinking/washing/dressing/grooming/using the toilet?
- Domestic activities: does the person have any problems with cooking/cleaning/shopping/laundry?
- Occupation: does the person have any problems with self-care/work/leisure activities?
- Daily routine: go through a daily/weekly timetable to highlight 'gaps' in service provision, occupational opportunities and social interaction;
- Physical environment: consider accommodation, access, layout, facilities, lighting, flooring, heating, and communication; both standard and in emergencies;
- Potential hazards and safety issues;
- Driving and community mobility: is the person still driving? If so, how often, and where to? What other forms of community mobility do they use to get to where they want to go?
- Equipment already provided/needed, including assistive technology;
- Social environment: consider other household members (including pets) and any support/social networks that are available.

Obviously, consideration must be given to coexisting physical and/or sensory impairment(s) within the occupational therapy process, but these are beyond the remit of this chapter. See Chapter 5 for a specific discussion about assessment and outcome measurement.

Occupational Therapy Assessment Tools

Many occupational therapists working with older people base their practice on the Model of Human Occupation (MOHO) (Kielhofner 2008) and use a range of MOHO-based assessments (Swinson et al. 2016), including the:

- Model of Human Occupation Screening Tool (MOHOST) (Parkinson et al. 2006);
- Modified Interest Checklist (https://www.moho.uic.edu/product);
- Occupational Self Assessment (OSA) (Baron et al. 2006);
- Volitional Questionnaire (VQ) (de las Heras et al. 1998);
- Assessment of Motor and Process Skills (AMPS) (Fisher 2003, 2006).

The AMPS is suitable for use with anyone, of any age, who experiences or is at risk of experiencing challenges with ADL task performance; it is sensitive to the smallest change in this. It has been shown to be reliable and valid for use with older people with dementia living in the community (Robinson and Fisher 1996) but it is not suitable for people who are unable to participate in the initial interview, activity selection and contract setting that is required before the two task assessments take place. It may therefore not be suitable for someone with more severe dementia (see https://www.innovativeotsolutions.com for up-to-date information on AMPS developments and resources).

Other assessments commonly used with older people include the (Swinson et al. 2016):

- Large Allen Cognitive Level Screen (LACLS): the LACLS uses a simple task, leather lacing, as a screening test. Interpretation using the Allen Cognitive Scale of levels and modes of performance (Allen 1999) determines the level of cognitive disability which enables the provision of appropriate environmental support and intervention. It originates from the cognitive disability model (Allen et al. 1992). The Allen Cognitive Level Screen was assessed as being appropriate to use with people with dementia (Wilson et al. 1989) and a further study established the validity of an enlarged version (the LACLS) designed for use with older people with impaired visual or manual dexterity (Kehrberg et al. 1992).

- Pool Activity Level (PAL): the PAL instrument (Pool 2012) was developed in the United Kingdom as a practical resource for carers of people with dementia to identify and capitalize on the person's abilities to enable their engagement in meaningful occupation while also providing the necessary assistance to meet their needs. Pool, an occupational therapist, used underpinning theory from the cognitive disability model (Allen et al. 1992). The instrument comprises a life history profile, a checklist, activity profile and an individual action plan for personal care activities.

The PAL checklist covers nine everyday activities and the results indicate the level of cognitive ability that an individual has reached in terms of being able to engage in the activity, be that at the planned, exploratory, sensory or reflex level. The PAL activity profiles outline the likely abilities and limitations of a person at that level and provide guidance on how best to engage and enable an individual. The PAL checklist has validity and reliability when used to assess older people with dementia (Wenborn et al. 2008). Although designed for caregivers' use, it is usually occupational therapists that introduce it into services and oversee its implementation in practice. It is used in many countries including the United Kingdom, Australia, Singapore, St. Helena, and the United States; and it has been translated into German, Spanish, Japanese and Lithuanian.

Creative Participation Assessment (CPA): the Vona du Toit model of creative ability (VdTMOCA), first conceptualized by South African occupational therapist Vona du Toit, is increasingly used to enable individuals to achieve their maximum potential through engagement in purposeful activity that is consistent with their level of creative ability (De Witt 2014). The CPA is one of three VdTMOCA assessments that may be used to determine an individual's level of motivation, and corresponding level of action (Casteleijn 2014).

OCCUPATIONAL THERAPY AND PEOPLE WITH DEMENTIA

Occupational therapists have a key role in enabling people with dementia to engage in personally meaningful occupations and maintaining independence.

In the United Kingdom the Memory Services National Accreditation Programme (MSNAP) Standards (RCOT 2020) require services to include an occupational therapist within the core team and to ensure that their input is sufficient to provide evidence-based interventions. These include: '... advice and support on assistive technology and telecare solutions designed to assist people with activities of daily living,' '... tailored psychosocial interventions for behaviour that challenges,' 'art/creative therapies,' and 'activities such as work, education and volunteering' amongst others that are relevant for occupational therapy provision.

Community-Based Occupational Therapy in Dementia

The community occupational therapy in dementia (COTiD) programme for older people with mild to moderate dementia and their carers was developed and evaluated in the Netherlands (Graff et al. 2006). The intervention aims to improve the service user's ability to carry out ADLs, improve the carer's supervision and problem-solving skills so as to increase their own sense of competence and decrease their burden of care, and improve the quality of life for both parties. The COTiD programme comprises ten 1-hour sessions of home-based occupational therapy provided over five weeks, with the occupational therapist working in partnership with the person who has dementia and their family carer. A single site RCT was conducted with 135 people and their family caregivers. The primary outcomes were that the person with dementia's ability to perform ADLs was enhanced, as was the carer's sense of competence. Secondary outcomes were enhanced quality of life, mood and general health status for both parties and carers' sense of control over their life. All scores improved significantly relative to baseline in the intervention group compared with the controls (Graff et al. 2006, 2007). The effect sizes of all primary outcomes were higher than those found in trials of medications or other psychosocial interventions and were still present at three months (Graff et al. 2006). The intervention was also found to be cost-effective in reducing usage of health and social care services (Graff et al. 2008). A subsequent study in Germany (Voigt-Radloff et al. 2011a) found no difference between providing COTiD or a single occupational therapy consultation. This highlighted the need to adapt complex interventions

before implementation and evaluation in other nations (Voigt-Radloff et al. 2011b).

Hence, a major research programme, Valuing Active Life in Dementia (VALID) was funded in England (Wenborn et al. submitted [Final report]; see www.ucl.ac.uk/valid for more details) to firstly translate and adapt the intervention to develop a UK version COTiD-UK (Hynes et al. 2015); and then to evaluate it through a RCT (Wenborn et al. 2016). The RCT ran in 15 sites across England, and people with mild to moderate dementia were recruited in pairs with a family carer and randomly allocated to either participate in the COTiD-UK intervention or continue with their usual care (TAU) which may or may not include occupational therapy. In total 468 pairs were recruited and data were collected by masked assessors at baseline and then at 12, 26, 52 and 78 weeks post randomization with the total BADLS score at 26 weeks being the primary end point. The intervention was delivered by 31 occupational therapists with moderate fidelity, albeit with variation between therapists and sites (Walton et al. 2019). At 26 weeks there was no statistical evidence of difference between the COTiD-UK and TAU groups in the primary or any of the secondary outcomes (quality of life, mood, resource use, carer sense of competence) (Wenborn et al. 2021). In contrast the qualitative interviews conducted with a purposive sample of seven occupational therapists and 22 pairs who had taken part in COTiD-UK reflected a very positive experience, with all interviewees valuing the occupational focus and the emphasis on working together to enable both the person with dementia and the family member to set and achieve individualized as well as joint goals. In addition, the 22 pairs reported that they felt better informed and thereby enabled to plan in the short and longer term to live well with dementia (Burgess et al. accepted).

COTiD is also being translated and adapted in other European countries, for example, a pilot study in France. Furthermore a prospective cohort study in Italy demonstrated positive effect on caregiver burden, as well as improved activities performance and satisfaction for people with dementia (Pozzi et al. 2019).

The Tailored Activity Programme (TAP), devised by Laura Gitlin in the United States, is a home-based occupational therapy intervention shown to reduce neuropsychiatric symptoms and caregiver burden (Gitlin et al. 2008, 2009) and be cost-effective (Gitlin et al. 2010). Within the United States, the TAP intervention has been adapted for use with veterans (Gitlin et al. 2018) and hospitalized populations (Gitlin et al. 2017). Elsewhere the intervention is being adapted, including a version for people with frontotemporal dementia in Australia (O'Connor et al. 2019), and translated, for example in Brazil where both a home-based version (Novelli et al. 2018) and an out-patient version (Oliveira et al. 2018) are being evaluated. Similarly, occupational therapy intervention has also been demonstrated to reduce neuropsychiatric symptoms as well as maintain cognition and ADLs and decrease carers' burden (Pimouguet et al. 2017)

The Journeying through Dementia (JtD) intervention was adapted from the Lifestyle Matters intervention in collaboration with people living with dementia (Wright et al. 2019). JtD is a manualized intervention consisting of 12 weekly facilitated groups with 8 to 12 participants in the early stages of their dementia journey. Each participant also receives four one-to-one sessions with one of the intervention facilitators, to pursue their individual goals, one of which happens before the group sessions start. The content aims to enable participants to develop skills and techniques to continue doing the things they enjoy for as long as possible and includes: ways of thinking about dementia, keeping physically well, memory, keeping mentally well, and in conclusion, a celebration of participants' achievements and planning how to move forward. People attending the programme could involve a supporter (usually a family member or friend) if they wished to. A multisite RCT conducted across the north of England tested the clinical and cost-effectiveness of JtD compared with usual care (Wright et al. 2019). In total 480 people with dementia and 350 supporters were recruited. Whilst there was a small increase in the primary outcome measure, Dementia-Related Quality of Life at eight months' post-randomization this did not reach statistical significance. However, the qualitative interviews with participants provided very positive accounts of taking part in the intervention and the impact it had.

OCCUPATIONAL THERAPY IN LONG-TERM CARE SETTINGS

As the numbers of older people and people with dementia increase, so too does the population of people residing in long-term care settings, often referred to as 'residential' or 'nursing' or 'care homes.' The majority of care home residents have cognitive impairment as well as physical and sensory impairments. Activity participation in care homes has been shown to improve residents' quality of life (Zimmerman et al. 2005), reduce levels of challenging behaviour and improve mood and function (Cohen-Mansfield 2005). The need to enable activity participation suggests a potential role for occupational therapy in care homes and two studies have sought to evaluate its effectiveness. The Care Home Activity Project (Mozley et al. 2007) tested the effectiveness of an occupational therapist working within a care home to increase participation in one-to-one and group activities and to reduce the severity of depression. Wenborn et al. (2013) evaluated the effectiveness of an occupational therapist-led programme to train and coach care home staff to increase activity provision to improve quality of life for residents with dementia. Neither study produced quantitative evidence for the efficacy of the intervention, but both produced qualitative findings that suggested residents who did receive enhanced occupational opportunities had a positive experience. These studies illustrate the challenges in evaluating complex interventions, such as occupational therapy, in the real life setting of care homes, not least of these being the difficulties related to management and staff cooperation with the interventions. They also highlight the need to develop outcome measures that more effectively measure the focus of the intervention, such as level of engagement and activity, especially for those residents with more severe dementia.

Occupational therapists certainly have a role within care homes, not only to facilitate activity participation, but also to enable residents to live as independently as possible. This can be done through the provision of rehabilitation and re-enablement programmes and specialist equipment to enhance function and/or maintain safety and comfort. This may include hoists, specialist seating and splinting (RCOT 2019a). These latter aspects become increasingly important as the person nears the end of their life and can be provided not only within residential settings but also to people still living at home. Occupational therapists may be based in the care home itself or provide an in-reach service, often as part of a multidisciplinary care home support team, or work in an advisory or consultancy capacity. As well as providing intervention directly to residents as outlined above, there is also a need to train and enable care staff to provide person-centred care, including opportunities to engage in personally meaningful occupations. The UK 'Living Well in Care Homes' toolkit outlines best practice in supporting residents to enjoy daily activities that support their health and well-being. It also provides ideas for activities and resources to support their provision devised for residents, family and friends, members of staff and care home managers (RCOT 2019b). Another key aspect is occupational therapists delivering interventions designed specifically to reduce the frequency and severity of behaviour that care staff can find challenging and difficult to deal with, thus reducing the level of antipsychotic medication prescribed and the number of falls whilst improving residents' quality of life and staff satisfaction (Manni et al. 2018).

MULTIDISCIPLINARY INTERVENTIONS USED IN COMMUNITY AND LONG-TERM CARE SETTINGS

There are a number of evidence-based treatment modalities that occupational therapists and other professionals use when working with people with dementia and their carers. These include cognitive stimulation, rehabilitation and training, life story work and multisensory interventions. Occupational therapists may use these interventions during the occupational therapy process or may provide advocacy and training to carers to include these modalities as part of a person with dementia's care package.

Cognitive Stimulation, Cognitive Rehabilitation and Cognitive Training

For cognitive symptoms, interventions can include cognitive stimulation therapy (CST), cognitive rehabilitation and cognitive training.

CST incorporates principles of reality orientation, reminiscence, validation and person-centred care delivered within a small group. The emphasis is on information processing and props are used to provide multisensory stimulation. A multicentre, RCT was conducted with 210 participants across 18 care homes

and 5 day centres. The intervention group experienced significant improvement in cognition, and improved quality of life, but there was no difference between the groups for depression, anxiety, behaviour and communication (Spector et al. 2003). A Cochrane review (Woods et al. 2012) found evidence of cognitive stimulation improving cognition in people with mild to moderate dementia and promising results for the impact on self-reported quality of life and well-being. Subsequent studies found that providing a maintenance CST (MCST) programme improved quality of life and improved cognition for those also taking acetylcholinesterase inhibitor medication (Orrell et al. 2014). In addition, studies also found that training family carers to provide individual CST (iCST) sessions had no effect on cognition or quality of life for people with dementia but appeared to enhance the quality of the caregiving relationship and carers' quality of life (Orrell et al. 2017).

Cognitive rehabilitation aims to improve daily functioning by working with the individual to set goals and then develop strategies to achieve them. The Goal-Oriented Cognitive Rehabilitation in Early-Stage Alzheimer's and related dementias RCT (GREAT) recruited 475 pairs comprising a person with mild to moderate dementia and their family carer across England and Wales. The results demonstrated statistically significant effects on goal attainment at three and then nine months although there was no difference to the standardized secondary outcome measures (quality of life, mood, self-efficacy, cognition, carer stress, health status) nor was it cost-effective (Clare et al. 2017).

Cognitive training, sometimes referred to as 'brain training', uses guided practice on structured tasks to improve or maintain specific cognitive functions, such as memory, attention and problem-solving. Traditionally, cognitive training was delivered using a paper-and-pencil format, but computerized versions are gaining popularity. The underlying premise is that improving cognitive skills will also improve functional ability although the evidence for this is limited. Cognitive training for people with mild to moderate dementia is probably associated with small to moderate positive effects on global cognition and verbal semantic fluency, and these benefits appear to be maintained in the medium term, although the strength of the evidence is considered low (Bahar-Fuchs et al. 2019).

Further studies are needed to evaluate the effectiveness of computerized cognitive training to maintain cognitive function in cognitively healthy people in midlife and thus delay or prevent the onset of dementia in later life, as currently the evidence to support this is weak (Gates et al. 2019).

There is mixed evidence to support the use of physical exercise to improve cognition and function and inconclusive evidence for using physical exercise to treat depression in people with dementia (Livingston et al. 2017; Lamb et al. 2018). Interventions designed to improve carers' communication skills and the delivery of person-centred care, engaging in personally meaningful and pleasurable activities, social engagement and sensory interventions have been shown to reduce the level of agitation (Livingston et al. 2017).

Multisensory Stimulation

All people need sensory stimulation to interpret and interact with their environment and sensory impairment or deprivation eventually results in physical and/or social disengagement. Sensory impairment can occur as part of normal ageing or due to conditions such as dementia and alters our sensory experience. People in institutional care may experience sensory deprivation through a lack of environmental stimulation and sensory opportunities. A sensory approach aims to maintain interaction with the environment and other people by providing a range of experiences to stimulate all the senses (i.e., smell, movement, touch, vision, hearing and taste) even if verbal communication is no longer possible.

The use of specialist multisensory rooms or environments originated in The Netherlands with the development of Snoezelen©, which literally translated means 'to sniff and doze.' Beneficial effects immediately after using such rooms have been noted (Livingston et al. 2014). Staff must be trained and users must be assessed to establish an agreed intervention plan. This ensures an appropriate level and type of stimulation is provided and avoids the dangers of sensory overload. However, a dedicated specialist room is not always necessary as many of the principles can be applied more generally. For example, using scented bath oils, background music and environmental props can turn a functional bath into a sensory experience. A range of sensory stimuli can be incorporated into the environment or used as an activity, such as rummage bags, sensory cushions and aprons, and these have been shown to effectively reduce challenging behaviour such as agitation (Livingston et al. 2014). Interventions such as animal-assisted therapy (Ming Lai et al. 2019) and using dolls and soft toys (Mitchell et al. 2014) are additional elements that can contribute to a sensory approach.

Music can be used in a variety of ways, as a group or individual intervention, and include active and/or receptive (or passive) musical elements. It can range from sessions with specific therapeutic goals delivered by an accredited music therapist to the more general use of music within an intervention, such as incorporating singing within CST or reminiscence sessions, or alongside care delivery, for example, playing personally meaningful music alongside other activities such as bathing and mealtimes. A Cochrane review identified 22 studies, of which 21 contributed data from 890 participants to a meta-analysis and found that providing people with dementia living in institutional care with at least five sessions of a music-based therapeutic intervention probably reduces depressive symptoms and improves overall behavioural problems at the end of treatment. Furthermore, it may also improve emotional well-being and quality of life and reduce anxiety but may have little or no effect on agitation or aggression or on cognition (van der Steen et al. 2018).

However, despite the large number of interventions developed and evaluated, a number of the studies are small and the quality of evidence moderate or low. Much as the 'gold standard' is seen as being an RCT there are inherent challenges in using this design to evaluate such complex interventions. Often the 'active' ingredients of an intervention are not sufficiently clearly defined or manualized to enable its replication. There are also challenges in how to adequately train and supervise those delivering the intervention to maximize its fidelity, bearing in mind the need to also tailor the intervention to best 'fit' the needs and preferences of the recipient(s), be that the person with dementia themselves, their family, or care staff (Van't Leven et al. 2019). It is obviously not possible to mask the research participants as to which intervention they have (or not) received and this therefore raises the risk of assessors being unmasked when collecting follow-up data, thus increasing the potential bias of the study results. Traditionally, dementia research has used outcome measures originally designed for use in pharmacological trials which inevitably focus on the level of impairment or deterioration experienced, and this does not reflect the positive person-centred care philosophy underpinning dementia care interventions and services. There has also been a reliance on proxy assessment of outcome rather than asking the person with dementia their opinion which was seen as not being a feasible or reliable method of collecting data but increasingly researchers are enabling the voice of people with dementia to be heard through the use of alternative data collection methods (Phillipson and Hammond 2018).

Life Story Work

Bearing in mind the emphasis on providing person-centred care that is tailored to the individual highlights the importance of knowing the individual's life story (Kitwood 1997). Indeed, life story work can constitute an intervention in its own right, which can improve the attitudes of care staff and their service delivery (Gridley et al. 2016). Ideally, the person with dementia will be involved in relating their own life story but it is often left to carers to do this on their behalf at a later stage. Benefits include enabling staff to know and better understand the individual person and their behaviour, informing the care planning process, providing personalized care, ensuring continuity of care and encouraging life review and reminiscence. It is potentially an activity that the individual, their family and staff can enjoy doing together, but it can also be an emotional activity that may need sensitive handling. Ensuring confidentiality is important as life story folders may contain personal information which the person or their relatives do not want to share with others.

Different formats of life story folders can be produced or purchased. It is a good idea to include a family tree, a list of significant dates, photographs and a frontispiece of current information about their home, family, likes and dislikes, emphasizing the more positive aspects. A memory box can also be created to contain objects of significance to represent the person's life. Increasingly, creative presentations are now possible utilizing technology such as digital picture frames. Also see Chapter 17 in which storytelling is used as an example of creative activity, and Chapter 20, which discusses personal narratives.

OCCUPATIONAL THERAPY PRACTICE

As well as the specific issues associated with working with older people with depression or dementia, there are some general points for occupational therapists to consider when working with older people. These concern mental capacity, assessing and managing risk, assistive technology and working with carers.

Mental Capacity

There will be instances when older people, particularly those with dementia, do not have the capacity to make and/or to communicate decisions regarding occupational therapy assessment and interventions. In the United Kingdom it is vital to be aware of the Mental Capacity Act (2005) and its implications for practice (see also Chapter 9). It has five statutory principles:

1. A person must be assumed to have capacity unless it is established that they do not;
2. A person is not to be treated as unable to make a decision unless all practicable steps to help him/her do so have been taken without success;
3. A person is not to be treated as unable to make a decision merely because they make an unwise decision;
4. A decision made, under this Act for, or on behalf of, a person who lacks capacity must be done their best interests;
5. Before a decision is made, regard must be given as to whether the purpose for which it is needed can be as effectively achieved in a way that is less restrictive of the person's rights and freedom of action.

The Act outlines how to establish that someone lacks capacity:

1. Does the person have an impairment of, or a disturbance in, the functioning of, the mind or brain (temporarily or permanently)?
2. Does the impairment or disturbance mean the person is unable to make this particular decision at this particular time? Can the individual:

- understand the information relevant to the decision?
- retain the information for long enough to reach a decision?
- use or weigh the information to make a decision?
- communicate a decision?

Occupational therapists must always ask for the person's consent before proceeding with an assessment or intervention and must re-check this on an ongoing basis. Capacity assessments must always be documented. There may be occasions when a person makes a decision that the occupational therapist considers to be unwise, such as refusing the installation of equipment or provision of community services or insisting on going home despite high levels of risk. There will be local procedures and guidance in place as to how to report, manage and document these decisions. There is further discussion about mental capacity in Chapter 7 (in relation to professional accountability) and in Chapter 10 (in relation to ethical practice.)

Assessing and Managing Risk

There are a number of potential risks that older people face. Depression or cognitive impairment can limit or decrease an individual's motivation or ability to undertake daily living skills, such as maintaining personal hygiene, meal preparation, using household appliances, shopping, medication compliance and managing finances. There is also the possibility of harming themselves or others through inadvertently flooding or setting fire to their home, or by driving dangerously. People who are disorientated in time or place can wander from their home and be at risk of accidents or hypothermia. People who are depressed are at risk of suicide. Older people may also experience physical health problems, which in turn impact on their safety, for example, reduced mobility, falls and infection. A person's home environment may become unduly cluttered or require adaptation to enable safe access. Older people are also vulnerable to physical or financial abuse by others, including informal and formal carers. In this instance, occupational therapists need to follow the locally agreed Safeguarding Vulnerable Adults policy. Occupational therapists have an important role in the identification and management of risk. A validated assessment of unmet needs such as the Camberwell Assessment of Need for the Elderly (Orrell and Hancock 2004) can be used to identify and prioritize potential risks. Many organizations use their own locally developed tool.

Health and social care staff can aim to minimize the level of risk but never totally remove it. Risk may be managed through the provision of equipment, assistive technology or support services. Redesign or adaptation of the environment, including the removal or adaptation of appliances, or to facilitate purposeful walking (as opposed to wandering) may also help.

As always, it is important to document all capacity and risk assessments and subsequent intervention, including any concerns about risk management recommendations made but declined by the individual. As discussed above, there is a difference between someone making what the practitioner thinks is an unwise decision and the individual not having the capacity to make an informed decision. In the first instance, the occupational therapist must respect the person's decision and do what they can to minimize the potential risk. In the latter case, any decision that the occupational therapist makes on the individual's behalf must be in their best interest.

Assistive Technology

Assistive technology includes anything that supports people to remain independent, manage their health or compensate for an impairment. It ranges from simple low-tech household devices such as walking frames to sophisticated sensors and computerized systems that are either standalone items or connected to a call system or centre to alert a response, which is often referred to as 'telecare' or 'telemedicine'. A range of assistive technology devices have been developed to support people with dementia and their carers to manage their daily activities and to enhance safety and includes:

- Time-orientation devices, such as large-faced clocks, digital calendar clocks, automated clock calendars;
- Alarm and monitoring systems to alert carers, such as fall alarms, passive alarm systems, and bed and chair monitors;
- Safety systems, such as automatic cooker switch-off, bath level/temperature monitor and control;
- Adapted telephones, and audiovisual/computer systems to facilitate social contact and occupation.

Assistive technology equipment can maintain safety, monitor and maintain health and enhance quality of life in several ways. It can remind people, provide them with something to do, point out or respond to danger, monitor activity, restrict access and egress and keep people in touch with each other. For example, sensors that activate when a person with dementia gets up at night and alert the carer are cost-effective in terms of preventing or delaying care home admission. They also enhance quality of life for the person with dementia (who is thus enabled to remain in their own familiar environment for longer) and reduce the psychological and physical stress experienced by the carer. Although assistive technology is accepted as being good practice (National Institute for Health Research 2018) and a domain of occupational therapy practice (World Federation of Occupational Therapists 2019), the number of studies evaluating its clinical effectiveness to support people with memory problems are still small with very limited good quality evidence, not least due to the challenges in evaluating what by definition need to be individualized solutions within the domestic home environment (van der Roest et al. 2017) so much more research is needed in this area. The ATTILA (Assistive Technology and Telecare to maintain Independent Living At Home for people with dementia RCT (Leroi et al. 2013) aims to: establish whether assistive technology and telecare interventions safely extend the time that people with dementia can continue to live independently in their own homes and whether this is cost-effective; establish whether these technologies can significantly reduce the number of incidents involving serious risks to safety and independent living, including acute admissions to hospital, reduce stress in family and other informal caregivers and increase quality of life for people with dementia and their caregivers; and collect qualitative and quantitative data from people with dementia, their formal and informal caregivers, about the experience of receiving these technologies.

Working with Carers

Often, a range of family and friends care for older people and occupational therapists have a key role in supporting them. Informal carers should be offered a carer's assessment and appropriate support provided in response to identified needs. As discussed, caring for a family member is a potential risk factor for depression (Rodda et al. 2011). Occupational therapists have a key role in educating and training carers. This may include training in coping strategies to enable the cared for person to continue doing certain things themselves, rather than the carer doing them on their behalf. It may also include techniques for enabling activity participation, using equipment and advising on benefits and direct payments. The COTiD and TAP interventions (described earlier) is a good example of an intervention that enables occupational therapists to engage in this educational/advisory/coaching role. Support can be provided to carers on a one-to-one or group basis. Occupational therapists also have a key role to provide training and advice to formal, paid carers on how best to enable older people to maximize function and maintain their engagement in daily activities and occupations, and how to use specialist equipment such as hoists.

SUMMARY

This chapter has described and illustrated, using evidence-based examples, the breadth of occupational therapy practice with older people. The importance of differentiating between the impact of normal ageing and impairment due to underlying pathology, and between dementia and depression, is highlighted. Occupational therapists' person-centred philosophy is often extended to include the older person's family carer as well, bearing in mind the number of informal carers supporting older people and the increasing dependence that a person with dementia will inevitably have on such supporters. It is also important to recognize the potential risk of carers becoming depressed, hence the need to offer them support to meet their own needs as well as those of the person that they care for.

It is interesting to speculate on what the future holds for occupational therapy services for older people. The current policy focus on enabling independence, choice and control, accords well with the occupational therapy philosophy and therefore may be seen as presenting an opportunity. However, the need to develop yet more robust evidence to demonstrate the value of occupational therapy intervention is a continuing challenge that occupational therapists must embrace.

QUESTIONS FOR CONSIDERATION

1. What services in your local area are provided exclusively for older people and their family and friends?
2. What guidance is available from the National Institute for Health and Care Excellence (NICE) that informs occupational therapy practice?
3. Dementia affects the person, their family and carers, as well as their friends. This means there are many sensitivities surrounding the treatment plans and diagnosis. What are some of the areas an occupational therapist must consider during the occupational therapy process with older people with dementia?
4. Highlight five of the most significant considerations you would have to make during assessments of older people and propose measures that you could implement to counteract the challenges.
5. Create a table of the measures used in the assessment of older people, the focus of the assessment and any specific considerations.
6. What role do you think an occupational therapy 'care coordinator' within long-term care facilities could play?
7. Plan and evaluate a multisensory stimulation intervention with one older person with dementia who you work with.

SERVICE USER COMMENTARY

My dad had long-term mental health issues and a diagnosis of Korsakoff syndrome/dementia from when he was fairly young. Many his age would be finalizing their working life and contemplating their retirement. My dad had not worked for many years, as his mental illnesses had affected his working life, dealing with the extreme highs and desperate lows of bipolar and clinical depression that often saw him bed bound for months or years. I was never sure if the alcoholism was to self-medicate his undiagnosed mental illness or his mental illness made him drink, excessively. Whatever it was, my childhood was filled with seeing him drunk and incapable, either through depression or drink, of functioning like other people were doing.

Following the death of my mum, he moved into supported care, which was quickly followed by needing nursing and caring support. The care home was a wonderful home, not like any of the stories I had read or heard about. It had regular occupational therapy sessions as well as other activities and visitors (even a visit from a donkey!) that the residents seem to get lots of benefit from.

Initially my dad loved to be involved and join in all the activities, but after a while he started to withdraw and then stated he no longer wanted to be involved in any of them. The occupational therapists did all they could to persuade him to join in, all to no avail. It got to the point where my dad would refuse to go anywhere near when they were about.

One day when I was there and my dad was sat in the quiet area whilst the sessions were on, I asked him what the problem was. It is important to remember my dad's diagnosis, and some days he was coherent and able to articulate what he wanted but others he did not make any sense at all. This was on a coherent day, so I knew he understood what was happening. He explained that he no longer wanted to take part because he often forgot things and it made him upset that he was getting like that. I said can you not just sit and watch? He stated that was what he wanted to do, but the occupational therapists insisted he join in. He was so upset and frustrated that he stopped going because the pressure to participate was too much.

I spoke with the staff and explained that my dad wanted to observe but not participate. 'Pestering' him to participate (his word not mine) had made him withdraw. The staff listened and agreed they would no longer ask him to join in and would let him enjoy the session by observing. This improved the quality of his life and was a huge step forward in his care, making the last years of his life so much more beneficial.

My story would be to remind occupational therapists that people can enjoy the sessions as observers. Yes, I know some people like encouragement to join in, but in my dad's case, he did not. He said it was 'annoying and the constant pestering' to join in meant he felt it best to not be involved at all. After listening to what my dad wanted, he was able to enjoy the sessions and gain some quality of life back.

Debbie Teale

REFERENCES

Age Concern and Mental Health Foundation. (2006). *Promoting mental health and well-being in later life. A first report from the UK Inquiry into mental health and well-being in later life.* London: Age Concern and The Mental Health Foundation.

Age UK. (2016). *Hidden in plain Sight: The unmet mental health needs of older people.* Available at: https://www.ageuk.org.uk/.

Age UK. (2019). *Later life in the United Kingdom 2019.* Available at: https://www.ageuk.org.uk/.

Alexopoulos, G. S., Abrams, R. C., Young, R. C., et al. (1988). Cornell scale for depression in dementia. *Biological Psychiatry*, *23*(3), 271–284.

Allen, C. K. (1999). *Structures of the cognitive performance modes.* Ormond Beach, FL: Allen Conferences.

Allen, C. K., Earhart, C. A., & Blue, T. (1992). *Occupational therapy treatment goals for the physically and cognitively disabled.* Bethesda, MD: The American Occupational Therapy Association.

American Psychiatric Association. (2013). *Diagnosis and statistical manual of mental disorders* (5th ed.). Washington, DC: American Psychiatric Association.

Bahar-Fuchs, A., Martyr, A., Goh, A., Sabates, J., & Clare, L. (2019). Cognitive training for people with mild to moderate dementia. *Cochrane Database of Systematic Reviews*, *3*, CD013069. https://doi.org/10.1002/14651858.CD013069.pub2.

Baron, K., Kielhofner, G., Iyenger, A., Goldhammer, V., & Wolenski, J. (2006). *Occupational self assessment (OSA) version 2.2.* Chicago, IL: University of Illinois. Available at: https://www.moho.uic.edu/products.aspx.

Bowling, A., Grundy, E., & Farquhar, M. (1997). *Living well into old age: Three studies of health and well-being among older people in East London and Essex.* London: Age Concern England.

Brooker, D. (2007). *Person-centred dementia care: Making services better.* London: Jessica Kingsley.

Bucks, R. S., Ashworth, D. L., Wilcock, G. K., et al. (1996). Assessment of activities of daily living in dementia: Development of the Bristol activities of daily living scale. *Age and Ageing*, *25*(2), 113–120.

Burgess, J., Wenborn, J., Di Bona, L., et al., submitted. Exploring the experiences of taking part in the community occupational therapy in Dementia (COTiD-UK) intervention from the perspective of people with dementia, family carers and occupational therapists.

Byrne, L. M., Wilson, P. M., Bucks, R. S., et al. (2000). The sensitivity to change over time of the Bristol activities of daily living scale in Alzheimer's disease. *International Journal of Geriatric Psychiatry*, *15*(7), 656–661.

Casteleijn, D. (2014). Using measurement principles to confirm the levels of creative ability as described in the Vona du Toit Model of Creative Ability. *South African Journal of Occupational Therapy*, *44*(1), 14–19. Available at: http://www.scielo.org.za/scielo.php?script=sci_arttext&pid=S2310-38332014000100004&lng=en&tlng=en.

Chatters, R., Roberts, J., Mountain, G., et al. (2017). The long-term (24-month) effect on health and well-being of the lifestyle matters community-based intervention in people aged 65 years and over: A qualitative study. *British Medical Journal Open*, 7, e016711. https://doi.org/10.1136/bmjopen-2017-016711.

Clare, L., Kudlicka, A., Bayer, A., et al. (2017). Goal-oriented cognitive rehabilitation in early-stage Alzheimer's and related dementias: Results from a multi-center, single-blind, randomised controlled trial (the GREAT trial). *Alzheimers Dementia*, *13*(7), 899–900 (Suppl.).

Clark, F., Azen, S. P., Zemke, R., et al. (1997). Occupational therapy for independent-living older adults: A randomised controlled trial. *Journal of the American Medical Association*, *278*(16), 1321–1326.

Clarkson, P., Hughes, J., Xie, C., et al. (2017). Overview of systematic reviews: Effective home support in dementia care, components and impacts – stage 1, psychosocial interventions for dementia. *Journal of Advanced Nursing*, *73*, 2845–2863.

Cohen-Mansfield, J. (2005). Non pharmacological interventions for persons with dementia. *Alzheimer's Care Quarterly*, *6*(2), 129–145.

Craig, C., & Mountain, G. (2007). *Lifestyle Matters: An occupational approach to healthy ageing.* Brackley: Speechmark.

Cuijpers, P., van Straten, A., Smit, F., et al. (2009a). Is psychotherapy for depression equally effective in younger and older adults? A meta-regression analysis. *International Psychogeriatrics*, *21*(1), 16–24.

Cuijpers, P., van Straten, A., Warmerdam, L., et al. (2009b). Psychotherapy versus the combination of psychotherapy and pharmacotherapy in the treatment of depression: A meta-analysis. *Depression and Anxiety*, *26*(3), 279–288.

De Witt, P. (2014). Creative ability: A model for individual and group occupational therapy for clients with psychosocial dysfunction. In *Occupational therapy in Psychiatry and mental health* (5th ed.) (pp. 3–32). Oxford: Wiley.

Drink Wise Age Well. (2019). *Drink Wise age well.* Available at: https://drinkwiseagewell.org.uk/ 20.01.2020.

Fisher, A. G. (2003). Amps: Assessment of motor and process skills. In (5th ed.). *Development, Standardization, and Administration manual* (Vol. 1) Three Star, Fort Collins, CO.

Fisher, A. G. (2006). Amps: Assessment of motor and process skills. In *Three star* (6th ed.). *User manual* (Vol. 2) Fort Collins, CO.

Folstein, M. F., Folstein, S. E., & McHugh, P. R. (1975). Mini mental state: A practical guide for grading the cognitive state of patients for the clinician. *Journal of Psychiatric Research*, *12*(3), 189–198.

Frost, R., Beattie, A., Bhanu, C., et al. (2019). Management of depression and referral of older people to psychological therapies: A systematic review of qualitative studies. *British Journal of General Practice*, 69 (680), e171–e181. https://doi.org/10.3399/njgp19X701297.

Gates, N. J., Rutjes, A. W. S., Di Nisio, M., et al. (2019). Computerised cognitive training for maintaining cognitive function in cognitively healthy people in midlife. *Cochrane Database of Systematic Reviews*, *3*, CD012278. https://doi.org/10.1002/14651858.CD012278.pub2.

Gilhooly, M., Phillips, L., Gilhooly, K., et al. (2003). *Quality of life and real life cognitive functioning. Growing older programme Project Summaries.* Swindon: Economic and Social Research Council.

Gitlin, L., Arthur, P., Piersol, C., et al. (2018). Targeting behavioral symptoms and functional decline in dementia: A randomized clinical trial. *Journal of the American Geriatrics Society*, *66*, 339–345. https://doi.org/10.1111/jgs.15194.

Gitlin, L., Hodgson, N., Jutkowitz, E., et al. (2010). The cost-effectiveness of a nonpharmacologic intervention for individuals with dementia and family caregivers: The tailored activity program. *The American Journal of Geriatric Psychiatry, 18*(6), 510–519. https://doi.org/10.1097/JGP.0b013e3181c37d13.

Gitlin, l., Marx, K., Alonzi, D., et al. (2017). Feasibility of the tailored activity program for hospitalized (TAP-H) patients with behavioral symptoms. *The Gerontologist, 57*(3), 575–584. https://doi.org/10.1093/geront/gnw052.

Gitlin, L., Winter, l., & Burke, J. (2008). Tailored activities to manage neuropsychiatric behaviors in persons with dementia and reduce caregiver burden: A randomized pilot study. *The American Journal of Geriatric Psychiatry, 16*(3), 229–239. https://doi.org/10.1097/JGP.0b013e318160da72.

Gitlin, L., Winter, L., Vause Earland, T., et al. (2009). The tailored activity program to reduce behavioral symptoms in individuals with dementia: Feasibility, acceptability, and replication potential. *The Gerontologist, 49*(3), 428–439. https://doi.org/10.1093/geront/gnp087.

Glass, T. A., Mendes de Leon, C., Marottoli, R. A., et al. (1999). Population based study of social and productive activities as predictors of survival among elderly Americans. *The British Medical Journal, 319*(7208), 478–483.

Graff, M. J. L., Adang, E. M. M., Vernooij-Dassen, M. J. M., et al. (2008). Community occupational therapy for older patients with dementia and their care givers: Cost effectiveness study. *The British Medical Journal, 336*(7636), 134–138.

Graff, M. J. L., Vernooij-Dassen, M. J. M., Thijssen, M., et al. (2006). Community based occupational therapy for patients with dementia and their care givers: Randomised controlled trial. *The British Medical Journal, 333*(7580), 1196–1201.

Graff, M. J. L., Vernooij-Dassen, M. J. F. J., Thijssen, M., et al. (2007). Effects of community occupational therapy on quality of life and health status in dementia patients and their primary caregivers: A randomised controlled trial. *The Journals of Gerontology. Series A, Biological sciences and Medical Sciences, 62*(9), 1002–1009.

Gregory, M. D. (1983). Occupational behavior and life satisfaction among retirees. *American Journal of Occupational Therapy, 37*(8), 548–553.

Gridley, K., Brooks, J., Birks, Y., et al. (2016). Improving care for people with dementia: Development and initial feasibility study for evaluation of life story work in dementia care. *Health Services and Delivery Research, 4*(23). https://doi.org/10.3310/hsdr04230.

de las Heras, C. G., Geist, R., Kielhofner, G., et al. (1998). *A user's manual for the volitional Questionnaire.* Chicago, IL: University of Illinois. Available at: https://www.moho.uic.edu/products.aspx.

Hynes, S., Field, B., Ledgerd, R., et al. (2015). Exploring the need for a new UK occupational therapy intervention for people with dementia and family carers: Community occupational therapy in dementia (COTiD). A focus group study. *Aging & Mental Health, 1*, 1–8. https://doi.org/10.1080/13607863.2015.1037243.

Jackson, J., Carlson, M., Mandel, D., et al. (1998). Occupation in lifestyle redesign: The well elderly study occupational therapy program. *American Journal of Occupational Therapy, 52*(5), 326–336.

Kehrberg, K. L., Kuskowski, M. A., Mortimer, J. A., et al. (1992). Validating the use of an enlarged, easier-to-see Allen cognitive level in geriatrics. *Physical & Occupational Therapy in Geriatrics, 10*(3), 1–14.

Kielhofner, G. (2008). *Model of human occupation: Theory and Application* (4th ed.). Philadelphia, PA: Lippincott Williams and Wilkins.

Kielhofner, G., Mallinson, T., Crawford, C., et al. (2004). *A user's manual for the occupational performance history interview, version 2.1 (OPHI-II).* Chicago, IL: University of Illinois. Available at: https://www.moho.uic.edu/products.aspx.

Kitwood, T. (1997). *Dementia Reconsidered: The person Comes first.* Buckingham: Open University Press.

Kroenke, K., Spitzer, R., & Williams, J. (2001). The PHQ-9: Validity of a brief depression severity measure. *The Journal of General Internal Medicine, 16*(9), 606–613 Sep.

Lamb, S., Sheehan, B., Atherton, N., et al. (2018). Dementia and physical activity (DAPA) trial of moderate to high intensity exercise training for people with dementia: Randomised controlled trial. *British Medical Journal, 361*, k1675. https://doi.org/10.1136/bmj.k1675.

Leroi, I., Woolham, J., Gathercole, R., et al. (2013). Does telecare prolong community living in dementia? A study protocol for a pragmatic, randomised controlled trial. *Trials, 14*(349). https://doi.org/10.1186/1745-6215-14-349.

Livingston, G., Huntley, J., Sommerlad, A., et al. (2020). Dementia prevention, intervention, and care: 2020 report of the Lancet commission. *Lancet, 396*, 413–446.

Livingston, G., Kelly, L., Lewis-Holmes, E., et al. (2014). Non pharmacological interventions for agitation in dementia: Systematic review of randomised controlled trials. *British Journal of Psychiatry, 205*, 436–442.

Livingston, G., Sommerlad, A., Orgeta, V., et al. (2017). The Lancet commission. Dementia prevention, intervention, and care. *Lancet, 390*, 2673–2734.

Manni, B., Federzoni, L., Lanzoni, A., et al. (2018). Occupational therapy in special respite care: A new multi-component model for challenging behaviour in people with dementia. *Geriatrics Care, 4*, 7649. https://doi.org/10.4081/gc.2018.7649.

McDermott, O., Charlesworth, G., Hogervorst, E., et al. (2019). Psychosocial interventions for people with dementia: A synthesis of systematic reviews. *Aging & Mental Health, 23*(4), 393–403.

Mental Capacity Act, 2005. HMSO, London.

Ming Lai, N., Mei Wern Chang, S., Shen Ng, S., et al. (2019). Animal-assisted therapy for dementia. *Cochrane Database of Systematic Reviews.* https://doi.org/10.1002/14651858.CD013243.pub2. Available at:.

Mitchell, G., McCormack, B., & McCance, T. (2014). Therapeutic use of dolls for people living with dementia: A critical review of the literature. *Dementia, 15*(5), 976–1001. https://doi.org/10.1177/1471301214548522.

Mountain, G., Mozley, C. G., Craig, C., et al. (2008). Occupational therapy led health promotion for older people: Feasibility of the lifestyle matters programme. *British Journal of Occupational Therapy, 71*(10), 406–413.

Mountain, G., Sprange, K., & Chatters, R. (2020). Lifestyle matters randomized controlled trial of a preventive health intervention for older people: Qualitative sub study with participants and intervention facilitators. *Clinical Interventions in Aging, 15,* 239–253. https://doi.org/10.2147/CIA.S232108.

Mountain, G., Windle, G., Hind, D., et al. (2017). A preventative lifestyle intervention for older adults (lifestyle matters): A randomised controlled trial. *Age and Ageing, 46,* 1–8. https://doi.org/10.1093/ageing/afx021.

Mozley, C. G., Schneider, J., Cordingley, L., et al. (2007). The care home activity project: Does introducing an occupational therapy programme reduce depression in care homes? *Aging & Mental Health, 11*(1), 99–107.

Nasreddine, Z. S., Phillips, N. A., Bedirian, V., et al. (2005). The Montreal cognitive assessment, MoCA: A brief screening tool for mild cognitive impairment. *Journal of the American Geriatrics Society, 53*(4), 695–699. Available at: www.mocatest.org.

National Institute for Health Research (NIHR). (2018). *Help at home: Use of assistive technology for older people.* NIHR Dissemination Centre, Themed Review. https://doi.org/10.3310/themedreview-03345.

National Institute for Health and Care Excellence (NICE). (2008). *Mental wellbeing in over 65s: Occupational therapy and physical activity interventions.* NICE Public health guideline [PH16].

National Institute for Health and Care Excellence (NICE). (2015). *Older people: Independence and mental wellbeing.* NICE guideline [NG32].

National Institute for Health and Care Excellence (NICE). (2020). *Mental wellbeing and independence in older people. NICE pathway.* Available at: https://pathways.nice.org.uk/pathways/mental-wellbeing-and-independence-in-older-people.

NeuRA. (2012). *Addenbrooke's cognitive examination-III (ACE-III).* Available at: www.neura.edu.au/frontier/research.

Nickel, F., Barth, J., Kolominsky-Rabas, P., et al. (2018). Health economic evaluations of non-pharmacological interventions for persons with dementia and their informal caregivers: A systematic review. *BMC Geriatrics, 18,* 69.

Novelli, M., Machado, S., Lima, G., et al. (2018). Effects of the tailored activity program in Brazil (TAP-BR) for persons with dementia: A randomized pilot trial. *Alzheimer Disease and Associated Disorders, 32*(4), 339–345.

O'Connor, C., Clemson, L., Brodaty, H., et al. (2019). The tailored activity program (TAP) to address behavioral disturbances in frontotemporal dementia: A feasibility and pilot study. *Disability & Rehabilitation, 41*(3), 299–310 doi:10.1080/09638288.2017.1387614.

Oliveira, A., Radanovic, M., Homem de Mello, P., et al. (2018). An intervention to reduce neuropsychiatric symptoms and caregiver burden in dementia: Preliminary results from a randomized trial of the tailored activity program–outpatient version. *International Journal of Geriatric Psychiatry* (34), 1301–1307 2019.

Orrell, M., Aguirre, E., Spector, A., et al. (2014). Maintenance cognitive stimulation therapy for dementia: Single-blind, multicentre, pragmatic randomised controlled trial. *British Journal of Psychiatry, 204*(6), 454–461. https://doi.org/10.1192/bjp.bp.113.137414.

Orrell, M., & Hancock, G. (2004). *Camberwell Assessment of need for the Elderly (CANE).* London: Gaskell.

Orrell, M., Yates, L., Leung, P., et al. (2017). The impact of individual cognitive stimulation therapy (iCST) on cognition, quality of life, caregiver health, and family relationships in dementia: A randomised controlled trial. *PLoS Medicine.* https://doi.org/10.1371/journal.pmed.1002269.

Oyebode, J., & Parvenn, S. (2019). Psychosocial interventions for people with dementia: An overview and commentary on recent developments. *Dementia, 18*(91), 8–35.

Park, S., Fisher, A., & Velozo, C. (1994). Using the assessment of motor and process skills to compare occupational performance between clinic and home settings. *American Journal of Occupational Therapy, 48*(8), 697–709.

Parkinson, S., Forsyth, K., & Kielhofner, G. (2006). *The model of human occupation screening tool (MOHOST), version 2.* Chicago, IL: University of Illinois. Available at: https://www.moho.uic.edu/products.aspx.

Patterson, C. The world alzheimer report 2018: The state of the art of dementia research: New frontiers. Alzheimer's disease international (ADI). London. Available at: https://www.alz.co.uk/research/world-report-2018.

Phillipson, L., & Hammond, A. (2018). More than talking: A scoping review of innovative approaches to qualitative research involving people with dementia. *International Journal of Qualitative Methods, 17*(1), 1–13. https://doi.org/10.1177/1609406918782784.

Pimouguet, C., Le Goff, M., Wittwer, J., et al. (2017). Benefits of occupational therapy in dementia patients: Findings from a real-world observational study. *Journal of Alzheimer's Disease, 56,* 509–517.

Pool, J. (2012). *The Pool activity level (PAL) instrument for occupational profiling: A practical resource for carers of people with cognitive impairment* (4th ed.). London: Jessica Kingsley. Available at: https://www.jackiepoolassociates.org/pool-activity-level-pal/about-pal/.

Pozzi, C., Lanzoni, A., Lucchi, E., et al. (2019). Community based occupational therapy for persons with dementia (COTID-IT program) and their caregivers: Evidence for applicability in Italy. *Aging Clinical and Experimental Research, 31*(9), 1299–1304. https://doi.org/10.1007/s40520-018-1078-7.

Robinson, S. E., & Fisher, A. G. (1996). A study to examine the relationship of the assessment of motor and process skills (AMPS) to other tests of cognition and function. *British Journal of Occupational Therapy, 59*(6), 260–263.

Rodda, J., Walker, Z., & Carter, J. (2011). Depression in older adults. *The British Medical Journal, 343,* 5219.

Royal College of Occupational Therapists (RCOT). (2019a). *Care homes and equipment: Guiding principles for assessment and provision.* Available at: https://www.rcot.co.uk/care-homes-and-equipment.

Royal College of Occupational Therapists (RCOT). (2019b). *Living well in care homes.* London: RCOT. Available at: https://www.rcot.co.uk/about-occupational-therapy/living-well-care-homes-2019.

Royal College of Psychiatrists. (2018). *Suffering in silence: Age inequality in older people's mental health care.* College Report CR221. Available at: https://www.rcpsych.ac.uk/improving-care/campaigning-for-better-mental-health-policy/college-reports/2018-college-reports/cr221.

Royal College of Psychiatrists. (2020). *Memory services national accreditation programme (MSNAP): Standards for memory services* (7th ed.). London: Royal College of Psychiatrists.

Spector, A., Thorgrimsen, L., Woods, B., et al. (2003). Efficacy of an evidence-based cognitive stimulation therapy programme for people with dementia: Randomised controlled trial. *British Journal of Psychiatry, 183,* 248–254.

van der Steen, J., Smaling, H., van der Wouden, J., et al. (2018). Music-based therapeutic interventions for people with dementia. *Cochrane Database of Systematic Reviews, 7,* CD003477. https://doi.org/10.1002/14651858.CD003477.pub4.

Storey, J., Rowland, J., Conforti, D., et al. (2004). The Rowland universal dementia assessment scale (RUDAS): A multicultural cognitive assessment scale. *International Psychogeriatrics, 16,* 13–31.

Surr, C. A., Griffiths, A. W., & Kelley, R. (2018). Implementing dementia care mapping as a practice development tool in dementia care services: A systematic review. *Clinical Interventions in Aging, 13,* 165–177. https://doi.org/10.2147/CIA.S138836.

Surr, C. A., Holloway, I., & Walwyn, R. E. (2020). Dementia care Mapping™ to reduce agitation in care home residents with dementia: The EPIC cluster RCT. *Health Technology Assessment, 24*(16), 1–172. https://doi.org/10.3310/hta24160.

Swinson, T., Wenborn, J., Hynes, S., et al. (2016). Community occupational therapy for people with dementia and their family carers: A national survey of United Kingdom occupational therapy practice. *British Journal of Occupational Therapy, 79*(2), 85–91.

Tullis, A., & Nicol, M. (1999). A systematic review of the evidence for the value of functional assessment of older people with dementia. *British Journal of Occupational Therapy, 62*(12), 554–563.

United Nations, Department of economic and social affairs population division, 2017. World Population Prospects, Key findings & advance tables; the 2017 Revision. Available at: https://www.ageinternational.org.uk and https://www.un.org/development/desa/publications/world-population-prospects-the-2017-revision.html.

Van der Roest, H., Wenborn, J., Pastink, C., et al. (2017). Assistive technology for memory support in dementia: Systematic review. *Cochrane Database of Systematic Reviews, 2,* CD009627. https://doi.org/10.1002/14651858.CD009627.

van Gelder, B. M., Tijhuis, M. A. R., Kalmijn, S., et al. (2004). Physical activity in relation to cognitive decline in elderly men: The FINE study. *Neurology, 63*(12), 2316–2321.

Van't Leven, N., de Lange, J., & Prick, A. (2019). How do activation interventions fit the personal needs, characteristics and preferences of people with dementia living in the community and their informal caregivers? *Dementia, 18*(1), 157–177.

Verghese, J., Lipton, R. B., Katz, M. J., et al. (2003). Leisure activities and the risk of dementia in the elderly. *New England Journal of Medicine, 348*(25), 2508–2516.

Voigt-Radloff, S., Graff, M., Leonhart, R., et al. (2011a). A multicentre RCT on community occupational therapy in alzheimer's disease: 10 sessions are not better than one consultation. *British Medical Journal Open, 1*(1) e000096.

Voigt-Radloff, S., Graff, M., Leonhart, R., et al. (2011b). Why did an effective Dutch complex psycho-social intervention for people with dementia not work in the German healthcare context? Lessons learnt from a process evaluation alongside a multicentre RCT. *British Medical Journal Open, 1.* https://doi.org/10.1136/bmjopen-2011-000094. e000094.

Walton, H., Tombor, I., Burgess, J., et al. (2019). Measuring fidelity of delivery of the community occupational therapy in dementia-UK intervention. *BMC Geriatr, 19,* 364. https://doi.org/10.1186/s12877-019-1385-7.

Wenborn, J., Challis, D., Head, J., et al. (2013). Providing activity for people with dementia in care homes: A cluster randomised controlled trial. *International Journal of Geriatric Psychiatry, 28*(12), 1296–1304. https://doi.org/10.1002/gps.3960.

Wenborn, J., Challis, D., Pool, J., et al. (2008). Assessing the validity and reliability of the pool activity level (PAL) checklist for use with older people with dementia. *Aging & Mental Health, 12*(2), 202–211.

Wenborn, J., Hynes, S., Moniz-Cook, E., et al. (2016). Community occupational therapy for people with dementia and family carers (COTiD-UK) versus treatment as usual (valuing active life in dementia [VALID] study): Study protocol for a randomised controlled trial. *Trials, 17,* 65. https://doi.org/10.1186/s13063-015-1150-y.

Wenborn, J., Mountain, G., Moniz-Cook, E., et al. (2019). *The development, evaluation and implementation of the community occupational therapy in dementia – UK version (COTiD-UK) intervention for people with mild to moderate dementia and their family carers: The valuing active life in dementia (VALID) research programme.* Submitted: Final Report.

Wenborn, J., O'Keeffe, Mountain, G., et al., (2021). Community occupational therapy for people with dementia and family carers (COTiD-UK) versus treatment as usual (valuing active life in dementia [VALID] study): A single-blind, randomised controlled trial. *PLOS Medicine, 18*(1): e1003433. https://doi.org/10.1371/journal.pmed.1003433.

Wilson, D. S., Allen, C. K., McCormack, G., et al. (1989). Cognitive disability and routine task behaviors in a community-based population with senile dementia. *Occupational Therapy Practice, 1*(1), 58–66.

Woods, B., Aguirre, E., Spector, A., & Orrell, M. (2012). Cognitive stimulation to improve cognitive functioning in people with dementia. *Cochrane Database of Systematic Reviews, 2,* CD005562. https://doi.org/10.1002/14651858.CD005562.pub2.

World Federation of Occupational Therapists. (2019). *Position Statement: Occupational therapy and assistive technology.* Available at: https://www.wfot.org/resources/occupational-therapy-and-assistive-technology.

World Health Organization. (2017). *Global action plan on the public health response to dementia 2017–2025.* Geneva: World Health Organization. Licence: CC BY-NC-SA 3.0 IGO. Available at: https://apps.who.int.

Wright, J., Foster, A., Cooper, C. et al., 2019. Study protocol for a randomised controlled trial assessing the clinical and cost-effectiveness of the Journeying through Dementia (JtD) intervention compared to usual care. *British Medical Journal Open* 9, e029207. doi:10.1136/bmjopen-2019-029207. Available at: https://bmjopen.bmj.com/content/9/9/e029207 (last accessed 28/11/19) www.bradford.ac.uk/dementia/research/journeying-through-dementia/#:~:text=Journeying%20through%20Dementia%20was%20a%20large-scale%20research%20study,of%20dementia%20to%20continue%20living%20healthy%2C%20fulfilling%20lives".

Yesavage, J. A., Brink, T. L., Rose, T. L., et al. (1983). Development and validation of a geriatric depression screening scale: A preliminary report. *Journal of Psychiatric Research*, *17*(1), 37–49.

Zigmond, A. S., & Snaith, R. P. (1983). The hospital anxiety and depression scale. *Acta Psychiatrica Scandinavica*, *67*(6), 361–370.

Zimmerman, S., Sloane, P. D., Williams, C. S., et al. (2005). Dementia care and quality of life in assisted living and nursing homes. *The Gerontologist*, *45*(S1), 133–146.

24 CHILDREN AND YOUNG PEOPLE

THEODORA MILDRED CHIKWANHA ■ JACKIE PARSONAGE
HARRISON[1]

CHAPTER OUTLINE

INTRODUCTION

Internationally, early identification and treatment of child and adolescent mental, emotional and behavioural problems are the focus of increased interest and attention (Patel et al. 2018). There is recognition of the multiple factors that influence mental health across the life course and an acknowledgment of the importance of intervention during the critical period of child and adolescent development (Patel et al. 2007; Kieling et al. 2011; Servili 2012; Patel et al. 2018; World Health Organization (WHO) 2018). Consistently, global surveys have shown that children and adolescents are at a higher risk of developing mental health problem compared to adults (WHO 2013). WHO (2018) estimates that 10% to 20% of the global population of children and adolescents experience a mental health problem by the age of 14 years, and three quarters of all mental illnesses begin by their mid-20s.

Multiple risk factors for developing mental health problems across the lifespan have been identified. These include social, economic and environmental factors such as poverty, parental mental illness, trauma, maltreatment, neglect, exposure to violence, abuse, natural disasters, or other humanitarian emergencies and additional disability (Kelly et al. 2011; Servili 2012; WHO 2013). Furthermore, the risk of developing a mental health problem increases when associated with the physical, emotional and social changes that occur during adolescence (Arain et al. 2013).

---

[1]With contributions from Sarah Crawley, Hannah Lukacs, Katie Macdonald, Emma Putman, Kevin Prince Stephen and Carly Watson.

Without access to the required treatment and rehabilitation services, mental health problems have a long lasting impact on skills development for adult roles, educational attainment, future economic potential and can also lead to marginalization, stigma, isolation, discrimination and shortened life expectancy (WHO 2013). Despite the recognized need for treatment, availability and access to appropriate treatment and services for this group of people remains poor as funding for mental healthcare and research is inadequate and disproportionate to the disease burden in all countries (Patel et al. 2018). The WHO has taken action to try to address the gap between need and appropriate treatment, including the Mental Health Gap Action Programme (mhGAP) (WHO 2017). An essential component of this programme was the development of management guidelines for mental health problems including those occurring in childhood and adolescence.

Child and Adolescent Mental Health Services (CAMHS) comprise of a wide range of agencies, services and individuals dedicated to the mental healthcare of children and young people aged between 0 and 18 years (NHS 2019). Occupational therapy is among the essential services provided in CAMHS to addresses the motor, psychological, cognitive and socio-emotional aspects of well-being through engagement in occupations (Gee et al. 2018). Despite the importance of occupational therapy in CAMHS, these services remain grossly underdeveloped in low- to middle-income countries (Juengsiragulwit 2015). The role of occupational therapy in CAMHS is to facilitate and enhance childhood occupations based on the following assumptions (Evans and Banovic 2014):

- Children and adolescents are occupational and social beings;
- The use of occupation is the foundation of occupational therapy and is equally important as means and end;
- Personal, environmental, social, cultural and temporal factors influence occupational performance;
- Occupational development is a dynamic and complex process.

OCCUPATIONAL PERSPECTIVE OF CHILDHOOD AND ADOLESCENCE

Childhood and adolescent development is multidimensional, encompassing physical, psychological, social and emotional well-being (UNICEF 2011; Servili 2012).

Development occurs in predictable stages, however, what is considered typical development varies across cultural, ethnic and religious groups (American Psychological Association (APA) 2018). The occupational perspective of development recognizes childhood (Kielhofner 2008) and adolescence (Widmark and Fristedt 2018) as critical periods of occupational transition facilitating development of competence and mastery required for later life stages and adult life. Mental health difficulties often start at an early age and can disrupt typical occupational development. Therefore occupational therapists are well placed to identify areas of occupational disruption and provide interventions to facilitate occupational development. Occupational therapists working with children and young people should consider the differences in developmental expectations and parenting styles which will impact the overall development of a child.

Working with Diagnostic Uncertainty

Difficulties in early detection and diagnosis of severe mental health conditions among children and young people remains, despite research efforts to identify early indicators such as the development of the Comprehensive Assessment of At Risk Mental States (CAARMS) tool (Oliver and Fusar-Poli 2017). Therefore professionals frequently work with diagnostic uncertainty and referrals are primarily based on assessment of need. The Diagnostic and Statistical Manual for Mental Disorders, 5th Edition, and the International Statistical Classification of Diseases and Related Health Problems, 11th Revision, are widely used to make clinical diagnosis in mental health across the globe. These clinical tools provide a common language for recording, reporting and monitoring mental health problems but do not reflect the dimensional nature or experience of mental health (Patel et al. 2018). In most cases, occupational therapists work within a team and are not expected to make a diagnosis on their own. Table 24.1 summarizes the primary clinical characteristics of the most commonly occurring childhood and adolescent mental, emotional and behavioural diagnoses that are usually referred for occupational therapy.

ACCESSING SERVICES, RESOURCES AND REFERRAL PATHWAYS

Internationally, the nature and scope of the support available to young people presenting with mental health difficulties varies considerably and services worldwide are significantly under resourced (Kieling et al. 2011; WHO 2013; Patel et al. 2018). There is also no uniform, standard referral or intervention pathway for mental health services; instead, the provision of care is shaped by the resources and political will of the country in which it is provided.

Children and adolescents may present with a wide variety of problems, some of which, although distressing for the young person, will resolve without

TABLE 24.1
The Primary Clinical Characteristics of the Most Commonly Occurring Childhood and Adolescent Mental, Emotional and Behavioural Problems that Are Usually Referred for Occupational Therapy

	Developmental Problems	Behavioural Problems	Emotional Problems
Commonly Associated Diagnoses	Autism Intellectual disability Psychosis	Attention deficit disorder Attention deficit hyperactivity disorder Conduct disorder Psychosis	Depression Anxiety Psychosis
Infants and Children (0–5 Years)	-Poor feeding -Failure to thrive -Poor motor tone -Delay in meeting expected age milestones (smiling, sitting, interacting with others, sharing attention, walking, talking and toilet training) -Disruption to social attachments -Disruption to emotional development -Difficulty in understanding the nature of objects and creation of categories -Disruption to language and self-control development	Excess over-activity: excessive running around, extreme difficulties remaining seated, excessive talking or moving restlessly	-Excessive crying -Clinging to a carer -Freezing (holding the body very still and being silent) and/or tantrums -Extreme shyness or changes in functioning (e.g., new wetting or soiling behaviour or thumb sucking) - Diminished initiation of play and social interaction - Sleep and eating difficulties
Middle Childhood (6–12 Years)	-Delay in reading and writing -Delay in self-care (e.g., dressing, bathing, brushing teeth) -Disruption to interpersonal relationship development -Disruption to cognitive process, specifically concrete thinking -Disruption to the development of 'sense of self' -Development of conceptual skills -Development of group play (Wright et al. 2009)	-Excessive inattention- absent-mindedness, repeatedly stopping tasks before completion and switching to other activities	-Recurrent, unexplained physical symptoms (e.g., stomachache, headache, nausea) -Reluctance or refusal to go to school -Extreme shyness or changes in functioning (e.g., new wetting or soiling behaviour or thumb sucking)
Adolescence (13–18 Years)	-Poor school performance -Difficulty understanding instructions -Difficulty in social interaction and adjusting to changes -Disruption to personal ideology development -Disruption to engagement with peer group -Disruption to sexual relationship exploration -Disruption to development of autonomous occupational choice	-Excessive impulsivity: frequently doing things without forethought -Repeated and continued behaviour that disturbs others (e.g., unusually frequent and severe tantrums, cruel behaviour, persistent and severe disobedience, stealing) -Sudden changes in behaviour or peer relations, including withdrawal and anger	-Problems with mood, anxiety or worry (e.g., irritable, easily annoyed, frustrated or depressed mood, extreme or rapid and unexpected changes in mood, emotional outbursts), excessive distress -Changes in functioning (e.g., difficulty concentrating, poor school performance, often wanting to be alone or stay home)

Continued on following page

TABLE 24				
The Primary Clinical Characteristics of the Most Commonly Occurring Childhood and Adolescent Mental, Emotional and Behavioural Disorders that Are Usually Referred for Occupational Therapy (Continued)				
	Developmental Problems		Behavioural Problems	Emotional Problems
All Ages	-Difficulty carrying out daily activities considered -Instructions; difficulty in social interactions and adjusting to changes; -Difficulties or oddities in communication restrictive/repetitive patterns of behaviours, interests and activities			-Excessive fear, anxiety or avoidance of specific situations or objects (e.g., separation from caregivers, social situations, certain animals or insects, heights, closed spaces, sight of blood or injury) -Diminished interest or participation in activities -Oppositional or attention-seeking behaviour

Adapted from WHO (2017) and Wright and Sugarman (2009).

support. Others, however, will require intensive long-term involvement from mental health services. This is because presentations can be transient, reactive or relate to development, for example, bereavement, bullying or social skills difficulties. Alternatively, a young person may experience early warning signs of a more severe and long-term mental illness, for example, behavioural changes suggesting a prodromal phase or acute episode of psychosis. A comparison of referral systems in the United Kingdom (high-income country) and in Zimbabwe (low-income country) will be used to show the differences that exist in different settings.

In the United Kingdom a needs-based, four-tier system is used to inform referrals to appropriate services. Those presenting with high levels of needs are referred to tiers 3 and 4 services such as CAMHS or acute inpatient services (UK Department of Health 2008). Over the past 25 years the UK government's health and education policies have reflected a commitment to improve the services and care offered to young people experiencing well-being and mental health difficulties. One of the more recent changes is the piloting and introduction of 'single point of access' (SPA) services in many mental health trusts. These services are a central hub into which anyone, including parents, teachers and youth services can refer a young person experiencing mental health concerns for a triage assessment before being directed on to other services for further

assessment, treatment and intervention. The SPA team working with the young person will consider their presentation and the level of need before deciding the most appropriate pathway for them.

Although most referrals into mental health services will come via SPA there are other routes such as accident and emergency (A&E) or police arrest. In many of these areas there are now specialist health professionals including occupational therapists, for example, youth justice liaison and diversion based within youth-offending teams (YOTs) and professionals based in A&E liaison teams. The aim of these services is to assess and identify unmet mental health and well-being needs and provide brief intervention or diversion to other support services.

The entry routes into mental health services are largely staffed generically, meaning that a nurse, a social worker or an occupational therapist can take on the role. Occupational therapists in such roles have been valued for bringing a holistic and occupation-focused approach to the role which can fit well with the presenting needs of young people. Specific referral for occupational therapy will depend on the resources, nature and set up of the service the young person is referred to.

In contrast, healthcare services in Zimbabwe are decentralized and can be accessed at primary, secondary, tertiary, central and quaternary levels of care. The primary healthcare system is the entry route into the healthcare system for children and adolescents at risk of developing mental health problems (Ministry of Health and Childcare for Zimbabwe 2016). However, occupational therapy services are not available at the primary care level and are part of specialist CAMHS services, which are still limited to tertiary and quaternary levels of care. A few institutions at the secondary level of care have occupational therapy services, which are provided by rehabilitation technicians. These rehabilitation technicians are mid-level workers trained to provide components of basic occupational therapy, physiotherapy and speech therapy services. The major challenges that arise as a result of this structuring of occupational therapy services is that service users have to travel long distances to access the services. There is also poor integration with the other services provided by the multidisciplinary team.

It can be helpful for occupational therapists working in children and adolescent mental health services to consider and develop their own occupational therapy pathway from referral to evaluation based on the occupational needs of their specific service user group. Pathways agreed with line managers can be used to prioritize and identify those who are most likely to benefit from the input of an occupational therapist. Pathways can maintain a clear occupational therapy focus and a standard that can be audited.

ASSESSMENT

Assessment is perhaps one of the most important parts of occupational therapy practice and provides the basis for an effective intervention. The assessment process aims to facilitate the creation of supportive environments, involving information gathering and problem identification, which informs goal setting, treatment planning, implementation and evaluation (see Chapters 3 and 6). Assessment is not a one-off action but an ongoing process that enables the occupational therapist to improve their understanding of the individual in context of their environment and the subsequent impact on their occupational performance. They may include 1:1 interactions with the child, task orientated observations, family and culture assessments as well as structured occupational therapy based interviews. The occupational therapist must also consider the developmental stage of the child and the level of family.

Establishing a Therapeutic Relationship

The critical starting point for any assessment or intervention with young people is to establish rapport and begin coconstructing an effective therapeutic relationship. Establishing and maintaining this relationship can be challenging and is often one of the most difficult parts of working with young people. The privilege of a working relationship with a young person carries the responsibility of influencing their development and recovery, potentially shaping who they become and influencing their interaction with other professionals in the future. Achieving developmentally and culturally appropriate interactions can be a precarious balancing act. Occupational therapists need to be aware of how children and young people's communication and social interaction skills are changing while they develop adult capabilities. Different groups of children and young people may require different approaches. In some groups it is necessary to be able to switch approaches rapidly and effortlessly to respond to fluctuating behaviour.

Adopting the following principles can help develop rapport:

- Be aware that it can take time to build trust and open up to a new person, especially if they have had difficult past experiences with adults;
- Try to understand and acknowledge their perspective regarding their experience;
- Look out for both verbal and nonverbal cues to what is going on;
- Remember that questions can feel intrusive and threatening and consider using creative approaches to assessment, especially with younger children;
- Be aware of the impact of illness on their mind and body performance and adjust assessment accordingly;
- Be aware of their sensitivities and perceptions of the reactions of others and ensure the approach is genuine, sincere, real, honest and authentic;
- Avoid being perceived as judgemental, particularly in youth justice areas where young people can feel judged by everyone, creating barriers to good engagement;
- Support and encourage self-reflection on their behaviour and choices;

- Support them to acknowledge potential fears, uncertainties and anxieties without losing face or feeling shame;
- Remember that for some young people and their parent this may be their first contact with mental health services; therefore always be clear about who you are and your role;
- Be clear about what you are going to do and who you are going to talk to; and if you said you are going to do it then do it;
- Wherever possible empower and involve them in decision-making and taking responsibility for their care plan;
- Consider the influence and impact of the environmental context on the individual during the assessment (e.g., in police custody or forensic settings a young person living in care service who is in trouble for the first time may be particularly anxious or distrusting around adults and as a result may find it difficult to take on board new information or be reluctant to open up about their experiences);
- Avoid healthcare terminology or jargon because a young person may not understand its meaning or may feel that what is described does not relate to them and their experience;
- Check understanding regularly, being careful to avoid embarrassment;
- Be willing to address the young person's questions or concerns before asking assessment questions;
- Depending on the age of the young person it may be helpful to take a bag of interactive tools for them to play with as part of the assessment process.

Using Occupational Therapy Models and Assessments

In practice, there is wide variation of occupation based clinical practice models and assessments used (models of practice are discussed in more detail in Chapter 3). In a recent UK survey of occupational therapists working with this population, the model of human occupation (MOHO) was found to be most commonly used (Brooks et al. 2018). MOHO is also advocated by the UK-based Royal College of Occupational Therapists for use with children and adolescents (Harrison

and Forsyth 2005) as it has multiple assessments to choose from including the specifically designed Child Occupational Self-Assessment (COSA). Other models include the Vona du Toit model of creative ability (Witt 2005), which has a developmental perspective; the Canadian model of occupational performance (Fearing et al. 1997) with a focus on client centredness and spirituality; the Kawa model with its symbolic representation of the experience of illness (Iwama et al. 2009); and the person environment occupation model with its focus on the importance of the environment (Law et al. 1996). In general most of the models used have not been specifically designed for this population, consequently model choice is often influenced by other factors such as those with assessments developed for children and adolescents, those advocated by their employer or those that are considered to work best for a specific client group in a particular setting.

Examples of some formal assessments used with children and young people include:

- COSA;
- Creative Participation Assessment and Activity Participation Outcome Measure (APOM);
- Canadian Occupational Performance Measure, which can be completed by either the child, the adolescent or their carer;
- Paediatric Activity Card Sort and the Adolescent and Young People Activity Card Sort.

Task-Oriented Observational Assessments

There are a wide range of standardized and non-standardized assessment tools to use in clinical practice and use is influenced by the practice setting, available resources as well as clinical expertise in using the available assessment tools. Most occupational therapists in low- to middle- income countries have no access to standardized tools and rely on observational assessments, while those in high-income countries may have access to a wide range of available assessments. Observational assessments use clinical judgement and theoretical principles (Stewart 1999) to assess the interaction of motor, psychosocial, socio-emotional and cognitive components of well-being, as well as to interpret how the sensory input and the environment (home, school, community) affect participation in everyday activities (Arbesman et al. 2013). The advantage of using observational assessment tools is that they allow a flexibility in the assessment that is not possible when using standardized tools (Corr and Siddons 2005). The downside to using observational tools is that the assessments are highly subjective and may be difficult to replicate. The assessments are done within the domains of play, leisure, activities of daily living (ADLs), education, sleep and rest as well as social participation. Case Study 24.1 illustrates the use of observation during activity as a method of assessment.

Family and Cultural Aspects of Illness

Family and Cultural Assessment

In the context of working with children and young people, families are critically important in providing information about both the history of the illness and the impact of illness on occupational performance. Families are also often the first to identify problems and are central to managing crisis. Consequently, the role of caring can be a considerable burden, causing both stress and anxiety for the whole family including other siblings. Effective timely support for the family can improve recovery outcomes for the young person and minimize potential problems for the family. It is therefore important that the occupational therapist ensures that the carers' needs are assessed, but also that the young person remains in control and at the centre of their care.

Understanding the environment and family culture should also form part of the assessment as it can significantly shape occupational expectations, affect attitudes to diagnosis, treatment and willingness to accept support from services, impacting treatment outcomes (APA 2018). Assessing cultural diversity requires a level of cultural awareness and sensitivity of not only our own cultural assumptions about mental illness and occupation, but also those of others.

Culturally sensitive working

Working in a culturally sensitive way means being aware of how children, young people, and their families may perceive or respond to mental health problems differently based on their values, beliefs, or culture. This awareness then creates opportunities for the therapist to engage in discussion about how occupational therapy can meet the family's unique needs. A brief description of some common issues follows.

Difference in Belief About What is Mental Illness

Western culture usually adopts a strongly medical approach to mental illness including lists of symptoms grouped into diagnostic labels with the aspiration of evidence-based treatments (Swaine 2011). In some cultures, hearing voices is seen as a gift that blesses the community, while in others it is viewed as a curse, witchcraft, or black magic. These beliefs are likely to affect when, how and if a young person comes into contact with mental health services. It is also likely to affect the willingness to engage with mental health systems and services. It is important to remember these beliefs may not be held by all family members, causing internal family conflicts.

Difference in Belief About How Mental Illness Should be Dealt With

The western approach to mental illness advocates a biopsychosocial approach typically advocating medication, psychological and some social interventions (McInerney 2002). In cultures where hearing voices is regarded as a gift, a person may be provided for and cared by their community and no attempt will be made to change their presentation as it is not viewed as problematic. In those cultures where an individual is seen as suffering from the effects of a Jinn, black magic or a curse a faith healer or religious leader may be asked to pray over a person or perform an exorcism.

Other religious traditions may not believe that mental illness is a curse but still believe in the power of God to heal and help an individual to recover. These viewpoints will affect the way that a child and their family respond to what is offered by mental health service and need to be responded to cautiously and sensitively (Mantovani et al. 2016).

Difference in How Communities Respond to a Person Presenting with Mental Illness

Stigma and feelings of shame are still commonplace across the world (Alonso et al. 2008). In some cases communities will shun and exclude those presenting with mental illness and their families. Consequently, families may choose to hide those who are unwell resulting in isolation and delays in appropriate treatment and interventions (Mantovani et al. 2016).

Difference in Cultural or Family Occupational Norms

It is also important to be aware of what the cultural and family norms and expectations are regarding occupation, such as gender norms, attitudes to study life balance, the value of family, acceptable leisure occupations and many others. Occupational norms and their associated value can sometimes be quite subtle or taken for granted but have a significant impact on intervention outcomes. Cultural issues are addressed in Case Study 24.2.

Intervention Types and Settings

Interventions are informed by the outcomes of the initial assessment and the service remit and its resources. The occupational therapist formulates aims and objectives in partnership with the child and family, structuring them according to the model chosen. For example, occupational therapists using MOHO, may formulate goals based on occupational performance areas such as volition, habituation or performance capacity. The goals should form the basis for the intervention plan and should also be meaningful and appropriate to the individual's level of ability.

Occupational therapists can choose from several general intervention types which include:

1. Occupation-focused individual sessions or therapy group sessions which provide psychoeducation, skills training and/or activity-based sessions;
2. Occupation-focused, community-based activities such as orientation to local environment or gradual desensitization to a specific setting (e.g., familiarization with the bus route to school);
3. Liaison with others such as social services, other mental health teams, families, school, or universities to facilitate and support future occupational engagement;
4. Assessment, adaptation or modification to the environment to enable specific occupations;
5. Support transitions, such as discharge from hospital back to the community or from one school to another;
6. Intervention through apps and virtual reality is also likely to become increasingly common;
7. Some occupational therapists may also have additional training that enables them to provide additional specialist input such as sensory integration or family therapy.

In High Income Countries such as the United Kingdom, United States, Canada and Australia, multiple specialist service types exist. Occupational therapy treatment and intervention will vary depending on the treatment setting. Below are some examples of UK clinical settings and the types of occupational therapy interventions that may be offered.

CAMHS: A multidisciplinary service that provides assessment and treatment to young people aged 3 to 18 years in the community. Occupational therapists' roles may include 1:1 sessions with a focus on psychosocial education, promoting appropriate occupational engagement and developing coping strategies. They may also offer skills based or behaviour change groups. The setting requires liaison with other agencies, especially schools, social services and other community agencies. Occupational therapists may also be involved in home assessments.

Early intervention services (EIS): A multidisciplinary evidence-based model for those experiencing their first episode of psychosis. Service models do vary and are typically offered for three to five years after the onset of the illness. The occupational therapist's role focuses on supporting the individual and family to cope with the trauma of psychosis onset, to adjust to the impact on occupational functioning and to support occupational recovery. The role is likely to include generic tasks. Typical interventions may include working on returning to school, supporting career aspirations and coplanning graded occupational engagement.

School liaison/In reach teams: Multidisciplinary school-based teams with a focus on reducing and preventing impact of mental illness on education performance. Services usually offer psychological support and also psychoeducation to help improve resilience and well-being.

Acute children and adolescent psychiatric inpatient units and psychiatric intensive care units: A multidisciplinary team, but one that often has specialist occupational therapy departments, that provides tier 4 care to those whose mental health places them at risk if they remained in the community. Stays are usually short lasting from four to six weeks. The occupational therapy role focuses on routine, education, social inclusion, self-care and other aspects of occupation whilst on the ward and can also include preparing for occupational engagement on discharge such home assessments and graded return to school planning.

Specialist eating disorders clinics or units: Works specifically with those who have an eating disorder. Admissions are usually longer than in other acute wards. The occupational therapist's role involves assessment of function with specific focus on occupational difficulties associated with eating. Groups are focused on behaviour change such as addressing occupational in balance and engagement in leisure activities. Activities such as cooking are graded dependent on individual's presentation and risks. Individual activities may include going out for snacks or eating out.

Forensic secure units and prison in reach: Work with young people using a community-based model of mental healthcare to address mental health needs within the prison environment. Occupational therapists may specifically focus on relaxation, emotion management, education and life skills. Some therapists also use sensory activities. Groups offered may include behaviour change groups such as healthy eating, creative groups such as music groups or skills base groups such as social skills training.

Home treatment teams: Work with a young person in their home during a period of crisis as an alternative to hospital admission or to facilitate earlier discharge. Occupational therapists in this role are likely to offer 1:1 sessions and to focus on supporting and encouraging the child to engage and participate in familiar activities within the home environment with their family and as appropriate with the wider community.

A&E liaison teams: Work with A&E departments to assess those presenting with acute mental health symptoms. The focus is on assessing and developing an emergency care plan and onward referral based on need. Consequently, interventions are brief and very short term. The role is often generic but occupational therapists are well suited to it because of their holistic approach and practical problem solving using an occupational focus.

YOTs and liaison and diversion: Work with young people in the criminal justice system to address multiple issues. Occupational therapists working in the generic role of liaison and diversion within YOTs provide a holistic assessment and then refer onto appropriate services. Occupational therapists have a unique perspective that can be useful in assessing needs and they may occasionally provide individual support whilst waiting for a referral to be accepted.

Family Interventions

Involvement with families varies dependent on need. It may involve psychoeducation to understand the diagnosis and symptoms or help to manage unhelpful behaviour and family dynamics. Support may also take the form of emotional support, such as stress management, providing the opportunity to talk about their own response to the situation or explaining how the mental health system works. This can happen informally such as a 1:1 with staff and formally through evidenced based approaches such as family therapy or family interventions. These interventions help family groups find better ways of coping and address areas of difficulty.

Other Alternative Interventions

Occupational therapists also draw on other complimentary treatment approaches. Many are developed for use across the lifespan rather than specifically for children and adolescents. Some of these approaches are specific to occupational therapy and others will cut across all the professional disciplines.

Sensory approaches: These include sensory processing strategies and Ayers sensory integration, strategies such as weighted vests, fidget toys and blankets.

Task-oriented techniques: These facilitate the development of functional skills in children with mental, behavioural and emotional disorders.

Behavioural approaches: These incorporate the principles of operant conditioning to elicit positive behaviour such as applied behavioural analysis. The occupational therapists utilize the Antecedent; Behaviour; Consequence; De-escalating, debriefing, deciding technique to determine why certain behaviours occur. The antecedent is what triggers the challenging behaviour, the behaviour is the response to the antecedent and the consequence is the caregiver's response to the behaviour. The consequence can reinforce or discourage the behaviour. De-escalating refers to what can be done to calm the situation, debriefing entails talking to someone about the incident. Therapists and caregivers also need to make decisions on what could be done differently in handling similar situations in future.

ADL training: This is aimed at establishing new functional skills, maintaining and modifying existing ones to address challenges with occupational performance.

Caregiver education and counselling: It is aimed at providing caregivers with information on the presenting problem based on scientifically proven strategies for promoting function and reducing disruptive behaviours as well as strengthening caregivers' coping skills. This can be done on an individual basis or within a group.

EVALUATION

Evaluation is an important part of the occupational therapy process in any clinical setting. It reviews the effectiveness of the intervention and an individual's progress against their set goals. Keeping good records of assessment, clearly documenting treatment goals and outcomes of intervention is important for building up the evidence base to support the profession, through identifying effectiveness and quality care. This topic is discussed in more depth in Chapter 6.

FACTORS INFLUENCING THE OCCUPATIONAL THERAPY PROCESS

Working as Part of a Wider Team

Occupational therapists commonly find that they are the only occupational therapist in a team. This can present specific challenges around maintaining professional identity and keeping interventions focused on occupation. Occupational therapists have an important part to play in the multidisciplinary team's (MDT's) decision-making and care planning, providing an occupational focus, including providing an insight into how personal occupational needs may be impacting health and well-being.

The intervention by the MDT should take into consideration information from clinical assessments, childcare or education settings as well as results from standardized instruments. The composition of the MDT varies from setting to setting and may include a paediatrician, child psychiatrist, occupational therapist, speech therapist, caregivers/parents and any other disciplines that are considered relevant depending on the identified abilities and needs of the client (Randal et al. 2018).

Occupational therapists can also use the occupational perspective to shape team process, service development and delivery. Aspects of generic working are also common in some of these roles requiring additional skill development such as capacity assessment, risk assessment and management and safeguarding.

Managing Risk and Promoting Resilience

The mental health of children and adolescents can be positively and negatively impacted by a variety of factors. Risk factors can be internal or external and relate to culture, economic situation or medical condition. Resilience on the contrary refers to factors which have a protective effect and can counterbalance risk factors (Schultze-Lutter et al. 2016). Occupational therapists may choose to focus on occupations which promote resilience such as assertiveness, problem solving, social skills and physical activity.

Occupational therapy assessments should focus on highlighting a child's strengths and needs, but any treatment and intervention plan will require the occupational therapist to also assess potential risks and consider how these will be managed. For example, when planning a ward-based cooking group, an occupational therapist needs to consider how to manage any use of knives in the group. Occupational therapists in some countries also have a legal duty to be observant for and report any safeguarding concerns. They may also have to contribute to generic risk management plans.

It is important to note that risk management strategies do vary across countries. High income countries typically have greater access to resources to manage serious risk of harm to self or others, for example, access to secure psychiatric hospital beds and rapid tranquilization. Low and Middle Income Countries often have fewer resources and, consequently, less options available to manage risks when faced with an individual who poses a serious risk to themselves and others. Priority must always be given to keeping a person safe whilst also protecting their human rights, and where restrain is absolutely necessary to prevent serious harm, universal principles of the least restrictive method available should be observed.

Contemporary Risk Issues

Culture has undergone rapid change and consequently there has been an evolution in the nature of some risks that young people face. Those working with young people need to be aware of these risks and challenges they face.

Young people may be in a gang or find themselves affected by gang behaviour such as knife crime or drug use. County lines, where gangs expand their operations to smaller towns by exploiting children and young people, is another particularly worrying trend in the United Kingdom (National Crime Agency 2019).

Another contemporary risk factor that young people face is social isolation. Children and adolescents are highly isolated and often connect to others via social media, which can leave them vulnerable to cyber bullying, unhelpful peer comparisons affecting self-esteem and grooming and exploitation.

A further factor impacting the mental health of young people is increased conflict leading to increased levels of trauma and displacement (Patel et al. 2018).

CASE STUDIES

The following case studies illustrate the occupational therapy process in this population and demonstrate the principles discussed in this chapter.

CASE STUDY 24.1

School Liaison/In Reach Teams

Referrer: School teacher

Reasons for referral: To make a general assessment and advise the teacher on how to enhance attention during classroom activities.

Case summary: Talent, aged 6, was referred to an outpatient child and adolescent service due to problems sustaining attention in classroom tasks. Talent stays with both parents in a rural area and has one younger sibling who is 4 years old. There is no occupational therapy department close to his home, and he has to travel to the central hospital (120 km away) to be seen by a multidisciplinary team. His parents are subsistence farmers.

Occupational therapy assessment: The occupational therapy assessment started with interviewing the parents using an institution designed semi-structured interview guide. This interview guide focused on identifying the occupational performance problems of the child as well as the caregivers' understanding of the child's problems. The parents reported that Talent was always running around, climbing trees around the family compound, and when he was not going to school, he spent the whole day outdoors playing with other children in the village; they had to go and look for him when it was time to go back home. The parents indicated that they knew their child was just 'naughty' and had never heard about attention deficit hyperactivity disorder (ADHD) until their son's teacher raised concerns that Talent was not performing well in school because he was not able to sit still in class and concentrate on his schoolwork during lessons. A review of the teacher's report indicated that Talent had an inability to complete written assignments given in class. His teacher also reported that he did not interacted well with a lot of children during play time, and, as a result, he did not have many friends. Observation during a structured play activity in which Talent was given step-by-step instructions showed that he was getting easily distracted during the structured play activity and kept leaving his seat and running around the occupational therapy playroom when expected to stay seated.

Occupational therapy intervention plan: The aims of the occupational therapy intervention were for Talent to develop the ability to attend to structured classroom tasks through use of structured play activities and to educate the parents about the child's condition. Occupational therapy was part of a multidisciplinary intervention that included a psychiatrist, a clinical psychologist and a social worker. The occupational therapist contacted the school teacher to discuss the following strategies that could be used in the classroom to enhance attention:

- Sitting Talent in the least distracting place where good eye contact could be maintained with the teacher, such as close to the teacher's desk;

- Sitting Talent near good role models in class;

Continued on following page

School Liaison/In Reach Teams (Continued)

- Giving Talent a list of the tasks that he had to complete in the classroom every morning before class;
- Signalling the beginning and ending of a lesson;
- Giving clear instructions to Talent and asking him to repeat them before remarking on a task;
- Setting clearly defined classroom rules.

Due to the long distances Talent's family had to travel to access occupational therapy services, a home programme was developed, which was reviewed on a monthly basis. For the parents to understand the home programme the initial step was to educate them about the child's condition. This was done through 1:1 counselling. The parents also took part in educational workshops in which they were taught various techniques. Talent's parents were given an attention training program in which they had to engage the child in structured play activities, which were agreed upon after considering the resources that were available in a rural setting.

Outcome: As a result of the intervention, the teacher reported that Talent's grades had improved as he became more focused on his schoolwork. His social skills also improved and he managed to make friends with most of his classmates. His parents became knowledgeable about his condition and were able to give him the necessary support to overcome the occupational performance problems related to ADHD.

Early Intervention Services

Case summary: Abdul is currently under the care of Early Intervention Services (EIS). He was born in Afghanistan and lived there with his grandparents until the age of 13, when he came to join his parents in the United Kingdom. His English language skills are poor. He was picked up by transport police for walking on the railway lines and was briefly admitted to hospital before being referred to EIS. Abdul denies any suicidal thoughts and cannot remember why he was on the train line. He believes he has human immunodeficiency virus (HIV) and that someone has hacked into his Facebook account and written that he is gay on his profile. Diagnostic tests indicate he does not have HIV, and his parents state that his account has not been hacked and no one has suggested that he is gay. He continues to present in a chaotic and odd manor. His family believes that he is misbehaving, and this causes regular conflicts with his father. Abdul is very concerned about what people think of him and rejects any suggestion of mental illness stating that he is not mad. Abdul is not in education or work and currently spends time watching TV. He used to play football in Afghanistan and believes that he used to be very good at it. He does not play now.

Occupational therapy assessment: An interpreter was used to complete a model of human occupation screening tool (MOHOST) assessment over several meetings with Abdul on his own. Information was also gathered from his family and medical notes.

Client-centred goals:

1. Abdul's immediate goals are to improve his English and play football again.
2. Abdul does not like the conflict with his family and agreed to work with the occupational therapist and with his family to help reduce conflict at home.

Occupational therapy intervention plan:

Abdul's family were provided with psychoeducation and support about psychosis. Strategies were discussed and a problem-solving approach was taken to try to reduce conflicts in the home. This was only partially successful as the father found it hard to accept that his son was ill and not just behaving badly.

CASE STUDY 24.2

Early Intervention Services (Continued)

Different interpreters where used at different times, some of which suggested that Abdul was talking normally; however, a second interpreter who was born in Afghanistan stated that Abdul was not speaking coherently or clearly and came across as thought disordered. The interpreter highlighted that sometimes those who have learned the language as second generation, whilst understanding the content, may not fully understand the subtly of the language and miss the presence of mild thought disorder. This meeting identified that Abdul had little understanding of his condition. Because of the language barrier, the occupational therapist liaised with the local GP who was born and grew up in Afghanistan. The GP agreed to work together with the occupational therapist to improve Abdul's understanding and, particularly, to try to destigmatise his opinions about mental health. Abdul was also supported to enroll in a local class for English to Speakers of Other Languages, which he enjoyed and attended regularly. He was also encouraged to join the local mental health football group,

and efforts were made to look for another local club for him to join. Abdul's mental health continued to fluctuate over the next couple of years, meaning that he went backwards and forwards towards his goals. After further assessment, the occupational therapist explored supported housing options because of the difficult relationships at home which was impacting the well-being of young family members and the need to provide Abdul with more support than the family were able to provide. The occupational therapist also continued to work with Abdul and his family as a care coordinator until he was transferred on to the adult community mental health team after three years with EIS.

Evaluation method: MOHOST was completed at various points to evaluate Abdul's current performance. Abdul and his family were regularly asked about his attendance at his English classes and football. Regular contact was maintained to see how he was doing at home as this fluctuated regularly.

CASE STUDY 24.3

Child and Adolescent Mental Health Services (CAMHS)

Case summary: Simon is a white British 15-year-old boy who was referred to Child and Adolescent Mental Health Services (CAMHS; tier 3) after expressing thoughts of ending his life because 'everyone hates him.' He has a brief history of self-harming behaviour, including making superficial cuts to his arm, and believes that he does not deserve anything. He is currently studying for his GCSE's and wants to be a mechanic. He enjoys sports, listening to music and playing on his PlayStation. Simon has a good relationship with both of his parents.

Occupational therapy assessment: An informal model of human occupation (MOHO)–based assessment was completed with Simon initially. With Simon's permission the occupational therapist also met with

his mother. At a further meeting the COSA was completed and discussed. Simon's progress was regularly reviewed.

Client-centred goals: Simon and his occupational therapist negotiated the following goals:

1. To support Simon to identify effective coping strategies for managing emotionally difficult situations that lead to suicidal thoughts;
2. To review Simon's daily time use and impact on emotional well-being to identify occupational related balance strategies to improve general mood;
3. To evaluate the school environment and explore reasonable adjustments to support Simon's ongoing engagement in his studies.

Occupational therapy intervention plan:

Continued on following page

CASE STUDY 24.3

Child and Adolescent Mental Health Services (CAMHS) (Continued)

Simon was supported to identify patterns of negative thinking and links to self-harm. Time was also spent identifying strategies for managing incidents of self-harming behaviour including identifying self-soothing actions that use the five senses and to identify distress tolerance strategies. A plan was then developed encouraging him to express his thoughts during meetings with his occupational therapist and between sessions by sharing them with his mother, trusted adults or by writing them down securely. He was also encouraged to seek help to dress and treat his self-harm wounds appropriately to reduce the risk of infection and promote healing and to keep an activity diary recording his daily activities and significant events including details about how he felt during the course of the day. He was also inspired to notice any events that happen preceding thoughts of self-harm. The diary was then used to identify patterns or triggers for self-harming behaviour, which were used by the occupational therapist to guide Simon to identify a variety of activities that he could use to distract him from self-harming thoughts, such as listening to a favourite piece of music. Simon and the occupational therapist also used the diary record to look at current patterns of behaviour and identify problem areas such as getting enough sleep and avoiding energy drinks. As Simon particularly liked sports, he was encouraged to engage in this more often as a way of helping him to improve his mood and manage his frustrations. The occupational therapist discussed with Simon at length about his experiences at school, and together they explored ways to improve his school experience. This included a variety of possible strategies such as identifying safe spaces, discussing ways to deal with bullies and planning how he would use non-class time. The occupational therapist discussed and agreed with Simon to jointly meet with his head of year to help the school better support him during the school day.

Evaluation method: COSA and goals were rated before and after intervention to identify levels of improvement.

CASE STUDY 24.4

Paediatric Practice

Referrer: Paediatrician

Reasons for referral: To facilitate improvement in the child's ability to participate in home, school and family activities.

Case summary:

Kyle is an 8-year-old boy diagnosed with autism spectrum disorder. He attends pre-school in a suburban area. He is the second child in a family with three children. He is dependent on his mother for his basic activities of daily living (ADLs). His parents became concerned when his speech did not develop at the age of 2 years; they visited the children's rehabilitation hospital and were seen by a paediatrician who then referred them for occupational therapy and speech therapy.

Occupational therapist assessment:

The occupational therapy assessment started with an interview of the parents to establish their reasons for bringing Kyle to occupational therapy. An occupational profile was conducted to ascertain Kyle's occupational history and experiences, patterns of ADLs, interests and values. His parents reported that, in addition to the delayed verbal communication, they were also concerned about Kyle's eating habits as he only enjoyed mashed potatoes with soup and brown rice with peanut butter. He also exhibited unusual reactions to typical activities such as crying when bathing and dressing, refusing to use the toilet and running outside church when the African drum was being played during praise and worship. He also did not enjoy playing in the sandpit or walking outside barefooted.

CASE STUDY 24.4

Paediatric Practice (Continued)

This was then followed by a review of previous evaluation reports from the Department of Education. According to Kyle's teacher, he only enjoyed art and computers. He sometimes had difficulties following instructions and appeared to be 'stubborn.' He had no friends and enjoyed being alone most of the time. The occupational therapists also observed Kyle's behaviour at home, school and in the occupational therapy department and confirmed what had been reported by Kyle's parents and his teacher.

Occupational therapy interventions:

The occupational therapy intervention was aimed at engaging the child in sensory-rich experiences that were designed to address his sensory needs. This intervention was based on the assessment findings and in consultation with Kyle's parents to ensure that the occupational therapy intervention addressed the concerns of Kyle's parents. The therapist engaged Kyle in various play activities that enhanced his ability to process and integrate sensory information to improve his functional independence and participation in play, ADLs, education and school.

Outcome:

Significant improvement was noted in Kyle's ability to participate in home, school and family activities. The goal attainment scale was used to document the intervention outcomes as well as to quantify and compare progress on each goal.

QUESTIONS FOR CONSIDERATION

1. What barriers might children and young people face in accessing occupational therapy services in your area?
2. What are the similarities and differences between the developmental, behavioural and emotional problems children may present with in middle childhood?
3. Identify the principles to develop rapport when establishing a therapeutic relationship that are most difficult for you. Write a reflection on these difficulties, and identify actions you might take to develop your therapeutic use of self.
4. Looking at the common difficulties faced when treating children in families with alternate beliefs to your own, how would you adapt your approach?
5. What support are you aware of for families of children with mental illness and psychosis in your local area?
6. Read Case Study 24.1. Based on Talent's parents' observations, which behavioural signs could his parents have identified earlier if they had better education about attention deficit hyperactivity disorder?
7. Read Case Study 24.2. Compare mental health beliefs and treatments in England and Afghanistan. Were there any other intervention plans that could have been suggested to improve progress for Abdul and his family?

SERVICE USER COMMENTARY

I grew up in a suburban area of the United Kingdom where it seemed that everybody had remarkably similar 9-to-5 lives. My friends and I might have resembled paper dolls, cut into an identical strip. Reading this chapter, it struck me how diverse the population of children presenting to occupational therapy can be. A 'heterogeneous population' is very often portrayed as a vast and challenging landscape for clinicians, but the chapter brings meaning to that statement. It invites the reader to zoom in to meet each child where they are at; young independent minds that, like each of us, hold dreams, humour, fears and favourites.

Throughout my childhood, I experienced both mental and physical disabilities (cerebral palsy, obsessive compulsive disorder and anorexia nervosa) for which I saw many professionals, including occupational therapists. I liked the section in this chapter on assessment. Most of my early memories of occupational therapy are clouded by not knowing who was sat opposite me or why. I remember fidgeting on brown plastic chairs, sitting opposite clipboards and pleated skirts, hoping that the questions would soon be over so that 'the lady' would get out the dolls or PlayDoh. Had I understood who was talking to me, and why, I might have paid attention. A great barrier to building trust was the sense that I was there because the adults saw me as broken, in need of a fix. I think the recommendations laid out in the chapter could help children to understand that assessments are not just another test to pass or fail.

I hope that anyone reading this pays close attention to the section on stigma and shame. I wasn't equipped with a good understanding of my needs and neither were my friends or family. My parents didn't particularly like the idea of engaging with 'mental health services' and weren't involved in my treatment. I think they may have felt differently if the goals being set meant more to us as a family. The embarrassment surrounding what was 'wrong' with me made me avoid difficult things. I think had I been offered the chance to set goals that mattered to me, I might have persevered more.

My worst experience was at age 15 and on the instruction of my occupational therapist, having to hand over a generic teacher assessment to my form tutor, which I knew included questions about 'the child's toileting capabilities.' It sat on her desk for days with my name highlighted at the top in piercing yellow ink. I felt like I had been reduced to a problem and swore never to return to occupational therapy. But a year later, living as an inpatient on an adolescent eating disorders unit, my mind was changed. Every Monday morning, six other patients and I sat on a squashy sofa with the occupational therapist to set weekly goals that, for once, weren't just about weight and food. Our occupational therapist saw us as people, not as 'troubled kids,' seeming genuinely interested in our opinions. She also noticed everything; prizing giant cushions from laps to confront body image issues, and coaxing us to sit back, rather than bolt upright – 'you deserve comfort.' In a similar way, this chapter encourages occupational therapists to be creative and look beyond the obvious, to see the person and their ambitions, which no manual or guideline can determine. That group challenged me beyond what I thought possible. From the child who was terrified of kitchen knives, food aromas, eating in public and saying the word 'chocolate' aloud, I have become an adult who loves to cook, lives independently and can strut down the street in shorts. Recovery restored my physical health, but occupational therapy brought colour to my life.

Hannah Harvey

REFERENCES

Alonso, J., Buron, A., Bruffaerts, R., et al. (2008). Association of perceived stigma and mood and anxiety disorders: Results from the world mental health surveys. *Acta Psychiatrica Scandinavica, 118.*

American Psychological Association (APA). (2018). Child and adolescent mental and behavioural health resolution. Available at: https://www.apa.org/about/policy/child-adolescent-mental-behavioral-health.

Arain, M., Haque, M., Johal, L., et al. (2013). Maturation of the adolescent brain. *Neuropsychiatric Disease and Treatment, 9,* 449–461.

Arbesman, M., Bazyk, S., & Nochajski, S. M. (2013). Systematic review of occupational therapy and mental health promotion, prevention, and intervention for children and youth. *American Journal of Occupational Therapy, 67,* 120–130.

Brooks, R., Monro, S., & Jones, J. (2018). Occupational therapy in children and young people's mental health: A UK survey of practice. *Children, Young people and Families Occupational Therapy Journal,* 9–14.

Corr, S., & Siddons, L. (2005). An introduction to the selection of outcomes measures. *British Journal of Occupational Therapy, 68,* 202–206.

Department of Health (DH). (2008). *Children and young people in mind: The final report of the national CAMHS review.* Available at: https://webarchive.nationalarchives.gov.uk/20090615071556/http://publications.dcsf.gov.uk/eOrderingDownload/CAMHS-Review.pdf.

Evans, S., & Banovic, J. (2014). Emotional health and wellbeing of children and young people. In W. Bryant, J. Fieldhouse, & K. Brannigan (Eds.), *Creek's occupational therapy and mental health* (5th ed.). London: Churchill Livingstone.

Fearing, V. G., Law, M., & Clark, J. (1997). An occupational performance process model: Fostering client and therapist alliances. *Canadian Journal of Occupational Therapy, 64,* 7–15.

Gee, B. M., Nwora, A., & Peterson, T. W. (2018). Occupational therapy's role in treatment of children with autism spectrum disorders. In M. Huri (Ed.), *Occupational therapy - therapeutic and creative use of activity.* IntechOpen. https://doi.org/10.5772/intechopen.72549.

Harrison, M., & Forsyth, K. (2005). Developing a vision for therapists working with in child and adolescent mental health services: Poised or paused for action? *British Journal of Occupational Therapy, 68,* 181–185.

Iwama, M. K., Thomson, N. A., & Macdonald, R. M. (2009). The Kawa model: The power of culturally responsive occupational therapy. *Disability & Rehabilitation, 31,* 1125–1135.

Juengsiragulwit, D. (2015). Opportunities and obstacles in child and adolescent mental health services in low- and middle-income countries: A review of the literature. WHO South East Asia J. *Public Health, 4,* 110.

Kelly, Y., Sacker, A., Del Bono, E., et al. (2011). What role for the home learning environment and parenting in reducing the socioeconomic gradient in child development? Findings from the Millennium Cohort study. *Archives of Disease in Childhood, 96,* 832–837.

Kielhofner, G. (2008). *Model of human occupation.* Lippincott Williams & Wilkins.

Kieling, C., Baker-Henningham, H., Belfer, M., et al. (2011). Child and adolescent mental health worldwide: Evidence for action. *Lancet, 378,* 1515–1525.

Law, M., Cooper, B. A., Strong, S., et al. (1996). The person-environment-occupation model: A transactive approach to occupational performance. *Canadian Journal of Occupational Therapy, 63,* 9–23.

Mantovani, N., Pizzolati, M., & Edge, D. (2016). Exploring the relationship between stigma and help-seeking for mental illness in African-descended faith communities in the UK. *Health Expectations, 20,* 373–384.

Mc Inerney, S. J. (2002). What is a good doctor and how can we make one? *The BMJ.*

Ministry of Health and Child Care of Zimbabwe. (2016). *The national health strategy for Zimbabwe 2016-2020, Equity and quality in health: Leaving no one behind.* Available at: https://malariaelimination8.org/wp-content/uploads/2017/02/National%20Health%20Strategy%20for%20Zimbabwe%202016--2020.pdf.

National Crime Agency. (2019). *County lines.* Available at: https://www.nationalcrimeagency.gov.uk/what-we-do/crime-threats/drug-trafficking/county-lines.

NHS. (2019). *Child and adolescent mental health services (CAMHS).* Crown Copyright. Available at: https://www.nhs.uk/using-the-nhs/nhs-services/mental-health-services/child-and-adolescent-mental-health-services-camhs/.

Oliver, D., & Fusar-Poli (2017). Meta-analytical prognostic accuracy of the comprehensive assessment of at risk mental states (CAARMS): The need for refined prediction. *European Psychiatry, 49,* 62–68.

Patel, V., Flisher, A. J., Hetrick, S., et al. (2007). Mental health of young people: A global public-health challenge. *Lancet, 369,* 1302–1312.

Patel, V., Saxena, S., Lund, C., et al. (2018). The Lancet commission on global mental health and sustainable development. *Lancet, 392,* 1553–1598.

Schultze-Lutter, F., Schimmelmann, B. G., & Schmidt, S. J. (2016). Resilience, risk, mental health and well-being: Associations and conceptual differences. *European Child & Adolescent Psychiatry, 25,* 459–466.

Servili, C. (2012). Organizing and delivering services for child and adolescent mental health. In R. Jm (Ed.), *IACAPAP e-textbook of child and adolescent mental health.* Geneva: International Association for Child and Adolescent Psychiatry and Allied Professions.

Stewart, S. (1999). The use of standardised and non-standardised assessments in a social services setting: Implications for practice. *British Journal of Occupational Therapy, 62,* 417–423.

Swaine, Z. (2011). Medical model. In J. S. Kreutzer, J. Delluca, & B. Caplan (Eds.), *Encyclopedia of clinical neuropsychology.* New York: Springer.

UNICEF. (2011). *The state of the World's children 2011, adolescence an age of opportunity.* Available at: http://www.ungei.org/SOWC-2011-Main-Report_EN_02092011.pdf.

Widmark, E., & Fristedt, S. (2018). Occupation according to adolescents: Daily occupations categorized based on adolescents' experiences. *Journal of Occupational Science, 26,* 470–483.

Witt, D. (2005). Creative ability- a model for psychiatric occupational therapy. In R. Crouch, & V. Alers (Eds.), *Occupational therapy in psychiatry and mental health* (4th ed.). London and Philadelphia: Wurr Publishers.

World Health Organization (WHO). (2013). *Mental health action plan 2013-2020.* Available at: https://apps.who.int/iris/handle/10665/89966.

World Health Organization (WHO). (2017). *mhGAP training manuals for the mhGAP intervention guide for mental, Neurological and substance use disorders in non-specialized health settings-version 2.0 (for field testing)*. Available at: https://apps.who.int/iris/bitstream/handle/10665/259161/WHO-MSD-MER-17.6-eng.pdf;jsessionid=01BA7F567945728C80401A1B47 47A942?sequence=1.

World Health Organization (WHO). (2018). *Mental health: Strengthening our response*. Available at: http://www.who.int/news-room/fact-sheets/detail/mental-health-strengthening-our-response.

World Health Organization (WHO). (2018). *Adolescent mental health*. Available at: https://www.who.int/news-room/fact-sheets/detail/adolescent-mental-health.

Wright, R., & Sugarman, L. (2009). *Occupational therapy and life course development: A work book for professional practice*. Singapore: Wiley-Blackwell.

25

INTELLECTUAL (LEARNING) DISABILITIES

ELSPETH CLARK ▪ EVA NAKOPOULOU

INTRODUCTION

This chapter provides an overview of occupational therapy in the United Kingdom (UK). The authors, both practicing occupational therapists, are aware of the limitations of this perspective and provide some insights into international practice when possible.

Healthcare provision varies across the UK as each country (England, Northern Ireland, Scotland and Wales) has its own system of publicly funding healthcare. Obviously, anyone working with people with intellectual disabilities must take into account the legalities of the health/social care system they work in. This chapter focuses on England, where the majority of healthcare is provided by the NHS. However, following the (UK wide), Health and Social Care Act (2012) private companies and non-profit organizations are also commissioned to run public health and social care services.

Working with people with intellectual disabilities often provides illuminating new perspectives on everyday problems and can be fun and life affirming. Whilst the chapter necessarily describes the discrimination and challenges facing people with intellectual disabilities, it also highlights the hope, resilience and joy woven into occupational therapy with this service user group.

Terminology

Individuals are described as having intellectual disabilities when they have a 'significant impairment of intellectual and social functioning which will affect them throughout their lives and which began before adulthood' (Department of Health (DH) 2001, p. 14). In the UK people who meet these criteria are commonly referred to as having a learning disability or learning disabilities (Emerson and Baines 2010; Williams 2013). Additionally, the term 'learning difficulties' is also sometimes used when referring to this client group. For example, in the UK the self-advocacy organization People First choose to use 'learning difficulties' (see Useful Resources list at the end of this chapter for link). However, in policy, research and practice worldwide the term intellectual disabilities is increasingly being used (Cluley, 2018), and is considered interchangeable with the term learning disability/disabilities (Emerson and Baines 2010). While the authors acknowledge that, currently in the UK, the term learning disabilities is often preferred by service users, for clarity, the term 'intellectual disabilities' will be used throughout the chapter, given the international readership of this book.

Terminology in this field has often been controversial, with labels associated with people with intellectual disabilities having developed as societal perceptions that have changed over time (Williams 2013). This was exemplified in the fifth edition of the Diagnostic and Statistical Manual of Mental Disorders (DSM-5) (American Psychiatric Association 2013) in the United States in which the term 'mental retardation' was replaced with 'intellectual disability.' While the replacement of outdated diagnostic terms is to be welcomed, Rapley (2004, p. 6) suggests 'intellectual disabilities remains a contested social identity for many.'

It is important to note that 'intellectual disabilities' is an umbrella term covering a range of abilities. According to the International Classification of Diseases for Mortality and Morbidity Statistics, 11th Revision (ICD-11) (World Health Organization (WHO) 2018), the diagnostic term used is 'disorders of intellectual development,' separated into sub-categories such as mild, moderate, severe and profound, with the difference between each sub-category being the intensity of the impact of the disability on daily functioning.

Prevalence and Prognosis

People with intellectual disabilities are estimated to make up 2% of the UK population (Di Lorito et al. 2018) and 1% to 3% of the worldwide population (WHO 2007), although international differences in data collection methods means this figure is an approximation. However, it is clear that people with intellectual disabilities experience poorer health throughout their lives than their non-disabled peers and die, on average, 20 years earlier than the general population (Heslop et al. 2013; Torjesen 2013). They are also more likely to have increased pre-disposition to heart disease (Emerson and Baines 2010), epilepsy (Mengoni 2015), early onset dementia (Chapman et al. 2018) and psychiatric problems (Cooper et al. 2007). Issues regarding working with people who have additional diagnoses are explored later in the chapter.

Historically people with intellectual disabilities and people with mental health conditions were placed in similar institutions (Goodman and Wright 2014) with their care governed by the same legislation. This has contributed to a shared history of exclusion and societal stigma. For both groups, the occupational therapy role is to help people tackle problems in living as opposed to treating a 'disorder.' This shared history and similarity in the occupational therapy role is the reason for this chapter being included in this textbook. It is, however, important to recognize some important distinctions between the two groups. An intellectual disability is a permanent condition that develops before adulthood (DH 2001, p. 14) and is not therefore something that can be recovered from. In contrast, mental health problems can affect people at any age and can be tackled through a wide range of psychosocial and psychiatric interventions. In this regard, it is worth noting that people with intellectual disabilities are pre-disposed to developing mental health problems, with the prevalence suggested to be as high as double of that of the general population (National Institute for Health and Care Excellence (NICE) 2016).

There is a range of health conditions that come under the umbrella term 'intellectual disabilities,' including autism, fragile X syndrome (FSX) and Down's syndrome (also known as Down syndrome).

Autism is a complex neurodevelopmental disorder, the prevalence of which is increasing throughout the world (Waye and Cheng 2018). The defining characteristics are impairments in social interaction and social communication combined with repetitive and restricted behaviours and interests (DePape and Lindsay 2015).

FSX is a genetic neurodevelopmental condition. It is the most common inherited cause of intellectual disabilities (Usher et al. 2019). In addition to cognitive impairments, people with FSX may also have short attention spans, sensory difficulties and can find social interactions challenging. This presentation is often described as being comparable to people with autism (Thurman et al. 2017), although they are two distinct conditions and it is possible to be diagnosed with both autism and FSX.

Down's syndrome is a genetic developmental disorder caused by an extra chromosome (trisomy 21). People with Down's syndrome have some level of intellectual disabilities, although this varies considerably from person to person, and many people with Down's Syndrome are able to live independently in the community. Having Down's syndrome does, however, increase the risk of other health conditions, including thyroid disease (Whooten 2018) and dementia (Hithersay et al. 2017).

People are described as having profound intellectual and multiple disabilities (PIMD) when they have a very severe cognitive impairment. Many people also have comorbid complex physical needs in additional to this related to atypical muscle tone and/or skeletal structure, a lack of ability to move or lack of voluntary movement, for example. These conditions can be linked to pain, pressure care needs, swallowing issues, and internal organ function problems (Robertson et al. 2018).

THE OCCUPATIONAL THERAPY ROLE

Best practice guidance in the UK suggests that occupational therapists working with adults with intellectual disabilities should support them to participate in the full breadth of daily activities (Royal College of Occupational Therapists (RCOT) 2019a), focusing on the enablement of skills development and participation in occupations. This should take into consideration key transitional life stages, such as moving from childrens' to adults' services (RCOT 2019a) or moving from an institution into the community. The transition from institutional to community living and the development of personal autonomy as part of this process are crucial areas in which occupational therapy input can make a significant difference (King et al. 2017). However, the degree of success in accomplishing this shift in service provision varies from country to country. In Scandinavian countries, for example, it is mostly complete, while in the United States and Australia it is still yet to be fully realized (Bigby et al. 2017).

In their seminal research exploring occupational therapy practice in the UK, Lilywhite and Haines (2010) suggest that occupational therapists in this field have both clinical and consultancy roles. This is still the case; the dual role being a feature of practice beyond the UK too, as highlighted in Johnson et al.'s (2019) examination of practitioners' roles in the United States.

A consultancy role may involve occupational therapists providing training and support to staff teams to develop their capacity to facilitate service users' participation in the day-to-day occupations they choose. Occupational therapists can also be expected to provide support to mainstream services when necessary. For example, in the UK there is a drive to optimize the inclusivity of mainstream education and community activities for people with intellectual disabilities (RCOT 2019a). An illustration of this is the Sport for Confidence (2020) organization, which is run by allied health professionals who are based at leisure centres and enables anyone who faces barriers to accessing a leisure centre to participate in meaningful physical activity (see also the Useful Resources list at the end of this chapter).

People with intellectual disabilities are less physically active and more socially excluded than the general population (Robertson 2000; Wilson et al. 2017). Roles and routines can be limited, and opportunities to access meaningful activities are often dependent on other people such as family/carers or paid support. This exclusion from activities can be defined as occupational deprivation, described by Whiteford (2010) as the 'state of preclusion from engagement in occupations of necessity and/or meaning due to factors that stand outside the immediate control of the individual' (p. 201).

The long-term effects of occupational deprivation can include poor physical and mental health, a higher risk of mortality and an increase in challenging behaviour (Channon 2014). The seriousness of this is acknowledged in official guidelines which suggest that, when considering a dementia diagnosis in individuals with intellectual disabilities, occupational deprivation should first be excluded as a contributory factor (Royal College of Psychiatrists & British Psychological Society 2015). Tackling this deprivation is a fundamental part of the occupational therapist's role. This can be done by determining what is experienced as a personally meaningful occupation by an individual and identifying strategies to support their participation in it and, if necessary, training their carers on how best to support this engagement (Mahoney et al. 2016).

RELEVANT UK LEGISLATION AND POLICY DEVELOPMENT

Occupational therapists working with adults with intellectual disabilities must have an understanding of relevant legislation and policy and the impact of key events that influence practice and shape the public's

perceptions of it. Although some positive reforms have taken place in the UK in the last two decades, progress towards less prejudiced societal attitudes regarding people with disabilities is still needed. According to research completed by Scope (the UK disability equality charity), one in three disabled people in Britain feel that they are still being discriminated against (Dixon et al. 2018). Fig. 25.1 shows significant UK events that have led to changes in legislation and impacted current practice. They are discussed more fully as the chapter unfolds.

During the 21st century it has become increasingly widely acknowledged that people with intellectual disabilities should have the same rights, independence and choices as the rest of the population (DH 2001). For example, Health Action Plans were introduced (DH 2002), which are personalized health plans aimed to improve access to healthcare for people with intellectual disabilities.

Impact of Avoidable Deaths and Service Failures

In the UK a significant reflection of the frequently poor care provided to people with intellectual disabilities has been the number of avoidable deaths of individuals while using services. For example, Mencap's (2007) *Death by Indifference* report (see Fig.

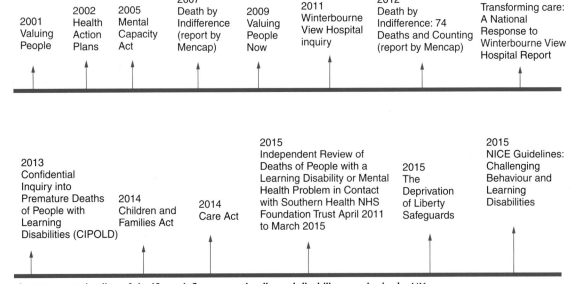

Fig. 25.1 ■ A timeline of significant influences on intellectual disability practice in the UK.

25.1) claimed that institutional discrimination within the NHS against people with intellectual disabilities had caused the deaths of six people with an intellectual disability. Whilst the UK government's Valuing People Now (DH 2009) strategy upheld the recommendations in the Mencap (2007) report, Mencap followed it up five years later with their *Death by Indifference: 74 Deaths and Counting* report (Mencap 2012).

A year later (2013) Connor Sparrowhawk (an 18-year-old man with intellectual disabilities, autism and epilepsy) suffered an epileptic seizure and drowned while left unsupervised in the bath following admission to an NHS assessment and treatment unit (ATU). A report commissioned by NHS England (Mazars 2015) found the Trust had failed to properly investigate the deaths of more than 1000 people with intellectual disabilities or mental health problems who had died in their care. This report identified significant service failures and recommended service improvements. In the same year, NICE published guidance on working with people with challenging behaviour (NICE 2015). The risk of avoidable deaths through negligent healthcare experienced by people with intellectual disabilities is not unique to the UK. O'Leary et al. (2018) systematically reviewed evidence of this problem from across the UK, Australia, Canada, and Scandinavia, for example.

Compounding the problem of avoidable deaths, there is also a risk of systemic service failure; that is, failure due to a flaw or flaws in the care provision system. In the UK the BBC television programme *Panorama* revealed a pattern of serious abuse taking place in an ATU for people with intellectual disabilities, autism and challenging behaviour run by a private company (BBC 2011), which led to the closure of the unit and the prosecution of staff. In response the government report, *Transforming Care: A National Response to Winterbourne View Hospital* (DH 2012) revealed systemic failures that led to the abuse and identified steps for service improvement.

Other Key UK Legislation

The main impact of the Children and Families Act (2014) was that adults with intellectual disabilities up to the age of 25 years would be able to access further education and training with more ease than before. Many more adults can now pursue their educational and vocational goals, because all further education establishments are expected to make reasonable adjustments to accommodate them. The Care Act (2014) has had a significant impact on how individuals access support. The aim has been to put people and their carers in control of their care and support, emphasizing personal health budgets (NHS 2020). These have proved controversial in the field of intellectual disabilities—and more widely—for being under-resourced and (because of the up-front allocation of resources) for failing to accommodate complex and/or increasing needs (Spandler 2004; Brindle 2011; Beddow 2014; Glasby 2014; Beresford 2016).

CONSIDERATIONS FOR PRACTICE

Risk Management

Risk assessment and management are an essential part of the occupational therapist's role when working with people with intellectual disabilities (Lillywhite and Haines 2010). Taking risks is a normal part of learning in everyday life, and occupational therapists should adopt a positive risk management approach to maximize skill acquisition. This means identifying, assessing and managing the potentially beneficial outcomes of taking certain risks, as opposed to being risk averse.

As a member of the multidisciplinary team occupational therapists are responsible for contributing to and updating the team-wide risk assessment and for conducting specific occupational therapy risk assessments. These assessments should be multidimensional and include environmental as well as individual risk factors (Blasingame 2018). When working in inpatient settings, there are specialist risk assessments that need to be completed, particularly in relation to violence, self-harm and suicide (Phillips 2004).

Consent to Treatment

The Mental Capacity Act (2005), which guides practice in England and Wales, states that every adult, whatever their ability, has the right to make their own decisions whenever possible and that, when an individual lacks capacity to make a decision, a best interest process is initiated. This requires people involved in the care of the individual (usually family and care professionals) to make a decision in what they perceive to be the person's best interest, including decisions relating to healthcare. In 2015 guidance on Deprivation of Liberty Safeguards (DH 2015) was published as a result of the Supreme Court judgments, which was an amendment to the Mental Capacity Act (2005).

Occupational therapists should always establish informed consent before work begins. However, depending on an individuals' cognitive impairment, it is not always possible to establish full, informed consent to conduct an assessment with the individual themselves, although this would always be preferable and should always be considered. With the five principles of the 2005 Mental Capacity Act in mind (Box 25.1), techniques should be used to support the person with intellectual disabilities to understand the therapist's role and the reason for referral. This could include using easy read resources, and/or meeting with the person and their carer/family member or advocate to discuss the referral. Case Study 25. 1 overleaf illustrates this process. If it is considered that an individual does not have the capacity to consent to intervention, the best interest process would need to be followed and recorded as such. Williams et al. (2014) have demonstrated inconsistencies in practice relating to consent and best interest across health services for people with intellectual disabilities, but the principles of the Mental Capacity Act (2005) should always be upheld.

BOX 25.1
FIVE PRINCIPLES GUIDING CONSENT AND BEST INTERESTS

1. Assume a person has capacity unless it is proved otherwise;
2. Do not treat people as incapable of making a decision unless all practicable steps have been tried to help them do so;
3. A person should not be treated as incapable of making a decision because their decision may seem unwise;
4. Always do things or take decisions for people without capacity in their best interests;
5. Before making a decision or acting on behalf of a person who lacks capacity, consider whether the outcome could be achieved in a less restrictive way.

CASE STUDY 25.1
Best Interest Process and Consent with Clara

Clara is a 26-year-old woman with intellectual disabilities. Her family have referred her to occupational therapy for support to develop her independent living skills.

During the first appointment (where the occupational therapist meets Clara and her parents), Clara struggles to understand what occupational therapy means and how this can help her become independent. The occupational therapist uses an accessible leaflet to explain occupational therapy and Talking Mats (Murphy and Cameron 2005), which use picture symbols to assist communication with/for people with communication difficulties, to give Clara an idea of areas they could work on, such as cooking, shopping, preparing for job interviews, etc.

Clara continues to struggle to understand what occupational therapy is, but through the use of Talking Mats, she agrees to work on budgeting, shopping, cooking and money skills but not interview skills. Her parents, who are present, agree to occupational therapy input for the goals that Clara has agreed to.

Later, the occupational therapist consults with other members of the community learning disability team where she works who confirm that input from occupational therapy would be likely to benefit Clara. Occupational therapy is thus agreed on and recorded under the best interest process on the basis that Clara has consented to the goals of therapy (as above) and has capacity to do so.

Communication

People with intellectual disabilities can encounter substantial barriers to being understood, and the therapist's communication skills can significantly affect the quality of any interaction (Griffiths 2009). Using easy read resources (which use plain English, short sentences and accompanying images), such as picture appointment letters, ensure that information is more accessible for people with intellectual disabilities (many of whom have limited reading skills). In the UK all publicly funded adult social care providers are legally required to ensure they meet the communication needs of people with disabilities, impairments or sensory loss as per the Accessible Information Standard (NHS England 2017). Suggested weblinks to resources that may help with this are included in the Useful Resources list at the end of the chapter.

There are additional communication techniques that occupational therapists could expect to be trained in. These include augmentative and alternative communication tools, such as Makaton, which is a language programme that uses signing alongside spoken language (Vinales 2013), Signalong (a sign-based programme based on British Sign Language), and Talking Mats (www.talkingmats.com), which is an interactive resource using picture symbols that has been shown to support effective communication (Murphy and Cameron 2008). Makaton, Signalong and Talking Mats provide adapted resources and training in different languages.

Eligibility Assessments

In the UK eligibility for accessing specialist health services such as community learning disability teams (CLDTs) and the intensive support teams (ISTs) varies according to locality. Some teams only offer input to adults with severe and profound intellectual disabilities, whereas other teams offer input to adults with any level of intellectual disabilities.

During the eligibility assessment phase, input from an occupational therapist may be requested as part of a team-wide process. In certain situations, specific occupational therapy input may be requested when, for example, an assessment of functional ability would help to determine whether the individual would qualify for input from the team.

Positive Behaviour Support

In the UK an international health service, providing support for adults with intellectual disabilities and complex distressed behaviour, has embraced a positive behaviour support (PBS) approach (Perez et al. 2012). Individuals' inappropriate behaviours can be hard to change because they are functional at some level; that is, they serve, or have served, a personal purpose. PBS aims to develop a deeper understanding of the motivations behind an individuals' distress and is underpinned by an international evidence base (Gore et al. 2013). Studies have shown its use can reduce the frequency of challenging behaviour and improve the quality of life for people with intellectual disabilities (Hassiotis et al. 2014).

The PBS approach is complemented by the holism and strengths focus of occupational therapy. Assessing how a person's disability affects their occupational performance and offering interventions to address challenges that can enhance the multidisciplinary team approach (Perez et al. 2012). For example, if an individual who demonstrates self-injurious behaviour by banging their head against walls when agitated is referred to the team, the occupational therapist conducts their assessments to identify any barriers to occupational engagement that may be influencing the person's behaviour and may also seek to identify what sensory feedback could also be a motivating factor. Depending on the personal factors unique to the situation, realistic activity alternatives could then be suggested to support the individual to self-calm before they become highly agitated and harm themselves.

SERVICE TYPES

Community Learning Disability Teams

Despite this chapter's adoption of the term 'intellectual disabilities' (as described earlier), the team title 'community *learning disability* team' is used here because that name (and the acronym 'CLDT') is still widely used in UK practice.

In the UK these teams were initially jointly commissioned and staffed by health and social care services and comprised social workers, nurses, psychiatrists, occupational therapists, psychologists, speech and language therapists and physiotherapists (National Learning Disability Professional Senate 2015). In many areas of the UK these teams are now commissioned and staffed by health services only. This has negatively impacted service provision by moving away from the kind of integrated health and social care that has always been strongly advocated for people with intellectual disabilities (National Learning Disability Professional Senate 2015). In some areas in England, multidisciplinary CLDTs are no longer commissioned, whilst, in other areas, CLDTs are providing a three-tier service offering different levels of support depending on individuals' needs. In the UK a three-tier service is the recommended configuration for serving people with intellectual disabilities, whereby Level 1 is a universal service, Level 2 is a targeted service supporting people to manage life stage transitions, and Level 3 focuses on adults with intellectual disabilities and complex needs, aiming to avoid hospital admission (RCOT 2019a) as shown in Fig. 25.2.

Intensive Support Teams

The aim of an IST is similar to that of a Level 3 service (see above) in that the team's focus is to support adults with intellectual disabilities and complex needs who are in crisis so they can to avoid a hospital admission. However, there can be wide variation in the names, configurations and operational approach of ISTs. These teams should ensure the best outcomes for people by working in partnership with individuals and families/carers, using person-centred approaches. They also have a liaison role supporting service users to access mainstream health services whenever possible and should be considered as an alternative to specialist inpatient services such as ATUs (Davison 2015; NICE 2015).

Assessment and Treatment Units

ATUs are specialist hospital wards for people with intellectual disabilities *and* severe mental health needs whose behaviour may be putting themselves or others at risk. Patients are admitted to an ATU when their needs cannot be appropriately met in general adult inpatient or community mental health services. Most

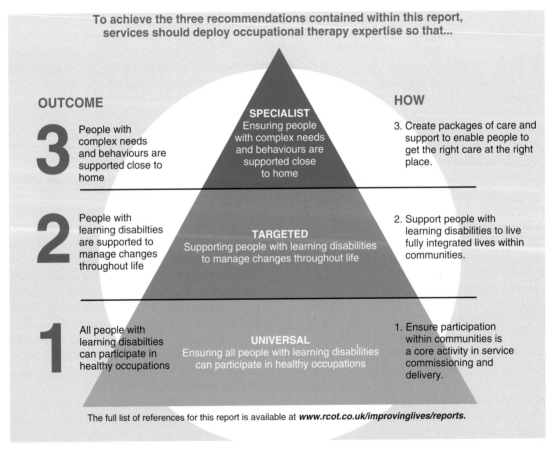

Fig. 25.2 ■ How a three-tier community learning disability team service should be implemented. (From Royal College of Occupational Therapists (2019a). *Leading fulfilled lives: Occupational therapy supporting people with learning disabilities.* Available at https://www.rcot.co.uk/promoting-occupational-therapy/occupational-therapy-improving-lives-saving-money.)

patients admitted to an ATU will be detained under mental health legislation, but this can change during their stay and they may instead become a voluntary patient. It is possible for a person to be admitted to an ATU as a voluntary patient, but this rarely happens.

ATU-based occupational therapists usually work as part of a multidisciplinary team comprising of nurses, psychologists and speech and language therapists. Some ATUs do not directly employ occupational therapists, however. Instead, therapists from the local community-based team (such as the CLDT or IST) may provide in-reach to the ATU, especially when people are getting ready for discharge back to the community.

Some ATUs came under scrutiny during the major investigations into abuse and neglect mentioned earlier. In England the national Transforming Care Programme (DH 2012) was designed to end over-reliance on inpatient care for people with intellectual disabilities and mental health needs. It focused on building up community capacity and reducing inappropriate hospital admissions (NHS England 2015).

Secure Settings

Individuals with a high level of forensic need requiring secure services are not usually admitted to an ATU. Instead they are admitted to one of the secure units across the UK that provide a service for people with intellectual disabilities (see Chapter 26: Forensic and Prison Services).

There is an over-representation of people with intellectual disabilities in prisons in the UK (Jones and Talbot 2010) and Europe (Søndenaa et al. 2008; Tort et al. 2016) and a growing recognition that offenders with intellectual disabilities require specialised rehabilitative care (Hellenbach et al. 2015). Some UK prisons employ occupational therapists directly, and therapists in community teams (such as CLDT and ISTs) may work with people who have recently been released from prison.

Specialist Colleges

The UK's Children and Families Act (2014) has led to an improvement in the access to further education opportunities for adults with intellectual disabilities. This is due to some specialist schools extending the time that young adults can stay in school (up to the age of 25), and

other specialist colleges—that would previously have only served people with physical disabilities (such as cerebral palsy and brain injury)—opening their doors to young adults with intellectual disabilities. There has also been a rise in specialist programmes for young adults with intellectual disabilities within mainstream colleges.

Some specialist schools and colleges employ occupational therapists who work with other health professionals and education staff, whereas mainstream colleges usually seek occupational therapy input by referring to the CLDTs/ISTs.

Having offered an overview of various types of services provided for people with intellectual disabilities, the chapter will now explore how occupational therapy operates within them.

THE OCCUPATIONAL THERAPY PROCESS

Referral

Referrals to an occupational therapy community team (such as a CLDT or IST) can be made by carers/family members, healthcare professionals or other agencies. Individuals can self-refer also, but most people with intellectual disabilities would probably need support to do this. New referrals are screened (or triaged) to ensure they meet the eligibility criteria for the service and that there is an appropriate occupational therapy need.

Occupational Therapy Assessment

Occupational therapy assessment is undertaken to obtain a comprehensive understanding of an individual's past, present and preferred future occupations and roles (Laver-Fawcett 2014) and the impact of an individual's intellectual disability on their occupational performance. A range of assessment tools is available to measure occupational performance and participation (Asaba et al. 2017), although only some of these are standardized to be used with adults with intellectual disabilities.

The Assessment of Motor and Process Skills (AMPS) is an example of a standardized method for conducting performance analysis (Fisher and Bray Jones 2011) and has been validated for use with adults with intellectual disabilities (Kottorp et al. 2003). Lilywhite and Haines (2010) showed that therapists working with people with intellectual disabilities found the AMPS helpful in highlighting service users' occupational performance strengths and difficulties. It can also be used for assessing eligibility to access specialist intellectual disability services (Mesa et al. 2014).

The Model of Human Occupation Screening Tool (MOHOST) (Parkinson et al. 2006) was designed to identify the factors that influence occupational participation (Kielhofner 2008) and has utility across a range of intellectual disability settings (Hawes and Houlder 2010). Participants in Lilywhite and Haines' (2010) study discuss how, when working with people who have profound and multiple intellectual disabilities, the MOHOST does not always detect subtle changes sufficiently to measure them. These concerns are reflected in the wider occupational therapy literature (Hawes and Houlder 2010). The authors of the MOHOST address these concerns (Parkinson et al. 2014), acknowledging that not all of its elements may be relevant for people with severe disabilities. However, a further assessment and outcome measure, based on the model of human occupation (MOHO)–related concepts, the MOHO-ExpLOR (Cooper et al. 2018) has been specifically designed for use when an individual's occupational performance and/or participation are severely impaired (Parkinson et al. 2017).

Other assessments that are commonly used in this field include the Interest Checklist (UK adapted version by McCormack 2014), the Pool Activity Level Instrument for Occupational Profiling (PAL) (Pool 2012), the Residential Environment Impact Survey (REIS) (Fisher et al. 2014) and the Vona du Toit Model of Creative Ability (VDTMoca) (De Witt 2014). Additionally, there are specialist assessments such as the Sensory Integration Inventory (Reisman and Hanschu 1992) which are employed when it is considered that a deeper understanding of an individual's sensory processing needs would be helpful.

Goal Setting

Setting effective goals is critical to successful therapy (Poulsen et al. 2014), and enabling people with intellectual disabilities to be involved in setting their own goals necessitates forming therapeutic relationships with the individual and with their carers and/or family members, which can take time (Lilywhite and Haines 2010). Due to the severity of an individual's disability, it will not always be possible to set goals with the person with intellectual disabilities themselves (although this should always be considered). In this circumstance, the therapist will work in partnership with the persons' carers and family members to identify and record meaningful goals.

Breaking down large goals into smaller, achievable actions can foster a sense of accomplishment while providing an overall sense of the long-term aim of occupational therapy. The visual scale employed in Goal Attainment Scaling (GAS) (Turner and Stokes 2009), or its simplified version GAS-Light, can be a useful tool when conceptualizing goals with people with intellectual disabilities; goals which can then be reviewed and used as an outcome measure to demonstrate progress made. Another goal-setting tool which can also be used as an outcome measure is the Life Star, which is based on the Recovery Star format used widely in mental health but which has been designed specifically for young people and adults with intellectual disabilities (Burns and MacKeith 2012).

Outcome Measurement

It can be challenging to identify outcome measures flexible enough to demonstrate the subtle changes that may occur when working with people with intellectual disabilities (Lilywhite and Haines 2010). Using more than one measure at a time can be beneficial to capture the diverse outcomes of occupational therapy (Doig et al. 2010). A recent online survey of occupational therapists who work with adults with intellectual disabilities in the UK and the Republic of Ireland identified that the MOHOST (Parkinson et al. 2006), the AMPS (Fisher and Bray Jones 2011) and GAS (Kiresuk et al. 1994) are being used most regularly in practice (Clark 2019). However, results also indicated that non-standardized measures are being used with the same frequency as the standardized ones. As non-standardized measures are not supported by research into their reliability and validity, their use can potentially undermine professional credibility (Laver-Fawcett 2014).

Adapting standardized outcome measures and assessment tools to make them more suitable for people with intellectual disabilities is described in the limited literature available on this topic (Lillywhite and Haines 2010; Perez et al. 2012). However, modifications to standardized measures may compromise the standardization of the measure itself (Wales et al. 2016), bringing the credibility of the results into question (Stigen et al. 2018).

Dear...,

Your social worker referred you to Occupational Therapy.

Since October 2021, we have worked on the following:

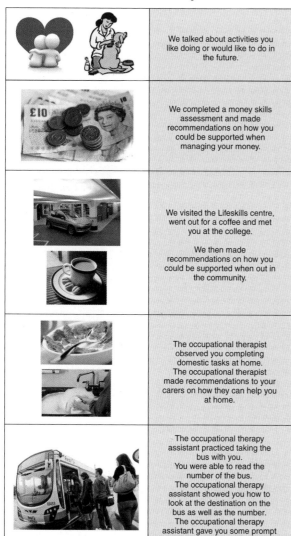

	We talked about activities you like doing or would like to do in the future.
	We completed a money skills assessment and made recommendations on how you could be supported when managing your money.
	We visited the Lifeskills centre, went out for a coffee and met you at the college. We then made recommendations on how you could be supported when out in the community.
	The occupational therapist observed you completing domestic tasks at home. The occupational therapist made recommendations to your carers on how they can help you at home.
	The occupational therapy assistant practiced taking the bus with you. You were able to read the number of the bus. The occupational therapy assistant showed you how to look at the destination on the bus as well as the number. The occupational therapy assistant gave you some prompt cards to help you with this.

We will now be discharging you from our caseload.
If at any point you wish to receive more Occupational Therapy input, please contact our team.

Best wishes,

Picture   Picture
Name   Name
Occupational Therapist   Occupational Therapy Assistant

Fig. 25.3 ■ Example of accessible discharge letter.

Discharge

It is important to have a plan for how carers can continue to support the service user to achieve their goals and develop their occupational performance once occupational therapy input has concluded. It is common practice to write a formal occupational therapy discharge report, which includes recommendations, including any onward referrals indicated (Fig. 25.3). If applicable, an accessible version of the report is produced for the service user, and, in their final meeting, the occupational therapist may go through this with them to help them understand that occupational therapy input has finished, to reinforce what has been achieved and to explain what happens next.

FEATURES OF OCCUPATIONAL THERAPY INTERVENTION

Skills Development

One of the most common interventions in this field of occupational therapy is skills development. This can range from supporting an individual to tolerate hair brushing and washing, to enabling learning how to shop for and prepare a healthy meal, to promoting the development of parenting skills, and facilitating the performance tasks under pressure at work (Case Study 25.2).

Often, the need for these skills is highlighted when the individual is going through a life transition, such as moving out of their family home or becoming a parent themselves. In Case Study 25.2, Ben has moved into supported living, where housing is provided within the local community (Watson et al. 2019) and there is greater potential (than residential care homes) for flexible person-centred support (Bigby et al. 2017) and independent living.

Environmental Adaptation and Provision of Equipment

Environmental adaptation (of both physical and social environments) is aimed at maximizing people's engagement in satisfying daily routines and life roles. In the UK NHS occupational therapists can prescribe certain pieces of equipment. This can include small items such as a raised toilet seat or specialised cutlery, or assistive technology (e.g., environmental control

CASE STUDY 25.2

Skills Development with Ben

Ben has a diagnosis of autism and mild to moderate intellectual disabilities. He is 25 years old and likes watching comedy shows on television and listening to heavy metal music. Ben has recently moved out of his parents' house into supported living, sharing a house with two other men who also have intellectual disabilities.

Ben has been referred to the occupational therapist in his local community learning disability team as his support providers feel his placement at his new house may be at risk. Ben has the skills to live more independently, but he has not been prepared to cook for himself or keep his own space in his new house clean. This is impacting his relationships with his new housemates.

The occupational therapist meets with Ben to discuss the referral. Through discussion, it emerges that Ben would like to have a girlfriend. He feels he needs to lose weight to feel more attractive, but he finds it difficult to use his cooker to prepare healthy meals. He is also accustomed to his mother doing most of the cooking for him.

The occupational therapist helps Ben to manage his weight by working with him to create an accessible recipe book of healthy meals. They use Ben's tablet computer to take pictures of Ben completing all the steps required to create each meal and use an app to compile them into a book format. Meal preparation also involves working together on money management, shopping and cleaning the kitchen.

Ben finds it hard to engage, however, saying 'I find money boring' and he does not like 'making a mess in the kitchen.' The occupational therapist decides to draw up an accessible contract with Ben. This is a written agreement that uses photos and large simple text to illustrate Ben's occupational therapy goals and the link between working on money skills, shopping and cooking and Ben's overall goal to lose weight and find a girlfriend. The contract is discussed with Ben at the beginning and the end of every session to assess his motivation to engage in the intervention and to jointly monitor progress with him.

---

systems, activity monitoring systems, etc.), sensory equipment (e.g., weighted blanket, vibro-acoustic seat, etc.) and moving and handling equipment (e.g., hoist, sling etc.). They may also recommend changes to the individual's home and/or work environment. Larger adaptations to the home may be funded through a disabled facilities grant (DFG), based on the recommendation of a local authority social services occupational therapist. The DFG is available from local councils in England, Northern Ireland, Scotland, and Wales. The amount available varies from country to country. It can be used to fund adaptions such as building a walk-in shower, making a home accessible to a wheelchair user or adaptions to address sensory qualities of the environment (such as noise levels, lighting and colours).

Providing Equipment and Specialist Training

Specialist advice and training input may range from teaching approaches on providing individual support (Case Study 25.3), to using equipment, to signposting people to relevant information and support

organizations. Occupational therapists are sometimes required to deliver training directly to service users (e.g., how to stay safe in the community, parenting skills, etc.) and to family members, paid carers and colleagues (such as how to support an individual with sensory processing difficulties). In Case Study 25.3, Maya lives in a residential care home, which, in the UK, indicates that she has a complex medical condition and is unable to live alone due to the level of support required regarding her self-care (NHS 2019).

Supporting Parenting Skills

In the UK the precise number of parents who have intellectual disabilities is not known. Estimates range from 23,000 to 250,000, and it is recognized that the number is rising (Working Together with Parents Network 2016). Internationally, studies have shown that women with intellectual disabilities who become pregnant should be considered a high-risk population, with raised levels of teen pregnancies, obesity and single parenthood compared to women without intellectual disabilities (Höglund et al. 2012). Indeed, adults with

CASE STUDY 25.3

Environmental Adaptation for Maya

Maya is 49 years old and has fragile X syndrome. She lives in a residential care home where she has recently withdrawn from activities she previously enjoyed, such as knitting items for family and friends. Maya has been referred to the occupational therapist on her local community learning disability team because staff at the care home have become concerned about this change in behaviour.

During the occupational therapist's initial visit it emerges that Maya has had several falls recently. Hearing Maya's story and through observation of her movement around the home (including being shown where the falls occurred), the occupational therapist refers Maya for an eye test, which shows her sight has deteriorated and she is likely to become partially-sighted.

The occupational therapist recommends to the care home that door thresholds and step edges are highlighted a different colour (using tape or paint) and indicates where additional lighting and support rails should be positioned. Maya (and other residents) are involved in choosing the colours and style of lighting to reflect the fact that it is their home.

With new prescription glasses Maya resumes knitting, but she finds it harder than before. The therapist supports Maya to attend a local knitting group where she enjoys the company and shares tips with others. However, Maya's speech impairment and her deteriorating vision means ongoing support to attend the group is needed. The occupational therapist provides specialist staff training to care home team members so they can continue to meet this need.

intellectual disabilities have experienced their children being taken away from them due to concerns about the children's welfare (Norah Fry Research Centre 2009). However, when advised by professionals who use a supportive stance, most parents have been able to show good parenting skills and keep their children (Norah Fry Research Centre 2009).

Support for parenting skills is therefore a growing area of practice, although not all health teams are commissioned to provide it. In some areas occupational therapists run adapted parenting groups with other professionals such as clinical psychologists or nurses or offer individual sessions at home with the child and the parents. Teaching is paced and tailored to meet the needs of the parents, accommodating a range of preferred communication styles and levels of understanding. Therapists often use visual aids, model specific tasks (such as changing a nappy) and offer step-by-step instructions. There are a variety of programmes, such as Mellow Futures (Mellow Parenting 2016), and apps, such as Baby Buddy (Best Beginnings 2014), which therapists have access to. It is also important to offer information about child health in accessible formats, along with signposting to adults regarding independent advocacy, mainly concerning child protection (Working Together with Parents Network 2016).

Addressing Profound Intellectual and Multiple Disabilities

Occupational therapy support for people with profound intellectual and multiple disabilities (PIMD) may include making environmental adaptations (such as installing a walk-in shower), and/or providing specialist equipment such as individualized seating or night-time supports. Providing training for family and carers on how to best support the individual is also important. These interventions aim to prevent physical deterioration and pain, increase comfort and promote good posture all of which support the individual's participation in occupation and enhance quality of life.

People with PIMD are often referred to occupational therapy for support to engage in day-to-day occupations (Lillywhite and Haines 2010) (such as cooking, cleaning and personal care) because their previous experience of daily life may be that everything has been done to or for them. Additionally, sensory needs may be addressed by supporting a person's engagement in activities (e.g., baking, hydrotherapy or aromatherapy massage etc.).

When working with carers who support people with PIMD, it is important to ensure that input will be sustainable and, given the likelihood that occupational therapy is time-limited, that the focus of the intervention is on facilitating a shift within the staff culture at the individual's place of residence (Haines et al. 2018).

Sensory Interventions

Sensory integration theory originated with Jean Ayres (2005) whose work was mostly conducted with children who had learning difficulties and additional motor skills disorders that influenced their ability to coordinate movements. 'Ayres Sensory Integration (ASI)' is now a registered trademark term covering Ayres' theory, assessments and intervention techniques and requires therapists to be trained to provide this intervention.

However, most occupational therapists adopt a sensory approach usually based on some post-qualification training linked to sensory integration theory. These types of intervention can sometimes be associated with people who display challenging behaviour. For example, when working with a person who removes their clothes and avoids most self-care activities due to tactile processing difficulties, the occupational therapist may set up desensitization activities to increase the person's tolerance, while also looking at alternative clothing and ways of carrying out self-care. Occupational therapists frequently offer sensory interventions in relation to engagement in occupations. For example, working with a service user who is motivated by the sensation they receive throughout the activity rather than the end result. It may be that the individual needs to move frequently, enjoys certain textures or seeks out deep pressure (such as through hugs). In this case the occupational therapist would look at the individual's daily routine and find ways for them to receive the desired input while maintaining their participation in activities of daily living.

It is important for occupational therapists using a sensory approach to consider the likely impact of specific activities on an individual's level of arousal. In some instances this may be the actual aim of the intervention: to engineer occupations so that the individual can be supported to become more alert or calmer. There are several programmes and tools that use this approach, for example the Alert Program (Williams and Shellenberger 1992).

Both ASI-trained and non-ASI–trained occupational therapists may offer training to family and carers on sensory strategies relevant to an individual.

Vocational Rehabilitation

The occupational therapy role in supporting people with intellectual disabilities with vocational training and employment coaching is widespread internationally (see Iwane et al. 2012; Terrana et al. 2016; Johnson et al. 2019).

In England the percentage of adults with intellectual disabilities in employment has declined (Public Health England 2016), and the role has shifted in emphasis from supporting people into employment to job retention (see also Chapter 20: Work). This may include facilitating meetings between the employer and the individual, perhaps offering training to the employer regarding environmental adaptations and reasonable adjustments (such as flexible working hours). It may also include confidence-building work with individuals. Occupational therapists may also support college leavers transitioning to supported living in which employment is part of a wider picture of independent living skills development.

Group Work

Occupational therapists in secure settings or ATUs frequently use group work (see Chapter 15: Client-Centred Groups). Some community-based occupational therapists (such as those within CLDTs or ISTs), when working with larger care homes or in more isolated areas, may also support care home staff to develop group sessions for their residents. A helpful resource in the UK is the Living Well in Care Homes toolkit (RCOT 2019b) designed to be used in care homes for the elderly but also with adults with intellectual disabilities.

Working with People Who Have Additional Diagnoses

Dementia

People with intellectual disabilities are more likely to develop dementia as they age compared to the general population (Strydom et al. 2013). Possible indications of this (indicating the need for occupational therapy assessment of daily living activities) might be apparent cognitive decline or a deterioration in skills-level, causing a person to withdraw from activities they previously enjoyed. If there are concerns about a possible dementia diagnosis (just as with people who do not have intellectual disabilities), all possible other causes, such as depression, sight loss or a urinary tract infection, should be excluded before dementia is considered.

Several assessments might be applicable in situations such as this. For example, the PAL (Pool 2012) could be used to identify the activity level at which staff and carers might best engage with the individual. Additionally, the REIS (Fisher et al. 2014) can assess how a person's environment impacts their performance, and The AMPS (Fisher and Bray Jones 2011) may be useful to establish a performance baseline and subsequent progress.

Occupational therapy interventions that may be beneficial would be similar to those used in the general population with this condition, including environmental adaptation (such as clear labelling or photos of contents on cupboards as memory prompts) and the creation of Life Story books as memory and communication supports.

As life expectancy for people with Down's syndrome has increased, many people with this condition are living into their 60s and 70s (Cipriani et al. 2018). People with Down's syndrome have an increased genetic risk of developing Alzheimer's dementia (Caraci et al. 2017), and referrals for occupational therapy assessment related to the dementia screening process for people with Down's syndrome are relatively common.

Mental Health Problems

People with intellectual disabilities are at greater risk of developing a mental health problem than the general population, especially depression (Cooper et al. 2007) and anxiety (NICE 2016). However, psychiatric diagnosing can prove difficult due to the individual's behaviour being attributed solely to their cognitive impairment. This is described as 'diagnostic overshadowing' (NICE 2016) and can lead to mental health conditions remaining untreated.

People with intellectual disabilities should be supported to access mainstream mental health services whenever possible. Some specialist community teams, such as the IST, provide intensive support to people with intellectual disabilities at risk of a psychiatric inpatient admission. If admission is required, mainstream adult mental health units are often used. The effectiveness of inpatient units specifically designed for adults with intellectual disabilities has been shown by Xenitidis et al. (2004). Whilst the duration of an admission tends be longer in these units, people are often discharged back into their local community and familiar support network.

Substance Misuse

Having mild intellectual disabilities and mental health problems increases the risk of substance misuse (Taggart et al. 2006; To et al. 2014). There are two main factors for this: adults with intellectual disabilities appear to have lower alcohol tolerance, and adults with mild intellectual disabilities struggle to access substance misuse services, as the expectation is that they will access mainstream services, which may be problematic (To et al. 2014). In the UK the problem is compounded because the mildness of of an individual's intellectual disability means the individual would not be eligible for input by specialist intellectual disabilities services, and mainstream addiction services are not well equipped to support people with intellectual disabilities (VanderNagel et al. 2011; Chapman and Wu 2012; To et al. 2014). Consequently, there are limited services available at present and the role of the occupational therapist in this setting remains to be developed.

CONCLUSION

Working with people with intellectual disabilities is a diverse area of practice that offers rich opportunities to engage individuals in occupational therapy across the lifespan. This chapter has described assessments and interventions and the breadth and variety of current practice. Despite the challenges highlighted, quality of life for people with intellectual disabilities is improving. Occupational therapists, with their philosophy of empowerment and their strengths-based approach, have a fundamental role in facilitating people with intellectual disabilities to fulfil their potential.

INSPIRATIONAL PEOPLE AND PROJECTS

To conclude, the Useful Resources list is the authors' selection of some inspirational projects and people who are challenging the stereotypes and limitations associated with intellectual disabilities, as follows:

- Misfits Theatre – A theatre, social group and training provider led by people with intellectual disabilities https://misfitstheatre.com/
- Stayuplate Charity – A charity working to ensure that people with intellectual disabilities should be supported to lead the lifestyle they choose www.stayuplate.org
- Alanna Julian and Ella Darling – Women with intellectual disabilities inspiring others to find work https://www.abc.net.au/news/2018-03-08/women-intellectual-disabilities-workforce-employment-job/9524936
- Isabelle Springmühl – The first fashion designer with Down's syndrome to be featured at London Fashion Week https://www.bbc.co.uk/news/world-latin-america-38132503
- Ángela Covadonga Bachille – Spain's first city councillor with Down's syndrome (since 2013) https://en.m.wikipedia.org/wiki/Ángela_Bachiller
- Pablo Pineda – Actor and the first European citizen with Down's syndrome with a university degree. He won the Concha De Planta award in 2009 at the San Sebastian film festival for his role in the movie *Yo, tambien.* https://www.loquedeverdadimporta.org/en/speaker/pablo-pineda/
- Chelsea Werner – Special Olympian and model: https://www.forbes.com/sites/lelalondon/2019/02/05/from-special-olympian-to-high-fashion-model-chelsea-werner-defies-all-down-syndrome-stereotypes/#24770a6072e0

USEFUL RESOURCES

Accommodation

- Supported living services: https://www.nhs.uk/conditions/social-care-and-support-guide/care-services-equipment-and-care-homes/supported-living-services/
- What is supported living and differences between supported living and residential care homes: https://www.choicecaregroup.com/can-we-help/care-and-support-packages/supported-living/what-does-supported-living-look-like/

- Care homes: https://www.nhs.uk/conditions/social-care-and-support-guide/care-services-equipment-and-care-homes/care-homes/
- Residential care: https://www.carehomeselection.co.uk/residentialcare/
- Nursing homes: https://www.carehomeselection.co.uk/nursingcare/
- Shared Lives scheme: https://www.nhs.uk/conditions/social-care-and-support-guide/care-services-equipment-and-care-homes/shared-lives-schemes/
- Therapeutic communities: https://www.therapeuticcommunities.org/what-is-a-tc/types-of-tcs/

Accessible Documents and Communication Difficulties

- Support to make documents accessible: https://www.changepeople.org/
- Easy read information on healthcare for people with intellectual disabilities: http://www.easyhealth.org.uk/
- Talking Mats: https://www.talkingmats.com/

Information on Intellectual Disabilities and Other Conditions

- The British Institute of Learning Disabilities: http://www.bild.org.uk/
- Mencap: https://www.mencap.org.uk/learning-disability-explained/what-learning-disability
- The Down's Syndrome Association: https://www.downs-syndrome.org.uk/
- National Autistic Society: https://www.autism.org.uk/about/what-is/asd.aspx
- Core and Essential Service Standards for Supporting People with PMLD: https://www.pmld-link.org.uk/wp-content/uploads/2017/11/Standards-PMLD-h-web.pdf

Other Resources

- Sport for Confidence: https://www.sportforconfidence.com/about-us/
- People First (Self Advocacy): https://peoplefirst-ltd.com/

QUESTIONS FOR CONSIDERATION

1. Why is it that people with intellectual disabilities typically suffer with poor health and shortened life expectancy?

2. What are the historic reasons for discrimination against those with an intellectual disability?

3. Are avoidable deaths of people with intellectual disabilities comparable with the higher mortality rate of those in other marginalized groups? Why/why not?

4. Regarding Case Study 25.1, if Clara is having such difficulty understanding what occupational therapy is and what therapists do, how might this be factored into working with her?

5. What kind of access is there to Makaton/Signalong/Talking Mats in the non-disabled population? What can be done to make this more widely understood?

6. How might an occupational therapist adapt a discharge report to be accessible to a service user with communication difficulties?

7. Regarding Case Study 25.2, what advice might you have given to Ben's parents (retrospectively) that could have helped with issues he faces now? What services, activities of daily living or goals might have been useful for his disabilities when he was developing life skills?

8. What could an occupational therapist work on with a person with an intellectual disability who has an interest in becoming a parent or is pregnant to help them prepare for childcare?

SERVICE USER COMMENTARY

I have campaigned in the past to change the terms 'mental handicap' and 'mental retardation' and championed the use of 'learning disabilities' or 'learning difficulties' personally by lobbying parliament. My occupational therapist at the time helped me write a letter to my MP. I feel the term 'intellectual disability' (used in this chapter) is not something I, or people like me, understand. Terminology has to be right for those who in the past didn't have a voice and whose choices were not considered relevant.

I see the occupational therapy role as facilitating people like me to have the confidence to decide things for themselves with the right support and consultation. Accessible information is vital to this process and should be discussed with service users to ensure understanding.

I was helped by occupational therapists when I left home more than 20 years ago; not only help with the decision to move to independent living but giving me the confidence and tools to take this big step. Since then they have helped me with physical assessments and bath aids, including getting handrails installed internally near the entrance to my flat. I have a trolley to move hot items around as I shake when carrying things. I struggled with packets of medication and remembering which pills to take and when; a dosette box was the answer.

These are practical solutions to my particular problems, but solving them allows me to live on my own and manage my own life for the most part to be as independent as I can.

As a service user teacher I try to educate students, including occupational therapy students, that their preconceived ideas about those with a learning disability need to be shaken up. There are many levels of disability and students need to have an open mind on how they can facilitate and address the issues in terms the service user can relate with. An occupational therapy assessment should be a two-way conversation where issues can be raised and resolved, hopefully, to all parties' satisfaction. Professional phraseology needs to be left to reports, offices and textbooks!

Kate Eldon

REFERENCES

American Psychiatric Association. (2013). *Diagnostic and statistical manual of mental disorders* (5th ed.). Washington, D.C.

Asaba, E., Nakamura, M., Asaba, A., & Kottorp, A. (2017). Integrating occupational therapy specific assessments in practice: Exploring practitioner experiences. *Occupational Therapy International*, 1–8 https://doi.org/10.1155/2017/7602805.

Ayres, A. J. (2005). *Sensory integration and the child* (25th Anniversary Edition). Los Angeles: Western Psychological Services (Original work published in 1976).

BBC. (2011). *Timeline: Winterbourne view abuse scandal.* Available at: https://www.bbc.co.uk/news/uk-england-bristol-20078999.

Beddow, T. (2014). *Direct Payments: 10 reasons for not using them. Socialist health association, 5.* Available at: https://www.sochealth.co.uk/2014/02/05/direct-payments-10-reasons-using/.

Beresford, P. (2016). *Personal budgets don't work. So why are we ignoring the evidence?.* The Guardian, 5 Available at: https://www.theguardian.com/social-care-network/2016/may/05/personal-budgets-health-care-nao-report.

Best Beginnings. (2014). *Baby buddy.* Available at: https://www.bestbeginnings.org.uk/baby-buddy.

Bigby, C., Bould, E., & Beadle-Brown, J. (2017). Conundrums of supported living: The experiences of people with intellectual disability. *Journal of Intellectual and Developmental Disability, 42*(4), 309–319.

Blasingame, G. D. (2018). Risk assessment of adolescents with intellectual disabilities who exhibit sexual behaviour problems or sexual offending behaviour. *Journal of Child Sexual Abuse, 27*(8), 955–971.

Brindle, D. (2011). *Are direct payments for social care still living up to their name? The guardian, 22.* Available at: https://www.theguardian.com/society/2011/jun/22/personal-budgets-social-care-choice-compromised.

Burns, S., & MacKeith, J. (2012). *The life star user guide and the life star: Organisation guide.* Hove: Triangle Consulting Social Enterprise Ltd.

Caraci, F., Iulita, M. F., Pentz, R., et al. (2017). Searching for new pharmacological targets for the treatment of Alzheimer's disease in Down syndrome. *European Journal of Pharmacology, 15*(817), 7–19.

Care Act 2014, c. 23. Available at: http://www.legislation.gov.uk/ukpga/2014/23/pdfs/ukpga_20140023_en.pdf.

Channon, A. (2014). Intellectual disability and activity engagement: Exploring the literature from an occupational perspective. *Journal of Occupational Science, 21*(4), 443–458. Available at: https://www.tandfonline.com/doi/abs/10.1080/14427591.2013.829398.

Chapman, S. L. C., & Wu, L. T. (2012). Substance abuse among individuals with intellectual disabilities. *Research in Developmental Disabilities, 33*(4), 1147–1156 Available at: https://www.ncbi.nlm.nih.gov/pmc/articles/PMC3328139/.

Chapman, M., Lacey, H., & Jervis, N. (2018). Improving services for people with learning disabilities and dementia: Findings from a service evaluation exploring the perspectives of health and social care professionals. *British Journal of Learning Disabilites, 46*(1), 33–44.

Children and Families Act 2014, c. 6. Available at: http://www.legislation.gov.uk/ukpga/2014/6/pdfs/ukpga_20140006_en.pdf.

Cipriani, G., Danti, S., Carlesi, C., & Di Fiorino, M. (2018). Aging with down syndrome: The dual diagnosis: Alzheimer's disease and down syndrome. *American Journal of Alzheimer's Disease & Other Dementias, 33*(4), 253–262.

Clark, E. (2019). *Perceptions and practice of outcome measurement in occupational therapy services for adults with intellectual disabilities: The OT-ID survey.* MSc dissertation, University of Plymouth.

Cluley, V. (2018). From "Learning disability to intellectual disability"—perceptions of the increasing use of the term "intellectual disability" in learning disability policy, research and practice. *British Journal of Learning Disabilites, 46*(1), 24–32.

Cooper, J. R., Parkinson, S., de las Heras de Pablo, C. G., Shute, R., Melton, J. M., & Forsyth, K. (2018). *A user's manual for the Model of Human Occupation Exploratory Level outcome Ratings (MOHO-ExpLOR), version 1.0.* Edinburgh: Queen Margaret University.

Cooper, S. A., Smiley, E., Finlayson, J., et al. (2007). The prevalence, incidence, and factors predictive of mental ill-health in adults with profound intellectual disabilities. *Journal of Applied Research in Intellectual Disabilities, 20*(6), 493–501.

Davison, S., McGill, P., Baker, P., & Allen, D. (2015). A national UK survey of peripatetic support teams for children and adults with intellectual and developmental disability who display challenging behaviour. *International Journal of Positive Behavioural Support, 5*(1), 26–33.

De Witt, P. (2014). Creative ability: A model for individual and group occupational therapy for clients with psychosocial dysfunction. In R. Crouch, & V. Alers (Eds.), *Occupational therapy in psychiatry and mental health* (5th ed.) (pp. 3–32). New Jersey: John Wiley & Sons, Ltd.

DePape, A. M., & Lindsay, S. (2015). Parents' experiences of caring for a child with autism spectrum disorder. *Qualitative Health Research, 25*(4), 569–583.

Department of Health (DH). (2001). *Valuing people - a new strategy for learning disability for the 21st century.* Available at: https://www.gov.uk/government/publications/valuing-people-a-new-strategy-for-learning-disability-for-the-21st-century.

Department of Health (DH). (2002). *Health action plans what are they? How do you get one? (A booklet for people with learning disabilities).* Available at: https://www.jpaget.nhs.uk/media/186362/health_action_plans.pdf.

Department of Health (DH). (2009). *Valuing people now.* Available at: http://webarchive.nationalarchives.gov.uk/20130105064234/http://www.dh.gov.uk/prod_consum_dh/groups/dh_digitalassets/documents/digitalasset/dh_093375.pdf.

Department of Health (DH). (2012). *Transforming care: A national response to winterbourne view hospital.* Available at: https://www.gov.uk/government/publications/winterbourne-view-hospital-department-of-health-review-and-response.

Department of Health (DH). (2015). *Department of health guidance: Response to the supreme court judgment/ deprivation of*

Liberty Safeguards. Available at: https://assets.publishing.service. gov.uk/government/uploads/system/uploads/attachment_data/ file/485122/DH_Consolidated_Guidance.pdf.

Department of Health (DH). (2015). *Deprivation of Liberty Safeguards*. Available at: https://www.gov.uk/government/ publications/deprivation-of-liberty-safeguards-forms-and-guidance.

Di Lorito, C., Bosco, A., Birt, L., & Hassiotis, A. (2018). Co-research with adults with intellectual disability: A systematic review. *Journal of Applied Research in Intellectual Disabilities*, 31(5), 669–686.

Dixon, S., Smith, C., & Touchet, A. (2018). *The disability perception gap. Policy report*. Available at: https://www.scope.org.uk/ campaigns/disability-perception-gap/.

Doig, E., Fleming, J., Kuipers, P., & Cornwell, P. L. (2010). Clinical utility of the combined use of the Canadian occupational performance measure and goal attainment scaling. *American Journal of Occupational Therapy*, 64(6), 904–914.

Emerson, E., & Baines, S. (2010). *Health inequalities and people with learning disabilities in the UK: 2010*. Available at: https://pure.strath.ac.uk/portal/files/7402206/vid_7479_ IHaL2010_3HealthInequality2010.pdf.

Fisher, A. G., & Bray Jones, K. (2011). Assessment of motor and process skills. *Development, standardisation, and administration manual* (Vol. 1). Fort Collins, CO: Three Star Press.

Fisher, A. G., Forsyth, K., Harrison, M., et al. (2014). *Residential Environment Impact Scale (REIS), version 4.0*. U.S.A.: The University of Illinois at Chicago.

Glasby, J. (2014). The controversies of choice and control: Why some people might be hostile to english social care reforms. *British Journal of Social Work*, 44(2), 252–266. Available at: https://academic.oup.com/bjsw/article/44/2/252/1713633.

Goodman, J., & Wright, W. (2014). Learning disabilities. In W. Bryant, J. Fieldhouse, K. Bannigan, & J. Creek (Eds.), *Creek's occupational therapy and mental health* (pp. 406–423). London: Churchill Livingstone.

Gore, N. J., McGill, P., & Toogood, S. (2013). Definition and scope for positive behavioural support. *International Journal of Positive Behavioural Support*, 3(2), 14–23.

Griffiths, C. (2009). The interface between communication and community living. In J. Goodman, J. Hurst, & C. Locke (Eds.), *Occupational therapy for people with learning disabilities: A practical guide* (pp. 69–84). London: Churchill Livingstone.

Haines, D., Wright, J., & Comerasamy, H. (2018). Occupational therapy empowering support workers to change how they support people with profound intellectual and multiple disabilities to engage in activity. *Journal of Policy and Practice in Intellectual Disabilities*, 15(4), 295–306.

Hassiotis, A., Strydom, A., & Crawford, M. (2014). Clinical and cost effectiveness of staff training in positive behaviour support (PBS) for treating challenging behaviour in adults with intellectual disability: A cluster randomised controlled trial. *BMC Psychiatry*, 219(14). Available at: https://link.springer.com/ article/10.1186/s12888-014-0219-6.

Hawes, D., & Houlder, D. (2010). Reflections on using the model of human occupation screening tool in a joint learning disability team. *British Journal of Occupational Therapy*, 73(11), 564–567.

Health and Social Care Act 2012, c. 7. Available at: http://www. legislation.gov.uk/ukpga/2012/7/pdfs/ukpga_20120007_en.pdf.

Hellenbach, M., Brown, M., Karatzias, T., & Robinson, R. (2015). Psychological interventions for women with intellectual disabilities and forensic care needs: A systematic review of the literature. *Journal of Intellectual Disability Research*, 59(4), 319–331. Available at: https://onlinelibrary.wiley.com/doi/ epdf/10.1111/jir.12133.

Heslop, P., Blair, P., Fleming, P., Hoghton, M., Marriott, A., & Russ, L. (2013). *Confidential inquiry into premature deaths of people with learning disabilities (CIPOLD) final report*. Available at: https://www.bristol.ac.uk/media-library/sites/cipold/migrated/ documents/fullfinalreport.pdf.

Hithersay, R., Hamburg, S., Knight, B., & Strydom, A. (2017). Cognitive decline and dementia in Down syndrome. *Current Opinion in Psychiatry*, 30(2), 102–107.

Höglund, B. ,, Lindgren, P., & Larsson, M. (2012). Pregnancy and birth outcomes of women with intellectual disability in Sweden: A national register study. *Acta Obstetricia et Gynecologica Scandinavica*, 91(12), 1381–1387.

Iwane, T., Yoshida, A., Kono, M., Hashimoto, H., & Yamamoto, S. (2013). Work support for persons with mental disabilities in Japan. *Work*, 45(2), 253–260.

Johnson, K. R., Blaskowitz, M., & Mahoney, W. J. (2019). Occupational therapy practice with adults with intellectual disability: What more can we do? *Open Journal of Occupational Therapy*, 7(2), 1–9.

Jones, G., & Talbot, J. (2010). No one knows: The bewildering passage of offenders with learning disability and learning difficulty through the criminal justice system. *Criminal Behaviour and Mental Health*, 20(1), 1–7. https://onlinelibrary. wiley.com/doi/abs/10.1002/cbm.746.

Kielhofner, G. (2008). In *Model of human occupation: Theory and application. MOHO* (4th ed.). Lippincott Williams & Wilkins, Baltimore, MD.

King, E., Okodogbe, T., Burke, E., McCarron, M., McCallion, P., & O'Donovan, M. A. (2017). Activities of daily living and transition to community living for adults with intellectual disabilities. *Scandinavian Journal of Occupational Therapy*, 24(5), 357–365.

Kiresuk, T., Smith, A., & Cardillo, J. E. (1994). *Goal attainment scaling: Applications, theory and measurement*. Hillsdale: Lawrence Erlbaum Associates.

Kottorp, A., Bernspang, B., & Fisher, A. G. (2003). Validity of a performance assessment of activities of daily living for people with developmental disabilities. *Journal of Intellectual Disability Research*, 47(8), 597–605.

Language skills of males with fragile X syndrome or nonsyndromic autism spectrum disorder. *Journal of Autism and Developmental Disorders* 47, 728–743.

Laver-Fawcett, A. (2014). Routine standardised outcome measurement to evaluate the effectiveness of occupational therapy interventions: Essential or optional? *Ergoterapeuten*, 4, 28–37.

Lilywhite, A., & Haines, D. (2010). *Occupational therapy and people with learning disabilities, Fndings from a research study*. London: College of occupational Therapists.

Mahoney, W. J., Roberts, E., Bryze, K., & Kent, J. A. P. (2016). Occupational engagement and adults with intellectual disabilities. *American Journal of Occupational Therapy, 70*(1), 1–6.

Mazars, L. L. P. (2015). *Independent review of deaths of people with a learning disability or mental health problem in contact with southern health NHS foundation trust april 2011 to March 2015.* Available at https://www.england.nhs.uk/south/wp-content/uploads/sites/6/2015/12/mazars-rep.pdf.

McCormack, A. (2014). *United Kingdom: Model of human occupation ClearinghouseInterest Checklist UK: Adapted version (v. 6.1).* Available at: https://www.moho.uic.edu/resources/files/InterestChecklistEasyReadVersionV1.1-2.pdf.

Mellow Parenting. (2016). Available at: https://www.mellowparenting.org/.

Mencap, 2007. Death by Indifference. Available at: https://www.mencap.org.uk/sites/default/files/2016-06/DBIreport.pdf.

Mencap. (2012). *Death by indifference: 74 deaths and counting.* Available at: https://www.mencap.org.uk/sites/default/files/2016-08/Death%20by%20Indifference%20-%2074%20deaths%20and%20counting.pdf.

Mengoni, S., Gates, B., & Durand, M. A. (2015). An intervention for people with learning disabilities and epilepsy. (Report). *Learning Disability Practice, 18*(2), 28–31.

Mental Capacity Act 2005, c.9. Available at: https://www.legislation.gov.uk/ukpga/2005/9/pdfs/ukpga_20050009_en.pdf.

Mesa, A., Heron, P., Chard, G., & Rowe, J. (2014). Using the assessment of motor and process skills as part of the diagnostic process in an inner-city learning disability service. *British Journal of Occupational Therapy, 77*(4), 170–173.

Murphy, J., & Cameron, L. (2005). *Talking mats: A resource to enhance communication.* Pub. University of Stirling.

Murphy, J., & Cameron, L. (2008). The effectiveness of Talking Mats[R] with people with intellectual disability. *British Journal of Learning Disabilites, 36*(4), 232–241.

National Institute for Health and Care Excellence (NICE). (2015). *Challenging behaviour and learning disabilities: Prevention and Interventions for people with learning disabilities whose behaviour challenges.* Available at: https://www.nice.org.uk/guidance/ng11.

National Institute for Health and Care Excellence (NICE). (2016). *Mental health problems in people with learning disabilities: Prevention, assessment and management.* Available at: https://www.nice.org.uk/guidance/ng54/evidence/full-guideline-pdf-2612227933.

National Learning Disability Professional Senate. (2015). *Delivering effective specialist community learning disabilities health team support to people with learning disabilities and their families or Carers.* Available at https://acppld.csp.org.uk/system/files/national_ld_professional_senate_guidelines_for_cldt_specialist_health_services_final_3_march_2015.docx.

NHS (2019). *Care homes.* Available at: https://www.nhs.uk/conditions/social-care-and-support-guide/care-services-equipment-and-care-homes/care-homes/.

NHS. (2020). *Personal health budgets.* Available at: https://www.england.nhs.uk/personal-health-budgets/.

NHS England. (2015). *Supporting people with a learning disability and/or autism who display behaviour that challenges, including those with a mental health condition.* Available at: https://www.england.nhs.uk/wp-content/uploads/2015/10/service-model-291015.pdf.

NHS England. (2017). *Accessible information standard specification.* Available at: https://www.england.nhs.uk/publication/accessible-information-standard-specification/.

Norah Fry Research Centre. (2009). Supporting parents with learning disabilities and difficulties. Stories of positive practice. Available at: https://www.choiceforum.org/docs/pppr.pdf.

O'Leary, L., Cooper, S. A., & Hughes-McCormack, L. (2018). Early death and causes of death of people with intellectual disabilities: A systematic review. *Journal of Applied Research in Intellectual Disabilities, 31,* 325–342.

Parkinson, S., Cooper, J. R., & De Las Heras De Pablo, C. G. (2017). Assessments combining methods of information gathering. In R. Taylor (Ed.), *Kielhofner's model of human occupation* (5th ed.) (pp. 291–298). Baltimore, MD: Lippincott Williams & Wilkins.

Parkinson, S., Cooper, J. R., De Las Heras De Pablo, C. G., & Forsyth, K. (2014). Measuring the effectiveness of interventions when occupational performance is severely impaired. *British Journal of Occupational Therapy, 77*(2), 78–81.

Parkinson, S., Forsyth, K., & Kielhofner, G. (2006). *The model of human occupation screening tool (MOHOST).* Chicago, IL: University of Illinois at Chicago.

Perez, M., Carlson, G., Ziviani, J., & Cuskelly, M. (2012). Contribution of occupational therapists in behaviour support. *Australian Occupational Therapy Journal, 59*(6), 428–436.

Phillips, J. (2004). Risk assessment and management of suicide and self-harm within a forensic learning disability setting. *Learning Disability Practice, 7*(2), 12–18.

Pool, J. (2012). *The pool activity level Instrument for occupational profiling: A practical resource for carers of people with cognitive impairment* (3rd ed.). Oxford: Blackwell.

Poulsen, A. A., Ziviani, J., Kotaniemi, K., & Law, M. (2014). I think I can: Measuring confidence in goal pursuit. *British Journal of Occupational Therapy, 77*(2), 64–66.

Public Health England. (2016). People with learning disabilities in england 2015: Main report. Available at: https://assets.publishing.service.gov.uk/government/uploads/system/uploads/attachment_data/file/613182/PWLDIE_2015_main_report_NB090517.pdf.

Rapley, M. (2004). *The social construction of intellectual disability.* Cambridge New York: Cambridge University Press.

Reisman, J., & Hanschu, B. (1992). *The sensory integration inventory: Revised for individuals with developmental disabilities.* Hugo, MN: PDP Press Inc.

Robertson, J., Baines, S., Emerson, E., Hatton, C., 2018. Postural care for people with intellectual disabilities and severely impaired motor function: A scoping review. *Journal of Applied Research in Intellectual Disabilities* 31(1), 11–28. Available at: file:///C:/Users/lydia/Downloads/Robertson_et_al-2018-Journal_of_Applied_Research_in_Intellectual_Disabilities.pdf.

Robertson, J., Emerson, E., & Gregory, N. (2000). Lifestyle related risk factors for poor health in residential settings for people with intellectual disabilities. *Research in Developmental Disabilities*, *21*(6), 469–486.

Royal College of Occupational Therapists (RCOT). (2017). *Occupational therapists' use of occupational-focused practice in secure hospitals. Practice guideline* (2nd ed.). Available at: https://www.rcot.co.uk/practice-resources/rcot-practice-guidelines/secure-hospitals.

Royal College of Occupational Therapists (RCOT). (2019a). *Leading fulfilled lives occupational therapy supporting people with learning disabilities*. Available at: https://www.rcot.co.uk/promoting-occupational-therapy/occupational-therapy-improving-lives-saving-money.

Royal College of Occupational Therapists (RCOT). (2019b). *Living well in care homes*. Available at: https://www.rcot.co.uk/about-occupational-therapy/living-well-care-homes-2019.

Royal College of Psychiatrists & The British Psychological Society. (2015). *Dementia and people with intellectual disabilities guidance on the assessment, diagnosis, interventions and support of people with intellectual disabilities who develop dementia*. Available at: https://www1.bps.org.uk/system/files/Public%20files/rep77_dementia_and_id.pdf.

Søndenaa, E., Rasmussen, K., Palmstierna, T., & Nøttestad, J. (2008). The prevalence and nature of ID in Norwegian prisons. *Journal of Intellectual Disability Research*, *52*(12), 1129–1137.

Spandler, H. (2004). Friend or foe: Towards a critical assessment of direct payments. *Critical Social Policy*, *24*(2), 187–209. Available at: http://clok.uclan.ac.uk/525/1/friend_or_foe_CSP.pdf.

Sport for Confidence. (2020). *What is sport for confidence all about?*. Available at: https://www.sportforconfidence.com/about-us/.

Stigen, L., Bjork, E., & Lund, A. (2018). The conflicted practice: Municipal occupational therapists' experiences with assessment of clients with cognitive impairments. *Scandinavian Journal of Occupational Therapy*, *4*, 1–12.

Strydom, A., Chan, T., King, M., Hassiotis, A., & Livingston, G. (2013). Incidence of dementia in older adults with intellectual disabilities. *Research in Developmental Disabilities*, *34*(6), 1881–1885.

Taggart, L., McLaughlin, D., Quinn, B., & Milligan, V. (2006). An exploration of substance misuse in people with intellectual disabilities. *Journal of Intellectual Disability Research*, *50*(8), 588–597. Available at: https://onlinelibrary.wiley.com/doi/epdf/10.1111/j.1365-2788.2006.00820.x.

Terrana, A., Dowdell, J., Edwards, B., Tahsin, F., Cacciacarro, L., & Cameron, D. (2016). Perspectives of key stakeholders about vocational training and rehabilitation in Trinidad and Tobago. *British Journal of Occupational Therapy*, *79*(11), 703–712.

The National LD Professional Senate. (2015). *Delivering effective specialist community learning disabilities health team support to people with learning disabilities and their families or carers*. Available at: https://acppld.csp.org.uk/documents/national-ld-professional-senate-briefing-paper.

Thurman, A.J., McDuffie, A., Hagerman, R.J., Josol, C.K., Abbeduto, L., 2017.

To, W. T., Neirynck, S., Vanderplasschen, W., Vanheule, S., & Vandevelde, S. (2014). Substance use and misuse in persons with intellectual disabilities (ID): Results of a survey in ID and addiction services in Flanders. *Research in Developmental Disabilities*, *35*(1), 1–9. Available at: https://www.sciencedirect.com/science/article/pii/S0891422213004526?_rdoc=1&_fmt=high&_origin=gateway&_docanchor=&md5=b8429449ccfc9c30159a5f9aeaa92ffb.

Torjesen, I. (2013). People with learning disabilities are more likely to die prematurely, inquiry finds. *The British Medical Journal*, *346*, f1853.

Tort, V., Dueñas, R., Vicens, E., Zabala, C., Martínez, M., & Romero, D. M. (2016). Intellectual disability and the prison setting. *Revista Española de Sanidad Penitenciaria*, *18*(1), 25–32.

Turner-Stokes, L. (2009). Goal attainment scaling (GAS) in rehabilitation: A practical guide. *Clinical Rehabilitation*, *23*(4), 362–370.

Usher, L. V., Dawalt, L. S., Greenberg, J. S., & Mailick, M. R. (2019). Unaffected siblings of adolescents and adults with fragile X syndrome: Effects on maternal well-being. *Journal of Family Psychology*, *33*(4), 487–492.

VanderNagel, J., Kiewik, M., Buitelaar, J., & DeJong, C. (2011). Staff perspectives of substance use and misuse among adults with intellectual disabilities enrolled in Dutch disability services. *Journal of Policy and Practice in Intellectual Disabilities*, *8*(3), 143–149. Available at: https://onlinelibrary.wiley.com/doi/abs/10.1111/j.1741-1130.2011.00304.x.

Vinales, J. J. (2013). Evaluation of Makaton in practice by children's nursing students. *Nursing Children and Young People*, *25*(3), 14–17.

Wales, K., Clemson, L., Lannin, N., & Cameron, I. (2016). Functional assessments used by occupational therapists with older adults at risk of activity and participation limitations: A systematic review. *PLoS One*, *11*(2), 1–20.

Watson, J., Fossey, E., & Harvey, C. (2019). A home but how to connect with others? A qualitative meta-synthesis of experiences of people with mental illness living in supported housing. *Health and Social Care in the Community*, *27*(3), 546–564.

Waye, M. Y., & Cheng, H. (2018). Genetics and epigenetics of autism: A review. *Psychiatry and Clinical Neurosciences*, *72*(4) 228–224.

Whiteford, G. (2000). Occupational deprivation: Global challenge in the new millennium. *British Journal of Occupational Therapy*, *63*(5), 200–204.

Whooten, R. (2018). Endocrine manifestations of Down syndrome. *Current Opinion in Endocrinology Diabetes and Obesity*, *25*(1), 61–66.

Williams, V. (2013). *Learning disability policy and practice: Changing lives?* Basingstoke: New York: Palgrave Macmillan.

Williams, V., Boyle, G., Jepson, M., Swift, P., Williamson, T., & Heslop, P. (2014). Best interests decisions: Professional practices in health and social care. *Health and Social Care in the Community*, *22*(1), 78–86.

Williams, M. S., & Shellenberger, S. (1992). *An introduction to "how does your engine run?"® the alert program® for self-regulation [booklet]*. Albuquerque, NM: TherapyWorks, Inc.

Wilson, N. J., Hayden, J., Amanda, J., & Brotherton, M. L. (2017). From social exclusion to supported inclusion: Adults with intellectual disability discuss their lived experience of a structured social group. *Journal of Applied Research in Intellectual Disabilities, 30*(5), 847–858.

Working Together with Parents Network. (2016). *The working together with parents network update of the DoH/DfES good practice guidance on working with parents with a learning disability (2007).* Available at: https://www.bristol.ac.uk/media-library/sites/sps/documents/wtpn/2016%20WTPN%20UPDATE%20OF%20THE%20GPG%20-%20finalised%20with%20cover.pdf.

World Health Organization (WHO). (2007). *Global resources for persons with intellectual disabilities.* Geneva, Switzerland: WHO Press.

World Health Organization (WHO). (2018). *International classification of diseases for mortality and morbidity statistics, 11th revision.* Available at: https://www.who.int/classifications/icd/en/.

Xenitidis, K., Gratsa, A., Bouras, N., et al. (2004). Psychiatric inpatient care for adults with intellectual disabilities: Generic or specialist units? *Journal of Intellectual Disability Research, 48*(1), 11–18.

26 FORENSIC AND PRISON SERVICES

NATHAN REEVE ■ TOM MILLS ■ STEVE TAYLOR

INTRODUCTION

This chapter introduces occupational therapy within a forensic environment, examining inpatient and community-based services and considering differences between public and private sector practice. It provides an overview of some widely used models of practice and assessment tools, considers the delicate balance between therapeutic relationship-building and risk management and reflects on particular aspects of forensic practice; namely, offence-specific work, vocational work, distinctions between acute and rehabilitation stages of intervention and issues around disclosure of sensitive information regarding risk and mental health. The overall focus is on UK forensic services in which the authors work in medium and low secure hospitals.

What Does Forensic Mental Health Mean?

In the United Kingdom 'forensic mental health' has replaced 'forensic psychiatry' as the most commonly used term in this field of practice, reflecting a move away from a medical/illness-orientated model and towards a health promotion/ill-health prevention model, which the World Health Organization (WHO; 1998) describes as the enablement of people to increase control over, and to improve, their health. It moves beyond a focus on individual behaviour towards a wide range of social and environmental interventions. Mullen (2000) defines forensic mental health as 'an area of specialisation that, in the criminal sphere, involves the assessment and treatment of those who are both mentally disordered and whose behaviour has led or could lead to offending' (p. 307).

The offence that leads to an individual's admission into forensic services is termed the 'index offence.' The nature and severity of an individual's index offence will determine the level of security needed for their care and treatment. For example, if a murder is committed, the offender will often be admitted to a medium secure or a high secure hospital depending on the level of ongoing risk. Over time, and with successful therapeutic interventions, it is hoped the person can move through progressively less restrictive environments until deemed safe to move into the community. In some cases in which there is high media interest, the Minister of State at the UK's Ministry of Justice (MoJ) may take a cautious approach, favouring more secure care for the purpose of public reassurance.

Forensic services straddle the criminal justice system and the mental healthcare system. A brief history of how the relationship between these two spheres has evolved in the United Kingdom may be helpful in illuminating particular challenges faced by practitioners in relation to assessing and managing risk and working within a stringent legal framework.

A Brief History of UK Forensic Services

In the United Kingdom the general understanding of mentally disordered offenders developed after a series of high-profile events in the 19th century (see Duncan 2008). In 1800 James Hadfield fired a pistol at King George III, and in 1843 Daniel McNaughton tried to murder the Prime Minister but killed his Private Secretary. In both cases lawyers argued that it was the men's delusional beliefs that led them to commit these actions; the latter case resulting in the 'McNaughton rules,' which clarified the judicial stance on diminished responsibility resulting from severe mental illness. Within a month of Hadfield's conviction the Criminal Lunatics Act (1800) was passed, which required those acquitted on the grounds of insanity to be held in custody. However, it was not until 1863 (following the Criminal Lunatics Asylums Act 1860) that the first special hospital/asylum—Broadmoor—was built.

Before this there was no specialist provision for mentally disordered offenders. There were only prisons or mental health asylums. With the creation of criminal lunatic asylums, the medical establishment took on board the care of mentally disordered offenders for the first time (Duncan 2008).

Christopher Clunis's fatal attack on Jonathan Zito on a London underground train platform in 1992 is considered by many to have been a watershed event in the development of forensic mental health services in England and Wales (Maden 2007). A detailed homicide inquiry highlighted two important issues: firstly, the need for better information regarding the assessment and treatment of forensic service users and improved continuity of care, and, secondly, the need to address the fear and concerns of the general public regarding potentially violent mentally ill people being in the community (Soothill et al. 2008).

What follows is an overview of the way UK forensic services are configured and delivered and how occupational therapy addresses the needs of service users.

AN OVERVIEW OF UK FORENSIC SERVICES

Referral to Forensic Services

Forensic services are provided for individuals with a variety of mental health problems such as psychotic disorders, personality disorders and neurodevelopmental disorders (including intellectual or learning disabilities and autistic spectrum disorders). Forensic services also provide care for mentally disordered offenders hearing impaired and those with an acquired brain injury.

This list of medical labels demonstrates that, even though there has been a reduction in emphasis on the medical model, psychiatry (as a medical profession) continues to have dominance over other professions in this field and over certain aspects of language. Similarly, the Mental Health Act (1983) uses the medicalized term 'disorder,' and the criminal justice system has medico-legal language embedded throughout it. Consequently, it is important for occupational therapists to be familiar with this language and to use it in multidisciplinary practice. Certain disorders, when classified as above, may give increased access to funding and support, enabling service users to have their social and occupational needs better met. McNeill and Brannigan (2014)

BOX 26.1
TERMINOLOGY WIDELY USED IN UK FORENSIC PRACTICE

Acquisitional offending is defined as an offence in which the offender derives material gain from the crime (e.g., shoplifting, burglary, theft and robbery).

Criminogenic is a system, situation or place causing or likely to cause criminal behaviour.

Criminogenic needs are an individual's characteristics, traits, problems or issues that directly relate to their likelihood to re-offend.

Criminal Justice System is the system of law enforcement that is directly involved in apprehending, prosecuting, defending, sentencing and punishing those suspected or convicted of criminal offences.

Desistance is defined as the cessation of offending or other antisocial behaviour.

Diminished responsibility exists when a person's unbalanced mental state is considered to make them less answerable to a criminal charge and to be grounds for a reduced charge.

HCR-20 The Historical, Clinical, Risk Management-20 (Webster et al. 2013) is an assessment tool that helps mental health professionals estimate the probability of an individual becoming violent.

Index offence is the offence listed in the Offence Classification Index for which the offender was convicted. The index includes a range of offences, such as murder, manslaughter, burglary, rape, stalking, arson, vehicle theft, etc.

Legal framework is a broad system of rules/laws that govern/regulate decision-making.

Pro-social behaviour is behaviour which is positive, helpful and intended to promote social acceptance and friendship. It includes voluntary behaviour intended to benefit other people or society as a whole.

Public protection means protecting the public from general offending and, importantly, from the serious harm caused by the offending and re-offending of violent and sexual offenders.

Recidivism refers to a person's relapse into criminal behaviour often after they receive sanctions or undergo intervention for a previous crime.

Resettlement involves work to secure the release of prisoners or service users in a secure hospital back to the community.

SVR-20 The Sexual Violence Risk-20 (Boer et al. 2018) is a set of structured professional judgement guidelines for assessing and managing risk for sexual violence.

The Secretary of State for Justice has overall responsibility for all Ministry of Justice business.

---

noted that forensic occupational therapists should familiarize themselves with terms such as 'criminogenic', 'index offence', 'public protection' and 'resettlement' (see terminology in Box 26.1) and develop a detailed understanding of the legal framework encompassing their practice. This means being familiar with the UK's Mental Health Act 1983, its 2007 amendment and the Mental Capacity Act 2005.

Most forensic services will require an access assessment to be completed by the multidisciplinary team (MDT) to establish (or otherwise) the person's suitability for forensic services. A forensic service MDT will usually comprise psychiatrists, nurses, psychologists, social workers and occupational therapists.

One of the distinguishing features of forensic (compared to general) mental health services is, of course, the presence of service users who present a risk to other people. It is the norm. It is unusual for individuals to present with a risk solely to themselves. The MDT assessment therefore includes information about the individual's mental disorder and their offending history or risk of offending. Typically, referrals will come from the criminal justice system (penal establishments, courts or police) or from secondary mental health services, such as acute psychiatric hospitals.

Types of Service

Occupational therapists work in a wide range of forensic settings. Forensic hospitals are divided into three levels of security: low, medium and high. Many localities may also have community forensic teams. Within some forensic hospitals and community teams there are healthcare professionals, including occupational therapy staff who are specialised in working with people with intellectual or learning disabilities (see Chapter 25).

The level of security that applies in a given setting impacts the type of work the occupational therapist can carry out there. Caution should be taken to maintain a balance between creating a therapeutic, caring environment (which enables service users to engage in valued occupations) and ensuring safety and security.

Low Secure Services

Low secure services provide treatment for those who present a significant risk of harm to others and whose escape from hospital must be prevented. In almost all cases, detention is authorized under the UK Mental Health Act (1983) and the law courts can stipulate the level of security. For example, even in a low secure setting, locked doors and fences are in place.

Low secure hospitals deliver MDT care for service users who suffer with complex mental health disorders. Offences (and risk) are not usually as high profile as those associated with medium and high secure services, however, it is possible, as part of service users' transitioning through descending levels of security/risk as their care progresses, that practitioners in low secure services will work with individuals who have committed serious acts, such as murder.

The function of low secure hospitals is to reintegrate service users back into the community or to less secure care. Due to the low risk, community leave may be accessed relatively often, and occupational therapists will focus their assessments and interventions on this external environment, developing a person-centred, recovery-orientated care plan with each service user.

Medium Secure Services

Medium secure services provide treatment to those adults who present a serious risk of harm to others and whose escape from hospital must be prevented. Again, detention in medium secure settings is authorized under the UK Mental Health Act (1983) and, compared with low secure care, all aspects of security are enhanced (see physical, procedural and relational security later and in Box 26.2).

Key functions of medium secure hospitals are to provide a step-down in security level from high secure and to provide additional assessment opportunities regarding service users' progress towards community integration. Medium secure services also have a significant role in the initial assessment and understanding of risk, so they have the most active role in terms of transitioning patients between settings. This work often involves specific training in risk assessment tools such as the Historical, Clinical, Risk Management-20 (HCR-20) (Webster

---

BOX 26.2
SUMMARY OF LEVEL AND FORMS OF SECURITY

PHYSICAL SECURITY

Physical security varies according to the level of security but involves:

- External or perimeter security (e.g., fences or walls)
- Entry security (e.g., locked door or airport-type security)
- Internal security (e.g., locked doors, secure window fittings and personal attack alarms for staff)
- Safe design of ward and off ward activity areas

PROCEDURAL SECURITY

Procedural security refers to the various control processes that are regular structures of life in secure environments which have been developed to minimize risk of harm to all individuals within the setting. Principally, there are three components to procedural security: control of communications, of items and of people.

RELATIONAL SECURITY

Relational security refers to the importance of the therapeutic relationship for continuing safety:

- Developing positive therapeutic relationships

- Management of violence and aggression
- Individual responses to therapeutic interventions
- Security intelligence

The 'See, Think, Act' (DH 2010) helps staff working in seunits to recognize relational security and the role that they have to play in ensuring a safe and effective environment. It describes relational security as the knowledge and understanding staff have of a person and the environment and how the knowledge and understanding is translated into appropriate response and care. The guide offers a person-centred model, identifying relevant factors:

- Team – boundaries and therapy
- Other patients – patient mix and patient dynamics
- Inside world – personal world and physical environment
- Outside world – outward connections and visitors

The goal is for all staff to observe what is going on in the environment, to recognize the importance of determining what the observed behaviour really means and to appreciate the importance of acting before something goes wrong.

Adapted from Duncan (2008) McNeil and Bannigan (2014).

et al. 2013) and the Sexual Violence Risk-20 (SVR-20) tool (Boer et al. 2018) (see Box 26.1) and a variety of other assessment tools that contribute to a comprehensive risk assessment. All professions within the MDT input into this process, too. Occupational therapists, for example, use occupations to observe and assess the risks service users pose when interacting with others and their environment. This occupation-focused assessment facilitates ongoing work towards providing care in a less secure, less restrictive environment.

High Secure Services

High secure services provide comprehensive MDT care for adults who demonstrate disturbed behaviour in the context of a serious mental disorder, such as paranoid schizophrenia, and have been assessed as presenting a grave and immediate danger to others (e.g., risk of homicide). In the United Kingdom high secure hospitals must be part of an NHS Trust approved by the Secretary of State (see Box 26.1) to provide high security psychiatric services.

Outside the United Kingdom people with a mental health diagnosis who pose a grave and immediate risk to the public may find themselves in prison and not receiving treatment in a secure mental health facility. Munoz et al. (2016) suggest occupational therapists in the United States are more likely to work in the community or in prisons, opposed to secure mental health facilities as in the United Kingdom. Across Europe the clinical challenges that are faced in treating forensic patients are the same, but the facilities they are treated in may vary from country to country. Seppanen et al. (2018) suggest that legislation causes significant differences at the service-patient interface, even among countries that have ratified and subscribed to the same human rights legislation and are subject to the same monitoring bodies.

High secure hospitals may sometimes resemble prisons from the outside, but inside treatment takes place within a therapeutic environment, focusing on increasing social interaction to counteract service users' tendency to withdraw, as well as skills development. Ozkan et al. (2018) suggest occupational therapists in high secure units focus on areas such as improving awareness of self, others and the environment; orientation to time, place and situation; cognitive abilities and skill acquisition to improve leisure time use and motivation. Pre-vocational skills may

be a likely progression step for some. For example, at Broadmoor high secure hospital in Berkshire, United Kingdom, occupational therapists provide a vocational skills service in which service users produce saleable goods such as cards, jewellery and craft items (West London NHS Trust 2018).

Prisons

A prison differs from secure services in that it is a custodial environment with limited therapeutic input. It is acknowledged that, whilst prisons are not therapeutic environments, some prisoners require a therapeutic approach during periods of vulnerability (Curran and Wilkinson 2010). Within the prison population in the United Kingdom, there is a high incidence of mental health problems, poor educational attainment, lack of employment, persistent alcohol and substance misuse and a lack of social support. Prisoners with learning disabilities, head injuries and personality disorders are encountered regularly and can become quickly institutionalised (Lovemore 2011).

Some prisons offer vocational and educational opportunities, but the staff providing these may have limited experience of mental health problems, and prisoners may struggle to make meaningful use of such input. Occupational therapists have an important role to play in prisons because of the inevitable occupational deprivation that occurs during incarceration, which can itself exacerbate mental health problems (Whiteford 2020). Occupational therapy in prisons might include health promotion activities, life skills programmes, interventions to help offenders gain insight into lifestyle choices which promote pro-social behaviours, and helping prisoners prepare for re-integration into the community, such as through educational and vocational rehabilitation programmes (Royal College of Occupational Therapists 2017).

Private Provision

In the United Kingdom secure services can be provided by the NHS or by private providers (with the exception of high secure services, which must be part of an NHS Trust). Private providers are nevertheless governed by the same commissioning standards and requirements as NHS services. The Care Quality Commission has a role in inspecting both the NHS and private providers to ensure consistent standards of care.

Liaison and Diversion Services

Liaison and diversion services identify people who have mental health problems, intellectual (or learning) disabilities, substance misuse problems, or other vulnerabilities when they first come into contact with the criminal justice system as suspects, defendants or offenders. The service can then support people through the early stages of the criminal system pathway, refer them for appropriate health or social care or enable them to be diverted away from the criminal justice system into a more appropriate setting, if required.

Liaison and diversion services aim to improve overall health outcomes for people and to support them to reduce re-offending. They also aim to identify vulnerabilities early on, which reduces the likelihood of mental health crises occurring and helps to ensure timely support is provided (NHS England 2019). In this role occupational therapists can be limited to specific parts of the occupational therapy process. For example, staff are frequently involved in the referral and assessment of individuals but less involved in the intervention phases, as they often refer onto other services/service providers for this aspect of care. This assessment phase is frequently a generic assessment of mental health that is completed by all members of the team.

Security

Forensic services use an approach incorporating three elements of security: physical, procedural and relational (see Box 26.2).

Physical Security

Forensic hospitals are carefully designed and equipped to reduce environmental hazards and risks. Furniture is often fixed to the floor or intentionally heavy so it cannot be easily picked up and is usually tamper proof, so it cannot be easily broken or dismantled into parts, which could then be used as weapons and pose a risk. Pictures are secured to walls and plastic used instead of glass in such fittings. The glass in windows is usually strengthened to protect against breakage and treated so that if it does break, it will break in to small pieces like a car windscreen or remain attached to an internal adhesive layer.

Although there is a focus on the risk to others presented by forensic service users, it is also important to remember the risk they may pose to themselves. Consequently, anti-ligature fittings are used in all areas.

For example, fixtures in bathrooms do not include taps which could be used to create a ligature.

Staff typically wear everyday clothing. In high secure hospitals, uniforms used to be worn but, generally, this appears to have been phased out (Pilgrim 2007). Ward environments may appear similar across all three levels of security with nursing office space, bedrooms in corridors with en-suite bathrooms, television lounges and quiet rooms. CCTV cameras are commonly used to maintain staff and service users' safety, monitoring entry and exit points and perimeter security.

Occupational therapists' work may take place on the ward, but they may also work in a separate space; the choice of venue often being influenced by risk assessment because time off the ward is something an individual will have more of as their recovery progresses.

Procedural Security

Many security and safety procedures involve the whole MDT, including occupational therapists. For example, on some wards, staff ensure they enter the bedroom corridors in pairs (as a minimum), never alone, and the occupational therapist will often count equipment and materials in and out at the beginning and end of sessions, such as paint brushes or sports equipment, as well as more obvious potential weapons such as cutlery and scissors.

A key element of procedural security is the establishment and maintenance of boundaries, and this can create a tension with the need to develop therapeutic relationships with service users (see Relational Security' in Box 26.2). The principle of 'least restrictive practice' aims to mitigate this tension by keeping various security procedures (such as locked doors and restrictions on what service users can do) to a minimum to promote service users' recovery and independence (Sustere and Tarpery 2019). This principle also informs referrers' decision-making, aiming to ensure service users are referred to the hospital setting which has the most appropriate (least restrictive) level of security possible.

There are entry/exit searches across all levels of security. One of the main differences is in high secure hospitals and prisons where service users, visitors and staff are usually subject to searches. Many items that are considered contraband in a secure hospital may actually be illegal in a prison, such as a mobile phone.

Across all levels of security, leave is conceptualized as being either within the hospital setting (the hospital building and its grounds) or in the local mainstream community. An MDT will jointly decide to grant access to the building prior to the grounds; community leave being significantly less common in a high secure hospital. A typical pattern of progressive amounts of leave is shown later in Table 26.2. In the United Kingdom, patients detained under Part 3 of the Mental Health Act 1983, also known as 'restricted sections,' will require approval from the Minister of Justice, which can slow down the process of receiving leave.

Relational Security

Relational security issues arise from the need to balance therapeutic relationship building with ongoing protection of the public. For example, the occupational therapist must balance the therapeutic gains an individual would experience if they were to cook some of their own meals, perhaps, against how this occupation (involving access to utensils) might be best managed if the service user's mental health is deteriorating and, as a consequence, risk is seen to be increasing. To manage this, the therapist's professional reasoning will incorporate in-depth knowledge of the individual, their own observations, positive risk management principles (see later) and wider MDT discussion and decision-making.

OCCUPATIONAL THERAPY PRACTICE

Theoretical Underpinning

The Model Of Human Occupation (MOHO) (Kielhofner 2008) is widely used in forensic occupational therapy. As well as offering a comprehensive evidence base to the profession, it also provides an invaluable array of standardized assessment tools (Ozkan 2018).

Other occupational therapy models of practice used in forensic settings include Kawa, which presents itself as offering increased cultural sensitivity (Leadley 2015), the Model Of Creative Ability (MOCA) (de Witt 2005) and the Canadian Model of Occupational Performance and Engagement (Townsend and Polatajko 2007).

The MOCA is widely applied, based on its elements of activity analysis and assessment of an individual's functional performance, which can be used to guide decisions about duration of session, complexity of task and suitability of group work (Sherwood et al. 2015).

Occupational Therapy Referral

In secure hospitals, there is usually a 'blanket' or open unspecified referral system whereby all service users are implicitly expected and supported to engage with occupational therapy. The various stages of the occupational therapy process presented here are illustrated with reference to Case Studies 26.1 (Colin) and 26.2 (Alex).

Assessment

Generalized Multidisciplinary Team Risk Assessment

Risk assessment and management is central to the work of forensic services and always involves multiprofessional assessment and decision-making by the whole MDT, with a specialist perspective being provided by the occupational therapist in relation to engagement in occupations (in which skills in activity grading, for example, can help mitigate risk). Risk assessment takes many forms, as presented in Table 26.1.

Positive Risk Management

Risk assessment and management minimizes risk but does not eliminate it and so the occupational therapist must remain mindful of this. Integral to recovery-oriented practice is positive risk management, and activities are frequently graded so that an individual can engage in an activity with alternative items and tools to minimize risk (as outlined later regarding graded access to sharp utensils). Thus a certain level of risk or uncertainty associated with an intervention is acknowledged but deemed to be an acceptable part of the skill acquisition or therapeutic process.

One of the considerations for occupational therapists in forensic services is the limited access to certain environments, equipment and materials because of risk. This limitation itself may even contribute to a service users' experience of occupational deprivation. For example, early-stage engagement work may take place where the service user resides, such as on an admission ward in a medium secure hospital where any materials or equipment used must be deemed safe and unlikely to be usable as weapons; although this constraint will reduce as the service user progresses and more varied environment/equipment options emerge.

By encouraging service users to participate in activity, the occupational therapist plays an important role in the assessment of a service user's readiness to engage with new environments, equipment and materials, and

TABLE 26.1		
Forms of Risk Assessment Undertaken by Forensic Occupational Therapists		
Form of Risk Assessment	Assessment Process	Source of Information
Unstructured Clinical Judgement	Decisions are based on the discretion of a professional who is deemed to have the appropriate qualifications and experience to make the judgement.	▪ Mental state examinations ▪ Summary of known risks ▪ Seclusion observation summaries ▪ Interest checklist ▪ Sharp utensil assessment
Actuarial Approach	Decisions are based on statistics, and an algorithm (or formula) works out the level of risk.	Research-based evidence and recorded data (e.g., rates of offending for certain crimes).
Structured professional judgement	An attempt is made to bridge the gap between actuarial, or statistics-based, approaches and unstructured clinical approaches (Judges 2016).	HCR-20 – violence risk assessment SVR-20 – sexual violence risk assessment (see Box 26.1)

grading service users' access to sharp utensils may be an integral part of that progression.

Graded Access to Sharp Utensils

There are two inter-connected strands to this dual assessment:

1. Establishing whether the service user poses a risk to themselves or others by deliberately using the sharp item as a weapon, particularly if the index offence involved a sharp weapon.
2. Establishing whether the service user has the required functional skills to avoid accidental injury in handling sharp tools/utensils when engaging in an activity; for example, crafting, cooking or gardening.

It can be a complex matter to assess, requiring ongoing consultation between the service user, the occupational therapist and the MDT. For example, there may be a psychological impact to the service user regarding handling an item associated with the index offence that needs to be considered. Usually, the whole MDT and the service user are involved in the assessment of point 1. It is not an assessment that should be made by the occupational therapist alone. However, the occupational therapist is well placed to lead the assessment of point 2.

A risk management plan for working in a kitchen will typically involve some or all of the following: sharp utensils being locked away and counted when handed back in, pre-selection of recipes that do not require cutting, adaptation of tasks to suit plastic cutlery and the preparation of certain ingredients prior to the cookery session starting. In subsequent sessions, sharp utensils may be gradually introduced according to the potential risk associated with each tool: a potato-masher could be followed by a tin-opener or pizza-cutter before sharp knives can be introduced, for example.

A cautious approach is required to consider risk in each specific context and to avoid generalizing decisions. For example, access to sharp utensils in a kitchen and in a gardening group may require individual risk assessments (e.g., one activity may involve an item previously used as a weapon while the other may not). Similarly, tool access arrangements agreed on between a service user and a particular therapist with an established therapeutic relationship may not be applicable to a staff member without this relationship.

Occupational Therapy Assessments

Occupational therapy initial assessment is increasingly happening at an early stage following admission and may include engaging with an individual in seclusion (Case Study 26.1 Colin). Depending on the practicalities of engaging an individual, the assessment may be a conversation between the service user and the occupational therapist (or with other MDT members, too, if the risk assessment indicates this). Alternatively, the assessment may begin during an activity-based session. For example, the occupational therapist may have little success in early attempts to engage in conversation with an individual but, when running a coffee morning quiz group, the service user may be interested in attending/participating.

CASE STUDY 26.1

Colin

ADMISSION

Colin, a 25-year-old male, has been admitted to a medium secure hospital (after being held on remand in prison) for assessment of his mental state and risk behaviour (which include verbal threats and occasional physical aggression to others). He is on an acute assessment ward with eight beds for males, a high ratio of staff (six per shift) and a high care/seclusion suite (i.e., a ward area where individual care can be provided within a low stimulus environment and which has controlled lighting/noise and no items/furniture that could be used as weapons).

Colin is detained under Section 48/49 of the Mental Health Act (1983), which allows the court to transfer an individual to a secure hospital rather than serve a custodial prison sentence. Colin was on remand because he recently stabbed his neighbour whom he had become paranoid about. Colin has a history of polysubstance use, which has led him to present as psychotic, appearing to experience auditory hallucinations that, according to him, are derogatory and persecutory.

WARD OBSERVATIONS

Ward nurses report that Colin has been accessing communal parts of the ward (rather than isolating himself in his bedroom) but often sleeps during the day and is up until the early hours, missing set meal and medication times. Colin has lots of energy but poor concentration, and he neglects personal hygiene and self-care (not washing/brushing teeth) and declines offers of fresh clothes despite a strong body odour.

OCCUPATIONAL THERAPY ASSESSMENT

Early engagement with occupational therapy is recommended and, whilst he is still in seclusion, Colin's initial assessment is conducted over three 15- to 20- minute 1:1 meetings, reflecting his poor concentration. The assessment indicates that Colin has a limited education, no formal qualifications, poor insight into his mental health difficulties and (prior to admission) much of his time was spent buying and selling drugs, which resulted in acquisitional offending (theft of money and/or goods to sell to purchase

drugs). The assessment also highlights Colin's interest in sports at school and in using the gym whilst in the hospital.

RISK ASSESSMENT

The HCR-20 assessment (see earlier) is completed by members of the multidisciplinary team (MDT), highlighting that Colin is a significant risk to others and himself and should have no access to sharp utensils for the foreseeable future. Currently, Colin has no access to the therapy centre due to his level of risk, and therefore activities/therapy sessions are offered solely on the ward.

ENGAGEMENT IN ACTIVITIES

Colin and the occupational therapist agree that he will be awake and out of his bedroom to attend at least one ward-based therapeutic activity each day; this will be with support. The aim is to provide daily structure and hopefully improve his sleep pattern. Other MDT interventions supporting this plan include sleep hygiene education by the nursing team and them prompting Colin to follow his activity programme.

For the occupational therapy intervention, all activities that Colin engages in undergo activity analysis by the occupational therapist, who then grades each one to the appropriate level for him. An example of this in relation to pizza-making is presented in Box 26.3. He is offered the following groups as part of his occupational therapy programme:

- 'Give It A Go' group – in which members are encouraged to try a variety of activities, some of which will be new to them, such as tee-shirt printing, making soap, gardening or artificial flower arranging in an environment without sharp utensils;
- Art group – in which the aim for members is to develop self-esteem and confidence through card-making, silk-painting, marbling, and mindful colouring in, for example, using crayons/pastels instead of (sharp) pens/pencils;
- Newspaper group – in which members discuss newspaper stories, grounding and orientating them to the outside world and providing opportunities for assessment of educational

Continued on following page

CASE STUDY 26.1

Colin (Continued)

ability/literacy. Newspapers are checked prior to the group to ensure content does not breach individuals' confidentiality (as service users may occasionally appear in the newspaper regarding a court appearance) or trigger risk behaviour (such as a news story about paedophilia triggering a violent reaction from an individual who has delusions that those around him are paedophiles);

■ Cookery group – in which members make pizza together, for example, providing opportunities for assessment of occupational performance skills such as motivation, concentration, initiation, sequencing and social skills such as turn-taking.

BOX 26.3

GRADING A PIZZA-MAKING GROUP ACTIVITY IN A FORENSIC SERVICE

A pizza-making group can be graded in different ways to accommodate any functional level and multiple group members (see Chapter 15 on Client-Centred Groups). Someone who has disordered thoughts as part of their psychosis is likely to have their performance of this task significantly impacted.

The occupational therapist will use their knowledge of the individuals' performance capabilities and their own activity analysis skills to construct a session which will push and stretch the service user whilst ensuring the task in hand is achievable. This may involve having a pre-bought pizza base and jar of sauce and pre-prepared toppings on the basis that more choices could be overwhelming and confusing. This way the service user is presented with a much-simplified task but one that will still result in a cooked pizza to eat.

As the individual's performance level improves, the complexity of the task, the number of stages involved, length of time taken and the degree of problem-solving required can all be manipulated/engineered by the therapist to maintain a 'just right' challenge.

Assessment wards often run groups with an open invitation designed to encourage service users to attend. Attendance of these groups, level of engagement and occupational performance then inform the assessment process.

Standardized Assessments

As noted earlier, MOHO (Kielhofner 2008) offers a battery of standardized assessments, observational, self-report and interview schedules (Ozkan et al. 2018). In the authors' experience the model of human occupation screening tool (MOHOST) is a widely used assessment in forensic hospitals. It is primarily used to evaluate service users' occupational participation (Parkinson et al. 2008).

In the Occupational Circumstances Assessment Interview and Rating Scale (OCAIRS) (Forsyth et al. 2005), questions have been specifically formatted to be relevant to service users in forensic settings. This can be useful in identifying patterns of pro-social behaviour and routines which helped individuals to stay well and maintain a well-balanced lifestyle before they committed offences (Connell 2016).

Intervention

Forensic practice is characterized by a multidisciplinary, client-centred approach with a sharp focus on supporting service users' constructive use of leisure time, aiming to improve quality of life, prevent relapse and reduce re-offending (Connell 2016). A programme of therapeutic activities is provided throughout all categories of secure care, and this is often seen as a specialist occupational therapy role.

Occupational therapy staff support service users to rekindle old interests or develop new ones, accessing occupations on the hospital ward, in the hospital's therapy centre and in the community-such as arts and crafts, woodwork, do-it-yourself tasks cooking, metalwork, sports, educational interventions, swimming, bowling, snooker and others. The expansion of service users' occupational engagement beyond the ward is essential within a restricted institutional environment where individuality, identity and autonomy may be compromised.

Typically, in low secure hospitals occupational therapists support service users towards community-based activities by using a hospital-based therapy centre, which may include a gym, art/craft room, and a computer room. Medium secure hospitals will often have a larger therapy centre because service users have less community leave due to increased risk. Resources may include a gym hall, a wood/metal workshop, an art room, horticulture space, classroom space, and vocational areas such as a café where service users can work as volunteers. In high secure hospitals where community leave is very limited, there may also be a swimming pool and a well-equipped gym.

In all settings, care should be taken by the occupational therapist to present activity at a level that challenges the service user but is achievable. Self-esteem and motivation can be fragile in this client group, and early failure can be both personally damaging and undermining of ongoing occupational therapy input. Grading and pacing are particularly important from the perspective of leave entitlement (see later). For example, offering more occupational opportunities than can be accommodated within Section 17 leave limitations would be detrimental, fostering frustration which may increase risk.

Service Users' Leave

In England and Wales, Section 17 of the Mental Health Act (1983) allows the responsible clinician to grant a service user (detained under part two of the Act) leave of absence from the hospital. For individuals under part three, the Minister of Justice is responsible for this.

Some service users such as those in prisons or high secure (and sometimes medium secure) hospitals will have no leave during their inpatient stay. Where leave has been risk assessed as appropriate, this is based on service users' ability to cope in the community, their behaviour on leave and their adherence to leave protocols (such as whether or not an individual has ever absconded). Taking these factors into account, leave is often introduced in a graded sequence (see Table 26.2).

Occupational therapists are involved in collaborative care planning regarding leave, which may be designated for specific occupations, such as swimming, gym use, accessing community support groups, doing voluntary work, or food shopping, for example. Service users' leave is therefore of particular interest to occupational therapists as it enables them to support engagement in mainstream community-based occupations, fostering an individual's independence and self-reliance.

TABLE 26.2
Example of a Graded Sequence of Steps for Leave Entitlement

Step	Leave Entitlement
1.	No leave off the ward
2.	Escorted leave within the building, for example, to a shared communal area or to parts of the therapy department (but probably not to workshops, initially)
3.	Escorted leave within the hospital grounds, starting with several staff escorts, perhaps, but progressing to a single staff member who will carry a radio
4.	Unescorted hospital ground leave
5.	Escorted community leave in which the locality is carefully considered (e.g., there may be an exclusion zone in a specific area where the victim of their previous offence lives) and staff will carry a mobile phone
6.	Unescorted community leave

Escorting a service user on leave provides opportunities for assessing life skills (such as budgeting, road safety, social interaction and use of public transport) in their real-life context, using observation and conversation. This informs MDT assessment and discharge planning, including gauging what level of support and what type of accommodation might best meet the service users' needs.

Recovery-Focused Practice in Forensic Settings

When applying recovery principles, occupational therapists working in forensic settings are, arguably, faced with additional barriers compared with practitioners in other mental health settings. Clearly, many of the security and risk considerations highlighted so far in this chapter locate a great deal of control over service users' lives with the service provider, with obvious implications for individuals' sense of empowerment or otherwise. This may include denial of access to certain items on the ward and being denied leave to access the community.

An important aspect of the occupational therapist's role, therefore, is to maximize the control the service user has in all aspects of their care experience and to provide opportunities to practise this. A first step may involve supporting service users to access recovery colleges/centres, promoting coproduction or engaging input from peers with lived experience.

Recovery colleges/centres involve service users in the planning and delivery of activities (Leach 2015), often presenting these in terms of education and training as opposed to therapy. For example, in the United Kingdom Dorset Healthcare University NHS Foundation Trust (2017) state in their recovery education centre prospectus, 'our courses are educational they are not therapy. We aim through education and the sharing of experiences to increase understanding' (Dorset Healthcare University NHS Foundation Trust, p. 6). Supporting a service user to engage with these courses will be factored into care planning and may open up access to a wider range of activities; for instance, a ukelele group, yoga session or a work placement in the therapy centre cafe. Some forensic hospitals are also implementing these principles into their therapeutic activity programmes. At the Discovery Centre, a recovery college situated in Langdon Forensic Hospital in Devon, United Kingdom which provides medium, low, and open levels of security, 75% of the courses are coproduced, and forensic service users have successfully progressed from the centre into voluntary positions and as peer support trainers in the community following discharge (Devon Partnership NHS Trust, 2017).

Working collaboratively with service users and their family/carers is valued in forensic services because of a growing recognition that the subjective experience of social exclusion and stigma can be linked to offending (De Luca et al. 2018). Regarding coproduction, occupational therapists must remain mindful of how easy it can be to adopt a (presumed) 'expert' professional position when discussing healthcare services with end point service users and of the inequity of power dynamics that are often implicit in such conversations. Box 26.4 presents some strategy options for working in this way.

Engaging peers with 'lived experience' (which may be an experience of mental health problems, addiction, trauma, learning difficulties and/or criminogenic behaviour) to work with forensic service users can also be beneficial (Drennan and Wooldridge 2014). Their input can foster a degree of trust and respect from service users that staff struggle to achieve, so this resource (from within the forensic service or from the wider community) should not be overlooked. For example, a current or former service user may become involved

---

BOX 26.4
STRATEGIES FOR COPRODUCTION

- Define problems/challenges and potential solutions jointly with service users, carers, and staff.
- Irrespective of who initiates an activity, recognize and draw upon everyone's expertise, strengths and skills – these may not be apparent at the outset and may emerge during the process of engagement once trust and confidence grow between those involved.
- Identify and articulate what can change as a result of coproduction based on knowledge of what has worked and not worked previously.
- The focus of the coproductive project will help to determine who needs to be involved; ensure that this includes staff from a range of backgrounds as well as service users and carers.
- Take time to build positive, trusting relationships between all involved, especially if people have had negative experiences of involvement in the past.

National Development Team for Inclusion 2016 Strategies for Coproduction Office.

---

in co-facilitating a therapeutic group, such as an art group. Safeguarding will have to be considered, and the peer will need to understand and agree to uphold levels of confidentiality regarding the information shared by the group members.

Addressing Criminogenic Behaviour

One of the distinctive features of occupational therapy in forensic services is that the offending behaviour which brought the person into the criminal justice system is addressed. For example, occupational therapists' knowledge and skills in group work can lead them to contribute to specialised interventions (along with other MDT members), such as psycho-educational groups, and interventions targeted at addressing recidivism. This may include anger management, dual diagnosis work and the Violent Offender Treatment Programme.

Related to this specialised inter-disciplinary input, a key function of forensic services is to assist service users to develop and lead personally meaningful, purposeful lives and to develop a positive sense of identity. This can also help reduce the risk of recidivism on discharge and re-admission to services; aspirations which lend themselves well to occupational therapy (Cronin-Davis 2017). Similarly, a lack of structured, meaningful occupation can be a contributory factor in individuals' substance misuse (Wasmuth et al. 2014), and occupational therapists are well placed to address this problem.

Some service users' lives show a pattern of offending throughout, while others, who may have no previous offending history, commit a single offence coinciding with the onset of mental health problems. The former may have a history of challenges in meeting occupational demands and have limited life roles and life skills available to draw on, whereas the latter may have more successful engagement in a number of meaningful occupations, fulfilling a variety of enriching life roles. The occupational therapist will consider this when developing a care plan to address criminogenic behaviours.

Coupled with the intrinsic benefits of occupation-focused interventions (such as enhancing self-esteem, self-efficacy, social skills and problem-solving capacity) occupational therapy provides opportunities for pro-social behaviour modelling (see Pro-social Behaviour in Box 26.1) to foster the values and habits of good citizenship and empathy amongst service users. Certain activities can help discourage, replace and erode often deep-rooted anti-social propensities and behaviours (Connell 2016). In this way, occupational therapy may focus on a wide range of activities designed to address and overcome previous occupational alienation and deprivation, which may have led to index offences (Table 26.3).

Vocational Rehabilitation

In secure settings it is recommended that occupational therapists find out service users' attitudes towards paid employment at the earliest opportunity and that real work, supported employment or prevocational training opportunities should always be considered (Cronin Davis 2017).

Various vocational services models were examined and the merits of Individual Placement and Support (IPS) highlighted in Chapter 20. However, it can be difficult to adhere strictly to IPS principles in the restrictive environment of secure hospitals, given that service users may have limited access to the community or perhaps none at all initially. Providing vocational opportunities, such as in-house cafés and shops, which aim to create a work-like environment, are vital ways of allowing service users to explore the 'worker' role and develop pre-vocational skills.

For service users with Section 17 leave (see earlier), voluntary work is often considered. This can develop/maintain vocational skills, which may be transferrable to other settings. Voluntary work may be easier to set up than paid work, and voluntary settings are often accepting of volunteers with a mental health problem and/or criminal record. This also provides an opportunity for the individual to practise disclosure of their history and to demonstrate the pro-social behaviour noted earlier by helping other people. Voluntary work also offers flexibility of work pattern, builds CV content (including helping to account for gaps in work history during inpatient stays) and can be a useful source for references.

Discrimination, Employment and Disclosure

The occupational therapist is well placed to become the advocate for employment with the service user and within the wider MDT. Stigma and prejudice are significant barriers to people with long-term mental health problems obtaining employment (Boardman and Khan 2017), and this problem can be compounded by the fact that many mental health professionals do not see employment as a focus for their work and, when considering employment options, are pessimistic about individual's abilities to obtain and retain work (Boardman and Khan 2017).

Furthermore, discrimination remains an obstacle even after discharge from a secure hospital where an individual may have to adapt to their new identity (in society's eyes) of being an 'ex-offender'; a label that can act as a constant reminder of their criminal histories. Disclosure is therefore a challenging issue for service users, especially in relation to accessing the community. It is also potentially damaging to the emergence of a positive sense of identity associated with a personal recovery journey. Disclosure may be formal or informal.

Formal Disclosure. Secure hospitals may have their own formal procedures regarding service users accessing external work and education opportunities. These are created for the benefit of community partners, such as voluntary work providers (e.g., city farms) or colleges, to inform them of potential risks and risk management strategies, criminal histories, relapse indicators and contact details of service users being referred.

TABLE 26.3		
Addressing Recidivism Through Occupational Therapy Interventions		
Encouraging desistence from harmful/antisocial behaviours (e.g., drug/alcohol misuse)	■ Engaging service users in high adrenaline activities as alternatives to the 'highs' from substance abuse (e.g., rock climbing, biking, go-karting, zip wire, canoeing) ■ Supporting service users to develop new pro-social lifestyles and to structure their lives differently to avoid returning to previous habitual anti social routines and relationships ■ Developing constructive leisure time in the community post-discharge is a key element	
Supporting community transition and integration	■ Promoting confidence and competence in community activities (e.g., using public transport, road safety, banking, money management) ■ Supporting service users to join community groups (e.g., chess clubs, football/pool teams, community walking groups)	
Promoting pro-social roles, attitudes and behaviour; hospitals will make individual decisions about payment to service users who undertake these roles	■ Ward or hospital environmental enhancement projects such as creating a sensory area in the garden or re-decorating the therapy room ■ Service user training for first aid courses qualifications ■ Pro-social work roles for service users, such as: 　■ cleaning/conducting supervised car checks regarding maintaining hospital pool vehicles 　■ office skills groups in which service users engage in jobs (creating posters; typing notices, newsletters, and timetables; etc.) 　■ setting-up a hospital library managed by service users 　■ clothes projects: redistributing donated clothes to their peers 　■ local dog-walking schemes or animal husbandry projects in city farms, etc. 　■ developing an interest in the wider environment (e.g., engaging in local volunteer nature conservation and community enhancement projects)	
Developing life skills	■ Personal growth through education (e.g., literary, numeracy, computer skills) ■ Do-it-yourself groups to develop home maintenance skills (e.g., changing a light bulb, mending a fuse, putting up shelves, painting/decorating, unblocking sinks, hanging pictures) ■ Developing confidence in social situations (e.g., eating out, going bowling, visiting museums/art galleries and places of interest on leave)	
Developing empathy/understanding other people's perspectives	■ Inviting positive role models to visit the hospital (e.g., former service users, recovering addicts, people who have triumphed over other adversities) to talk to service users ■ Promoting understanding of diverse faiths (e.g., celebrating festivals, cooking culture-specific cuisine) ■ Raising money for nominated charities at fairs/fetes, focusing certain service user activities (e.g. arts, crafts, baking) on making items to sell	
Coproduction	■ Using service user's expertise through lived experience to fulfill meaningful roles as well as engage positively with the mental health system, whereas previously they may have been disengaged or at odds with it ■ Involving service users in: 　■ the staff recruitment interview process 　■ planning/running groups 　■ planning/running social events and sport competitions, etc.	

The UK's Rehabilitation of Offenders Act (1974) allows most convictions and all cautions, reprimands, and final warnings to be spent after a certain period. There is no legislation compelling the disclosure of information regarding mental health problems, but criminal convictions have to be disclosed. This, along with other areas of formal disclosure, can be daunting and should be explored with reference to the specifics of each individual and their context. Occupational therapists and other healthcare professionals who support/advise service users regarding spent convictions and disclosure in formal processes, such as filling in employment application forms, should seek professional advice from agencies such as the National Association for the Care and Rehabilitation of Offenders in the United Kingdom.

A helpful approach in formal disclosure may be to consider using a cover letter alongside a CV or application form. In this letter a service user may explain the context of their offence and how circumstances have changed (emphasizing how 'that was then, but this is now'). They may explain that they have 'recovered' and would appreciate a second chance; emphasizing their personal motivation to do the job and, perhaps, expressing their remorse and empathy.

Informal (Social) Disclosure. In the community, service users from secure settings may encounter personal questions from the people they casually meet who are naturally curious. In day-to-day social interactions service users may suddenly find themselves in conversations in which they feel compelled to reveal information about their mental health or criminal history. The occupational therapist may help the service user develop personal strategies to manage this, using debrief/reflection on real life situations, perhaps, or role play. Case Study 26.2 highlights disclosure issues that service users from secure hospitals may encounter in the community.

CASE STUDY 26.2
Alex

ADMISSION

Alex is a 23-year-old man convicted of grievous bodily harm after he attacked a friend with a knife, believing his friend had evil powers. Alex was not known to the mental health services at the time, and his index offence was deemed to have occurred in the context of psychosis and polysubstance misuse. After six months in prison Alex was given a diagnosis of paranoid schizophrenia and transferred to an admissions ward in a medium secure hospital for assessment and treatment under Sections 47 and 49 of the Mental Health Act (1983), which was later changed to a Section 37/41 detention order.

WARD OBSERVATIONS

On the rehabilitation ward, Alex made steady progress and was eventually granted ground and community leave (see Table 26.2), leading to short periods of unescorted ground leave. However, despite his attendance in the hospital's Narcotics Anonymous group, Alex tested positive in random urinary drug screening, (having seemingly obtained crack cocaine on the grounds on unescorted leave) and his leave was rescinded.

Following this setback, Alex continued to engage in his occupational therapy programme together with exploratory work into the origin and nature of his index offence (in music psychotherapy and psychology sessions). This resulted in Alex rebuilding trust with the multidisciplinary team and having his leave reinstated. This opportunity enabled him to study GCSE English and Maths at a local further education (FE) college. Alex's stated aspirations were to have a girlfriend, a flat and a job.

College attendance required liaison between his occupational therapist and college staff, adhering to the hospitals outside work and education policy and formal disclosure and risk management processes. Alex was informed and fully consented to this process.

Alex's course went well, and his attendance was good. However, during conversation with two fellow students (who Alex had befriended), Alex revealed that he was currently being detained in a forensic psychiatric hospital, despite guidance from his care team to be cautious in situations where social disclosure might occur. He was shocked when his college friend said, 'Are you telling us, you're a nutter?.' He was upset and stopped attending his course. Subsequently Alex obtained drugs, disengaged from hospital-based therapies, too, and appeared to lose hope and direction.

Gradually, Alex became more settled and after 9 months started working in the hospital café, run by the occupational therapy team and spoke about doing voluntary work in the community at a city farm. As part of the application/referral process, risk information was shared and Alex also wrote a cover letter. Role-playing scenarios related to social disclosure also helped Alex prepare for working at the farm. The placement went well, and Alex was eventually discharged into supported accommodations. An occupational therapy referral to an employment coach ultimately led to Alex getting paid for employment as a kitchen porter.

SERVICE USER COMMENTARY

During my time in prison, it was up to me to find my own thing to do, so, often, I went to the gym. But during my time in a high security hospital setting there has been a big involvement with occupational therapists. They always seem to take an interest in what you want to do, and this is a big motivator for me. I often take part in occupational therapy activities such as cooking, playing games and crafts, and I have learnt I can't function properly without a structure, so it's really important for me to have things to do.

By taking part in occupational therapy assessment groups, I have carried out a number of different activities and learnt new skills. Recently, I have started to sew patchwork, with the aim of creating a cushion. The occupational therapists are good because they motivate you but don't push you too far. I have learnt, for example, that I can only cope with doing a vocational activity for a short period of time. During these assessment groups I have often spent half an hour sewing and then chosen to play a board game such as Scrabble. I like that the therapist encourages me to do this, recognizing my preferences.

The occupational therapists have also referred me to other areas within the hospital. I have enjoyed attending music sessions where I have learnt how to read and write music. They have also referred me to work in the shop and the café, which also gives me structure to my week. I find it really important for my mental health to know what I am doing each week.

There was also an occupational therapy team in the medium secure setting I attended. The difference was that, here, you were encouraged to make your own structured plan of activities to do throughout the week, though you were not left on your own. There was always something to do, even at the weekends, which helped too, and there were often game days or social functions that were held on the ward. I cooked ward meals sometimes and attended game competitions. You could always get involved, which was great. The occupational therapists weren't involved as much in these activities, but they always showed their faces every day and were always interested. There was frequently the opportunity to join occupational therapy groups. Also, in the medium secure setting, the occupational therapists could refer you for trial leave, which was always my aim.

Overall the occupational therapy interventions I have received in both medium and high secure settings have definitely benefitted me. They were very motivating and flexible, which is important to me. I never thought I would say, 'I enjoyed sewing.' I have nothing bad to say about occupational therapists.

Mark Booth

CONCLUSION

This chapter has considered what forensic mental health means and outlined its evolution as a distinctive field of practice. It has presented various types of forensic service, exploring different levels of security and the implications this has for occupation-focused practice. The occupational therapy process has been traced with particular reference to positive risk management, rehabilitation and recovery, using two case studies (Colin and Alex) as illustrative examples of how occupational therapists work.

In the previous edition of this book it was suggested that referring to practitioners as 'forensic occupational therapists' was somewhat misleading, as it implied that occupational therapists working in this field somehow employed a unique skill-set. Whilst this chapter has highlighted the relevance of core occupational therapy skills to forensic practice and the elements it shares with mental health work generally, the authors would argue that the emphasis placed on addressing criminogenic behaviour and reoffending remains a distinctive feature for occupational therapists working in secure hospitals and prisons.

ACKNOWLEDGEMENTS

The authors gratefully acknowledge the assistance and advice of the following colleagues:

- Julie Mills, Occupational Therapist
- Rebecca Knight, Occupational Therapy Team Leader
- Naomi Morgan, Occupational Therapist
- Elizabeth O'Mahony, Consultant Psychiatrist
- Rachel Wiltshire, Team Administrator
- Seamus O'Reilly, Registered Mental Nurse and Clinical Security Lead

QUESTIONS FOR CONSIDERATION

1. What challenges may an individual face on discharge from secure services as they start to re-integrate back into society?
2. Are you aware of any high-profile offences that resulted in a service user accessing some kind of secure service and which received media coverage? What issues did the media coverage or public debate raise?
3. What precautions or considerations should an occupational therapist make when working with prisoners for their own health and safety as well as the service users?
4. Introducing sharp utensils to an occupation may be part of positive risk taking; how can it benefit an offending service user, especially when their index offense may have involved a knife or weapon?
5. How might you explain the hospital ward system to Colin (see Case Study 26.1) or to his friends and family that is reassuring, avoids jargon, and links his issues to a recovery-orientated intervention plan?
6. What possible assessment tools might an occupational therapist use to determine whether leave could be suitable for an individual?
7. Research which employers have consistently supported the employment of ex-offenders and consider the occupations which users of secure services may find most beneficial in developing their own vocational skills.
8. What kind of guidance (if any) should be given to the public (such as the local FE college in Case Study 26.2) about forensic psychiatric detainees and leave?

Acknowledgments

Steve Taylor retired shortly after completing the work on this chapter and sadly passed away before publication. We were pleased and privileged to coauthor this chapter with him.

REFERENCES

Boardman, J., & Khan, M. (2017). Employment and mental health. *Occasional paper OP101*. London: Royal College of Psychiatrists.

Boer, D. P., Hart, S. D., Kropp, P. R., & Webster, C. D. (2018). *Manual for the sexual violence risk–20 v2: Professional guidelines for assessing risk of sexual violence*. Vancouver: Mental Health, Law, and Policy Institute.

Chia-Wei, F., Morley, M., Graham, M., Henseman, D., & Taylor, R. (2016). Examining changes in occupational participation in forensic patients using the MHOST. *British Journal of Occupational Therapy*, 79(12), 727–733.

Connell, C. (2016). Forensic occupational therapy to reduce the risk of reoffending: A survey of practice in the United Kingdom. *The Journal of Forensic Psychiatry & Psychology*, 27(6), 907–928.

Connor, D., Edworthy, E., Holley, J., et al. (2017). A mixed-method study exploring the characteristics and needs of long-stay patients in high and medium security settings in England: Implications for secure organisation. *Health Service and Delivery Research*, 15, 11 NIHR Journals Library, Southampton (UK).

Cordingley, K. (2015). *How do occupational therapists practising in forensic mental health know?* PhD thesis submitted. London:

Department of Social Sciences, Media and Communications. Brunel University.

Cronin-Davis, J. (2017). Forensic mental health: Creating occupational opportunities. In *Occupational therapy evidence in practice for mental health* (2nd ed.) (pp. 139–163). Oxford: Willey-Blackwell.

Curran, A., & Wilkinson, C. (2010). *Development of regional forensic mental health occupational therapy services*. Belfast: Northern Ireland OT Managers Forum.

Davies, S., Clarke, M., Hollin, C., & Duggan, C. (2007). Long-term outcomes after discharge from medium secure settings; a cause for concern. *British Journal of Psychiatry*, 191, 70–74.

De Luca, J., Mulay, A., O'Donovan, K., & West, M. (2018). Forensic psychiatric experiences, stigma and self concept: A mixed method. *The Journal of Forensic Psychiatry & Psychology*. https://doi.org/10.1010/8014789949.2018.1425.473.

Department of Health (DH). (2010). *Your Guide to Relational Security: See, Think, Act*. London: UK Gov/DH. Available at: https://assets.publishing.service.gov.uk/government/uploads/system/uploads/attachment_data/file/320249/See_Think_Act_2010.pdf.

Devon Partnership NHS Trust. (2017). *The Discovery centre (recovery college based at Langdon hospital) – Devon partnership NHS trust*. Available at: http://positivepracticemhdirectory.org/adults/discovery-centre-recovery-college-based-langdon-hospital-devon-partnership-nhs-trust/.

de Witt, P. (2005). Creative ability: A model for psychosocial occupational therapy. In R. Crouch, & V. Alers (Eds.), *2005. Occupational therapy in psychiatry and mental health* (4th ed.) (pp. 20–53) London.

Dorset HealthCare University NHS Foundation Trust. (2017). *Recovery education centre prospectus.* Available at: https://www. dorsethealthcare.nhs.uk/application/files/5214/9881/9242/ Annual_Prospectus_2016_2017.pdf.

Douglas, K. S., Hart, S. D., Webster, C. D., & Belfrage, H. (2013). *HCR-20V3: Assessing risk of violence – user guide.* Burnaby, Canada: Mental Health, Law, and Policy Institute, Simon Fraser University.

Drennan, G., & Alre, D. (Eds.). (2012). *Secure recovery: Approaches to recovery in forensic mental health settings.* London: Routledge.

Drennan, G., & Wooldridge, J. (2014). Making recovery a reality in a forensic setting. In *Implementing Recovery through Organisational Change (IMROC). 4*th *Annual conference presentation. (Realities and possibilities for recovery focused practice in secure settings).* Centre for Mental Health Network NHS Confederation.

Duncan, E. A. S. (2008). Forensic occupational therapy. In J. Creek, & L. Lougher (Eds.), *Occupational therapy and mental health* (forth ed.) (pp. 514–535). Edinburgh: Churchill Livingstone.

Forsyth, K., Deshpande, S., Kielhofner, G., et al. (2005). *The Occupational Circumstances Assessment Interview and Rating Scale (OCAIRS) version 4.0.* Chicago, IL: Model of Human Occupation Clearinghouse.

Information Commissioners Office. (2008). *Annual report 2007/2008.* London: House of Commons. The stationery office.

Judges, R. (2016). A critique of historical clinical risk – 20, version 3, risk and assessment instrument. *The Journal of Forensic Psychology Practice, 16*(4), 304–320.

Kielhofner, G. (2008). *Model of human occupation: Theory and application* (4th ed.). Baltimore: Lippincott, Williams and Wilkins.

Leach, J. (2015). *Five things you might like to know about recovery colleges.*

Leadley, S. (2015). The Kawa model: Informing the development of a culturally sensitive, occupational therapy assessment tool in Aotearoa- New Zealand. *New Zealand Association of Occupational Therapists, 62*(2), 48–53.

Lovemore, D. (2011). Making best use of limited options. *Occupational Therapy News, 19*(1), 24.

Maden, T. (2007). *Treating violence: A guide to risk management in mental health.* Oxford: Oxford University Press.

McNeill, S., & Bannigan, K. (2014). Forensic and prison services. In J. Creek, & L. Lougher (Eds.), *Occupational therapy and mental health* (5th ed.) (pp. 424–438). Edinburgh: Churchill Livingstone.

Mullen, P. E. (2000). Forensic Mental Health. *British Journal of Psychiatry, 176*(4), 307–311.

Munoz, P., Moreton, E., & Audra, M. (2016). The Scope of practice of occupational therapy in US. Criminal justice settings. *Occupational Therapy International, 23*(3), 241–254. https://doi. org/10.1002/Oti1427.

National Development Team for Inclusion. (2016). *Strategies for coproduction office.* Available at: ndti.org.uk.

NHS England. (2019). *National liaison and diversion service specification.* NHS England.

Royal College of Occupational Therapists (RCOT). (2017). Occupational Therapist's Use of occupation-focused practice in secure hospitals: practice guideline (2nd ed.). London: Royal College of Occupational Therapists.

Open University. Available at: https://www.open.edu/openlearn/ health-sports-psychology/health/health-studies/mental-health/ five-things-you-might-know-about-recovery-colleges.

Ozkan, E., Belhan, S., Yaran, M., & Zarif, M. (2018). Occupational therapy in forensic settings. Occupational therapy – therapeutic and creative use of activity. *Meral Huri, Itechopen,* 51–70. https://doi.org/10.5772/Intechopen.79366.

Parkinson, S., Chester, A., Cratchley, S., & Rowbottom, J. (2008). Application of the model of human occupation screening tool (MOHOST) in an acute psychiatric setting. *Occupational Therapy in Health Care, 22*(2–3), 63–75. https://doi. org/10.10800738057801989465.

Pilgrim, D. (Ed.). (2007). *Inside ashworth.* Professional Reflections of Taylor and Francis Ltd.

Seppanen, A., Tormanen, L., Shaw, C., & Kennedy, H. (2018). Modern forensic psychiatry hospital design: Clinical, legal and structural aspects. *International Journal of Mental Health Systems, 12,* 58. https://doi.org/10.1186/s13033-01800238-7.

Sherwood, W., White, B., & Wilson, S. (2015). *The vona du Toit model of creative ability: A practical guide for acute mental health occupational therapy practice.* London: Vona du Toit Model of Creative Ability Foundation.

Soothill, K., Rogers, P., & Dolan, M. (2008). *Handbook of forensic mental health.* Devon: Willan publishing.

Sustere, E., & Tarpey, E. (2019). Least restrictive practice: Its role in patient independence and recovery. *The Journal of Forensic Psychiatry & Psychology, 30*(4), 614–629.

The College of Occupational Therapists. (2012). *Scottish prison service: Women in custody – a consultation response from the college of occupational therapists.*

Townsend, E. A., & Polatajko, H. J. (2007). *Enabling occupation II: Advancing an occupational therapy vision for health, well-being and justice through occupation.* Ottawa, ON: CAOT Publications ACE.

Wasmuth, S., Crabtree, J. L., & Scott, P. J. (2014). Exploring addiction-as-occupation. *British Journal of Occupational Therapy, 77,* 605–615.

West London NHS Trust. (2018). *Winter 2018 @ West London (West London NHS trust).* Available at: https://www.westlondon. nhs.uk/wp-content/uploads/2018/12/@WL-Winter-2018- Interactive.pdf.

Whiteford, G., Jones, K., Weekes, G., et al. (2020). Combatting occupational deprivation and advancing occupational justice in institutional settings: Using a practice-based enquiry approach for service transformation. *British Journal of Occupational Therapy, 83*(1), 52–61.

World Health Organization (WHO). (1998). *The WHO health promotion Glossary.* Geneva: WHO.

27 SUBSTANCE USE

JENNY LANCASTER ■ CLEMENT NHUNZVI ■ ROSHAN GALVAAN

CHAPTER OUTLINE

INTRODUCTION

According to the 2020 World Drug Report (United Nations (UN) 2020) it is estimated that 35.6 million people worldwide use drugs to an extent that requires treatment; yet, only one in eight suffering from drug disorders received treatment. Occupational therapists in all fields of practice are likely to meet service users who have challenges with substance use. This chapter is a starting point for occupational therapists who focus on or encounter people with substance use disorders (SUDs) during their practice. It focuses on the nature and extent of substance use, offering an occupational perspective to some of the reasons why people use substances and the challenges that individuals may experience as a consequence. The occupational therapy process is also outlined, with the role of the therapist highlighted. Clinical and recovery-oriented approaches in occupational therapy are described.

Defining Substance Use Disorders

The American Psychiatric Association's (2013) Diagnostic and Statistical Manual of Mental Disorders, 5th ed. (DSM-5) identifies two categories of substance-related disorders. These are Substance Use Disorders (SUDs) and substance-induced disorders. This chapter focuses on substance use disorders and their impact on occupational performance. SUDs are defined as a problematic pattern of substance use resulting in clinically significant impairment and distress, largely evident as health concerns, disability and occupational dysfunction. A diagnosis of SUD is based on risky or impulsive use of the substance in question, social impairment, impaired self-control and presence of biological markers (American Psychiatric Association 2013). The level of severity of SUD is usually based on the number of diagnostic criteria a person meets and is described as mild, moderate or severe. The category of substance(s) used includes alcohol, tobacco, cannabis, hallucinogens, opioids, among others. The most diagnosed SUD varies globally by region (UN 2020).

Four key concepts to understand when working with people with substance dependence include:

Tolerance: This is when the user has developed largely a neurobiological need to use an increased amount of the substance of choice to achieve the same desired effect as with a lower dose in the past. It can also be a case of the same amount of a substance being used now having less of an effect.

Intoxication: A reversible substance-specific syndrome following a recent ingestion of a substance (American Psychiatric Association 2013) that is usually seen as behavioural/psychological changes secondary to effects of the substance on the central nervous system. The changes can present as perceptual disturbances, neurocognitive impairments and disturbances in psychomotor behaviour and interpersonal behaviour. The other key criterion is that the disturbances should not be due to another medical condition.

Craving: A strong desire or urge to use a substance, sometimes so great that the person cannot think about or do anything else.

Withdrawal: A syndrome with clear evidence of recent cessation or reduction of substance use after usually chronic, pathological use of the substance in very high doses. The withdrawal state can further be specified according to a particular substance and its known features of withdrawal. Symptoms and signs should not be accounted for by other medical conditions present.

Historical and Cultural Context

Patterns of substance use are constantly changing with the emergence of new substances such as fentanyl and synthetic cannabinoids. The harmful use of psychoactive substances includes the use of alcohol, illicit drugs and the hazardous use of medication. For example, in Zimbabwe and South Africa the abuse of codeine-containing cough syrups is common. Such drugs are often also used to make drug concoctions (Zimbabwe Civil Liberties and Drug Network (ZCLDN) 2018). In addition, patterns of substance use are influenced by drug trading routes. For example, Africa is moving from being a passage for cocaine and heroin distribution to also being a consumer (World Health Organization (WHO) Regional Office for Africa 2017). Patterns of substance use are mediated by factors such as age, gender, socio-economic group and culture. Similarly, different regions and groups have had different histories of substance use across the world (UN 2020).

The use of addictive substances has been entwined with human occupation throughout humankind's history. Archaeological evidence exists for the use of alcohol in ancient Egypt from as early as 6000 BC (Nunn 1996). In Britain in the 17th century, due to the lack of drinking water, beer and gin were commonly drunk by the whole population throughout the day, starting at breakfast (Tyler 1995; Allen 2001). One-third of England's farmland was devoted to growing barley for beer, and one in seven buildings was a tavern. In the second half of the century 2000 coffee houses sprang up in London. This had a sobering effect on the population. Instead of getting drunk in taverns, coffee houses provided a safe place to read, play games and engage in political debate. Indeed, the first ballot box was used in the Turk's Head Coffee House in London. This change from the use of a depressant substance (alcohol) to a stimulant (caffeine in coffee) has been associated with increased literacy, political change, and improved standards of living (Allen 2001). However, during the Industrial Revolution alcohol use dramatically increased in response to changes in the occupational lives of workers—toiling in factories and mines—and increasing urbanization (Tyler 1995).

The establishment of a slave society in the Cape colony in South Africa draws attention to the pervasive influence of colonization on substance abuse. The 'dop (tot) system' was introduced in the Cape Winelands in the 1650s and remained lawful into the late 1800s. This system involved providing slaves, working as farm labourers, with alcohol as full or partial remuneration

(Williams 2016). These wine rations were usually given at regular intervals during the day. This and similar practices continued even after the abolition of slave trade with the consequences still reflected in the statistic that South Africa has the highest prevalence of foetal alcohol spectrum disorders worldwide (Olivier et al. 2016) and a high prevalence of binge drinking in the farmworker community in the Cape (Lesch and Adams 2016). The influences of colonization and substance use are intergenerational and evident in the lives of many young children (Cloete and Ramaugondo 2015).

SUBSTANCE USE

The chronic and/or pathological use of substances often leads to substance-related disorders (APA 2013). Substances that are commonly misused or abused may be legal (e.g., over-the-counter or prescription medication) or illegal (e.g., cocaine) and are subject to restrictions according to age, culture, and varying legislatures in different countries. Substance use can lead to social, psychological, physical or legal problems, mostly related to intoxication or regular excessive consumption and/or dependence (National Treatment Agency for Substance Misuse 2002). These negative consequences not only affect the individual, but also their family and community members. The effects may be related to emerging health, social, cultural, spiritual, family, economic and political problems. The economic and societal costs of substance abuse have been recognized in that it may lead to income poverty, but also is often used as a means of coping when relative poverty exists. The health and social consequences of commonly used substances are comprehensively summarized in *A Summary of the Health Harms of Drugs* (Department of Health (DH) 2011).

Frequently, people develop substance use problems in an attempt to deal with problems in their lives such as the breakdown of a relationship, unemployment or mental health problems. Contexts with few economic and further opportunities for participation are recognized as places where substance use is prevalent. Examining the relationship between the individual and the environment in relation to their occupations is a core component of occupational therapy. When working with service users using substances, occupational therapists consider how the substance use (or abstinence from a previously habitually used substance) affects a person's occupations. For example, an individual's alcohol consumption may increase due to changes in their work environment, or an ex-heroin user who, having given up a large network of drug-using friends, may feel they do not have the confidence to engage in new leisure activities alone.

Substance misuse has been described as a chronically relapsing condition (NTA 2002). Research indicates high relapse rates (40% to 60%) following an episode of substance misuse treatment (National Institute on Drug Abuse 2020). There is evidence for the effectiveness of some substance use treatments like the Alcoholics Anonymous (AA) and other 12 step facilitation programmes for alcohol use disorder (Kelly et al. 2020). Conversely, there is no high-quality evidence to support other interventions, for example, cognitive behavioural therapy (CBT) for amphetamine-type stimulant use disorders (Harada et al. 2018).

Effects of Substance Abuse on the Person

Alcohol and drugs act on specific centres of the brain, leading to physiological changes which may be temporary or permanent. These changes in turn may affect occupational performance. For example, opiates (such as heroin) act on the opiate receptor in areas of the brain such as the limbic system, specifically the nucleus accumbens and the ventral tegmentum (Carter 1998). Changing the state of these receptors by using drugs creates pleasurable experiences. Alcohol has a variety of complex actions but is generally a nervous system depressant. The reason alcohol appears to produce euphoria is that it depresses frontal cortex functioning, resulting in loss of inhibition.

Dopamine Theory of Addiction

Many drugs are known to act on the dopamine system (Solinas et al. 2019). Dopamine is a chemical messenger which plays an important role in the brain's reward centre. It is released when we do pleasurable things, such as eating good food or having sex. Drugs such as cocaine and heroin cause a massive surge of dopamine to be released, creating the sensation of pleasure. Over time, repeated drug use can lead to dopamine receptor sites in the brain being reduced or shut down (Solinas et al. 2019). Therefore the drug user finds less effect from using a drug, which leads to an increase in the amount used. The other significant effect is that the drug user may experience a decreased ability to feel pleasure or satisfaction in activities of daily life (Whitten 2009). This can lead to further drug use or thrill-seeking activities. Service users who have recently stopped using drugs and have reduced dopamine levels may struggle to feel satisfaction from their participation in occupations.

Alcohol-Related Brain Damage

Alcohol-related brain damage (ARBD) is an umbrella term that covers the various cognitive and psychoneurological conditions that are associated with long-term alcohol misuse and related vitamin deficiencies (Royal College of Psychiatry 2014). ARBD includes a wide range of conditions, some related directly to the effects on long-term heavy alcohol on the brain and others more indirectly, for example, as a consequence of poor diet and traumatic brain injury through falls and fights whilst intoxicated.

ARBD is associated with cognitive memory problems such as short-term memory loss, poor concentration, difficulty processing new information, confabulation, apathy and depression and physical problems such as poor balance and coordination, a shuffling gait and numbness and pins and needles in the limbs due to peripheral neuropathy (Alcohol Concern 2014).

However, if people can sustain abstinence from alcohol, there is hope for recovery. Broadly, 25% make a complete recovery, 25% make a significant recovery, 25% make a slight recovery and 25% make no recovery (Smith and Hillman 1999). Recovery can occur in the first two years of abstinence (Cox et al. 2004 cited in Alcohol Concern 2014).

The potential role of rehabilitation and occupational therapy with this client group is significant. As Alcohol Concern (2014) points out 'research suggests that recovery is enhanced by developing a rehabilitation programme specific and relevant to each patient, helping them to acquire (or regain) the skills they need to manage their own lives and their own environment' (Alcohol Concern 2014, p. 11). For example, occupational therapists can support clients to practise memory management techniques in activities of daily living (ADLs) and engage in meaningful occupations.

New Psychoactive Substances

Over recent years a new trend for the use of novel psychoactive substances has emerged. These are new substances designed to replicate the effects of an illegal substance whilst remaining legal. Hence the term sometimes used as 'legal highs.' However, as quickly as drugs are identified and prohibited, new substances are being developed. Between 2009 and 2016, 739 new drugs were reported (UN 2017). This means that the potential harms of these newly synthesized drugs are poorly understood. Despite the continual changes in the synthetically produced drug market, the increasing use of synthetic cannabinoids or 'synthetic cannabinoid receptor agonists' often known as 'spice,' are causing particular concern amongst many communities, in particular amongst the UK prison community (Abdulrahim and Bowden-Jones 2016; Ralph et al. 2017). Although the harms and effects of these types of substance are still being understood, it is complicated by the fact that the active ingredients are often unlisted and therefore unknown by the user. Use of spice or synthetic cannabinoid is associated with psychotic symptoms, tremor, and ataxia. Users, however, report feelings of euphoria and relaxation (Rassoul 2011; Spaderna et al. 2013).

Occupational Performance Disruptions from Substance Use

Substance use consequences are diverse and include biological, psychological, and social areas of a person or the family's life (Nordfjern et al. 2010; APA 2013). The occupational performance and identity of the user, the family and society are all affected by substance use, making them primary focus areas in occupational therapy and recovery (Martin et al. 2008; Bell et al. 2015; Duncan et al. 2020).

Usually, the valuable roles, tasks, habits and activities which allow meaningful use of time and resources are lost as substance use takes the organizing place in a person's life. This disruption in occupational performance will consequently give rise to ill-health and social problems (Helbig and McKay 2003; Nhunzvi et al. 2019). Substance use may affect a person's occupational performance through neglect and diminished engagement in socially valued and meaningful occupations such as schooling, work, and self-care. People also experience loss of life skills and diminished satisfaction with life roles with the quality of performance in occupations negatively affected (Peloquin and Ciro 2013; Stone 2017; Nhunzvi et al. 2019). Leisure and free time use are another challenge for people with SUD since the contexts of these occupations are where intoxicating substances are most commonly used. Many people who have become dependent on substances will have little or no awareness of leisure activities other than those that involve substance use.

Substance use is closely tied to human occupational behaviour. Some of the reasons for substance use can be categorized under the headings below, but it is important to note that each individual drug user will have their own specific reasons for taking drugs.

- Enabling occupation: by reducing tension, removing inhibition, stimulating mental alertness, or through imitating others' drug use;
- Avoiding occupation: through intoxication, stimulus seeking, denial of responsibility or through escape into drug culture;
- As a coping mechanism: to counter anxiety, relieve pain, mask distress, increase confidence and peer acceptance or as self-medication for mental health problems;
- To alter perception: to develop a wider understanding of life, for desired spiritual attainment, as part of a religious ritual, to assist creativity, to enjoy drug-induced perception;
- To develop meaning in life: through the ritual and habits of drug-taking behaviour, the routine of obtaining drugs or drug-dealing, the excitement of illegal activities, or through interacting and sharing a culture with associates in a drug-using network;
- To enhance occupations: by celebrating positive events, enhancing good feelings, or removing negative emotional states;
- To manage occupational risk factors: to cope with occupational deprivation and/or boredom ('killing time') or coping with occupational imbalance such as the pressure of too many demands on one's time.

Transition into Recovery

There is a novel body of knowledge emerging in occupational science and occupational therapy, conceptualizing substance use as an occupation with both negative and positive outcomes (Kiepek and Magalhaes 2011; Wasmuth et al. 2014; Nhunzvi et al. 2019). A study conducted in Zimbabwe by Nhunzvi and colleagues (2019) to explore the recovery journeys from substance abuse among young adults suggested that substance use/abuse could be viewed and experienced as an occupation with meaning and purpose in its own right. Similarly, in a study with pregnant mothers in South Africa, alcohol consumption was experienced as an occupation that was perpetuated through intergenerational poverty (Cloete and Ramugondo 2015). Since substance use may be experienced as an occupation in and of itself, recovery from substance abuse should be viewed from an occupational perspective. The change process during recovery from substance use can best be understood as an occupational transition which involves abandoning and modifying substance abuse occupations followed by the adoption of contextual and adaptive occupations (Nhunzvi et al. 2019). Adapting and rebuilding one's occupational identity from a life dominated by substance use is primary in this transitioning into recovery.

The term 'recovery' in the field of addiction generally has a different meaning to the way it is used in general mental health practice, and it remains a controversial term according to different treatment approaches. According to the 12 step approaches, there is an emphasis on defining oneself as being 'in recovery' or as 'a recovering addict' once one has become completely abstinent from *all* drugs and alcohol. The UK Drug Policy Commission (UKDPC 2008) created a description of recovery, drawing on different approaches to addiction and the model of recovery in mental health: the process of recovery from problematic substance use is characterized by voluntary control over substance use which maximizes well-being and participation in the rights, roles and responsibilities of society (UKDPC 2008). The notion of someone with controlled substance use being 'in recovery' is likely to be considered an anathema from a 12 step perspective.

DUAL DIAGNOSIS

Dual diagnosis is defined by WHO as comorbidity or the cooccurrence in the same individual of a psychoactive SUD and another psychiatric disorder (WHO 2020). However, it is important to acknowledge that many people have multiple and complex needs, for example, physical health needs and homelessness (Turning Point 2016; DH 2017). Mental health problems may be induced by drug use or drugs can be used to self-medicate the symptoms (Findings 2020). When alcohol and drugs are used by people with mental health problems, they can severely exacerbate symptoms and disrupt treatment. Mental health problems are experienced by most people in treatment for drug or alcohol problems, and this is associated with poorer outcomes (Public Health England (PHE) 2017). However, despite this knowledge, those with dual diagnosis who are often excluded from treatment many have unmet needs. To address this, approaches such as 'Everyone's job' and 'No wrong door' are being promoted (PHE 2017). Traditional treatment has been 'sequential' (e.g., treatment for alcohol dependence followed by mental health). However, given the increasingly recognized reciprocal relationship between mental health and substance misuse, a more integrated approach is now advocated (PHE 2017). Thankfully, this approach sits well with occupational therapy with the focus on occupation as opposed to symptoms. Occupational therapy literature has focused on occupational needs and engagement with this client group, examining issues such as leisure participation (Hodgson et al. 2001; Roy et al. 2017).

TREATMENT OF SUBSTANCE USE

Drug and alcohol treatment services are operated by health and social services, prisons, private clinics and the voluntary (non-profit) sector. People with alcohol and drug problems are frequently referred for treatment by their general practitioner, self-refer or are referred after a substance-related physical problem is identified, such as in A&E. Others are referred from within the criminal justice systems. Some referrals come from employers or employee assistance programmes. Treatment settings include hospital and community locations, and treatment can commence in either of these.

Entry into treatment is usually triggered by a crisis. For example, an individual is caught committing burglary to fund a growing crack cocaine habit or loses his or her job after work performance suffers due to heavy drinking. This can provide a window of opportunity to encourage engagement in treatment. Consequently, treatment services often target crises for this reason. For example, specialist alcohol nurses may assess people attending A&E services, or drug users may be assessed while in police custody or in the criminal justice system.

The earliest papers describing occupational therapy with people addicted to alcohol highlight areas of concern similar to those identified within modern evidence-based practice. For example, Hossack (1952, cited by Rotert 1989) highlighted the reduction in former interests, activities and social connections; difficulty concentrating; tension and family problems and suggested that the individual must aim to develop a more fully rounded life with a balance of activity. Doniger (1953, cited by Rotert 1989) suggested unpredictability, elusiveness, relationships, leisure and motivation as areas for concern. The issues raised by these two pioneers of occupational therapy in the field of addiction remain fundamental to the occupational therapy/addiction knowledge base.

Occupational therapy can have a significant impact on enabling people to develop meaningful occupations, routines and skills that support abstinence and recovery and reduce the risk of relapse. Substance dependence has an inherently occupational basis since people spend a great deal of time on the activities necessary to obtain the substance, use the substance, and then recover from its effects. In addition, substance dependence leads to the reduction or giving up of important social, work or leisure activities (American Psychiatric Association 1994). Many people with substance misuse problems, after being completely focused on their drug/alcohol use, experience a vacuum in their day-to-day lives when they become abstinent or engage in treatment. This can leave them feeling de-skilled, vulnerable and bored. Occupational therapy can help people to develop skills and coping strategies, as well as a more satisfying, balanced lifestyle. McIntosh and McKeganey (2000) found that it was not enough for ex-users to 'keep busy,' but that finding purposeful, meaningful and rewarding activities, which restored personal identity and fostered positive life roles, was essential.

Some of the issues occupational therapy can address may be categorized under the three occupational performance areas: work, self-care and leisure. However, these are not entirely separate domains and may all be addressed simultaneously through engagement in meaningful occupation.

ASSESSMENT

Multidisciplinary Assessments

Assessment of an individual needs to be tailored, needs-led and part of an ongoing process (NTA 2002). Many guidelines stress the importance of expressing empathy and a non-judgmental manner (DH et al. 2007; National Institute for Health and Care Excellence (NICE; 2011), recognizing both the stigma that service users feel as well as ambivalence about change that is common at the beginning of treatment. A number of assessment techniques may be used, including screening assessments, structured questionnaires, interviews, risk assessment, observation (including for signs of physical withdrawal) and physiological assessments (e.g., urine and blood analysis, electrocardiogram).

Screening Assessments

A number of screening assessments are available. For alcohol, NICE recommends the Alcohol Use Disorders Identification Test (NICE 2011). Health and social care professionals should be competent to identify harmful drinking and alcohol dependence and competent to initially assess the need for an intervention (NICE 2011). For opiate misuse, it is important to screen for withdrawal symptoms (Edwards 1987) using assessments such as the Clinical Opiate Withdrawal Scale (Wesson 2003). Many clinical guidelines stress the importance of a comprehensive assessment across many domains as cornerstone of successful treatment (DH 2017). Table 27.1 lists common screening tools.

Structured Questionnaires and Interviews

Structured questionnaires aim to investigate the severity of dependence, the range and complexity of problems associated with substance use (including the effects of drug-using behaviour on dependent children) and motivation to engage in treatment or to change substance use behaviour. Interviews should also cover the number of different drugs used, the amount used, a typical day of use and a history of use, including the first drug use occasion and changes in use over time. There may also be assessment of anxiety or depression.

Occupational Therapy Assessment

Focus of Assessment

All categories of occupation, such as ADLs, leisure, self-maintenance and work/productivity, can be affected by substance use. As described earlier, occupational therapists are concerned that substance dependence disrupts the balance of work, self-care and leisure (Rotert 1989; Chacksfield 1994; Morgan 1994; Martin et al. 2008). Quantitative research by occupational therapists such as Mann and Talty (1990), Scaffa (1991), Stoffel et al. (1992) and Chacksfield and Lindsay (1999) has highlighted use of leisure time by alcohol-dependent service users as a key problem area. Work and productive occupations are also known to be negatively affected by substance abuse.

Successful engagement in all performance areas requires abilities in terms of sensorimotor, cognitive, psychosocial and psychological components. Drug action can have both short- and long-term effects on performance components. Occupational therapy research has suggested that low motivation and low self-esteem are significant in substance misusers (Viik et al. 1990; Stoffel et al. 1992). Research by Martin et al. (2008) with homeless substance misusers admitted to a residential recovery programme explored performance capacity issues, as well as their impact on quality of life, using a variety of ratings, including the Occupational Performance History Interview II (OPHI-II) (Kielhofner 2008). Positive changes in occupational competence (based on OPHI-II scores) were associated with recovery at the six-month follow-up after a dip in scores at three months, which the authors attributed to the impact of the environment. The research appears to suggest that occupational competence is a key factor in recovery from addiction.

Research into cue exposure (Drummond et al. 1995) shows that environmental cues can trigger addictive behaviour in individuals. Someone returning to an alcohol- or drug-orientated environment on discharge is likely to re-experience the same cues as before and may relapse back into substance use without developing coping strategies to counteract the environmental effects.

TABLE 27.1
Common Screening Tools

Tool	Patient Population	Substance Type	How it Is Administered	Number of Items	Time it Takes	Availability
CAGE (Cut down, Annoyed, Guilty, Eye opener) (Ewing 1984)	Adults	Alcohol	Clinician	4	2 min	Free http://pubs.niaaa.nih.gov/ publications/inscage. htm (NIAAA).
CAGEAID (CAGE Adapted to include drugs) (Brown and Saunders 1995)	Adults	Alcohol and other drugs	Clinician	4	2 min	Free http://adai.uw.edu/instruments/ pdf/CAGE-AID.pdf.
The Alcohol Use Disorders Identification Test (AUDIT) (WHO 1992)	Adults	Alcohol	Clinician	10	10 min	Available http://whqlibdoc.who.int/ hq/2001/WHO_MSD_ MSB_01.6a.pdf (WHO).
Brief Screener for Alcohol, Tobacco, and other Drugs (BSTAD)	Adolescents	Alcohol, tobacco and other drugs	Self or clinician	12	5 min	Online http://pubs.niaaa.nih.gov/ publications/Practitioner/ YouthGuide/YouthGuide.pdf.
The Alcohol, Smoking and Substance Involvement Screening Test (ASSIST) Version 3. (WHO 2002)	Adolescents and adults	All substances	Clinician	8	5–10 min	Available http://www.who.int/substance_ abuse/activities/en/ASSIST%20 V.3-%20Guidelines%20for%20 use%20in%20primary%20care_ TEST.pdf (WHO, ASSIST v.3).
Drug Use Disorders Identification Test (DUDIT) (Bernan et al. 2005)	Adults	Drugs	Self-administered	11	10 min	http://www.sciencedirect.com/ science?_ob=RedirectURL&_ method=externObjLink&_ locator=url&_issn=03064603&_ origin=article&_zone=art_ page&_plusSign=%2B&_tar getURL=http%253A%252F% 252Fwww.emcdda.europa. eu%252Fattachements. cfm%252Fatt_10455_EN_ DUDIT.pdf.

Occupational Therapy Assessment Tools

Occupational therapists may wish to supplement the standard initial interview with open questioning to obtain information about how substance use is impacting the individual's occupational performance areas, components and contexts. The Occupational Circumstances Assessment Interview and Rating Scale (Forsyth et al. 2005) is a semi-structured interview often used for this purpose. Other appropriate tools include:

■ Occupational Self-Assessment,
■ Rosenberg Self-Esteem Inventory,
■ Self-Efficacy Scale,

- Volitional Questionnaire,
- Coping Responses Inventory,
- Interest Checklist,
- Role Checklist,
- Assessment of Motor and Process Skills,
- Internal/External Locus of Control Scale, and
- OPHI-II.

INTERVENTIONS

Intervention is usually via individual work and group work aimed at developing performance components in a range of contexts, for example, learning to cope with anxiety without alcohol or saying 'no' if offered drugs. Group contexts and community locations can provide the chance to rehearse performance components. Individual work can focus on enhancing specific components through goal setting. As described earlier, substance misuse is typically a chronically relapsing condition. Interventions often do not follow a linear path, and the stages of change model is useful in assessing treatment readiness and in selecting the most appropriate intervention.

Many people with substance misuse problems struggle to engage with treatment services. Feelings of ambivalence, anxieties about change, fluctuating levels of motivation and a chaotic lifestyle are factors in this. Enhancing engagement is pivotal in achieving positive treatment outcomes (NTA 2004; DH 2007; NICE 2011), and the importance of establishing rapport and empathy and of using motivational enhancement techniques following assessment must not be underestimated (NTA 2004).

People with drug and/or alcohol problems frequently present with complex needs. They may be clinically depressed, have poor physical health and be homeless. Therefore it is important that treatment plans are comprehensive, involving other disciplines and agencies as needed (Edwards 1987; DH 1996). People can also feel that they are overwhelmed and controlled by their addiction. Therefore it is important to emphasize empowerment and hope in overcoming substance problems or dependence.

NICE (2010) recommends that brief interventions (Bien et al. 1993) are offered in a range of settings including primary care and A&E designed to help people reduce alcohol use to less harmful levels. Those with less severe alcohol problems and binge drinkers may opt for controlled drinking. This means keeping alcohol consumption within safe levels by adhering to a set of personal rules, such as not drinking alone, not having more than two drinks a day and not drinking on consecutive days.

After becoming abstinent or successfully controlling alcohol consumption, NICE (2011) recommends that people are offered:

- CBT (discussed more fully in Chapter 15), which is often provided in the form of a relapse prevention (RP) approach;
- Behavioural therapies such as cue exposure, whereby a person is repeatedly exposed to learnt cues to drink alcohol until they habituate to those cues and the cravings to drink are extinguished;
- Social network and environment-based therapies, whereby an individual is supported to build a network of family and friends that are supportive of a change in drinking. Recreational, social and vocational activities can be encouraged on the basis that developing a non-substance–using network and developing a role or a positive identity may be key factors in preventing relapse (McIntosh and McKeganey 2000);
- Behavioural couples therapy. This is a manual-based method combining CBT with methods that address relationship problems caused by the alcohol use.

Withdrawal and Stabilization

Medically assisted withdrawal (commonly known as detoxification or detox) followed by abstinence is recommended for people who are physically dependent on alcohol. This usually occurs in the community but may need to be on an inpatient basis if there is a risk of withdrawal seizures. Similarly, the first stage of treatment for opiate users is stabilization using substitute prescribing (such as methadone or buprenorphine). This aims to stop the user experiencing unpleasant withdrawal symptoms but does not provide a 'high.' The rationale behind substitute prescribing is that the drug user no longer has to inject street heroin with its associated health risks or be involved in illegal activities to fund a habit. Long-term prescription of methadone, or methadone maintenance, aims to allow users to stabilize their drug use and therefore their lives and, combined with psychological and social support, make positive lifestyle changes. It requires close monitoring due to the risk of overdose or harm related to illicit drug or alcohol use.

In practice this stabilization can take a long time to achieve due to, for example, a longstanding chaotic lifestyle, the social environment of drug-using friends and the continued desire to use drugs to escape from reality. Many service users also have physical, social, legal and psychological problems which need to be addressed as part of a comprehensive treatment plan. Once an individual has achieved stability in their lives, they may consider a 'detox' from substitute opiate medication. This is normally followed by a period of rehabilitation, or rehab, usually in a residential or day programme.

Multidisciplinary Approaches to Intervention

There are numerous models of substance misuse treatment, and it is beyond the scope of this chapter to cover all of them. However, those of most relevance to occupational therapists will now be described. These approaches are recommended in national guidelines (NICE 2007, 2011).

The Stages of Change Model

Before considering drug and alcohol treatment, a transtheoretical model of change that can be used with individuals with any addictive behaviour (or anyone working towards behaviour change) is presented. The stages of change model is a useful tool for guiding treatment goal-setting and interventions which can be targeted to help service users progress through the stages of change (Prochaska et al. 2013).

Prochaska and DiClemente (1982, 1986) and Prochaska et al. (1992) first developed this model with cigarette smokers, who they found reported progression through different stages of change as they attempted to give up. The model continued to evolve and today is widely used in treatment planning and goal setting for substance dependence, eating disorders and mood disorders (Krebs et al. 2018). It reflects the reality that it is normal for an individual to go through all the stages several times before achieving lasting behaviour change. Most of us can relate to attempting behaviour changes, such as dieting, exercising regularly or

stopping smoking perhaps, where we have not succeeded in maintaining the change at the first attempt. In fact, the smokers in Prochaska and DiClemente's initial study went around the cycle between three and seven times before finally giving up smoking permanently.

The relapses associated with addiction (a chronic relapsing condition) may be seen as normal events that can be learned from, rather than being seen as indications of failure. Although represented as a cycle, it is now conceptualized as a spiral acknowledging that each time the person goes through the stages, they are learning from the experience of previous attempts to change.

The central concept of this model is that behaviour change takes place through the following discrete stages (Krebs et al. 2018), also illustrated in Fig. 27.1:

- Precontemplation: In this stage people do not recognize that they have a problem and only present for treatment because they are put under pressure by others. However, when they do, it is to assuage the concerns of others.
- Contemplation: In this stage the person recognizes that their behaviour is problematic and considers doing something about it. This change is

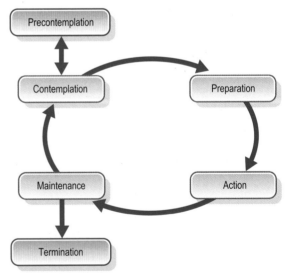

Fig. 27.1 ■ **A model of change.** (Reprinted and adapted from Prochaska, J.O., DiClemente, C.C., 1986. Towards a comprehensive model of change. In: Miller, R.J., Heather, N. (Eds.), Treating Addictive Behaviours: Processes of Change. Plenum, London, with permission from Springer Science + Business Media.)

characterized by ambivalence. Motivational enhancement therapy or motivational interviewing is a useful, evidence-based approach to use during this stage.

- Preparation: The person prepares to change in the near future, and starts making small changes.
- Action: This stage is about making changes to experiences, behaviour or the environment and implementing a plan. This phase can last anywhere between one day and six months.
- Maintenance: This is about sustaining the change and integrating it into the individual's lifestyle. For people with SUDs, the maintenance stage may last a lifetime.

In this model, a person may slip back a stage or exit the cycle into precontemplation at any time. Establishing at which stage the individual is enables the therapist to select the most appropriate intervention. This is important because interventions should be matched to the person's readiness for change (Edglow and Cramm 2020). For example, a service user in the maintenance phase may benefit from learning stress management techniques and developing satisfying day-to-day occupations, which are important in boosting confidence and preventing relapse. However, these strategies are likely to be wasted on a 'precontemplator,' who still needs to develop an awareness of the need to change their substance use behaviour.

Despite the widespread use of this model there is mixed evidence to prove the efficacy of matching treatment to the patient's stage of change (e.g., Norcross et al. 2011; Krebs et al. 2018). Some authors suggest that the model of change may oversimplify complex motivational states (i.e., it is impossible to definitively determine what change an individual is in) (Norcross et al. 2011), while others recommend specific tools for measuring readiness for change (Edgelow and Cramm 2020). The model is also criticized for a lack of emphasis on the importance of the social and physical environment surrounding an individual (Norcross et al. 2011).

Twelve Step Interventions

One of the most well-known interventions is the '12 step' approaches of AA and its associate, Narcotics Anonymous (NA). The 12 step approach is a self-help movement that offers an extensive support network of group meetings for substance users and their families.

In this approach an individual achieves recovery by progressing through the 12 steps with the support of a sponsor (mentor).

Criticism has been levelled at the requirement that those who attend AA or NA must adhere to the idea that dependence is a disease and must constantly remind themselves that they are alcoholic, even when they have been abstinent for many years. Additionally, criticism is directed at the idea that a higher power is responsible for an AA or NA member's abstinence, suggesting that this removes the responsibility for sobriety from the individual. Recent research has found that it is the supportive social network provided by the 12 step approaches—rather than the associated belief system—that generates good outcomes. This research recommends that treatment providers de-emphasize the philosophy of the 12 step approaches but encourage attendance as a means of gaining social support that promotes abstinence. Studies show that changing one's role from being someone in need of help to someone who provides help to others and takes an active role in meetings (such as simply making coffee, initially) was associated with positive outcomes, more so than just attending (Pagano et al. 2004; Weiss et al. 2005).

A growing, secular alternative to 12 step approaches is SMART recovery (Smart Recovery UK 2010), which is a programme offered online that includes a network of meetings and volunteers based on motivational enhancement therapy, CBT and rational emotive behaviour therapy.

Relapse Prevention

RP is a widely used intervention based on CBT. Marlatt and Gordon (2005) describe RP as a self-management programme designed to enhance the maintenance phase of the stages of change model. NICE (2007) recommends that this approach is only routinely offered to those with coexisting anxiety and depression. However, as described earlier in relation to dual diagnosis, it is likely that most service users will present with these additional problems. RP focuses on 'self-management and the techniques and strategies aimed at enhancing maintenance of habit change.' It is 'a self-control programme that combines behavioural skills training, cognitive interventions and lifestyle change procedures' (Wanigaratne et al. 1990, p. 1). There is a growing body of evidence supporting the effectiveness of RP interventions (Grant et al. 2017).

The RP approach uses cognitive behavioural strategies to help people learn how to anticipate and cope with situations and problems that might lead to a relapse (Wanigaratne et al. 1990). It focuses on the notions of high-risk situations and coping strategies available to the individual.

Research shows that people who are aware of potential relapse situations and who use specific strategies to, for example, manage stress, can effectively reduce their risk of relapse (Andersson et al. 2019). Boredom and negative mood states are most likely to precipitate a relapse. Second comes social pressure and being offered, or talking about, drugs. Other risk factors include interpersonal conflict and environmental cues.

Initial stages of RP focus on enabling the individual to develop a good awareness of internal and external triggers to craving, such as through diary-keeping. Service users are encouraged to identify their own possible relapse triggers and to work on these with the therapist. The therapist, either in a group setting or individually, helps the individual to analyse these situations. The person will also be taught how to analyse situations on their own. Structured problem-solving techniques are used as well as roleplay or rehearsal of relapse situations.

There are specific cognitive behavioural techniques (Wanigaratne et al. 1990; Marlatt and Gordon 2005) used to assist people in preventing relapse, such as problems of immediate gratification. These techniques see craving as being caused by high-risk situations and external cues. Marlatt (2010) proposes a method for managing urges called 'urge surfing'. This is based on mindfulness and the facilitation of detachment, whereby the thought 'I notice I am feeling the urge to drink' replaces the act of immediately drinking, on the understanding that the urge will arise and then subside. Coping with the urge by not responding to it at its peak starves it. Coping strategies such as relaxation methods, distraction, biofeedback or other approaches may assist this technique.

RP also stresses the importance of global lifestyle change, which aims to enable people to:

- arrive at a balanced lifestyle,
- learn effective time management (to fill up the vacuum left by giving up the substance),
- discover and take up positive activities, and
- identify and change unhealthy habit patterns.

It can be seen from these approaches that RP fits well with occupational therapy, particularly because it focuses on individuals' lifestyles and the day-to-day situations that cause relapse. In such work, occupational performance areas, components and contexts are critical to treatment success. Developing psychological performance components, such as self-esteem and volition, can help an individual cope with environmental triggers to relapse.

Contingency Management

This is a behavioural approach based on operant conditioning, whereby incentives are offered, often in the form of vouchers that can be exchanged for goods or services. Giving the voucher is contingent on drug tests being negative regarding illicit drug use. In the contingency management approach the value of vouchers increases with increasing periods of continuous abstinence. There is potential for these vouchers to be used to support occupational and recovery-focused goals such as paying for gardening equipment, art materials or sessions in a sports centre. Despite a clear evidence base demonstrating the cost-effectiveness of this approach (Lussier et al. 2006), it has not been adopted in many countries possibly due to the resource implications of funding the vouchers, drug testing, as well as a possible moral reluctance to being seen to 'pay' drug users to engage in treatment.

Motivational Interventions

NICE recommends that for those with alcohol problems a 'motivational intervention' is carried out using key elements of motivational interviewing, such as helping people to recognize the problems caused by their drinking, resolving ambivalence, encouraging belief in the ability to change and being persuasive and supportive rather than confrontational (NICE 2011).

Harm Reduction Approaches

Since the advent of human immunodeficiency virus (HIV) and the development of structured methadone maintenance programmes, treatment for opiate use has traditionally adopted a harm reduction or harm minimization approach. This is designed to reduce the risk of infection with blood-borne viruses through sharing injecting equipment, as well as avoiding the risks associated with using contaminated, adulterated street heroin. These approaches include providing needle exchange schemes and education for drug users on safer injecting methods and prescribing medical substitute opiates such as methadone. This has undoubtedly been successful in preventing an epidemic of HIV among injecting drug users, and substitute prescribing has enabled many drug users to live productive lives whilst continuing to be prescribed an opiate drug. However, these approaches have caused much debate over what constitutes successful treatment and recovery. There is a longstanding disagreement and debate in the field of drug treatment between supporters of 'harm reduction' approaches and those that follow 12 step approaches (AA 2002), which are based on total abstinence.

Occupation-Centred Interventions

The growing research and practice evidence base in occupational therapy, mental health and occupational science continues to assert the central role played by meaningful occupational participation in facilitating recovery. This role is founded on the undeniable occupational disruptions and impairments on occupational performance associated with SUD (Cruz 2019). Stone (2017) study found out that substance abuse negatively affected occupational functioning and was correlated with seven key domains of occupational disruption, dominating habits and routines, social context, family disapprobation, residual strengths and self-medicating or sleep. Occupational therapists' education, knowledge and skills position them well to apply evidence-based interventions, which put special emphasis on enabling the affected groups to engage in occupations, participation in community living and ultimately contributing to wider society (Amorelli 2016). Using occupation, occupational therapy works to improve and maintain performance and participation for mental health service users, including those with addictions (Rojo-Mota et al. 2017) and other SUDs (Peloquin et al. 2018). The occupational areas most targeted for intervention include leisure, work/productivity and self-care.

Leisure

The importance of leisure as an effective component of RP for psychiatric disorders has been highlighted in a wide range of research literature, including occupational therapy literature (Sarsak 2018). Health-promoting leisure activities are particularly useful in restructuring habits and routines for meaningful and productive use of time as well as reducing the frequency of negative thoughts and cravings (Rojo-Mota 2017; Sarsak 2018). Providing access to meaningful leisure has also been reported as a role of occupational therapists in facilitating recovery from addictions and

SUDs, with the ultimate goal of promoting occupational justice (Sy et al. 2018).

The use of physical activities in particular for a variety of therapeutic goals is described in the research literature (Rojo-Mota et al. 2017) and provides a small but promising evidence base despite the quality of studies informing this. Recent occupational therapy and science literature cements that a balanced pattern of occupations inclusive of physical leisure activities should be promoted to enhance health and fulfill the

---

CASE STUDY 27.1

Using Art with a Service User with an Opiate Dependency

This case study concerns a service user in treatment for opiate dependence. This intervention involved substitute prescribing, one-to-one occupational therapy and participation in creative art workshops run by the occupational therapy service in partnership with a local community arts organization. The workshops culminated in an art exhibition displaying artwork from various projects, which was opened by the service user with a speech in which she said, 'When I came to my clinic I was not the person I am today. I wanted to give up drugs, but every attempt had failed miserably. I had been with a treatment clinic before, but all they gave us was medication, and after a few months I was using again. Since I have been with this clinic, I have had huge support and help from everyone who has worked with me, but especially my occupational therapist …. From the day I met my occupational therapist my life has got better and better. … The occupational therapy artspace project helps in ways you wouldn't even imagine: something as simple as getting you out of the house and facing life, instead of sitting alone brooding which in turn creates boredom or depression, both of which can lead straight back to drugs or alcohol … Giving people a routine to stick to and a goal to aim for is one of the most basic things that will put someone on the track to recovery, and a new and better life. Not only does it help in that way, but, meeting people and socializing also gives confidence and self-belief, all of which is taken for granted in most people. But they can be the hardest things to instill into someone whose life has been on the fringe of society for the length of their addiction, which in most cases is years if not decades' (Lancaster 2008, pp. 12–13).

participation and inclusion needs of individuals, families and communities including those affected by SUD (Reitz and Scaffa 2020). Ussher et al. (2000) describe the development of a physical activity programme as part of occupational therapy within a community alcohol service. Sport and fitness-related activities raise self-esteem and confidence and counteract individuals' negative affect. Discovering or rediscovering leisure can help develop motivation for positive change (see Chapter 14 regarding the impact of physical activities).

Leisure intervention may form an important part of family therapy, where family-oriented leisure has been involved with or affected by substance use. In the authors' clinical experience, activities that help a substance user to engage in adaptive interactions with family members are often highly successful. This is especially so when the individual enjoys and can remember the activity and when it stimulates both service user and family member. Examples include cooking group meals, group creative arts, swimming, playing racket sports, bowling and visiting theatres, cinemas or art galleries, even practising magic tricks. Activities that individuals can take up as a hobby and talk about with the family are similarly effective.

Work/Productivity

There are three domains within which to consider work and productivity in the field of substance use:

- Work-based substance use – where there is drug use during the working day in (legal) employment;
- Substance-based productivity – where drug use or drug-dealing follow a similar pattern to paid work and provide similar rewards and meaning to life;
- Vocational interventions – helping service users gain employment.

Case Study 27.2 illustrates how opportunities for work may interface with substance use as an occupational transition.

CASE STUDY 27.2

Tinashe is a 34-year-old university graduate with a teaching qualification and living in Zimbabwe. Born in a family of two, his father died when he was young. He grew up with his mother in a strict Catholic family. He started to experiment with marijuana when he was in high school, mainly out of peer pressure and the need to fit in. He managed to hide this away from his mother until the end of high school. Tinashe passed and qualified to go to university, but his grades were not as good as was expected of him. While at university, he narrates the ordeal of having too much freedom without hope and going deeper in his substance use practices. Upon completion of his studies, Tinashe was forced to join the many 'educated, skilled and unemployed' young men in Zimbabwe. With the frustrations, stress and pressure of an anticipated productive life, Tinashe like many others, reached for the low hanging fruits of maladaptive coping. He went deeper into substance use to a point where his life became defined by substance engagements, that is, in the use of his time and energy resources. This involved looking for substances, doing piece jobs in exchange for marijuana and alcohol, looking for company to drink and smoke with and using anything intoxicating to drown the stresses of reality. However, unlike his peers, Tinashe succumbed to substance-induced psychosis. After a violent episode at home, he was admitted to one of Zimbabwe's mental health institutions. This would be the start of a chronic and relapsing journey involving abuse of alcohol, marijuana and codeine-containing cough syrup. In one of the many admissions, Tinashe was referred to an occupational therapist who applied an occupational perspective to the case.

Despite Tinashe's health crisis, substance use remained a meaningful engagement for him. It served as a coping mechanism for unemployment-related stress, enhancing socialisation and maintaining his identity to continue to fit into his friendship circles. Substance use had become an occupation with both positive and negative outcomes. A detoxification program was initiated to support him to move into sobriety as a primary goal. This was a shared goal for Tinashe, his family and the mental health team. By considering substance use as an occupation, dropping it needed to be followed by other socially valued and 'healthy' occupations to fill in the void. The occupational therapist was to explore ways of sustaining this.

For Tinashe, this meant an occupational transition to recovery involving abandoning substance use occupations, modifying occupations which used to sustain substance use and adopting new occupations to sustain recovery. Using his acquired teaching

CASE STUDY 27.2 (CONTINUED)

qualification, a multisectoral and collaborative programme was initiated by the occupational therapist to get Tinashe into formal employment. He started with intensive work skills retraining programme. This was done with the help of a headmaster from a school on which he had done his teaching practice. The journey was long and recursive but premised on internal motivation for change from Tinashe and a very supportive family, some obstacles were movable. After three years of occupational therapy focusing on getting him into paid work, Tinashe finally got a teaching job at the school he had done his teaching practice. This also took political buy in to convince the authorities to open the post for him as part of his rehabilitation. He has maintained sobriety and continues to receive on-the-job support from occupational therapy. In one of his visits to see to occupational therapist, in a reflective manner, he had this to say: '… at last I am occupied productively, I am now positioned to be useful. This is a better way to stay "dry," than just talk and yet the problems won't go away with talk….'

Where substances are used during a job, this can be subtle and often either linked to peer pressure or to coping with work pressure. Substance use can be considered a part of work when, for example, the entertainment of business clients is part of the working day. Substances are often used covertly at work. Initial experiences of high achievement may reinforce a pattern of substance use, but errors of judgement usually ensue and crises may occur.

Jobs are often affected negatively or lost altogether once substance misuse patterns become established. Other non-paid work, such as housekeeping and voluntary work, are similarly affected. Occupational therapy focuses on helping a person cope with work without using the drug and develop resistance to relapse triggers in work settings. This may involve liaison with an employer to develop graded re-entry into work.

Where maintaining a drug habit becomes 'work,' an individual's efforts can be directed to obtaining a regular supply of the substance, selling the substance or engaging in regular criminal activity to fund the addiction. These behaviours may display characteristics that are similar to legal employment. Occupational therapy focuses on identifying habit-maintaining skills and transferring these to non-drug–related activities such as voluntary work, training or paid employment.

There is an increasing focus within treatment services on helping service users gain employment. Most developed governments such as the UK government have a target of reducing the number of people receiving welfare benefits and acknowledge the positive link between employment and recovery from SUD (Dietz and Schriber 2017; Kirsh et al. 2019; Duncan et al. 2020).

There is significant evidence that employment, training and education for people with substance use problems enhance clinical outcomes by reducing rates of relapse, restricting time of use, and reducing criminality and parole violation (Walton and Hall 2016). Pre-vocational skills (such as confidence, interpersonal skills, time-keeping and budgeting) are reported in research as necessary to improve employment outcomes among persons with SUD (Amorelli 2016). The importance of 'soft outcomes' or pre-vocational skill development is also emphasized in the facilitation of recovery—a function that blends well with occupational therapists as specialists in developing pre-vocational skills using creativity and building on ADLs.

Education, employment or training goals should therefore be included in all treatment plans. Occupational therapists, alongside employment specialists (where present) can act as vocational leads within the multiprofessional team, assessing vocational and pre-vocational skills and developing individualized plans.

Self-care

Self-care activities tend to decrease as substance use increases. The compulsion to use a drug eventually supersedes any awareness of nutrition, health, cleanliness, safety or responsibility for finances. Consequently, daily living becomes chaotic. Drug users, once abstinent or stabilized in treatment, often feel particularly de-skilled in relation to day-to-day household activities such as budgeting or basic time management.

Dental problems and loss of teeth are common consequences of SUDs (Cuberos et al. 2020); the effect that this has on self-image can pose a barrier to achieving occupational and social goals. Development of public health strategies involving dental health professionals could be a critical step towards improving the quality of life and recovery among those affected. Remedial dental work can be a helpful early goal included in a treatment plan to help them construct a 'non-addict identity' and remove perceived barriers to social interaction caused by concerns about appearance (Robinson et al. 2005). By focusing on ADLs, occupational therapy delivers preventative measures for improving oral hygiene and reduction of the risk and burden of dental problems in the population of persons with SUD.

Evaluation of Outcomes

Outcome measurement is possible through a wide range of occupational therapy–specific and other questionnaires or assessment tools. Some of these are described in the assessment section of this chapter. Most of those described are used before and after phases of intervention. It should remain foundational that the outcome measures used should reflect the personal concerns of the patients and include other biopsychosocial variables of interest (Alvens et al. 2017). Others can be used on a sessional basis, such as the General Health Questionnaire-28 as applied among patients with addictions (Ardakani et al. 2016).

SUMMARY

This chapter has focused on the range of issues affecting people who misuse substances and the intervention strategies that are available to address these. Clearly, there is considerable scope for occupational therapists to contribute to substance misuse interventions. Substance misuse occurs at the very centre of human occupation in work, leisure and self-care, and it gradually takes over as the most central driver of occupational behaviour, changing and damaging performance components as it progresses.

Occupational therapy methods work well with the key clinical approaches already developed in the field of addiction. Furthermore occupational therapists can enhance practice by tackling the subtle and complex challenges to day-to-day living that service users experience. Further reading is recommended in this area as is further education, especially as substance use exists within all areas of mental health practice and is more likely to increase than decrease in everyday practice.

REFERENCES

Abdulrahim, D., Bowden-Jones, O., & On Behalf of NEPTUNE Group. (2016). *Harms of synthetic cannabinoid receptor agonists (SCRAs) and their management.* London: Novel Psychoactive Treatment UK Network (NEPTUNE).

Alcohol Concern. (2014). All in the mind. *Meeting the challenge of alcohol-related brain damage.*

Alcoholics Anonymous (AA). (2002). *Twelve steps and twelve traditions.* New York: Alcoholics Anonymous World Service Inc.

Allen, S. L. (2001). *The Devil's Cup – coffee's driving Force in history.* New York: Ballantine Books.

Alves, P., Sales, C., & Ashworth, M. (2017). Does outcome measurement of treatment for substance use disorder reflect the personal concerns of patients? A scoping review of measures recommended in Europe. *Drug and Alcohol Dependence, 179,* 299–308.

American Occupational Therapy Association (AOTA). (2008). Occupational therapy practice framework: Domain and process, second ed. *American Journal of Occupational Therapy, 62*(6), 625–683.

American Psychiatric Association. (2013). Diagnostic and statistical manual of mental disorders, (DSM-V), 5th ed. Washington: American Psychiatric Association.

Amorelli, C. (2016). Psychosocial occupational therapy interventions for substance-use disorders: A narrative review. *Occupational Therapy in Mental Health, 32*(2), 167–184. https://doi.org/10.1080/0164212X.2015.1134293.

Andersson, H. W., Wenaas, M., & Nordfjærn, T. (2019). Relapse after inpatient substance use treatment: A prospective cohort study among users of illicit substances. Addict. *Beyond Behavior, 90,* 222–228.

Ardakani, A., Seghatoleslam, T., Habil, H., et al. (2016). Construct validity of symptom checklist-90-revised (SCL-90-R) and general health questionnaire-28 (GHQ-28) in patients with drug addiction and diabetes, and normal population. *Iranian Journal of Public Health, 45*(4), 451.

Ashworth, M., Gerada, C., & Doyle, M. (2008). Addiction and dependence: Alcohol. In T. Davies, & T. Craig (Eds.), *ABC of mental health* (2nd ed.). Chichester: Wiley-Blackwell.

BBC News website, 2000. 'Cambridge Two' vow to fight on Available at: http://news.bbc.co.uk/1/hi/uk/1083446.stm.

BBC News website, 2007. Drug services make slow progress. Mark Easton. Available at: http://news.bbc.co.uk/1/hi/uk/7068572.stm.

Bennett, L. W., Cardone, S., & Jarczyk, J. (1998). Effects of a therapeutic camping program on addiction recovery: The algonquin relapse prevention program. *Journal of Substance Abuse Treatment, 15*(5), 469–474.

Berridge, V. (2005). *Temperance: Its history and impact on Current and future alcohol policy.* York: Joseph Rowntree Foundation.

Bien, T. H., Miller, W. R., & Tonigan, J. S. (1993). Brief interventions for alcohol problems: A review. *Addiction, 88*(3), 315–335.

BMA Board of Science. (2008). *Alcohol misuse: Tackling the UK epidemic.* London: BMA.

Buijsse, N., Caan, W., & Davis, S. F. (1999). Occupational therapy in the treatment of addictive behaviours. *British Journal of Therapy and Rehabilitation, 6*(6), 300–307.

Burling, T. A., Seidner, A. L., Robbins-Sisco, D., et al. (1992). Batter up! Relapse prevention for homeless veteran substance abusers via softball team participation. *Journal of Substance Abuse, 4*(4), 407–413.

Cabinet Office. (2004). *Harm reduction Strategy for England.* London: Cabinet Office.

Carter, R. (1998). *Mapping the mind.* London: Seven Dials, 68–69.

Chacksfield, J. D. (1994). Occupational therapy: The whole in one treatment for alcohol dependent clients. Paper presented at the world Federation of occupational therapists, 11th International Congress. *Congress Summaries, 3*, 995–997.

Chacksfield, J. (2003). Forensic addictive behaviours. In L. Couldrick, & D. Aldred (Eds.), *Forensic occupational therapy.* London: Whurr.

Chacksfield, J. D., & Forshaw, D. M. (1997). Occupational therapy and forensic addictive behaviours. *International Journal of Therapy and Rehabilitation, 4*(7), 381–386.

Chacksfield, J. D., & Lindsay, S. J. E. (1999). The reduction of leisure in alcohol addiction. *Paper presented at College of occupational therapists Conference,* 1999, personal communication.

Chandler, D., Meisal, J., Jordan, P., et al. (2004). Substance abuse, employment and welfare tenure. *Social Service Review, 78*, 1–19.

Cheung, C., Lee, T., & Lee, C. (2003). Factors in successful relapse prevention among Hong Kong drug addicts. J. Offender Rehabil. Special issue: Treating substance abusers in correctional contexts: *New Understandings, New Modalities, 37*(2–4), 179–199.

Cloete, L. G., & Ramugondo, E. L. (2015). I drink": Mothers' alcohol consumption as both individualised and imposed occupation. *South African Journal of Occupational Therapy 45*(1), 34–40.

Cornish, R., Macleod, J., Strang, J., et al. (2010). Risk of death during and after opiate substitution treatment in primary care: Prospective observational study in UK. *The British Medical Journal, 341,* c5475.

Cruz, T. (2019). *Identifying occupational therapy role for individuals in substance abuse and addition recovery programs.* Available at: soar.usa.edu.

Cuberos, M., Chatah, E. M., Baquerizo, H. Z., & Weinstein, G. (2020). Dental management of patients with substance use disorder. *Clinical Dentistry Reviewed, 4*(1), 1–8.

Davidson, R. (2001). The cycle of change -thematic review. *Drug & Alcohol Findings, 5,* 19–24.

Department of Health (DH). (1996). *The task Force to Review services for drug misusers: Report of an Independent Review of drug treatment services in England.* London: Department of Health.

Department of Health (DH). (2002). *Mental health policy Implementation Guide: Dual diagnosis good practice Guide.* London: Department of Health.

Department of Health (DH). (2007). *Scottish Office Department of health, Welsh Office, Department of health and social Security in Northern Ireland. Drug misuse and dependence: Guidelines on clinical management.* London: Stationery Office.

Department of Health (DH). (2011). *A summary of the health harms of drugs.* Liverpool: Department of Health.

Department of Health (DH). (2017). *Clinical guidelines on drug misuse and dependence Update 2017 Independent Expert working group. Drug misuse and dependence: UK guidelines on clinical management.* London: Department of Health.

Dietz, J., & Schriber, E. (2017). *Intensive Outpatient program for substance abuse: Occupational therapy guideline to recovery.* Available at: commons.und.edu.

Donaghy, M. E., & Mutrie, N. (1999). Is exercise beneficial in the treatment and rehabilitation of the problem drinker? A critical review. *Physical Therapy Reviews, 4*(3), 153–166.

Doniger, J. M. (1953). An activity program with alcoholics. *American Journal of Occupational Therapy, 7*(3), 110–112.

Donmall, M., Jones, J., Davies, L., et al. (2009). *Research report 23: Summary of the key findings of the drug treatment outcome research study (DTORS).* London: Home Office.

Drake, R. E., Becker, D. R., Bond, G. R., et al. (2003). A process analysis of integrated and non-integrated approaches to supported employment. *Journal of Vocational Rehabilitation, 38*(1), 51–58.

Drake, R. E., Essock, S. M., Shamer, M. D., et al. (2001). Implementing dual diagnosis services for clients with severe mental illness. *Psychiatric Services, 52*(4), 469–476.

Drug and Alcohol Findings, 2010. Commentary on Jones A., Donmall M., Millar T (2009) The Drug Treatment Outcomes Research Study (DTORS): final outcomes report. Available at: http://findings.org.uk/count/downloads/download.php?file=Jones_A_4.txt.

Drugscope. (2009). *Drug treatment at the crossroads: What it's for, where it's at and how to make it even better.* London: Drugscope.

Drummond, D. C. (1992). Problems and dependence: Chalk and cheese or bread and butter? In M. Lader, G. Edwards, & C. Drummond (Eds.), *The nature of alcohol and drug related problems* (pp. 61–82). Oxford: Oxford University Press.

Drummond, D. C., Tiffany, S. T., Glautier, S., et al. (1995). *Addictive behavior: Cue exposure, theory and practice.* New York: Wiley.

Duncan, A., Lee, S., Ratti, S., Pickles, C., & Rakshit, H. (2020). The lived experiences of people with substance use issues seeking care from a rapid access clinic: An occupational perspective. *Occupational Therapy in Mental Health, 36*(1), 68–84.

Edgelow, M., & Cramm, H. (2020). Developing an occupation-centred framework for trauma intervention. *Occupational Therapy in Mental Health, 36*(3), 270–290. https://doi.org/10.1080/0164212X.2020.1808148.

Edwards, G. (1987). *The treatment of drinking problems*. Oxford: Blackwell Scientific.

Edwards, R. (2010). The dental aspects of treating a patient with substance misuse problems. In *Substance misuse management in general practice*. Resource library. Available at: www.smmgp.org.uk/html/others.php.

Edwards, G., Arif, A., & Hodgson, R. (1981). Nomenclature and classification of drug-and alcohol-related problems: A WHO memorandum. *Bulletin of the World Health Organization*, 59(2), 225–242.

Edwards, G., & Gross, M. M. (1976). Alcohol dependence: Provisional description of a clinical syndrome. *The British Medical Journal*, 1(6017), 1058–1061.

Forsyth, K., Deshpande, S., Kielhofner, G., et al. (2005). *The occupational Circumstances assessment interview and rating scale (OCAIRS) Version 4.0*. IL: University of Illinois at Chicago.

Gerada, C., & Ashworth, M. (2008). Addiction and dependence: Illicit drugs. In T. Davies, & T. Craig (Eds.), *ABC of mental health* (2nd ed.). Chichester: Wiley-Blackwell.

Ghodse, H. (2002). *Drugs and addictive behaviour – a Guide to treatment*. Cambridge: Cambridge University Press.

Goldberg, D. (1986). Use of the general health questionnaire in clinical work. *The British Medical Journal*, 293(6556), 1188–1189.

Gossop, M. (1990). The development of the short opiate withdrawal scale (SOWS). *Addictive Behaviours*, 15(5), 487–490.

Gossop, M. (2000). *Living with drugs* (5th ed.). Aldershot: Ashgate.

Gossop, M., Darke, S., Griffith, P., et al. (1995). The severity of dependence scale (SDS): Psychometric properties of the SDS in English and Australian samples of heroin, cocaine and amphetamine users. *Addiction*, 90(5), 607–614.

Grant, S., Colaiaco, B., Motala, A., et al. (2017). Mindfulness-based relapse prevention for substance use disorders: A systematic review and meta-analysis. *Journal of Addiction Medicine*, 11(5), 386.

Gutman, M., McKay, J., Ketterinus, R., et al. (2003). Potential barriers to work for substance abusing women on welfare: Findings from the CASAWORKS for families pilot demonstration. *Evaluation Review*, 27(6), 681–706.

Harada, T., Tsutomi, H., Mori, R., & Wilson, D. B. (2018). Cognitive–behavioural treatment for amphetamine–type stimulants (ATS)–use disorders. *Cochrane Database of Systematic Reviews*, 12, CD011315. https://doi.org/10.1002/14651858.CD011315.pub2.

Heather, N., Gold, R., & Rollnick, S. (1991). *Readiness to change questionnaire: User's manual. Technical report 15*. Kensington, Australia: National Drug and Alcohol Research Centre, University of New South Wales.

Helbig, K., & McKay, E. (2003). An exploration of addictive behaviours from an occupational perspective. *Journal of Occupational Science*, 10(3), 140–145.

HM Government. (2010). *Drug: Strategy 2010: Reducing demand, restricting supply, building recovery, supporting people to live a drug free life*. London: HM Government.

Hodgson, S., Lloyd, C., & Schmid, T. (2001). The leisure participation of clients with a dual diagnosis. *British Journal of Occupational Therapy*, 64(10), 487–492.

Hossack, J. R. (1952). Clinical trial of occupational therapy in the treatment of alcohol addiction. *American Journal of Occupational Therapy*, 6(6), 265–266.

Hunt, W. A., Barnett, L. W., & Branch, L. G. (1971). Relapse rates in addiction programs. *Journal of Clinical Psychology*, 27(4), 455–456.

Institute of Alcohol Studies. (2010). *Binge drinking – nature, prevalence and causes. IAS Factsheet*. Available at http://www.ias.org.uk/resources/factsheets/factsheets.html.

Jenner, M. (1998). Harm minimization outcomes for methadone recipients: Role of employment. *Journal of Substance Misuse*, 3(2), 114–118.

Kang, S. Y., Magura, S., Blankertz, L., et al. (2006). Predictors in engagement in vocational counselling for methadone treatment patients. *Substance Use & Misuse*, 41(8), 1125–1138.

Kelly, J. F., Humphreys, K., & Ferri, M. (2020). Alcoholics Anonymous and other 12-step programs for alcohol use disorder. *Cochrane Database of Systematic Reviews*, 3, CD012880. https://doi.org/10.1002/14651858.CD012880.pub2.

Kielhofner, G. (2008). *Model of human occupation: Theory and Application*. Baltimore, MD: Lippincott, Williams and Wilkins.

King's College. (2012). *Contingency management in addiction treatment*. Available at http://www.kcl.ac.uk/iop/depts/addictions/research/drugs/contingencymanagement.aspx.

Kirsh, B., Martin, L., Hultqvist, J., & Eklund, M. (2019). Occupational therapy interventions in mental health: A literature review in search of evidence. *Occupational Therapy in Mental Health*, 35(2), 109–156.

Krebs, P., Norcross, J. C., Nicholson, J. M., & Prochaska, J. O. (2018). Stages of change and psychotherapy outcomes: A review and meta-analysis. *Journal of Clinical Psychology*, 74(11), 1964–1979. https://doi.org/10.1002/jclp.22683.

Lancaster, J. (2008). Art comes to life. *Drink and Drug News*, 11(Feb), 12–13 London.

Lesch, E., & Adams, A. R. (2016). Couples living with and around alcohol abuse: A study of a farmworker community in the Cape Winelands, South Africa. *Social Science & Medicine*, 156, 167–174.

Lussier, J. P., Heil, S. H., Mongeon, J. A., et al. (2006). A meta-analysis of voucher-based reinforcement therapy for substance use disorders. *Addiction*, 101(2), 192–203.

Mann, W. C., & Talty, P. (1990). Leisure activity profile: Measuring use of leisure time by persons with alcoholism. *Occupational Therapy in Mental Health*, 10(4), 31–41.

Marlatt, G. A. (2010). *Surfing the urge. Report of an interview with Dr Marlatt. Inquiring mind*. Available at: http://www.inquiringmind.com/Articles/SurfingTheUrge.html.

Marlatt, G. A., & Gordon, J. R. (2005). In *Relapse prevention: Maintenance strategies in the treatment of addictive behaviors* (2nd ed.). New York: Guilford Press.

Marsden, J., Farrell, M., Bradbury, C., et al. (2007). *The treatment outcomes profile (TOP): A structured interview for the evaluation of substance misuse treatment*. London: National Treatment Agency for Substance Misuse.

Martin, L. M., Bliven, M., & Boisvert, R. (2008). Occupational performance, self-esteem, and quality of life in substance addictions recovery. *OTJR (Thorofare N J)*, 28(2), 81–88.

McIntosh, J., & McKeganey, N. (2000). The recovery from dependent drug use: Addicts' strategies for reducing the risk of relapse. *Drugs*, *7*(2), 179–192.

McKeown, O., Forshaw, D. M., McGauley, G., et al. (1996). Forensic addictive behaviours unit: A case study (part I). *Journal of Substance Misuse*, *1*, 27–31.

Milkman, H., Weiner, S. E., & Sunderwirth, S. (1984). Addiction relapse. *Advances in Alcohol & Substance Abuse*, *3*(12), 119–134.

Morgan, C. A. (1994). Illicit drug use: Primary prevention. *British Journal of Occupational Therapy*, *57*(1), 2–4.

Morganstern, J., McCrady, B. S., Blanchard, K. A., et al. (2003). Barriers to employability among substance dependent and non substance affected women on federal welfare: Implications for programme design. *Journal of Studies on Alcohol*, *64*(2), 239–246.

National Institute for Health and Care Excellence (NICE). (2007). *CG51 drug misuse: Psychosocial interventions*. London: NICE.

National Institute for Health and Care Excellence (NICE). (2010). *PH24 alcohol-use disorders: Preventing harmful drinking*. London: NICE.

National Institute for Health and Care Excellence (NICE). (2011). *NICE clinical guideline 115. Alcohol Use disorders: Diagnosis, assessment and management of harmful drinking and alcohol dependence*. London: NICE.

Nhunzvi, C., Galvaan, R., & Peters, L. (2019). Recovery from substance abuse among Zimbabwean men: An occupational transition. *OTJR (Thorofare N J)*, *39*(1), 14–22.

National Institute on Drug Abuse (NIDA). (2020). *Principles of drug addiction treatment: A research-based Guide* (3rd ed.). Available at: https://nida.nih.gov/publications/principles-drug-addiction-treatment-research-based-guide-third-edition/preface.

Norcross, J. C., Krebs, P. M., & Prochaska, J. O. (2011). Adapting psychotherapy to the individual patient: Stages of change. *Journal of Clinical Psychology*, *67*(2), 143–154.

National Treatment Agency for Substance Misuse (NTA). (2002). *Models of care for the treatment of adult drug misusers – Part Two: Full reference report*. London: NTA.

NTA. (2004). *Research into practice no. 5 – engaging and Retaining clients in drug treatment*. London: Department of Health.

NTA. (2006). *Models of care for the treatment of adult drug misusers: Update 2006*. London: NTA.

Nunn, J. F. (1996). *Ancient Egyptian medicine*. London: British Museum Press.

Olivier, L., Viljoen, D. L., & Curfs, L. M. G. (2016). Fetal alcohol spectrum disorders: Prevalence rates in South Africa: The new millennium. *South African Medical Journal*, *106*(Suppl. 1), 103–106.

Pagano, M. E., Friend, K. B., Tonigan, J. S., et al. (2004). Helping other alcoholics in alcoholics anonymous and drinking outcomes: Findings from project MATCH. *Journal of Studies on Alcohol*, *65*(6), 766–773.

Peloquin, S. M., & Ciro, C. A. (2013). Self-development groups among women in recovery: Client perceptions of satisfaction and engagement. *American Journal of Occupational Therapy*, *67*(1), 82–90.

Peloquin, S. M., Ciro, C. A., Fingerhut, P., & Patterson, T. (2018). Population-centered groups for women recovering from substance abuse: Satisfaction, engagement, and lessons learned. *Occupational Therapy in Mental Health*, *34*(2), 138–150.

Platt, J. J. (1995). Vocational rehabilitation of drug abusers. *Psychological Bulletin*, *117*(3), 416–433.

Platt, J. J., Widman, M., Lidz, V., et al. (1998). The case for support services in substance abuse treatment. *American Behavioral Scientist*, *41*(8), 1050–1062.

Principles of Effective Treatment. Available at: https://www.drugabuse.gov/publications.

Prochaska, J. O., & DiClemente, C. C. (1982). Transtheoretical therapy: Towards a more integrative model of change. *Psychotherapy Theory Research Practice*, *19*(3), 276–278.

Prochaska, J. O., & DiClemente, C. C. (1986). Towards a comprehensive model of change. In R. J. Miller, & N. Heather (Eds.), *Treating addictive behaviours: Processes of change*. London: Plenum.

Prochaska, J. O., DiClemente, C. C., & Norcross, J. C. (1992). In search of how people change: Applications to addictive behaviors. *American Psychologist*, *47*(9), 1102–1114.

Prochaska, J. O., Norcross, J. C., & DiClemente, C. C. (2013). Applying the stages of change. *Psychotherapy in Australia*, *19*(2), 10–15.

Project MATCH Research Group. (1993). Project MATCH: Rationale and methods for a multisite clinical trial matching patients to alcoholism treatment. *Alcoholism: Clinical and Experimental Research*, *17*(6), 1130–1145.

Public Health England (PHE). (2017). *Better care for people with Co-occurring mental health and alcohol/drug Use conditions: A Guide for Commissioners and service providers*. London: Crown Publishing.

Ralph, R., Williams, L., Askew, R., & Norton, A. (2017). Adding spice to the porridge: The development of a synthetic cannabinoid market in an English prison. *International Journal of Drug Policy*, *40*, 57–69.

Rassoul, G. H. (2011). *Understanding addiction behaviours: Theoretical & clinical practice in health and social care*. Basingstoke: Palgrave Macmillan.

RCPsych. (2014). *Alcohol and brain damage in adults*. RCPsych Publication 2014, CR185.

Reitz, S. M., & Scaffa, M. E. (2020). Occupational therapy in the promotion of health and well-being. *American Journal of Occupational Therapy*, *74*(3), 7403420010p1–7403420010p14.

Rojo-Mota, G., Pedrero-Pérez, E. J., & Huertas-Hoyas, E. (2017). Systematic review of occupational therapy in the treatment of addiction: Models, practice, and qualitative and quantitative research. *American Journal of Occupational Therapy*, *71*(5), 7105100030p1–7105100030p11.

Room, J. A. (1998). Work identity in substance abuse recovery. *Journal of Substance Abuse Treatment*, *15*(1), 65–74.

Rotert, D. (1989). Occupational therapy and alcoholism. *Journal of Occupational Medicine*, *4*(2), 327–337.

Sarsak, H. I. (2018). Overview: Occupational therapy for psychiatric disorders. *Journal of Psychology & Clinical Psychiatry, 9*(5), 518–521.

Scaffa, M. E. (1991). Alcoholism: An occupational behaviour perspective. *Occupational Therapy in Mental Health, 11*(2/3), 99–111.

Scottish Executive. (2001). *Moving on: Education, training and employment for recovering drug users.* Edinburgh: Effective Interventions Unit.

Simpson, D. D., Joe, G. W., & Brown, B. S. (1997). Treatment retention and follow-up outcomes in the Drug abuse treatment outcome study (DATOS). *Psychology of Addictive Behaviors, 11*(4), 239–260.

Skodbo, S., Brown, G., Deacon, S., et al. (2007). *Research report 2. The drug interventions programme (DIP): Addressing drug Use and Offending through 'Tough choices.'* London: Home Office.

Smart Recovery UK, 2010. Available at: http://www.smartrecovery.org.uk/.

Smith, I., & Hillman, A. (1999). Management of alcohol Korsakoff syndrome. *Advances in Psychiatric Treatment, 5,* 271–278.

Solinas, M., Belujon, P., Fernagut, P. O., et al. (2019). Dopamine and addiction: What have we learned from 40 years of research. *Journal of Neural Transmission, 126,* 481–516. https://doi.org/10.1007/s00702-018-1957-2.

Spaderna, M., Addy, P. H., & D'souza, D. C. (2013). Spicing things up: Synthetic cannabinoids. *Psychopharmacol Heidelberg, 228*(4), 525–540.

Stephens, R., & Cottrell, E. (1972). A follow-up study of 200 narcotic addicts committed for treatment under the narcotic addict rehabilitation act (NARA). *British Journal of Addiction, 67*(1), 45–53.

Stoffel, V. C., Cusatis, M., Seitz, L., et al. (1992). Self-esteem and leisure patterns of persons in a residential chemical dependency treatment program. *Occupational Therapy in Health Care, 8*(2/3), 69–85.

Stone, M. (2017). *Understanding the impact of substance abuse on occupation using the lifestyle history questionnaire.* Available at encompass.eku.edu.

Strategy Unit. (2003). *Alcohol harm reduction project: Interim Analytical report.* London: Cabinet Office.

Sy, M. P., Ohshima, N., & Roraldo, M. P. N. R. (2018). The role of Filipino occupational therapists in substance addiction and rehabilitation: A Q-methodology. *Occupational Therapy in Mental Health, 34*(4), 367–388.

Turning Point. (2016). *Dual Dilemma: The impact of living with mental health issues combined with drug and alcohol misuse.* London: Turning Point.

Tyler, S. (1995). *Street drugs.* London: Hodder and Stoughton.

UK Drug Policy Commission (UKDPC). (2008). *The UK drug policy Commission recovery Consensus group: A vision of recovery. Policy report.* London: UKDPC.

United Nations (UN). (2020). *World drug report 2020 (United Nations publication, Sales No. E.20.XI.6).*

United Nations (UN) Office on Drugs and Crime. (2017). *Global synthetic drugs assessment.*

Ussher, M., McCusker, M., Morrow, V., et al. (2000). A physical activity intervention in a community alcohol service. *British Journal of Occupational Therapy, 63*(12), 219–231.

Valliant, G. E. (1998). What can long term follow up teach us about relapse and prevention of relapse addiction? *British Journal of Addiction, 83*(10), 1147–1157.

Viik, M. K., Watts, J. H., Madigan, M. J., et al. (1990). Preliminary validation of the assessment of occupational functioning with an alcoholic population. *Occupational Therapy in Mental Health, 10*(2), 19–33.

Walton, M. T., & Hall, M. T. (2016). The effects of employment interventions on addiction treatment outcomes: A review of the literature. *Journal of Social Work Practice in the Addictions, 16*(4), 358–384.

Wanigaratne, S., Pullin, J., Wallace, W., et al. (1990). *Relapse prevention for addictive behaviours – a manual for therapists.* London: Blackwell.

Wasmuth, S., Crabtree, J. L., & Scott, P. J. (2014). Exploring addiction-as-occupation. *British Journal of Occupational Therapy, 77,* 605–613. https://doi.org/10.4276/03080221 4X14176260335264.

Wegner, L., Blake, L., Jupp, L., Nyabenda, F., & Turner, T. (2015). Clients' perceptions of an occupational therapy intervention at a substance use rehabilitation centre in the Western Cape. *South African Journal of Occupational Therapy., 45*(2), 10–14.

Weiss, R. D., Griffin, M. L., Gallop, R. J., et al. (2005). The effect of 12-step self-help group attendance and participation on drug use outcomes among cocaine-dependent patients. *Drug and Alcohol Dependence, 77*(2), 177–184.

Wesson, D. R., & Ling, W. (2003). The clinical opiate withdrawal scale (COWS). *Journal of Psychoactive Drugs, 35*(2), 253–259.

Whitten. (2009). Receptor complexes link dopamine to long-term neuronal effects. *Nida Notes, 22*(4), 15–16.

Williams, G. (2016). Slaves, workers, and wine: The 'dop system' in the history of the Cape wine industry, 1658–1894. *Journal of Southern African Studies, 42*(5), 893–909.

World Health Organization (WHO). (2020). *Lexicon of alcohol and drug terms.* Available at: https://www.who.int/substance_abuse/terminology/who_lexicon/en/ 01/10/2020.

World Health Organization (WHO), Regional Office for Africa (2017). *Substance abuse.* Available at: https://www.afro.who.int/health-topics/substance-abuse.

Zimbabwe Civil Liberties and Drugs Network, 2018. Zimbabwe Civil Liberties Drugs Network April Update. Available at: https://idpc.net/profile/zcldn.

28

EATING DISORDERS

CLARE LAWRENCE ■ SARAH MCAULEY

CHAPTER OVERVIEW

This chapter describes the clinical features, causes and impacts of eating disorders and the treatment settings and services in which occupational therapists work. It considers some theoretical materials, skills and tools used by occupational therapists and explores widely used occupational therapy interventions. With the huge impact that an eating disorder can have on occupation and function, the field is, unsurprisingly, an area of growing input and specialism for occupational therapists.

INTRODUCTION

Eating disorders are serious mental health problems characterized by an individual's preoccupation with, or overvaluation of, food and their own weight and body shape (Lydecker et al. 2017; Rodgers et al. 2019), or with fears related to the act of eating, such as fear of choking (Ornstein et al. 2017). This frequently

TABLE 28.1
Eating Disorder Symptoms and Associated Medical Complications

Symptom	Medical Complication
Restricting food intake	Altered metabolism with hypothermia, cognitive impairment, dizziness, hypotension, bradycardia, orthostasis, amenorrhea, oedema, fatigue
Binging on food	Obesity, hypertension, hyperlipidaemia, insulin resistance, joint deterioration, dyspnoea, sleep apnoea, gall bladder disease
Vomiting	Electrolyte imbalance (hypokalaemia), arrhythmias, esophagitis/gastritis, gastroesophageal reflux disease, dental caries, dehydration, alkalosis, parotid/submandibular gland hypertrophy
Laxative abuse	Cathartic colon, dehydration, electrolyte imbalance, metabolic acidosis, alkalosis
Diuretic abuse	Dehydration, electrolyte imbalance
Appetite suppressant abuse	Hypertension, tremor, arrhythmias
Ipecac (emetic) abuse	Myopathy, cardiomyopathy
Water loading	Hyponatremia, headache, nausea, dizziness, seizure
Compulsive exercise	Severe bradycardia, joint deterioration, stress fractures, overuse syndromes

From Jahraus, J., 2018. Medical complications of eating disorders. Psychiatr. Ann. 48 (10), 463–467.

prevents the attainment or maintenance of a normal body weight.

Eating disorders are also associated with significant medical complications (Klump et al. 2009) arising from dermatological, cardiovascular, gastrointestinal, musculoskeletal, genitourinary and cognitive changes (Table 28.1). These problems frequently predicted by the nature of, and time spent on, specific eating disordered behaviours (Jahraus 2018) and their impacts range from comparatively minor to life-threatening. Indeed, anorexia nervosa has the highest mortality rate of any mental disorder (Jahraus 2018).

Eating disorders are recognized in a range of cultures and societies, and it is noted that, despite the thinking around 'a Western body ideal,' anorexia nervosa 'has been observed in every non-Western region in the world' (Keel and Klump 2003, p. 754). Studies do, however, suggest there is greater prevalence of eating disorders in the West or in areas with strong Western influences (Makino et al. 2004), although whether this is related to influences such as population demographics, media exposure, social circumstances or, conversely, a lack of recognition of eating disorders or a cultural bias in instruments or diagnostic criteria is uncertain.

Eating disorders can occur at any age but most commonly develop during adolescence (13–17 years) (National Institute for Health and Care Excellence (NICE) 2017). Although eating disorders are more common among women, up to a quarter of people with eating disorders are men (Sweeting 2015; Keski-Rahkonen 2016). The introduction of the Diagnostic and Statistical Manual of Mental Disorders, 5th Edition (DSM-5) (American Psychiatric Association (APA) 2013), provides greater opportunity for more accurate recognition of eating disorders in adults, young people and children and a likelihood of a changing picture of prevalence (Dahlgren and Wisting 2016).

CLINICAL FEATURES OF EATING DISORDERS

The terms 'anorexia nervosa' and 'bulimia nervosa' have long been widely known in relation to eating disorders. However, the range of symptoms and behaviours exhibited by many people with eating disorders are not adequately accommodated under these labels and may have been more accurately described, based on the DSM-IV criteria (APA 2000), as having an 'eating disorder not otherwise specified' (EDNOS). To better reflect people's experience and behaviours, the DSM-5 (APA 2013) has expanded the diagnostic categories of eating disorders, removing EDNOS, including binge eating disorder, making modifications to the diagnoses of anorexia nervosa and bulimia nervosa and adding three further categories: avoidant/restrictive food intake disorder, rumination disorder and pica (Table 28.2). Despite clear differences in the descriptors of each disorder, most are characterised by the individual having an overvaluation of their weight and shape. The case studies (Suzanne, Lizzie, Catherine and Daniel) presented later in the chapter aim to illustrate some of the differing presentations associated with eating disorders.

CAUSES OF EATING DISORDERS

As in Suzanne's case (Case Study 28.1), a person with an eating disorder may identify a significant event or time when problems began, such as the beginning of a 'normal' weight loss diet that elicited compliments from significant others. However, eating disorders are unlikely to relate to one discrete cause, but rather to a complex interaction of internal and external factors, one of which may be highlighted as responsible for 'triggering' the disorder.

Whether or not there was a significant event, it is likely that vulnerability to an eating disorder pre-dates its onset (Leon et al. 1993) and there is a growing understanding of predisposing experiences common in those with eating disorders, which include:

TABLE 28.2	
Eating Disorder Descriptors Recognized in the Diagnostic and Statistical Manual of Mental Disorders, 5th Edition (DSM-5)	
	DSM-5 Criteria
Anorexia Nervosa	A. Persistent restriction of energy intake leading to significantly low body weight in the context of age, sex, development, physical health B. Intense fear of gaining weight/becoming 'fat' or persistent behaviour that interferes with weight gain (even though significantly low weight) C. Disturbance in the way body shape/weight is experienced, undue influence of body shape/weight on self-evaluation or persistent non-recognition of seriousness of low body weight. Subtypes: Restricting type; binge-eating/purging type
Bulimia Nervosa	A. Recurrent episodes of binge eating, characterized by both of the following: ■ Eating, in a discrete period of time, a larger amount than most people would eat during a similar period under similar circumstances ■ A sense of lack of control over eating during this period B. Recurrent inappropriate compensatory behaviour to prevent weight gain (e.g. self-induced vomiting, misuse of laxatives/diuretics/other medications, fasting, excessive exercise) C. The above both occur, on average, at least once a week for three months D. Self-evaluation unduly influenced by body shape/weight E. The disturbance does not occur exclusively during episodes of anorexia nervosa
Binge Eating Disorder	A. Recurrent episodes of binge eating (above) associated with three or more of the following: ■ Eating much more rapidly than normal ■ Eating until feeling uncomfortably full ■ Eating large amounts of food when not feeling physically hungry ■ Eating alone due to feelings of embarrassment about the amount one is eating ■ Feeling disgusted with oneself, depressed or very guilty afterwards ■ Marked distress regarding binge eating B. Binge eating occurs, on average, at least once a week for 3 months C. Binge eating is not associated with the recurrent use of inappropriate compensatory behaviours (as in bulimia nervosa) nor exclusively during the course of bulimia nervosa or anorexia nervosa methods of compensation (e.g., self-induced vomiting)
Pica	A. Persistent eating of non-nutritive substances for a period of at least 1 month B. The eating of non-nutritive substances inappropriate to the person's developmental level C. The eating behaviour is not part of a culturally supported or socially normative practice D. If it occurs in the presence of another mental disorder or medical condition, it is severe enough to warrant independent clinical attention

Continued on following page

	TABLE 28.2		
	Eating Disorder Descriptors Recognized in the Diagnostic and Statistical Manual of Mental Disorders, 5th Edition (DSM-5) (Continued)		
	DSM-5 Criteria		
Rumination Disorder	A. Repeated regurgitation (rechewed/reswallowed/spat out) of food for at least 1 month B. The above is not due to a gastro-intestinal or other medical condition C. The above does not occur exclusively in the course of another eating disorder D. If occurring in the presence of another mental health problem, symptoms are severe enough to warrant independent clinical attention		
Avoidant/ Restrictive Food Intake Disorder	A. An eating/feeding disturbance manifested by persistent failure to meet appropriate nutritional and/or energy needs associated with one (or more) of the following: ■ Significant weight loss (or failure to gain expected weight/faltering growth in children) ■ Significant nutritional deficiency ■ Dependence on enteral feeding or oral nutritional supplements ■ Marked interference with psychosocial functioning B. Behaviour is not better explained by limited food availability or normalized in the person's culture C. Behaviour does not occur during the course of another eating disorder nor is there evidence of a disturbance in the subjective experience of body weight/shape D. The above is not attributed to a medical condition or better explained by another mental health problem or, if it does occur in the presence of another condition/disorder, it exceeds norms and warrants additional clinical attention		
Other Specified Feeding/Eating Disorder (OSFED)	A. Feeding or eating behaviours that cause clinical distress or impairment in areas of functioning but do not meet the full criteria for any other feeding/eating disorders B. A diagnosis might then be made that specifies a reason why the presentation does not meet the criteria of another disorder (e.g., bulimia nervosa - low frequency).		
Unspecified Feeding/ Eating Disorder	A. Feeding or eating behaviours that cause clinical distress or impairment in areas of functioning but do not meet the full criteria for any other feeding/eating disorders B. Used when clinicians do not specify the reason that the presentation does not meet the criteria of another disorder, including times when there is insufficient information to make this diagnosis.		

CASE STUDY 28.1

Suzanne

Suzanne is a 52-year-old woman who has been overweight for much of her life, with her highest body mass index (BMI) being 46. She has four children, the youngest of whom is 22 and left home the previous year to go travelling. Up until last year Suzanne was working as a PA for a large manufacturing firm, where she had been since her children were young. Suzanne was widowed 5 years ago and remarried 2 years ago to Clive. Prior to the wedding she embarked on a weight loss programme and successfully reached her target weight for which she received lots of positive feedback from friends and family. At this point, however, she was reluctant to work on maintaining her weight and persisted in significantly restricting her food and fluid intake. This ongoing restriction has resulted in physical symptoms requiring investigations through her GP and local outpatient departments.

■ Negative affect and reduced psychosocial functioning, such as facing challenges in forming supportive relationships (Stice et al. 2017);

■ Difficulties in early attachment/adverse childhood experiences (Lejonclou et al. 2014);

■ History of eating disorders within the family home (Watkins et al. 2012);

■ Genetic influences (Zerwas and Bullik 2011);

■ History of trauma, particularly childhood sexual abuse (Lejonclou et al. 2014);

■ Internal and societal pressure of slimness/body ideal, although it is noted that this is associated with predictors of binge eating disorder and bulimia nervosa, not anorexia nervosa (Stice et al. 2017);

■ Participation in sports in which a particular weight or shape may offer a competitive advantage (Joy et al. 2016).

THE IMPACT OF EATING DISORDERS

Recovery from an eating disorder is a challenging and time-consuming process (Biddiscombe 2018). From an occupational therapy perspective, the eating disorder can dominate every part of the individual's life, stripping away or altering an individual's habitual occupations.

When living with an eating disorder, the balance between self-care, productivity and leisure becomes distorted, with some occupations being over-valued while others are considered insignificant. This can result in a collection of unhelpful roles, routines and behaviours, leaving a void to be filled before recovery can occur. Examples of such changes are illustrated, in relation to Lizzie (Case Study 28.2) in Fig. 28.1.

CASE STUDY 28.2

Lizzie

Lizzie is 18 years old with a current body mass index (BMI) of 15. She has a diagnosis of obsessive compulsive disorder (OCD). She lives at home with her parents, where her older sister returns during university holidays. She completed school, achieving her A levels with all A-grades. Since leaving school she has lost contact with her friends and previous boyfriend. She is unemployed and spends at least 5 hours of her day walking or running. Much of her other time is spent cleaning and engaging in OCD-related rituals. She weighs herself multiple times a day, including before and after eating. Her diet consists of yoghurt, crackers, and hot water or hot chocolate.

EATING DISORDER SERVICES AND SETTINGS

The Multidisciplinary Team

Typically, in eating disorder services within the United Kingdom (UK), the multidisciplinary team (MDT) includes nurses, healthcare assistants, medical staff, dietitians, psychologists, psychotherapists, occupational therapists, family therapists art or drama therapists, and social workers. Due to the intensity and long-term nature of the MDT work, good communication within the team is essential along with an awareness of each clinician's specialist role. It is important for the occupational therapist to be confident, clear and assertive about the role of occupational therapy, including its assessments and interventions.

Accessing Services

NICE guidelines (NICE 2017) recommend that individuals with an eating disorder be treated, as far as possible, in the community; usually under the care of a GP, a mental health nurse and a dietician or a specialist eating disorders community team if one exists locally. However, if the severity of a person's condition requires it, hospitalization is recommended. In the UK, this may involve being detained in the hospital for assessment and/or treatment under the Mental Health Act (1983, updated 2007) (Department of Health 2007).

Compared to other eating disorders, anorexia nervosa prompts the highest proportion of hospital admissions (Schmidt et al. 2013). Hospital treatment is usually

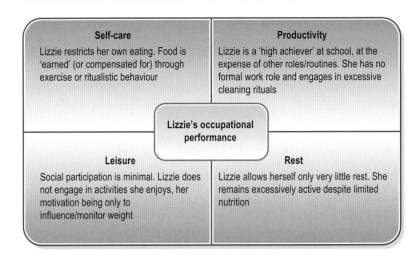

Fig. 28.1 ■ The impact of Lizzie's eating disorder on her occupational performance (see Case Study 28.2).

required at least once during an individual's period of care, requiring supervision, containment and access to an MDT of experienced professionals (Abraham 2008). Alternatively, a day service environment may be more appropriate, whereby individuals continue living at home and attend a clinic each day for treatment.

In the UK the type of intervention settings and treatment offered is subject to significant geographical variation (Parliamentary and Health Service Ombudsman 2017). Some areas of the United Kingdom are served by specialist eating disorder services (offering inpatient, outpatient and day services) whilst other areas may be served only by non-specialist mental health crisis and recovery teams. This may result in individuals having to travel long distances or move from home to access support. Additionally, the waiting times to be seen by an eating disorder specialist can be up to, and are sometimes in excess of, six months; by which time it is not uncommon for the individual's condition to have deteriorated, requiring more intensive care than if support had been timely. The different types of intervention settings will now be explored.

Inpatient Units

These usually form part of a larger psychiatric or general hospital and care for male and female service users from the age of 18 years who are diagnosed with an eating disorder. The individual lives on the ward (with agreed periods of leave) and the duration of stay depends on their personalized care programme.

Admissions

As noted earlier, eating disorder inpatient settings accommodate individuals who are engaging in treatment of their own volition and those being compulsorily detained for the purpose of assessment and/or treatment under the Mental Health Act (1983/2007).

An agreed safe weight for each individual is often identified by the care team based on the individual's body mass index (BMI), which is calculated by dividing the person's weight (in kilograms) by the square of their height (in metres) (Lacey et al. 2007). A BMI below 17.5 is deemed to be in the 'underweight' range and below 13.5 is deemed 'severely malnourished,' with a healthy adult weight falling between 18.5 and 24.9 (World Health Organization 2019). A Mental Health Act (1983/2007) assessment may be required if concerns exist for the

person's health and safety, such as following a drop in body weight to a dangerously low BMI. A programme of supervised, weight-increasing meals aims to restore the individual's weight to within a safe range. Recommended rates of weight gain are 0.5 to 1 kg/wk in an inpatient setting and 0.5 kg/wk in an outpatient setting (Marzola et al. 2013). To achieve this the individual will be encouraged to eat small, regular meals with the ultimate aim being to encourage the return to a normal diet (Lacey et al. 2007).

If an individual is unwilling to eat the meals provided and their weight is deemed to be at a dangerous level, then nasogastric tube feeding may occasionally be used whereby the individual is fed via their nose into their stomach. Sometimes an individual may be more accepting of this than eating food, just as they may be more accepting of a nutritional drink than solid food. However, if a person is refusing to eat and also refusing to allow a nasogastric tube, then compulsory treatment under the Mental Health Act (1983/2007) may be considered. This is deemed a last resort due to the importance placed on the therapeutic alliance between the individual and the clinical team to support recovery (Lacey et al. 2007).

Initial Assessment

The initial assessment will often be completed by a nurse, doctor or mental health practitioner of any profession, acting as first point of contact. This assessment will focus on mental and physical health, including current weight and eating behaviours, risks, health history, social situation and motivation for change. Occupational therapy assessment will occur after the initial assessment, commonly after an MDT discussion and review and usually after a period of sustained nutrition and weight stabilization, but this is dependent on the individual and their care goals.

No standardized occupational therapy eating disorders assessment tool currently exists. So, often, occupational therapists will use an assessment tool that is linked to their chosen model of practice with an emphasis on the impact of the individual's eating and food behaviour on their occupational performance, components and contexts.

Inpatient Care

Inpatient settings adopt a multidisciplinary approach, encompassing a combination of medical and psychosocial approaches. Weight restoration and medical stabilization will be a significant early aim of the care plan followed by psychological work and occupational therapy, depending on the individuals' progress and their recovery goals. It is common for individuals to transition to a day service to step-down and complete their care programme, but this depends on the availability of local services.

Inpatient Facilities

The inpatient service will feature communal areas such as a lounge or recreational area where activities take place (such as board games, crafts, reading, watching television), a dining area, kitchen, bathrooms, and sleeping accommodation, which usually consists of single rooms, each with a sink and access to a shared bathroom. Additionally, there are rooms for clinical and therapeutic sessions and staff areas. The individual's care plan will specify whether they are able to leave the ward or not, so the environment must provide appropriate stimulation for service users who have to stay on the ward.

The work that takes place in the dining room on an eating disorder ward or in a day clinic is often challenging. Here the service user is expected to sit and eat three meals and three snacks during the course of the day (see examples in Table 28.3). In doing so, they are also encouraged to behave in a socially acceptable manner. Consequently, it is common for the dining room to have different tables, each with a particular level of support, monitoring and encouragement being provided. With this level of bespoke support in place, common eating disorder–related behaviours/habits such as spoiling, hiding or regurgitating food (see Interventions section) can be tolerated, as an oral diet is preferred for an individual compared to nasogastric feeding.

It is common for all members of the MDT to participate in these therapeutic eating interventions, which are based on a broadly behavioural approach involving the modelling of appropriate eating behaviours by staff (who eat the same meal at the same tables as service users) and encouragement and support to service users to express their feelings verbally rather than through eating disorder–related behaviours. It is also an opportunity to observe how each individual is managing with their meal plan. Not surprisingly, the dining room can be an emotionally charged and stressful place to be. Maladaptive eating disorder–related behaviours are witnessed alongside individual's obvious distress regarding food and drink. Consequently, staff support and reflection is vital for team members to understand and manage their own feelings and thoughts and to look after themselves.

A period of sustained starvation, as characterized by anorexia nervosa and/or deregulated eating for bulimia nervosa and some other eating disorders, can have an impact on an individual's brain (Van den Eynde et al. 2012; Treasure and Schmidt 2013), causing adverse effects in cognitive function and emotional regulation amongst other kinds of neural damage. Therefore a period of regular nutritional intake and stabilized eating will be advantageous for the care plan as a whole because it optimizes overall functionality, and, hence, the utilization and ultimate efficacy of the occupational therapy and other psychologically informed interventions (which may be offered by any MDT member, including occupational therapists).

The prime focus of occupational therapy input may be, for example, to enable an individual to successfully shop for, cook and eat their (so called) fear foods, that is, foods thought by the individual to lead to weight gain (Biddiscombe et al. 2018). However, for

TABLE 28.3	
An Example of a Weight Restoration Meal Plan	
Breakfast	Corn flakes with full-fat milk, banana, two pieces of toast with butter and jam, cup of tea or coffee with milk, glass of water or fruit juice
Lunch	Cheese sandwich (made with two pieces of bread and butter, one tomato, three slices of cucumber), full-fat yogurt, slice of cake or cookie, glass of squash
Evening Meal	Shepherd's pie with vegetables, sponge cake and custard, glass of squash
Three Snacks (AM, Mid-PM, and Bedtime)	Two bourbon biscuits, cup of tea/coffee and milk or hot chocolate at bedtime

a psychologist the aim may be to help the individual understand the cause of their eating disorder. Fear foods is a term created by individuals with eating disorders which has been adopted by clinicians and services, often referring to food perceived as high calorie or indulgent or food which was previously binged on.

Additionally, a more 'light touch' or diversional group program (that is, a range of groups based on occupations not directly related to eating behaviours but aiming to create routine and/or promote social engagement) is available to all service users at different stages of treatment. It is usual for the occupational therapist to be fully involved in the group programme alongside their MDT colleagues.

Day Services

Eating disorder day services offer a part-hospitalization approach whereby the full range of medical and therapeutic MDT input (regarding intensity and duration) is combined with the flexibility of the individual returning home each day. Weight restoration will often be the primary aim, running parallel with psychological work and occupational therapy to address eating disordered habits, as described earlier.

The combination of daily hospital attendance and home living enables the individual to develop their skills and confidence in independent living, such as eating out and managing food shopping, and support for this is a key feature of the day service occupational therapy role. However, being a day service attendee also requires high levels of motivation to attend the service during the day and to adhere to an agreed food and meal plan when away from it. A day service may be used as a step-down from inpatient care or a step-up from community settings to help people transition successfully.

Community Care

Community care is the least restrictive intervention setting and thus regarded as current best practice if the individual can be treated safely (Madden et al. 2015; NICE 2017). This setting generally involves once-or twice-weekly sessions with a practitioner from any discipline who will manage and oversee the individual's care, receiving input from other clinicians. The focus remains on weight restoration alongside psychological and occupational therapy input. Not all eating disorder services offer care coordination, so this role may be undertaken by a practitioner from a more generic community mental health team, whose care planning will incorporate specialist input from the community worker in the eating disorder service.

Adolescents and Eating Disorders

In the UK, following a Health Select Committee (2014), inquiry into systemic problems with young people's mental health services, NHS England (2015) stipulated that young people with a probable eating disorder should be seen within a month of referral, that urgent cases should be seen within a week and emergencies within 24 hours.

The most cost-effective treatment for anorexia nervosa is reported to be delivered by community-based eating disorder services for children and young people (CEDS-CYP) as opposed to generic Child and Adolescent Mental Health Services (CAMHS) (Byford et al. 2007). Consequently, across the UK new standalone services have been set up, supported by NICE (2017) guidelines for eating disorders (see overleaf). However, as with adult services there are huge geographical variations in service provision.

CEDS-CYP teams offer intensive home treatment, family-based interventions, individual therapy (psychology or psychotherapy), family therapy, occupational therapy, therapeutic groups (e.g., focusing on body image, social eating practice, meal cookery, relaxation), parent support, medical monitoring and liaison with tier 4 CAMHS for an inpatient stay if home treatment does not improve the situation.

Clinicians working with young people use weight for height measurements rather than BMI when calculating healthy weight ranges. This is because, when working with young people with anorexia, age and gender are important to take into consideration, which BMI does not. Therefore the Royal College of Psychiatrists (2012) recommends using percentage BMI (BMI/Median BMI for age and gender ×100). A typically healthy weight range for a young person is 95% to 105% weight for height or, in females, when periods consistently return.

Junior MARSIPAN (Royal College of Psychiatrists 2012), an acronym for 'management of really sick patients with anorexia nervosa,' is a risk assessment tool to help clinicians assess physical and psychological risk areas such as cardiovascular health, temperature, self-harm, muscle weakness, and disordered eating behaviours. This is important because young people with eating disorders can often become medically compromised and present at accident and emergency or paediatric departments where professionals can feel deskilled due to the complicated and covert nature of their presenting symptoms.

NICE (2017) guidelines recommend the use of anorexia nervosa–focused family therapy for children and young people, which emphasizes the role of the family in helping the person to recover and includes psychoeducation aimed at the young person and their family regarding nutrition and the damaging effects of starvation. The guidelines also highlight the importance of support regarding the distress felt by families. Consequently, services have set up support groups where parents can seek support from each other and learn how vital their role is in helping the young person recover.

As noted previously, when an individual has an eating disorder their previous healthy roles and occupations fade and their primary occupations become those associated with the eating disorder, such as the many rituals and behaviours required to maintain it. Where a young person once engaged in a variety of occupations, such as attending school, socializing with friends, engaging in hobbies and spending time with family, these are replaced by 'the eating disorder,' which becomes the main focus of the person's life. Occupational therapy uses practical interventions to assist young people to reestablish healthy occupations and roles and the life balance they once had, using activity analysis and graded therapeutic activity to address these occupational performance deficits. Establishing a connection to meaningful occupations helps individuals change the way they think about themselves, their environment and their potential for recovery.

For example, part of an anorexia nervosa–focused family therapy approach involves parents being told to take back control of food planning/preparation and then to gradually give this responsibility back to the young person. They are asked to challenge food fears, eating disorder rituals and behaviours. Occupational therapists are uniquely positioned to use their skills of assessing, adapting, grading, goal setting and engaging in activity to support this (Gardiner and Brown 2010). Interventions may include 'snack out' practise (eating in social settings, such as coffee shops, fast food chains or public areas such as parks), meal cookery practise (in the home or hospital setting) and social eating with peers at school and/or in restaurants.

Although the work of an occupational therapist within eating disorder services necessarily covers all aspects of a person's life, there is obviously a focus on food, challenging the food-related maladaptive behaviours and supporting the person to tolerate their negative feelings about food. This may involve working closely with schools/colleges to help the individual achieve a healthy balance between schoolwork and other areas of life. Typically, an individual may use schoolwork as a distraction and over-perform. Occupational therapy interventions may be designed to challenge perfectionism, encouraging the belief that things can be 'just okay'; perhaps using a craft activity as a medium for this. When appropriate it is important to include the family/carers in the intervention.

A core occupational therapy skill is group work (see Chapter 15), and this is an integral part of adolescent service provision in both inpatient and community settings. Leisure-based group work aims at facilitating social skills and engagement in appropriate levels of leisure and exercise activities to promote a healthy and balanced lifestyle (Gardiner and Brown 2010) without the eating disorder being 'used' as a coping mechanism. Self-care–based groups aim to challenge a young person to look after themselves and take care of their body and mind; examples might include mindfulness, nail painting and massage.

Independent or Private Treatment

Treatment from the private sector (from a psychologist, psychotherapist, occupational therapist and/or nurse) is a growing area in the UK. This could reflect individual preference or be prompted by the lack of services in some parts of the country and the long waiting times, as noted earlier. Occupational therapists working independently will usually insist a service user has completed psychological work (such as psychotherapy or other talking therapies to address underlying causes of the eating disorder) and/or is under the care of a medical professional (for weight and physical health management) before beginning occupational therapy.

THEORETICAL CONTEXTS

This exploration of the theoretical context for occupational therapy with people who have an eating disorder includes consideration of models of practice and approaches.

Using a Model of Practice

As noted earlier, occupational therapists often use assessment tools that are linked to particular models of practice. The Model of Human Occupation (MOHO) (Taylor 2017) is concerned with how occupations are motivated, patterned and performed within given social and physical environments. It is frequently used by occupational therapists working in eating disorder services, but it is by no means the only model used in this field. The 'referral' section of the occupational therapy process illustrated in Case Study 28.3, Part 1, uses MOHO principles to consider Catherine's presentation at the point of referral to an eating disorder inpatient unit, and Catherine's progress is also charted to illustrate subsequent stages.

Assessment tools linked to the MOHO that fit well for this service user group include the Model of Human Occupation Screening Tool (MOHOST), the Occupational Self-Assessment (OSA), the Child Occupational Self-Assessment (COSA), the Occupational Circumstances Assessment Interview and Rating Scale

---

CASE STUDY 28.3, PART 1
Catherine (The Occupational Therapy Process)

REFERRAL

Catherine is a 22-year old woman living in supported housing for people with mental health difficulties and is currently unemployed. She has reduced volition attributed to the anorexia nervosa heavily influencing all cognitive processes. Catherine's thought patterns are dominated by obsessive ideas about food, weight and eating behaviours. In terms of habituation, Catherine's daily routines are maladaptive as they are controlled by the cycle of binging and vomiting and by obsessive-compulsive disorder rituals, such as hand washing and constantly re-arranging her possessions. On assessment, Catherine does not appear to have any functional roles or routines in her day-to-day life. Regarding performance capacity, Catherine is cognitively and physically compromised due to a low body weight, which impacts her functionality. However, she does have a successful school and employment history. The physical and social environments influence occupational behaviour by generating both opportunities and constraints (Taylor 2017). Catherine has a disruptive, unsupportive family milieu, and recent living conditions have led to isolation and a limited social circle. Both of these environments can be understood in terms of their constraining influence on Catherine's occupations. For example, she has not developed any friendships in her accommodation where she further isolates herself.

ASSESSMENT (USING THE MOHOST)

The occupational therapist meets Catherine twice for approximately 40 minutes each time. Catherine is forthcoming. She describes her challenges with meal planning, food shopping and preparation and her eating disorder–related behaviours. The occupational therapist completes the MOHOST rating scale and cocreates a care plan with Catherine.

CARE PLANNING

See Case Study 28.3, Part 2 for details.

EVALUATION

A post-intervention MOHOST will be used as an outcome measure, the results being recorded in clinical notes and shared with Catherine. Treatment goals will be finalized, progress updated and all results included in Catherine's discharge summary. This information is a feature of accountable and transparent professional practice, evidence (for Catherine) of her own progress and a means of communicating the role of occupational therapy across the multidisciplinary team.

DISCHARGE

The occupational therapist meets Catherine to reflect on her achievements and the challenges weathered. A plan is cocreated to support the transfer of Catherine's skills to new accommodation and social environments. Catherine says 'goodbye' to her groups, and, in the ward meeting, reads a poem about her experiences with the service and her recovery journey to date.

(OCAIRS) and the Single Observation MOHOST (Taylor 2017). The MOHOST benefits from including clinical observations and notes as part of the assessment process and a rating scale, which means the tool can be used as an outcome measure also. Both the OSA and OCAIRS require the client to be cognitively and emotionally able to participate in the interview.

Using an Approach/Frame of Reference

A cognitive-behavioural approach is widely used to inform eating disorder interventions. The way an individual thinks about a phenomenon affects the way they feel about it, of course, which influences their behaviour towards it. For people with an eating disorder, eating can carry strong negative associated thoughts and, similarly, an 'empty stomach' can bring feelings of happiness and power, which may lead to a person restricting their food intake.

A cognitive-behavioural approach informs group work (including personal skills development groups, projective art groups and relapse prevention groups, for example) and diary-keeping to record feelings and actions. Service users are helped to examine and modify unhelpful attitudes towards food, dieting and body image and to identify triggers for these with the aim to replace them with positive realistic expectations. This involves encouraging service users to recognize

the antecedents and consequences of behaviour and be 'retrained' in new dietary and eating habits. This may involve complementing the cognitive-behavioural approach with a more purely behavioural one. Service users are encouraged to stop all abnormal eating patterns and reach a safer and stable weight through adaptive eating behaviour. For example, during an admission it is expected that meals are eaten in the dining room with health professionals present to model appropriate eating behaviour, as described previously. Once the target weight for an individual is achieved and sustained, systematic de-sensitization might be used, by gradually introducing the feared stimulus of food through a meal cookery group (see intervention section).

Using the Transtheoretical Model of Change

The transtheoretical model of behaviour change, or stages of change model (Prochaska and DiClemente 1983), is commonly used in eating disorders services as a tool to assist in assessing an individual's attitude to, and readiness for, change and to support their motivation. The model conceptualizes behaviour change as a cyclical process, with pre-contemplation (where there is no desire to change) preceding contemplation of change, as depicted in Fig. 28.2.

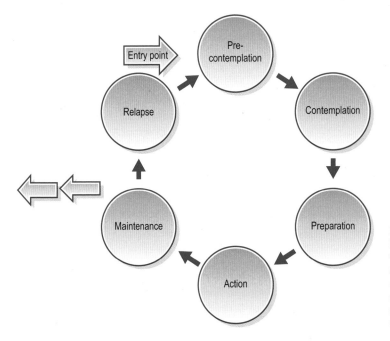

Fig. 28.2 ■ **The transtheoretical model of behaviour change.** (From Prochaska, J., DiClemente, C., 1983. Stages and processes of self-change in smoking: toward an integrative model of change. J Consult. Clin. Psychol. 51 (3), 390–395. Available at: https://psycnet.apa.org/doiLanding?doi=10.1037%2F0022-006X.51.3.390.)

An individual in the contemplation (or 'maybe') phase may be ambivalent about change and be offered psychoeducational interventions coupled with a motivational interviewing approach to prompt them into planning and preparation for change. In the action stage active work is central, so an individual may engage in meal cookery aimed at promoting adaptive eating habits and patterns and addressing their fear foods, for example. Relapses are common, but crucially they are regarded as an integral part of the change process, an experiential learning opportunity rather than a failure, whereby new learning by the individual (about themselves and/or their condition) can be carried forwards with them as they go around the cycle again. During maintenance, relapse prevention is actively supported, and if stability is achieved, individuals may exit the process at that stage.

THE OCCUPATIONAL THERAPY PROCESS

What follows, using Case Study 28.3 as an illustration, is a description of a typical service user pathway through an eating disorder service mapped against the stages of the occupational therapy process: referral, assessment, care-planning, evaluation and discharge.

Referral

Within inpatient and day care services there is usually a 'blanket' or unspecified referral process whereby all service users are assessed and seen by the occupational therapist as part of their care pathway. Occupational therapists working in independent or private practice receive referrals from professional colleagues or from the individual themselves who feels motivated and ready to embark on more practical elements of recovery. In a community team setting referral for occupational therapy will come from within the team when input is required.

Assessment

As described earlier, the occupational therapist will choose their assessment tool depending on the service user's presentation and their own preferred model of practice, or in some settings a format devised by the occupational therapy service may be used.

Assessment data is gathered from case notes, from discussion with other MDT members when possible and from a face-to-face interview with the individual, in which both information-gathering and observation is crucial. This meeting is often the first contact and provides an opportunity to build a therapeutic rapport, which is vital. The occupational therapist must be familiar with the interview questions and all areas of functioning to be covered so the interview can be conducted in a conversational, flexible, person-centred way.

The assessment may be completed in one session or in two parts; usually anything more than an hour's duration creates fatigue for the interviewee. It is also good practice to share assessment data across the MDT to minimize the risk of fatigue caused by duplicate questions from multiple clinicians' assessments.

The Eating and Meal Preparation Skills Assessment (EMPSA) (Lock et al. 2012) is a specialist occupational therapy eating disorder outcome measure used to measure clients perceived ability and motivation to perform tasks related to eating self-prepared, cooked meals with a dessert. On the basis that the client has one session with the occupational therapist (plus one independent practise session in their own residence) each week and that this intervention may last between six months to a year, the EMPSA can be completed at the first, tenth, and final meal cookery sessions, for example (Lock et al. 2012).

Additionally, an interest checklist and sensory processing measures are commonly adopted by occupational therapists to further enhance the assessment of a client. Ascertaining a person's sensory preferences can inform self-care or distress tolerance activities. For example, an individual may be encouraged to explore ways of giving themselves strong sensory feedback (by holding ice cubes, by snapping elastic bands on the wrist or splashing the face with cold water, for instance) as alternative responses to distress than their customary self-harm behaviours.

Care Planning

Assessment focuses not only on the service user's areas of difficulty, but also on their strengths and wishes for the future. Treatment goals are then cocreated to reflect this, combined with the professional reasoning of the occupational therapist. To begin treatment goals may be simple to encourage engagement and motivation by adapting and grading an activity to fit the service user's current level of functioning, for example, and will be subject to regular review to maintain momentum towards recovery.

Case Study 28.3, Part 2, presents an example of occupational therapy treatment goals for Catherine and the occupational therapist's professional reasoning as Catherine progresses along her care pathway. Commonly used eating disorder interventions are presented in more detail in the next section of the chapter.

Interventions

Research-based evidence for occupational therapy for people with eating disorders is currently limited. However, Clark and Nayar (2012) note the global influence of eating disorders on occupational performance and how occupations can support or maintain recovery or, conversely, may sustain the eating disorder itself, thus indicating a need for occupational therapy input in the treatment of eating disorders. Indeed, occupational therapists' experiential knowledge and practice wisdom attest to the relevance of an occupational perspective when helping individuals address the maladaptive behaviours caused by an eating disorder and the void they can create in people's lives. As described earlier, although a primary occupational therapy focus is likely to be on eating and food-related behaviour, an eating disorder impacts all areas of living. Supporting change can be challenging because, in many instances, an individual's damaging or unhelpful behaviour will have begun as a coping strategy, albeit a maladaptive one, and thus may be hard to change.

CASE STUDY 28.3, PART 2

Catherine (Occupational Therapy Care Plan)

Stage of Occupational therapy process	Cocreated goal	Occupational therapist's professional reasoning
Early stage of inpatient admission	Catherine will read a book for ½ hr/day	• To encourage a chosen leisure pursuit which Catherine has not engaged in for a long time • To encourage Catherine to sit and rest her body in sedentary normal activity
	Catherine will attend a weekly open art group for 6 weeks	• To attend a diversional group to establish routine engagement in a leisure pursuit and social interaction with others • Review after 6 weeks indicates that Catherine enjoys the art as a leisure pursuit and appreciates the structure it provides, enabling her to establish a routine
Safe weight achieved and engaging with treatment programme	Catherine will access local shops to buy self-care items as required	• To develop independent living skills and practise accessing the community (Catherine struggles to spend money on items for herself such as self-care items – e.g., hair products/make-up) • The occupational therapist will accompany Catherine initially, and the destination/purchases will be pre-agreed, but grading will lead to unaccompanied trips, and to it being a social outing with friends
	Catherine will join a cookery group, aiming to start eating meals with her peers	• To attend a meal cookery group to practise planning for, shopping for, preparing, and eating meals without exhibiting 'problem eating behaviours'

For the intervention types now described, intervention can take the form of group or one-to-one work, or both, depending on the client and setting, and in each case occupational therapy must occur alongside physical management (including weight and other physical monitoring) of the individual, as previously described.

Psychoeducation

Psychoeducation is the provision of education and information to individuals with a mental health condition and to their families so they can understand and cope with it better. Psychoeducation has been shown to be beneficial in the treatment of mental health conditions generally (Ashcroft et al. 2016; Cho et al. 2016), and Andrewes et al. (1996) have shown that more formal psychoeducational initiatives show favourable results for people with eating disorders.

The importance of psychoeducation within eating disorders services can be underestimated due to it frequently being done in an informal way as and when opportunities present themselves, as well as in more formal planned intervention. It permeates all the interventions described in this chapter to varying degrees.

Service users may need education on the eating disorder itself, on its impact on health and well-being, on the risks of disordered eating and self-damaging behaviours on nutrition and regarding what is deemed 'normal' in terms of food consumption and one's relationship with food. This is because many service users may have had limited opportunities to engage in normal eating or lack role models that demonstrate a healthy or adaptive relationship with food. Information around the ineffectiveness of purging and laxatives on weight control, as well as the dangers of these behaviours (see Table 28.1) is essential, as is the involvement of the individual's family and/or supporters.

Service users, particularly those presenting for the first time, may need information on the specialized services and support available. Families and supporters may value this information, too, as well as education on how the eating disorder may impact relationships and how they may support the person on their recovery journey, which has been demonstrated to be significant in service users' experience (Geller at al. 2018). It is crucial to ensure that individuals are aware of how to access support themselves, given the nature of the condition and the impact on the family and social environment.

Diversional Activities

The word 'diversional' may be a misnomer in this treatment context because diversional activities in an eating disorder service have several specific purposes. Not only do they introduce the individual to leisure occupations unrelated to eating-related behaviours, they also encourage them to establish an adaptive daily routine and to tolerate their own difficult feelings (for periods of time) without adopting eating disordered behaviours.

These activities may in themselves be a challenge for the service user. For instance, Lizzie (see Case Study 28.2) may have great difficulty tolerating a sedentary activity (such as a board game or reading) because she would usually spend much of her free time 'earning' her food through very active pursuits. In contrast, Daniel (Case Study 28.4) may be unused to engaging in these types of activities without the inclusion of alcohol or large quantities of food.

Diversional activities could include arts and crafts, games, self-care, music or any other activity suitable for the client group, with consideration for age and social/cultural appropriateness. The occupational therapist may frequently use these activities in a group setting to offer greater opportunities for reflection and challenge, but they can be adapted as one-to-one sessions when individuals are on bed rest, for instance. Person-centred care planning is vital. A diversional activity focused on self-care, for example, which uses pampering products may challenge the individual who struggles with self-esteem and feels they do not deserve to indulge themselves in that way. These difficult feelings can be explored with support from the occupational therapist or other members of the MDT.

Emotional Regulation and Communication Skills Development

There is a strong correlation between having an eating disorder and having significant difficulties in managing one's emotions (Haynos et al. 2015). Indeed, the eating disorder itself can be understood as a seemingly effective yet maladaptive way of coping with and regulating emotions. There is also a strong correlation between having an eating disorder and other maladaptive means of coping such as substance use, self-harm, and/or obsessive-compulsive behaviours (Gregorowski et al. 2013; Wang et al. 2018), all of which may serve a similar function regarding emotional regulation.

Removing the maladaptive 'coping' behaviours on which a service user has become reliant can, understandably, feel frightening for individuals who are used to a quick means of reducing the felt impact of difficult emotions rather than fully experiencing or 'sitting with' them. Occupational therapists play an important role in helping service users manage these experiences by equipping them with more adaptive self-management skills, such as anxiety management, distress tolerance, problem solving or assertiveness. These interventions can be performed using a combination of psychoeducation, discussion, and facilitated reflection and feedback along with an experiential component such as role play, goal-setting and homework tasks in which skills are practised outside the one-to-one or group therapy setting, such as within their home environment or in the community. This 'real world' experiential aspect of the intervention provides further opportunities for reflection and feedback to consolidate learning, to identify appropriate supports and to gradually build confidence.

Communicating difficult emotions verbally (rather than through habitual maladaptive behaviours) may feel very demanding, so the occupational therapist may use creative media (such as art) to offer service users an alternative means of self-expression and a non-threatening context and prompt for initiating discussion about their experiences. For individuals who have had little opportunity to use positive forms of communication previously, this is likely to still feel uncomfortable initially, and the eating disorder–related behaviour may at times continue to appear to the individual as a more effective short-term way of managing difficulties.

Reflective Discussion Groups

This intervention is based loosely on the principles of Marlatt and Gordon's widely used relapse prevention model (George 1989), which adopts cognitive-behavioural strategies to help service users prevent relapse. Group members participate by offering a verbal reflection on an event or incident relevant to their eating disorder that happened to them during the week. With the assistance and support of peers, the individual reflects on eating disorder triggers and management of the event/incident, the challenges experienced and the successes they achieved. It is the role of other group members, with the support and facilitation of the occupational therapist, to offer different perspectives, questioning and challenging each other in a supportive environment.

Participation in this kind of group requires commitment to sharing personal experience, openness to group discussion and seeing things from a new, unfamiliar perspective (including being challenged) and a capacity to offer support to peers. The group will include individuals at different stages in their recovery journey, which can be challenging but also motivating. As the name suggests, this is primarily a group intervention but one-to-one discussion along similar lines can also be effective.

Independent Living Skills Development

This intervention aims to build and support occupational performance focusing on self-care, productivity, and leisure. Skill deficits or maladaptive habits are identified, and a plan is cocreated to address dysfunction and develop appropriate, healthy living skills. This is an important intervention because it is common for people with an eating disorder to adopt harmful or self-punishing day-to-day habits that reflect low self-worth, such as only allowing themselves cold showers, standing whilst watching television or reading, or refusing to spend money on basic self-care needs.

The intervention comprises psychoeducation, self-reflection, goal-setting/homework and graded experiential exposure. Activity analysis and grading are widely used by the occupational therapist to assist skill acquisition related to all kinds of activities such as watching a film at home with a friend, applying for a job or creating a personal care routine.

Community Skills Development

This intervention builds on independent living skills work, but it focuses on doing so in the context of the mainstream community. Examples of skill areas include going to the cinema, booking a visit to a hairdresser and using public transport.

Food/Eating-Related Interventions

Disordered eating and maladaptive participation in food-related occupations such as planning meals and shopping and preparing food inevitably form a large component of occupational therapy. This work is largely experiential, and it is important to plan and structure these activities to maximize opportunities to challenge areas of dysfunction, reflect on experiences, and consolidate learning.

Overall, interventions around food and eating aim to support service users to move from rigid/inflexible or unrestrained attitudes to food to having a more relaxed, responsible attitude and improved skills. Given the intractable and prominent position food and eating has during a normal day, this shift would then allow a significantly improved quality of life. Biddiscombe (2018) suggests that experiential groups, whether involving outings centred around food or meal cookery groups, are a useful intervention in challenging disordered eating and applying new skills to real life situations.

A starting position for the occupational therapist and service user may be to encourage the individual to consider and rate their own fear foods. These ratings may be unique to the individual, or there may be similar themes noted across service users or diagnostic groups. For example, Lizzie (see Case Study 28.2) may include high-fat/high-calorie foods at the top of her fear foods list and would choose to avoid them completely. On the contrary, Daniel (see Case Study 28.4) may eat these foods regularly but fear them due to his difficulties in stopping at a 'normal' portion size. In addition, Lizzie might rate salad as a 'safe' food, whereas Daniel might fear this due to his difficulty tolerating hunger and worry that this may not be satisfying or worthwhile. Suzanne (see Case Study 28.1) may have a wider range of foods that she will eat but not feel able to eat a prescribed portion size.

Interventions usually take place over a series of sessions and, as the service user progresses, the therapist

---

CASE STUDY 28.4

Daniel

Daniel is 30 years old and works as a mental health nurse on a hospital ward for people with dementia. His weight is normal. He is well-liked by his colleagues and has a wide circle of friends. Daniel does not eat at all during his shifts at work, but on his way home he will shop for food to binge on, such as loaves of bread, fizzy drinks, blocks of cheese, and packets of biscuits/crisps. He eats alone, consuming large quantities in single sittings, and repeatedly vomits afterward until he is confident his stomach is empty. He also regularly uses excessive amounts of over-the-counter laxatives. Daniel drinks up to two bottles of wine most evenings. He rewards himself for his food restriction on workdays by enjoying meals out with friends on his days off.

Daniel, in discussion with his occupational therapist, has identified self-care as one of his priorities, including the personal goal of eating regular healthy meals, following discharge, in his work environment. Together, they agree on the following graded plan:

- Daniel will plan meals in advance to take to work. Initially these will be microwaved meals or packaged sandwiches, but he will progress towards preparing home-made meals to take in.
- Daniel will identify supports at work, and, because his manager is approachable, he decides he will talk to her about his difficulties, sharing his goal to take his meal break daily and asking her to prompt him if she notices this has not happened. He identifies a supportive colleague too but defers involving them until his return to work.
- Daniel and the therapist agree on a location away from the ward to eat meals, and the therapist agrees to join him on the first day to model a suitable pace of eating and to provide emotional support regarding the difficult feelings likely to arise afterward.
- Daniel agrees to use the toilet prior to the meal, setting a goal to not use the bathroom for an hour after the meal to reduce the risk of being tempted to purge.
- To consolidate this, Daniel decides to ask his manager for tasks directly after his meal break that will keep him busy.
- To prepare for this on the ward, Daniel joins a group with the music therapist which takes place immediately after lunch to assist in distracting him from purging behaviour.
- To address the habit of purchasing food for binges on his way home from work, Daniel considers shopping online each week, but, due to concerns about having large quantities of food in the house, Daniel and the therapist agree to plan meals in advance each week and to go into the shops daily with a shopping list. He recognizes that being hungry when he shops can be triggering and so decides to change his shopping time to the morning, before his afternoon shift.

continues to grade the intervention to incorporate a flexible 'just right' challenge for the person at any given time. Keeping a record of previous sessions and goals (such as the fear foods tackled) and reflecting on this with the service user can be a useful motivational tool in an individual's recovery process. Table 28.4 outlines some of the challenges and considerations that may need to be taken into account during goal setting.

Evaluation

Throughout the individual's occupational therapy care pathway, ongoing evaluation is performed, informally with the person (via reflective conversations to review progress and goal attainment) and formally using tools such as the Single Observation MOHOST. Based on evaluation, an individual's goals and care plan will be modified as required.

If relevant, a post-intervention outcome measurement will be made, for example, using the MOHOST or the EMPSA, the results of which inform the discharge summary and are shared with the service user. Outcome measurement can be evidence for the individual of their progress and supports the accountability and transparency of the occupational therapy provided.

Discharge

Successful discharge requires careful consideration and planning time if it involves additional areas of occupational therapy support, such as preparing for new accommodation or applying for education, training or employment. This will be incorporated into the treatment goals and one-to-one sessions.

It is good practice to offer a 'closing' of occupational therapy input, which is an opportunity to reflect on

TABLE 28.4	
Challenges and Considerations Associated with Treatment Goal Setting	
Challenges	**Considerations for Goal Setting**
Planning Meals	■ Separating emotion from meal choice (e.g. eating excessively for comfort following a difficult day or a restrictive option as punishment if self-worth is low) ■ Considering a wide range of foods ■ Planning balanced meals ■ Tackling fear foods, possibly from a pre-prepared list
Shopping for Food	■ Spending an appropriate amount of time in the supermarket (i.e. not rushing to avoid associated emotion/behaviours or lingering excessively) ■ Not excessively label checking (e.g. calories, fat content) ■ Considering brands (e.g. always choosing a 'luxury' brand to make food seem more worthwhile or a 'budget' brand due to beliefs around being undeserving) ■ Accepting the need to spend money on food ■ Being mindful of budgeting/payment method (e.g. paying in cash to cap spending) ■ Shopping in only one or two shops (i.e. accepting what is available as good enough rather than spending excessive time trying to find the right ingredients or brands)
Preparing a Balanced Meal	■ Addressing rules around cutting out food groups (e.g. carbohydrates) ■ Including all aspects of a balanced meal (e.g. fats) ■ Difficulty identifying normal portion size/adhering to prescribed portion sizes ■ Exploring the foundations of dietary preferences (e.g. veganism as a positive choice versus motivation being to avoid eating a balanced diet) ■ When dietary preferences exist, ensuring that a balanced diet is still achieved ■ Recognizing that meal preparation needs to be in the context of other meals and snacks (i.e. this may not be the case if the individual is not used to eating regularly or adopts a pattern of restriction before or after eating a balanced meal) ■ Being able to prepare a meal in a room with others present or where others are preparing food for themselves ■ Cooking for others ■ Being in a room where someone else is preparing food for you ■ Allowing use of 'extras' such as sauces or a calorific drink with a meal

Continued on following page

TABLE 28.4	
Challenges and Considerations Associated with Treatment Goal Setting (Continued)	
Challenges	**Considerations for Goal Setting**
Eating Adaptively	■ Avoiding rituals around eating, such as cutting food into tiny pieces, using inappropriate cutlery (e.g. a teaspoon for a main meal) or spoiling food (e.g. excessive pepper/sauces/burning to reduce the guilt around eating) ■ Challenging preferences that have become rules (e.g. leaving favourite mouthful until last) ■ Eating at an appropriate pace ■ Finishing prescribed portions ■ Comparing food with others (e.g. guilt if perceiving others as having a 'healthier' option or envy/satisfaction if observing a more 'indulgent' option)
Socializing Around Food	■ Being present, avoiding distracting oneself with activities (e.g. watching television) ■ Having conversations ■ Being seen eating and seeing others eating
Tolerating Difficult Feelings	■ 'Sitting with' difficult feelings ■ Avoiding compensatory behaviours (e.g. laxatives, purging, over-exercise, restricting meals later in the day) or other behaviours (e.g. binging, excessive hand washing, brushing teeth or smoking after a meal to get rid of the taste) to manage distress ■ Tolerating new physical sensations (e.g. feeling full or not being uncomfortably full) ■ Verbalize difficulties instead of using maladaptive behaviours

Transferring to Everyday Environments	■ Transferring new skills from the clinical setting to everyday environments:
	  ■ Home environment
	  ■ Family meals
	  ■ Public spaces (e.g. picnic in a park, snacking at a cinema)
	  ■ Eating on the go/take-aways
	  ■ Restaurants/cafés
	  ■ Being cooked for by friends/family and cooking for them

achievements and recovery milestones and to consider an action plan for how these will transfer and support transition to new environments and the next phase of the individual's journey. The service user is offered the opportunity to say goodbye to the groups they have attended and to reflect with their peers on their shared experience. It is customary for other clinicians to hold similar closure/goodbye sessions in their work and for the service user to mark their departure in the MDT meeting or ward round if circumstances permit (see Catherine's 'goodbye' in Case Study 28.3, Part 1).

An MDT discharge summary (including occupational therapy input) is distributed to relevant external agencies and to the service user. Additionally, the occupational therapist may create a specific occupational therapy summary if discharge is to a service that also offers occupational therapy to provide continuity of care.

CONCLUSION

This chapter has provided an overview of the role of occupational therapy within eating disorder services,

primarily in the UK. The prevalence of eating disorders is great, spanning demographics, as illustrated by the case studies of Suzanne, Lizzie, Catherine and Daniel. It is a mental health condition that is growing and changing in its presentation, and the great variety of services offers much scope for occupational therapy input.

The role of occupational therapy is vital in supporting an individual with an eating disorder in their recovery journey, whatever form that may take. To that end it is an area that requires more research to enhance the evidence base and expand and strengthen clinical tools.

ACKNOWLEDGMENTS

The authors would like to thank the following people for their support in creating this chapter:

Dr Bryony Bamford, Aine Loi, Abigail Cardwell and Claire Main. We would also like to offer special thanks to Alexis Hutton for contributions to the adolescent section.

QUESTIONS FOR CONSIDERATION

1. List some of the potential triggers in Case Study 28.1 that, together, have led to disordered eating behaviours.
2. Regarding Case Study 28.2, what effects will this limited diet have on Lizzie's body?
3. Regarding Case Study 28.2, suggest some possible diversional activities that could allow Lizzie to address some of her difficulties.
4. What percentage of children (under 18 years of age) are recognized as experiencing some kind of eating disorder in the United Kingdom?
5. Consider some intervention activities that challenge perfectionism.
6. Consider what comparative advantages/disadvantages there may be in using the OCAIRS and the MOHOST.
7. Why is first contact so important to building a therapeutic rapport with service users with eating disorders?
8. Can you suggest alternative activities which could further benefit Catherine based on Case Study 28.3?

SERVICE USER COMMENTARY

This chapter highlights the complex nature of eating disorders and how occupational therapy can be considered as a holistic approach towards understanding and treating this mental health problem. In this commentary I will reflect on my own lived experience of anorexia nervosa and the treatment I have received to comment on some key points that I have drawn from this chapter.

There is a great focus on the role of occupation in the chapter. An eating disorder impacts on the most basic human needs, depriving the individual of food, water and rest needed to survive. When I was in the depths of anorexia, it was the most important thing in my life. I was constantly engaging in eating disorder-related behaviours and thoughts that ultimately gave me meaning and purpose. Occupations that I once enjoyed like exercise became disordered and compulsive. I was having to continually do more to keep up with the demands of anorexia. My occupational therapist showed me how to recognize the value of being 'in the present'; that I was capable of being and becoming who I wanted to be without my eating disorder and its unattainable demands.

This chapter does a great job in highlighting the role that occupational therapy plays within eating disorder treatment. However, there is a gap that I cannot ignore from both a personal and professional perspective, which is about the timeliness of intervention. Occupational therapy can provide an invaluable contribution to early intervention and prevention. It is readily available in inpatient hospital settings, but the individual is often in psychological crisis and medically unsafe at this point. In my experience of being hospitalized, I did not have the mental capacity, nor the level of distress tolerance needed to engage. I did not want to 'get better' or rather, with hindsight, I did not want to lose the very thing that had helped me cope with so many challenges and past experiences.

Surely intervention would be invaluable before the individual reaches this point. It is important to provide outpatient occupational therapy that is accessible within the community, particularly when it is so difficult to access inpatient treatment due to the strict clinical criteria applied, the lack of beds and the geographical variations in service provision. Earlier intervention positively impacts an individual's recovery and reduce the risk of relapse. Environment is a vital component for occupational performance, thus grading daily occupations such as food shopping and cooking with therapeutic support outside of a hospital environment would be beneficial to recovery.

Hospital wards offer limited real-life occupations which can be problematic when discharged; something that I believe contributed to my relapse. We are all occupational beings, but I did not know how to 'live' outside of hospital. I lost all sense of doing, being and becoming and, like many, turned to my eating disorder to cope. Early intervention is vital to prevent and limit the occupational disruption caused by eating disorders. There is scope for occupational therapy in outpatient eating disorder services, yet from my first-hand experience and research, this appears to be almost absent in practice.

Shannan Rugg

REFERENCES

Abraham, S. (2008). *Eating disorders* (6th ed.). Oxford University Press.

American Psychiatric Association (APA). (2000). In *Diagnostic and statistical manual of mental disorders* (4th ed.). Washington, DC: Text Revision. American Psychiatric Association.

American Psychiatric Association (APA). (2013). In *Diagnostic and statistical manual of mental disorders* (5th ed.). Arlington, VA: (DSM-5). American Psychiatric Association.

Andrewes, D. G., O'Connor, P., Mulder, C., et al. (1996). Computerised psychoeducation for patients with eating disorders. *Australian and New Zealand Journal of Psychiatry*, *30*(4), 492–497. Available at: https://www.researchgate.net/publication/14318632_Computerised_Psychoeducation_for_Patients_with_Eating_Disorders.

Ashcroft, K., Insua-Summerhays, B., & Schurter, C. (2016). Evaluating the evidence for online interventions in mental health care. *Psychiatric Annals*, *46*(10), 584–588. Available at: https://www.researchgate.net/publication/14318632_Computerised_Psychoeducation_for_Patients_with_Eating_Disorders.

Biddiscombe, R. J., Scanlan, J. N., Ross, J., Horsfield, S., Aradas, J., & Hart, S. (2018). Exploring the perceived usefulness of practical food groups in day treatment for individuals with eating disorders. *Australian Occupational Therapy Journal*, *65*(2), 98–106.

Byford, S., Barrett, B., Roberts, C., et al. (2007). Economic evaluation of a randomised controlled trial for anorexia nervosa in adolescents. *British Journal of Psychiatry*, Available at: https://www.researchgate.net/publication/14318632_Computerised_Psychoeducation_for_Patients_with_Eating_Disorders.

Cho, S. H., Torres-Llenza, V., Budnik, K., & Norris, L. (2016). The integral role of psychoeducation in clinical care. *Psychiatric Annals*, *46*(5), 286–292. Available at: https://www.researchgate.net/publication/14318632_Computerised_Psychoeducation_for_Patients_with_Eating_Disorders.

Clark, M., & Nayar, S. (2012). Recovery from eating disorders: A role for occupational therapy. *New Zealand Journal of Occupational Therapy*, *59*(1), 13–17.

Dahlgren, C. L., & Wisting, L. (2016). Transitioning from DSM-IV to DSM-5: A systematic review of eating disorder prevalence assessment. *International Journal of Eating Disorders*, *49*(11), 975–997.

Department of Health (DH). (2007). *Mental health act*. London: HMSO.

Gardiner, C., & Brown, N. (2010). Is there a role for occupational therapy within a specialist child and adolescent mental health eating disorder service? *British Journal of Occupational Therapy*, *73*(1), 38–43.

Geller, J., Iyar, M., Srikameswaran, S., Zelichowska, J., Zhou, Y., & Dunn, E. C. (2018). The relation between patient characteristics and their carers' use of a directive versus collaborative support stance. *International Journal of Eating Disorders*, *51*(1), 71–76.

George, W. H. (1989). Marlatt and Gordon's relapse prevention model: A cognitive-behavioral approach to understanding and preventing relapse. *Journal of Chemical Dependency Treatment*, *2*(2), 125–152. Available at: https://www.researchgate.net/publication/14318632_Computerised_Psychoeducation_for_Patients_with_Eating_Disorders.

Gregorowski, C., Seedat, S., & Jordaan, G. P. (2013). A clinical approach to the assessment and management of co-morbid eating disorders and substance use disorders. *BMC Psychiatry*, *13*, 289. Available at: https://www.researchgate.net/publication/14318632_Computerised_Psychoeducation_for_Patients_with_Eating_Disorders.

Haynos, A. F., Roberto, C. A., & Attia, E. (2015). Examining the associations between emotion regulation difficulties, anxiety, and eating disorder severity among inpatients with anorexia nervosa. *Comprehensive Psychiatry*, *60*, 93–98. Available at: https://www.researchgate.net/publication/14318632_Computerised_Psychoeducation_for_Patients_with_Eating_Disorders.

Health Select Committee. (2014). Third Report: Children's and adolescents' mental health and CAMHS. Available at: https://publications.parliament.uk/pa/cm201415/cmselect/cmhealth/342/34202.htm.

Jahraus, J. (2018). Medical complications of eating disorders. *Psychiatric Annals*, *48*(10), 463–467. Available at: https://www.healio.com/psychiatry/journals/psycann/2018-10-48-10/%7B357052a4-a663-4a4d-a73b-e5d737caff44%7D/medical-complications-of-eating-disorders.

Joy, E., Kussman, A., & Nattiv, A. (2016). 2016 update on eating disorders in athletes: A comprehensive narrative review with a focus on clinical assessment and management. *British Journal of Sports Medicine*, *50*(3), 154.

Keel, P. K., & Klump, K. L. (2003). Are eating disorders culture-bound syndromes? Implications for conceptualizing their etiology. *Psychological Bulletin*, *129*(5), 747–769. Available at: https://content.apa.org/record/2003-99991-005.

Keski-Rahkonen, A., & Mustelin, L. (2016). Epidemiology of eating disorders in Europe: Prevalence, incidence, comorbidity, course, consequences, and risk factors. *Current Opinion in Psychiatry*, *29*(6), 340–345. Available at: https://journals.lww.com/co-psychiatry/Abstract/2016/11000/Epidemiology_of_eating_disorders_in_Europe_.5.aspx.

Klump, K. L., Bulik, C. M., Kaye, W. H., Treasure, J., & Tyson, E. (2009). Academy for eating disorders position paper: Eating disorders are serious mental illnesses. *International Journal of Eating Disorders*, *42*, 97–103.

Lacey, H., Hinton-Craggs, C., & Robinson, K. (2007). *Overcoming anorexia*. Sheldon Press.

Lejonclou, A., Nilsson, D., & Holmqvist, R. (2014). Variants of potentially traumatizing life events in eating disorder patients. *Psychological Trauma*, *6*(6), 661–667.

Leon, G. R., Fulkerson, J. A., Perry, C. L., & Cudeck, R. (1993). Personality and behavioral vulnerabilities associated with risk status for eating disorders in adolescent girls. *Journal of Abnormal Psychology*, *102*(3), 438–444. Available at: https://psycnet.apa.org/record/1993-45864-001.

Lock, L. C., Williams, H. A., Bamford, B., & Lacey, J. H. (2012). The St George's eating disorders service meal preparation group for inpatients and day patients pursuing full recovery: A pilot study. *European Eating Disorders Review*, 20(3), 218–224.

Lydecker, J. A., White, M. A., & Grilo, C. M. (2017). Form and formulation: Examining the distinctiveness of body image constructs in treatment-seeking patients with binge-eating disorder. *Journal of Consulting and Clinical Psychology*, 85(11), 1095–1103.

Madden, S., Hay, P., & Touyz, S. (2015). Systematic review of evidence for different treatment settings in anorexia nervosa. *World Journal of Psychiatry*, 5(1), 147–153. https://doi.org/10.5498/wjp.v5.i1.147.

Makino, M., Tsuboi, K., & Dennerstein, L. (2004). Prevalence of eating disorders: A comparison of western and non-western countries. *Medscape General Medicine*, 6(3), 49. Available at: https://www.ncbi.nlm.nih.gov/pmc/articles/PMC1435625/.

Marzola, E., Nasser, J., Hashim, S., Shih, P., & Kaye, W. (2013). Nutritional rehabilitation in anorexia nervosa: A review of the literature and implications for treatment. *BMC Psychiatry*, 13, 290. https://doi.org/10.1186/1471-244X-13-290.

National Institute for Health and Care Excellence (NICE). (2017). *Eating disorders: Recognition and treatment NICE guideline [NG69]*. Available at: https://www.nice.org.uk/guidance/ng69.

NHS England. (2015). *Access and waiting time standard for children and young people with an eating disorder: A Commissioning Guide*. Version1.0.

Ornstein, R. M., Essayli, J. H., Nicely, T. A., Masciulli, E., & Lane-Loney, S. (2017). Treatment of avoidant/restrictive food intake disorder in a cohort of young patients in a partial hospitalization program for eating disorders. *International Journal of Eating Disorders*, 50(9), 1067–1074.

Parliamentary, & Health Service Ombudsman. (2017). Ignoring the alarms: How NHS eating disorder services are failing patients. Available at: https://www.gov.uk/government/publications. https://www.ombudsman.org.uk/sites/default/files/page/FINAL%20FOR%20WEB%20Anorexia%20Report.pdf.

Prochaska, J., & DiClemente, C. (1983). Stages and processes of self-change in smoking: Toward an integrative model of change. *Journal of Consulting and Clinical Psychology*, 51(3), 390–395. Available at: https://psycnet.apa.org/doiLanding?doi=10.1037%2F0022-006X.51.3.390.

Rodgers, R. F., Dubois, R., Thiebaut, S., et al. (2019). Structural differences in eating disorder psychopathology after history of childhood abuse: Insights from a bayesian network analysis. *Journal of Abnormal Psychology*, 128(8), 795–805. Available at: https://pubmed.ncbi.nlm.nih.gov/24991159/.

Royal College of Psychiatrists. (2012). *Junior MARSIPAN: Management of really sick patients under 18 with anorexia nervosa (college Report CR168)*. Royal College of Psychiatrists

(pdf) Available at: https://www.rcpsych.ac.uk/docs/default-source/improving-care/better-mh-policy/college-reports/college-report-cr168.pdf?sfvrsn=e38d0c3b_2.

Schmidt, U., Renwick, B., Lose, A., et al. (2013). The MOSAIC study - comparison of the Maudsley model of treatment for adults with anorexia nervosa (MANTRA) with specialist supportive clinical management (SSCM) in outpatients with anorexia nervosa or eating disorder not otherwise specified, anorexia nervosa type: Study protocol for a randomized controlled trial. *Trials*, 14, 160. https://doi.org/10.1186/1745-6215-14-160.

Stice, E., Gau, J. M., Rohde, P., & Shaw, H. (2017). Risk factors that predict future onset of each eating disorder: Predictive specificity in high-risk adolescent females. *Journal of Abnormal Psychology*, 126(1), 38–51. Available at: https://pubmed.ncbi.nlm.nih.gov/24991159/.

Sweeting, H., Walker, L., MacLean, A., Patterson, C., Raisanen, U., & Hunt, K. (2015). Prevalence of eating disorders in males: A review of rates reported in academic research and UK mass media. *International Journal of Men's Health*, 14, 2. Available at: https://www.ncbi.nlm.nih.gov/pmc/articles/PMC4538851/.

Taylor, R. (2017). *Kielhofner's model of human occupation: Theory and application* (5th ed.). Lippincott Williams and Wilkins.

Treasure, J., & Schmidt, U. (2013). The cognitive-interpersonal maintenance model of anorexia nervosa revisited: A summary of the evidence for cognitive, socio-emotional and interpersonal predisposing and perpetuating factors. *Journal of Eating Disorders*, 1, 13. https://doi.org/10.1186/2050-2974-1-13.

Van den Eynde, F., Suda, M., Broadbent, H., et al. (2012). Structural magnetic resonance imaging in eating disorders: A systematic review of voxel-based morphometry studies. *European Eating Disorders Review*, 20(2), 94–105. https://doi.org/10.1002/erv.1163.

Wang, S. B., Pisetsky, E. M., Skutch, J. M., Fruzetti, A. E., & Haynos, A. F. (2018). Restrictive eating and nonsuicidal self-injury in a nonclinical sample: Co-occurrence and associations with emotion dysregulation and interpersonal problems. *Comprehensive Psychiatry*, 82, 128–132. Available at: https://pubmed.ncbi.nlm.nih.gov/24991159/.

Watkins, B., Cooper, P. J., & Lask, K. B. (2012). History of eating disorder in mothers of children with early onset eating disorder or disturbance. *European Eating Disorders Review*, 20(2), 121–125.

World Health Organization (WHO)(2020). Health Topic: Body mass index (BMI). Available at: http://www.euro.who.int/en/health-topics/disease-prevention/nutrition/a-healthy-lifestyle/body-mass-index-bmi.

Zerwas, S., & Bulik, C. M. (2011). Genetics and epigenetics of eating disorders. *Psychiatric Annals*, 41(11), 532–538. Available at: https://pubmed.ncbi.nlm.nih.gov/24991159/.

29 WORKING ON THE MARGINS

MADELEINE DUNCAN ■ JENNIFER CREEK

CHAPTER OUTLINE

INTRODUCTION

A margin is the part of an area that is adjacent to the edge. To marginalize someone is to move them 'to the margin of a sphere of activity, make economically marginal, impoverish' (Shorter Oxford English Dictionary 2002). The margins of society may be geographical places or social spaces where marginalized people congregate. Margins represent opportunities for occupational therapists to contribute to social development and public mental health through occupation-centred practice. Occupational therapists target the occupational dimensions of health and human well-being by working alongside marginalized people in generating practical solutions to the challenges of everyday life that compromise their mental well-being and development due to social exclusion.

This chapter commences with a brief overview of the characteristics of margins: why they exist and persist, how they are experienced and how they impact peoples' occupations. Global mental health challenges on the margins in developed and developing countries are considered, followed by a summary of the World Health Organization (WHO; 2013) Health Action Plan 2013–2020. The story of Ms H is used to illustrate the practical solutions that occupational therapists can contribute to the challenges of mental distress as a feature of life on the margins. The chapter concludes by describing how occupational therapists working on the margins might orientate themselves, using a number of direction pointers.

UNDERSTANDING THE MARGINS

In this section, a discussion of margins as a sociological concept is structured through a series of questions.

Why Do Margins Exist?

Margins exist because human difference is used as the basis for oppression and exclusion. There are many vectors and combinations of perceived and imposed differences involving complex constructs such as gender, race, class, ethnicity, ability, sexual orientation and other intersectional dimensions of identity including mental health. When differences become socially significant, they cause social stratifications and divisions in which some people are elevated over others, giving them a disproportionate amount of resources, power and prestige. Young (2000) identified five faces of oppression: exploitation, marginalization, powerlessness, cultural imperialism and violence.

Exploitation

Relations of power and inequality are enacted through the social process of exploitation, which occurs when the results of the labour of one social group are regularly transferred to benefit another. The powerful get to make the social rules about what work is, who does what for whom and how work is compensated. For example, farm workers on some wine estates in South Africa used to be paid through the *dop* system, which entails wages in the form of alcohol rather than money (see Chapter 27). The term 'modern slavery' is sometimes used to refer to the exploitation of labour through coercion, force or deception. In the UK, for example, the main types of modern slavery identified by the government are labour exploitation and sexual exploitation (HM Government 2019).

Marginalization

Marginalization is the process by which 'a whole category of people is expelled from useful participation in social life' (Young 2000, p. 41). To be marginalized means to be discriminated against, excluded, considered unequal and potentially subjected to material deprivation or even extermination. As individuals, we all experience social marginality or exclusion at times; however, for some categories of people such as immigrants; refugees; gay, lesbian and transgendered people; people with disabilities; the homeless and the elderly, being marginalized is a part of daily life. Worldwide, people with mental disorders are marginalized by stigma, social exclusion and injustice (Krishnan et al. 2015). They experience discrimination in all aspects of their daily living, especially when trying to access mental healthcare and employment (Mental Health Foundation 2019).

Powerlessness

Powerlessness is a process by which 'people come to lack authority, status, a sense of self' (Young 2000, 57). People's social positioning influences the level of power they can exert; for example, women with mental illness face particular forms of marginalized identity and powerlessness that are associated with their gender (Gujendragad 2015; Van Den Tillaart et al. 2009). Similarly, mental illness and poverty are closely linked and interact in a complex negative cycle of powerlessness. In a seminal study of the experiences of poor people in 58 countries in the developing and transitional world, Narayan and colleagues (2000, 2) identified 10 interlocking dimensions of powerlessness and ill-being associated with poverty:

- The body is hungry, exhausted, sick and poor in appearance.
- Capabilities are weak because of a lack of information, education, skills and confidence.
- Security is lacking in both protection and peace of mind.
- Livelihoods and assets are precarious, seasonal and inadequate.
- Gender relations are troubled and unequal.
- Places of the poor are isolated, risky, un-serviced and stigmatised.
- Social relations are discriminating and isolating.

- Behaviours of the more powerful are marked by disregard and abuse.
- Institutions are disempowering and excluding.
- Organizations of the poor are weak and disconnected.

Cultural Imperialism

Cultural imperialism occurs when the 'dominant group in society imposes their own experiences, values, goals and achievements as the social norm' (Young 2000, p. 43). When people deviate from socially imposed norms, they are treated as inferior, or their ways of doing and being are negated, marking them as the *other*. Being *othered* reinforces social differences and marginalization by imposing dominant discourses, lifestyles and worldviews. For example, the biomedical model of psychiatry dominates Western medicine and has been critiqued as a form of cultural imperialism because it is not universally accepted that mental illness has physical causes (Miller 2014). The 'othering' of indigenous peoples' wisdom and traditional healing methods, which link mental illness to social and spiritual causes, limits opportunities to learn from different cultures on how they address psychological distress.

Violence

Violence is 'the intentional use of physical force or power, threatened or actual, against oneself or another person or against a group or community that either results in or has a high likelihood of resulting in injury, death, psychological harm, maldevelopment, or deprivation' (Krug et al. 2002, p. 5). This definition includes threats, intimidation, neglect and abuse (whether physical, sexual or psychological), as well as acts of self-harm and suicidal behaviour. The inclusion of power in a definition of violence expands on the conventional understanding of the term to a social practice in which the societal context makes it possible, even acceptable, to act violently against certain categories of people, including the mentally ill. In public perception, mental illness is often conflated with dangerousness and violence. Societal bias contributes to the stigma faced by those with a psychiatric diagnosis, which contributes to non-disclosure of the mental illness and decreased treatment-seeking (Varshney et al. 2016).

Why Do Margins Persist?

Margins persist where inequality exists. Inequality refers to the uneven distribution of opportunities and resources in a given society to different categories of persons based on characteristics such as power, religion, ability, kinship, prestige, race, ethnicity, gender, age, sexual orientation and class. Inequality is perpetuated by global economic and geopolitical dynamics. In his text, *Why the West rules - for now*, historian Ian Morris (2010) argues and scientifically demonstrates that the current 40 years will prove to be the most important in global history, with top priorities being the avoidance of nuclear war, slowing down global ecological deterioration and managing mass human mobility. In this scenario the scope of need created by marginalized populations will exponentially increase across the globe. The development surge associated with globalisation will be evidenced by three major social changes (Morris 2010):

- Large-scale urbanisation as people migrate in search of work, education and healthcare or to seek relief from violence, famine, disease and poverty
- Increased energy use that will exacerbate current levels of climate change and environmental degradation
- Advances in information technology that will speed up globalisation and the proliferation of war-making capacity and violence.

Most of the world's poorest people live in an 'arc of instability' (Morris 2010, p. 602), which is what the US National Intelligence Council calls the region stretching from central Africa in a rainbow-shaped arc across the Middle East to South-East Asia. Much of what happens environmentally, politically and socially in this region reverberates worldwide. For example, food and water insecurities have been identified as drivers of conflict and cross-border migration in countries such as Syria and the Democratic Republic of the Congo (United Nations (UN) 2018, p. 138). Civil unrest, natural disasters and declining harvests in the regions of the arc are expected to unleash an estimated 200 million famine and climate migrants across the globe, many times larger than the world's entire refugee population in 2018.

How Are Margins Experienced?

Margins are experienced subjectively in uniquely different ways. There is, for example, no single way of experiencing a psychotic episode, being a woman, being a person of colour or being poor. We should, therefore, avoid conflating people's social positions, identities and world views and refrain from essentialising their experiences of marginalization. Essentialising is a form of cultural imperialism in which dominant constructions of the world and of particular groups of people come to be reiterated, solidified and accepted as reality. It involves generating 'internal categories of personhood that are unchanging and timeless, that come to be inescapable, and that bear a determining influence of sorts on the person in question' (Parker 2004, p. 140). Therapists may essentialise when they impose models of practice or standardized protocols to draw conclusions about people's experiences of being marginalized. The ability to make informed clinical judgements about a person's mental state or level of functioning should not be conflated with understanding their experience. The latter is something that only the person or people concerned can voice (Trevedi 2014).

How Do People on the Margins Respond?

How people respond and what they are able to do (i.e., what they are capable of) depends on personal, social and structural circumstances, such as the amount of freedom they have to act to their advantage, their ability to transform resources into valuable activities, the distribution of opportunities within society and the balance of materialistic and non-materialistic factors affecting their welfare. Philosopher Martha Nussbaum (2000), in her seminal writing about human capabilities and development, argues that adequate food and shelter are prerequisites for bodily health; safety and security are necessary for bodily integrity; affiliations with other people depend on being respected; and having some control over one's environment requires access to personal, material and political resources. Individual and collective forms of agency, resilience and resistance characterize people's responses and capabilities on the margins.

Agency

Agency is the ability to take action towards a desired end or to produce an effect (Shorter Oxford English Dictionary 2002). An agent is someone who acts and brings about change, whose achievements can be evaluated in terms of his or her own values, objectives and functioning. The aetiology of mental illness may erode a person's motor drive and psychological volition and therefore their level of agentic functioning. Agency also depends on whether or not economic, social and/or political barriers impede a person's ability to pursue substantive freedoms; that is, the things they need and want to do that give expression to their being (Mooney 2016). Discerning the two dimensions of agency is crucial in the assessment of a mentally ill person's capabilities on the margins of society, where access to personal, material and political resources is likely to be restricted.

Resilience

Resilience is the dynamic process that enables an individual to adapt successfully over the life course to severe adversity such as prolonged exposure to physical and/or psychological pain, deprivation or abuse. It involves the use of a range of protective mechanisms that enable people to withstand the potentially damaging effects of stress associated with adversity and mental ill-health. Understanding the psychology and neurobiology underlying resilience can help occupational therapists develop occupation-centred strategies aimed at preventing psychopathology during or after exposure to intractable adversity (Rutter et al. 2013). A word of caution is indicated. Implicit in some discourses of agency and resilience is a tacit acceptance of and therefore complicity with the oppressive ways in which society functions (Duncan et al. 2011b, p. 68). Acknowledging and strengthening the resilience and agency of people on the margins should not divert attention away from also resisting social inequality and diminishing the adversities to which they are exposed.

Resistance

To resist is to strive against, oppose, refuse to yield to and refuse to comply with (Oxford English Dictionary 2002). Resistance can take various forms: individual or collective, passive or active, violent or non-violent. People facing similar forms of oppression and social injustice may resist by mobilising civic action for their rights through various forms of activism, including campaigning, lobbying, boycotting, protesting, taking direct action and even rioting (Corbett 2017). A ground swell of mental health activism through social movements can bring about substantive shifts in policy formulation, resource distribution and power alignment (Rose 2018).

How Do Margins Affect Human Occupation?

Of the numerous ways in which the occupations of persons with mental ill-health can be affected by marginalization, three aspects are mentioned here.

Occupational Injustice

Prevailing socio-political and economic influences determine the form and degree of occupational injustice that exists amongst different groups of marginalized people. Hence, occupational deprivation, alienation, imbalance and other forms of occupational injustice manifest differently in different societies and contexts. For example, ethnic minorities with mental illness in Sweden are not established in the labour market and seldom in paid employment. They face difficulties in terms of support for meaningful occupations and lack of access to occupation-based rehabilitation services (Pooremamali et al. 2017). People with psychiatric disability in rural areas of South Africa face social stigma, have limited access to basic mental health services and are disadvantaged by structural and chronic poverty that narrow the type and range of occupations that they can engage with, meaning that the likelihood of them developing their potential is curtailed (Watson 2013).

Intergenerational Perpetuation of Occupations

People develop shared identities and consciousness of their social class over generations, because parents confer their social position and associated repertoire of occupations on their children (Eberharter 2012). For example, low education may be perpetuated across generations, with illiterate or semi-literate parents being under-equipped to help their children learn or affect their children's occupational preferences. Parental mental health is also associated with lasting effects on a child's educational attainment, choice of occupation to secure future household income and the probability of having criminal convictions (Johnston et al. 2012).

Inequity of Occupational Choice

Unemployment, poverty, lack of infrastructure—such as decent housing, sanitation and transport—and other social determinants of health, such as civil unrest, food insecurity and climate change can keep people trapped on the margins. There, they are forced by circumstances beyond their control to make choices about what they do every day simply to survive. Consider, for example, people who live on the garbage dumps of large cities; the forced labour of child soldiers; or people bound by caste, disability or economic necessity to engage in occupations such as refuse collection, begging, drug peddling and prostitution. The unjust socio-political dispensation of *apartheid* (separateness) in pre-1994 South Africa created geo-spatial dispersions between different race groups, resulting in restricted occupational choice for Black youth currently living in historically segregated communities (Galvaan 2012). Likewise, apartheid created generational circumstances in which women living and working on wine farms continue to be socially conditioned to participate in entrenched excessive drinking. Cloete and Ramugondo (2015) refer to this behaviour as an imposed occupation, pointing out its contribution to the prevalence of foetal alcohol syndrome (FAS) in the wine-producing regions of South Africa.

WHY WORK ON THE MARGINS MATTERS

Bridging the Mental Health Gap

The WHO (2013, p. 7) expressed the view that the 'determinants of mental health and mental disorders include not only individual attributes such as the ability to manage one's thoughts, emotions, behaviours and interactions with others, but also social, cultural, economic, political and environmental factors such as national policies, social protection, living standards, working conditions, and community social supports.' The WHO (2013, p. 15) has also drawn attention to the mental health needs of populations exposed to extreme stressors, 'including isolated, repeated or continuing conflict, violence and disasters.' While mental, neurological and substance use (MNS) disorders are common in all regions of the world, affecting every community and age group across all countries, people in low-income countries are less likely to have access to the treatment they need (WHO 2018). Writing about mental health services in low- and middle-income countries (LAMIC), Murthy (2011, p. 333) stated:

> ... development of mental health services all over the world, countries rich and poor alike, have been the product of larger social situations, specifically the importance society gives to the rights of disadvantaged/marginalised groups. Economically rich countries have addressed the movement from institutionalised care to community care, building on the strengths of their social institutions. LAMIC have begun this process in a different way and have made significant progress. There is a need to continue the process by widening the scope of the mental health interventions, increasing the involvement of all available community resources, and rooting the interventions in the historical, social and cultural roots of countries.

The service gap between what is needed to promote public mental health and prevent the onset of MNS disorders and what is available to reduce the burden through treatment and recovery-orientated rehabilitation remains considerably wide. To address some of these inequalities, the WHO (2013) produced a comprehensive *Mental Health Action Plan 2013–2020*. The six cross-cutting principles and approaches that underpin the plan provide sub-headings for the rest of this section.

Universal Health Coverage

In 2015 the UNs' *Sustainable Development Goals* (SDGs) were extended to include the prevention and treatment of mental disorders.

> To promote physical and mental health and well-being, and to extend life expectancy for all, we must achieve universal health coverage and access to quality health care. No-one must be left behind... We are committed to the prevention and treatment of

> non-communicable diseases, including behavioural, developmental and neurological disorders, which constitute a major challenge for sustainable development.
>
> *UN 2015, p. 11*

> SDG number 3, which is to ensure healthy lives and promote well-being for all ages, includes a commitment to 'Achieve universal health coverage including financial risk protection, access to quality essential healthcare services and access to safe, effective, quality and affordable essential medicines and vaccines for all' (UN 2015, p. 20). Occupational therapy adds distinct value to mental health promotion, prevention, and intervention across the lifespan and in diverse settings with diverse populations (American Occupational Therapy Association 2016).

Human Rights

A strong link is made between human rights violations and mental ill-health in the WHO mhGAP action programme:

> Almost three quarters of the global burden of neuropsychiatric disorders is in countries with low and lower middle incomes. The stigma and violations of human rights directed towards people with these disorders compound the problem, increasing their vulnerability, accelerating and reinforcing their decline into poverty, and hindering care and rehabilitation. Restoration of mental health is not only essential for individual well-being, but is also necessary for economic growth and the reduction of poverty in societies and countries.
>
> *WHO 2008, p. 12*

Many therapists have adopted a human rights perspective on health and healthcare provision, acknowledging that they both have a role in protecting human rights in the interests of health and a moral obligation to advocate for people's right to access the occupations they need and want to do (Sakellariou and Pollard 2017). This obligation is articulated in the World Federation of Occupational Therapists' (WFOT) position statement on human rights as: 'a professional responsibility to identify and address occupational injustices and limit the impact of such injustices experienced by individuals' (WFOT 2019).

Evidence-Based Practice

Basing services and interventions on the best available scientific evidence and/or best practice enables programme planners, policy makers and clinicians to know what they should target for the best possible outcomes. However, the *Mental Health Action Plan* (WHO 2013) notes that cultural considerations should be considered: what is best practice in one country may not be so in another. The research agenda to establish evidence for mental health occupational therapy on the margins requires greater commitment to transdisciplinarity and strategic positioning of the profession within global-national-local research consortiums (Swarbrick and Noyes 2018; Richardson and Duncan 2013).

Life-Course Approach

A life-course approach acknowledges that MNS disorders either begin or manifest early in life (Veldman 2016). The risk of developing these disorders can be averted by building mental capital, which is defined as 'the cognitive and emotional resources that influence how well an individual is able to contribute to society and experience a high quality of life' (Collins et al. 2011, p. 28). Early interventions aimed at developing mental, emotional and occupational capital have been shown to interrupt the downward social drift of mentally vulnerable youth and maintain their viable engagement in employment (Veldman 2016). Working within communities and in collaboration with community-based organizations, occupational therapy is increasingly locating itself as a mental health promotion and prevention service concerned with facilitating the optimal person-occupation-environment interface (Watson 2013; American Occupational Therapy Association 2016).

Multisectoral Approach

A multisectoral approach to mental healthcare in marginal settings implies a comprehensive and coordinated response from multiple public sectors working in partnership, including health, education, employment, judicial, housing, social and other relevant sectors, as well as the private sector (Rathod et al. 2016; WHO 2013). Occupational therapy contributes to the prevention and reduction of MNS disorders and other health conditions by extending its role across sectors to underserved and neglected populations such as people in refugee camps, migrant hostels, slums, prisons, orphanages, homeless shelters, first people's and third nation reserves, shelters for abused women and children and facilities for child soldiers, asylum seekers, people displaced by natural disasters, civil unrest and war, and other marginalized groups (Sakellariou and Pollard 2017).

Empowerment

The *Mental Health Action Plan* (WHO 2013, p. 12) states that 'persons with mental disorders and psychosocial disabilities should be empowered and involved in mental health advocacy, policy, planning, legislation, service provision, monitoring, research and evaluation.' An empowerment perspective indicates a wider vision than the remediation of illness or disability; however, important functional outcomes might be for individuals and their families. Therapists have to be prepared to work flexibly and tailor their actions to the circumstances. Empowerment involves sharing professional skills rather than applying them as experts (Creek and Cook 2017).

The next section illustrates some of the ways in which these six cross-cutting principles and approaches are being applied by occupational therapists at a service for homeless people in Cape Town, South Africa.

CASE EXAMPLE: HOMELESSNESS

Because of the relative nature of culture and language, definitions of homelessness vary worldwide. However, a common thread among the definitions is the difficulty in locating and retaining permanent residence and integrating into normative society.

People with poor mental health are more susceptible to three main factors that can lead to homelessness: poverty, disaffiliation and personal vulnerability. Because they often lack the capacity to sustain employment, they have little income. Delusional thinking may lead them to antagonise or withdraw from friends, family and other people. Loss of social support leaves them with fewer coping resources in times of trouble. Mental illness can also impair a person's ability to be resilient and resourceful; it can cloud thinking and impair judgment. For these and other reasons, people with mental illness are at greater risk of experiencing homelessness.

Homelessness, in turn, exacerbates poor mental health. The stress of experiencing homelessness may precipitate or intensify previous mental illness by causing anxiety, fear, depression, sleeplessness and substance use. In the UK, for example, the proportion of homeless people diagnosed with a mental disorder is almost double that of the general population (Homeless Link 2014). Furthermore, people with severe mental illnesses may become homeless when they are discharged from hospitals and jails without proper community supports in place.

The needs of people experiencing homelessness include: physical safety, education, transportation, affordable housing, affordable medical/dental treatment and longitudinal psychosocial support. Community-based mental health services play an important role in helping find appropriate, supportive housing and other necessary community supports for people with severe mental illness. Housing outreach services that provide a safe place to live are a vital component in stabilising illness and helping individuals on their journey to recovery. U-Turn is an example of a service that uses a phased rehabilitation programme (Table 29.1) designed to meet the needs and address the challenges of clients at each phase in their restoration journey, from the street back into the mainstream society.

U-Turn is the first non-profit organization (NPO) in the homelessness public social services sector in Cape Town, South Africa to employ occupational therapists instead of social workers.

People living on the street enter the phased Service Centre Programme of their own volition, thereby endorsing their human right to dignity and self-determination. They access daily meals, clothing and toiletries, which may be purchased with vouchers earned by attending activity groups offered by previously homeless people who are further along the rehabilitation journey at easily accessible U-Turn premises. Clients are slowly introduced to a daily, structured programme that facilitates a transition from begging to working towards meeting their basic needs (food,

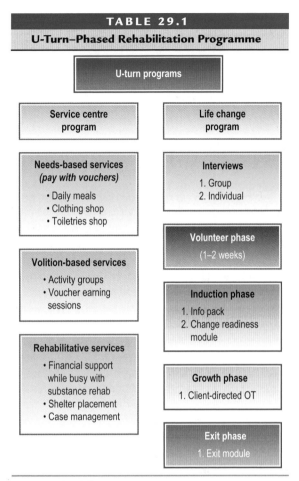

TABLE 29.1

U-Turn–Phased Rehabilitation Programme

OT, Occupational therapy.

shelter, ablution). The programme uses peers to inspire hope for change as an empowerment strategy. The occupational therapist as case manager gets to know each client's story, and together they plan the first steps on the restoration journey towards dignity. Clients may be financially supported to access multisectoral development resources such as specialised substance abuse rehabilitation, shelter placement and public health services that form part of universal health coverage.

Once the client feels ready, they may apply to join the phased Life Change Programme that aims to teach vocational and life skills. Group and individual interviews are conducted to screen and orientate clients, who are encouraged first to volunteer for one to two weeks before contracting to commence the Induction Phase that involves attending a Change Readiness

Module. Monitored work hardening and work readiness occur by working in U-Turn's second-hand clothing business. Clients attend a life skill training day once a week, including an individual occupational therapy session. While clients follow a structured curriculum during the Growth Phase, the occupational therapist makes constant adaptations depending on each client's needs and level of creative ability based on the Vona du Toit Model of Creative Ability (de Bruyn and Wright 2017; Schulz and Buys 2011). When clients feel ready to re-enter mainstream society, they transition into the Exit Phase, during which critical aspects of sustainable life change are reinforced though a structured exit module, which may be repeated when necessary.

CASE STUDY 29.1

Ms H's Story

Ms H left school at a young age as she was groomed into a local gang. In this 'gang family,' she was socialised to submit to higher ranking members without question, to never show weakness, to always revenge perceived wrongs, to take blood before yours is spilled, to not feel or show emotion and to manipulate and threaten to get what you want. Gang members trained Ms H to become a successful drug merchant, the only vocation she ever knew, a job for which formal school qualifications were unnecessary. A serious crime resulted in Ms H being given an 18-year prison sentence. Before her release from prison, Ms H made up her mind to leave the world of drugs and crime behind. However, she found that good intentions are not easily realized. It was not easy to overcome her addiction to methamphetamine, and, with her background, it was almost impossible to find an honest job. Ms H was unable to return to her biological family, as she had long ago been alienated from them. She did not want to return to her 'gang family,' as she wanted to live a drug and crime-free life. She found herself homeless.

Living on the street is dangerous for single women, so Ms H started a romantic relationship with a homeless man for protection. Drug use was part of the daily routine of the homeless group to which Ms H and her boyfriend belonged. Despite her best intentions, she relapsed. Ms H and her boyfriend sold pens and begged for money at a traffic light during the day. After 6 months of living on the street, one day Ms H was given a U-Turn voucher by a driver. That evening she attended the U-Turn soup kitchen, where she learned that she could earn more vouchers by attending daily voucher-earning activities and educational groups. Since it was winter and the U-Turn Centre offered some warmth, she joined the activities the following day. While busy with the voucher-earning activities, Ms H struck up a conversation with the man leading the session. She soon found that he, too, was a U-Turn client. He told her his story of homelessness and drug use and how U-Turn was sponsoring his shelter fees and transport to attend a drug and alcohol rehabilitation programme. He also told her that he was hoping to be accepted into U-Turn's Life Change Programme after completing his drug rehabilitation. Ms H could relate to this person's story and later said that it kindled hope for her own rehabilitation.

She was excited to tell her boyfriend about what she had learned that evening. He was angry with her for not earning money with him at the traffic lights that day and told her not to return to U-Turn. She argued with him and he beat her. Ms H did not want to lose his protection on the streets so she returned to begging at the traffic light. Ms H and her boyfriend continued to attend the evening meal at U-Turn, using vouchers that they begged for from passing drivers. After three more months of begging, drug use and abuse at the hands of her boyfriend, as well as continuous supportive conversations with U-Turn staff, Ms H knew that she had to choose between her boyfriend and the life she aspired to live. That evening, she told one of the U-Turn staff members that she was ready to move off the street and start attending drug rehabilitation.

U-Turn found Ms H space in a shelter and referred her to the addiction rehabilitation centre, which she attended during the day, volunteering at the voucher-earning activities and soup kitchen in the late afternoons and evenings. She also narrated her story to new clients, wanting to inspire hope in them as had happened for her. She met with the occupational

Continued on following page

Ms H's Story (Continued)

therapist on a weekly basis to discuss her progress and any problems. After 3 months, she graduated from addiction rehabilitation and was accepted into the Life Change programme.

For the first week, Ms H was placed in a U-Turn second-hand clothing shop in the position of a sales assistant. Ms H found that the long periods of standing around waiting for customers made her anxious. She started having flashbacks to traumatic incidents from her past. After 3 days, she walked out of the shop in the middle of the day, telling the manager that she was quitting. The store manager informed her occupational therapist, who contacted Ms H and asked her to come for a consultation the following day. After assessment, the occupational therapist referred Ms H for assessment by a doctor. She also moved Ms H to the laundry where all the clothing sold in the shops is prepared, as this is a fast-paced workspace with very little idle time. After visiting the clinic, Ms H was diagnosed with post-traumatic stress disorder (PTSD) and anxiety disorder and placed on medication. The occupational therapist referred Ms H to an external counsellor.

Ms H was very reluctant to take medication as she was afraid of becoming addicted to it. She was also afraid that the medication would make her crazy, a general misperception in her community. The occupational therapist spent a number of sessions educating Ms H about PTSD, anxiety disorder and how the medication works. After each session, the occupational therapist gave Ms H questions related to PTSD, anxiety disorder and her prescribed medication to research on the Internet (accessed at U-Turn Centre for free). They discussed Ms H's research findings each week. Ms H eventually started taking her medication. After a number of sessions with the occupational therapist, Ms H started becoming quite emotional during sessions. She made excuses for her crying and said that she had never felt or displayed such strong emotions. When the occupational therapist asked about her feelings, she was unable to name them. Over time, Ms H's emotional vocabulary grew as the occupational therapist helped her reflect on and name the emotions she experienced in different situations.

Ms H attended the Change Readiness Module that covered topics such as understanding your environment, understanding yourself within your environment (personality, sensory profile and reaction to tasks), taking ownership, stress-handling techniques, common pitfalls in the recovery journey and goal setting. Ms H experimented with different stress management techniques and found that high-impact exercise had a calming effect; this led to her joining a running and soccer club. She also found that deep breathing and praying helped her calm down when she started feeling anxious.

From time to time, Ms H's manager would report to the occupational therapist that she threatened another client or that she made life difficult for a client she had argued with. When confronted about her behaviour, Ms H would often say, 'This is all so new to me. All I know is how the gang taught me to behave. I don't know how people on the outside deal with things.' The occupational therapist gave Ms H research assignments on healthy conflict management and used role play to practise healthy responses. The occupational therapist also mediated between Ms H and another client to give Ms H opportunities to practise healthy conflict management and to guide her towards mindful responses when dealing with interpersonal problems.

After a year in the Life Change Programme, Ms H learned enough coping and interpersonal skills for the occupational therapist to suggest placing her in a shop again. Before Ms H moved to a shop, the occupational therapist helped her prepare for situations that she might find difficult. After Ms H started working at the shop, the occupational therapist continued to meet her once a week to discuss her progress and help her solve any problems. Ms H also phoned the occupational therapist between weekly sessions when she needed extra support. After Ms H successfully worked at a shop for 3 months, the occupational therapist agreed that she was ready to start looking for a job in the open labour market. She completed the Exit Module, which prepared her for job hunting and interviews. Ms H eventually secured a position as a sales assistant in a retail store and has maintained her sobriety and dignity for the past 4 years.

In the next section, a way of working on the margins is proposed based on the application of several pointers for thinking and action.

THINKING AND ACTING ON THE MARGINS

Occupational therapy practice on the margins aims to address both individual and social forms of development (Duncan 2016). A development focus requires different forms of professional reasoning, as the occupational therapist needs to consider the impact of biography (personal stories), history (a society's story) and structure (prevailing governance systems and social environments) on people's occupations, as well as the conditions of society that pose major barriers to their functioning and participation (Cole and Creek 2016). The pointers offered here are not intended to give a comprehensive overview of the current state of knowledge or to be a definitive guide to practice on the margins. They provide a starting point for therapists to add to and refine their own compass when tackling some of the social conditions that impact their clients.

- **Sociological imagination** about the biographies, history and structure associated with individuals and social groupings;
- **Reflexivity** as a way of 'being' that locates the therapist as an active co-participant in social change;
- **Values** to support a socially just practice;
- **Partnership** with stakeholders concerned with particular public issues;
- **Theory** that is contextually relevant for practice, education and research;
- **Policy** orientation with knowledge of current local, national and international developments;
- **Occupation** as a route to health, well-being and social inclusion; and
- **Self-care** by the therapist to maintain good mental health and avoid burnout.

Sociological Imagination

C. Wright Mills (1916–1962), a social thinker during the first half of the last century, was an American Marxist and sociologist who introduced the concept of sociological imagination (Mills 1967). Sociological imagination is a quality of mind that discerns the intricate connections between individual stories and the stories of the particular society and history within which individuals are located. As a way of thinking, sociological imagination recognizes how the social contexts within which people live contribute to the creation and perpetuation of their personal problems. Mills believed that neither the life of an individual nor the history of a society can be understood without recognizing their dialectical interaction. For Mills (1967, p. 4), sociological imagination transforms personal problems into public and political issues; doing so helps people become agents of social change. By linking biography, history and structure, the interconnectedness between individuals and society becomes obvious, thus enabling people to identify critical points of action. Mills suggested that practitioners, therefore, keep their eyes open to both human variety and the social norms of the time: '... many personal troubles cannot be solved merely as troubles, but must be understood in terms of public issues—and in terms of the problems of history making' (Mills 1967, pp. 225–226; orig. 1957).

Sociological imagination guides occupational therapists in drawing links between individual biographies; the social structures that determine people's occupations; and the unfolding public issues that shape history, such as politics, policy and resource distribution. It helps therapists to see individual troubles or triumphs in relation to the wider social context, that is, to think about personal problems as problems of society and vice versa. The challenges faced by individuals experiencing mental health problems must be *understood* and *addressed* within prevailing socio-historical contexts. Sociological imagination opens up avenues for occupational therapists to recognize and address the occupational dimensions of social structures that compromise health, including mental well-being.

Consider, for example, cases of post-traumatic stress disorder and attempted suicide amongst ex-combatants. Sociological imagination compels considering the prevailing socio-historical conditions that precipitate and perpetuate mental ill-health in the biographies of these individuals. The creation of occupation-centred recovery pathways for traumatised ex-combatants must enable them to resolve deep trauma by reframing a dignified and purposeful place in the society that sent them to war in the first place (Nell and Shapiro 2012, p. 27; Fossey 2012, pp. 21–23).

Reflexivity

Reflexivity refers to the bidirectional relationships between cause and effect. Both therapist and client (individual, group, community) are shaped by the circumstances of their lives and the ways that they respond to the opportunities and challenges presented to them. A reflexive occupational therapist understands and actively engages with the two-way influence between the self and the other. Active engagement implies partnering with marginalized people in thinking through the interconnectedness between their individual and collective lives and the social structures within which they are embedded, and, in so doing, imagining and co-creating realistic alternative futures (Duncan 2016).

Occupational therapists are trained to assess, interpret and address individual biographies that are affected by processes of mental ill-being, in particular people's functioning and participation in valued occupations. Clinical reasoning involves a biopsychosocial interpretation of illness behaviour and the identification of practical solutions to personal problems in collaboration with the person concerned. Reflexivity in the context of development practice requires different forms of professional reasoning (Cole and Creek 2016). As mutually accountable actors, everyone in the field of action on the margins knows—equally but differently—each person's contribution, adding value to the emergent tasks at hand. Working in partnership with various stakeholders, occupational therapists become occupation-focused activists, addressing the social structures and determinants of health. In doing so, they think and act sociologically and politically (Cole and Creek 2016). A reflexive and socio-political way of thinking is believed to provide occupational therapists with four general benefits:

- An ability to challenge commonly held assumptions about occupation and humans as occupational beings;
- An ability to discern opportunities for and constraints on occupational engagement;
- A means for becoming critical, imaginative and active in relation to human occupation; and
- A lens for understanding how human differences and human suffering influence what people do every day and for recognizing the relative strengths and challenges of diverse lifestyles.

Values

Values are culturally defined standards by which people assess desirability, goodness and beauty, and which serve as broad guidelines for social living (Macionis and Plummer 2008). The values of a particular culture or marginalized group tell us what they believe to be morally right and indicate how they expect outsiders to act to bring about beneficial outcomes. Working on the margins requires occupational therapists to subject their personal and professional values and principles to critical examination to determine what constitutes 'good.' They must guard against inadvertently reflecting 'local preconceptions and prejudices, which may not survive reasoned confrontation with others not restricted by the same parochialism' (Sen 2009, p. viii). For example, when we work to increase the wealth of a particular group of people, is this at the expense of another group whose needs are equally pressing? Such critical scrutiny and reflexivity can enable occupational therapy practice, education and research to resist cultural imperialism, avoid ideological dominance and be aligned with culturally defined standards for social living.

Partnership

Partnership is a complex process that best unfolds through longitudinal, mutual engagement. Occupational therapy partnerships focus on social inclusion through the interface between individual and collective occupation (Ramugondo and Kronenberg 2015). Occupational therapists who wish to promote occupational justice must build on their abilities in working co-operatively and in partnership with communities (Kohrt et al. 2018; Sakellariou and Pollard 2017). However, communities are contested sites of meaning in which constant change and complex social processes create all sorts of margins, boundaries, borders and stratifications that may confound cooperation and partnerships. To meet these challenges, occupational therapists practicing on the margins make use of a range of participatory methods that enable vulnerable individuals and groups to make occupational choices that promote health and participation in safe, productive and socially acceptable activities (Galvaan 2012).

Occupational therapists also use a range of professional reasoning approaches that support and enable partnership working. For example, a South African occupational therapist, Theresa Lorenzo (2016), identified a collaborative reasoning process through which the occupational therapist could 'generate capacity for reciprocal learning among persons with disabilities, their families, and service providers' (p. 99). This process is based on the five elements of radical collaboration identified by Tamm and Luyet (2004): identify the intention to collaborate, build trustworthiness and openness, create safe spaces where people can share, seek deeper self-awareness and awareness of others and foster self-responsibility and acceptance of responsibility. Lorenzo described collaboration as 'a powerful, consensual way of working' (op cit, p. 99).

Policy

Policy includes national and international legislation, conventions, position statements and practice guidelines pertinent to different stakeholder groups, for example, the WHO *Mental Health Action Plan 2013–2020*, which was described above. The WFOT has produced position papers and manuals on a number of issues to give occupational therapists some of the knowledge and resources needed to work in different areas. Examples relevant to the field of mental health include: *Ethics, sustainability and global experiences* (WFOT 2016); *Occupational therapy and community-centred practice* (WFOT 2019a); and *Occupational therapy for displaced persons* (WFOT 2019b).

Being familiar with the appropriate policies for a particular context enables occupational therapists to frame mental health occupational therapy services in ways that will be recognized and promoted by governing structures.

Occupational therapists can lobby for more effective policies to promote social justice at the local and national levels by aligning themselves with diverse communities, such as mental health consumer and family organizations and governmental structures (Mirza et al. 2016). Occupational therapists can also promote the access of marginalized constituencies to high-quality care, including those services offered by the profession, by joining research consortiums that are concerned with the social determinants of mental health (Richardson and Duncan 2013).

Occupation

Although the conditions necessary for social inclusion may be enhanced by the institutions of government, such as social services and welfare provision, people must feel and be actively engaged as citizens rather than passively supported if they are to experience inclusion (van Bruggen 2016). Occupational therapy on the margins uses occupation as both a means and an end to enable social inclusion at the individual and community levels. At an individual level, occupation provides the primary means for learning how to participate or regaining confidence in participating in society; for example, buying food from the local market, cooking a meal with friends or playing a team sport. At the community level, occupation creates interactive spaces where people can experience a feeling of connectedness with others, such as safety, trust in others and having the opportunity to grow. People participate in their communities through collective occupation, for example, by working, voting, socialising or volunteering. Collective occupation provides the biographical, historical and structural context through which people can share the same rights, privileges and activities (Kronenberg and Ramugondo 2015). As an end in itself, occupation can be used developmentally to work against discrimination, exclusion and marginalization in several ways and on many levels (Sakellariou and Pollard 2017).

Self-Care

Working with people who are experiencing trauma or extreme events can be stressful for occupational therapists, even those who have years of experience.

Working on the margins can add an additional layer of stress, as the therapist may have limited access to support, supervision and debriefing. It is, therefore, important for the occupational therapy practitioner to have in place strategies for self-care, coping and recovery before going to work on the margins.

The term 'secondary trauma' is sometimes used to refer to the negative effects of witnessing or hearing about trauma in others (Sodeke-Gregson et al. 2016). This can manifest as burnout, compassion fatigue or secondary traumatic stress. The WFOT has addressed this issue, identifying the risks and offering practical tools for the therapist to safeguard their own health and well-being, such as ways to build emotional resilience, tools for recognizing signs of secondary trauma and strategies for maintaining a positive outlook (WFOT 2019c).

SUMMARY

This chapter provides an overview of some of the social dynamics that shape people's position in society, influence their choices and opportunities for occupational engagement and compromise or mediate their mental health. It described approaches aimed at bridging global mental health service gaps, and used a case example of homelessness to illustrate how occupational therapy can contribute to the social inclusion of mentally ill and marginalized people. Sociological imagination and reflexivity were introduced as ways of thinking on the margins. The importance of remaining grounded in values, including social justice and human rights, was confirmed as was the role of theory, policy and partnerships in contextually relevant, occupation-centred practice.

In conclusion, individuals who take a stand against social injustice can mobilise social change. When occupational therapists stand in solidarity with marginalized groups and communities, new horizons beyond traditional hospital and social care practice settings begin to emerge. Taking a step back from the familiar ways of conducting mental health occupational therapy implies questioning taken-for-granted perspectives on what the profession has to offer to society and exploring how a different skill set can be used to address people's needs and aspirations through occupation.

Acknowledgement

The authors would like to acknowledge Anneke Buys, principal occupational therapist, U-Turn, Cape Town, South Africa for providing the case example. See www.homeless.org.za.

QUESTION FOR CONSIDERATION

1. What margins can you identify that exist in your context/society today?
2. Do you face marginalization, and if so, how does it impact you?
3. Why should occupational therapists be vigilant about cultural imperialism?
4. In which ways can different forms of violence be inflicted within a person's own marginalized community? Why may violence be an occupational therapy issue?
5. What is the difference between 'values and principles' and 'moral obligations?' How would an occupational therapist know which is which when working on the margins?

SERVICE USER COMMENTARY

OCCUPATIONAL THERAPY AND SOCIAL INCLUSION

It is a pleasure to read a thoughtful and insightful piece of work that is actively thinking through the complicated aspects of social inclusion. This chapter demonstrates how some societies and cultures are trying to move on from less sensitive and, consequently, more authoritarian perspectives that both simultaneously colonize and exclude individuals from their own lives. Often, this is done with good intentions through the damaging axiom 'for their own good.'

We have a comfortable illusion of thinking the 'we' have moved away from problematic ways of doing things. As cultural landscapes change, so do the means of exclusion. Searching for how social inclusion needs to be enacted requires a dynamism of thought, which can adapt to the changing configurations and circumstances.

This work opens up important vistas of human experience. It clarifies nuanced understandings of how the circumstances of oppression can be and are structured into society. It indicates how some outcomes are used as a basis of difference and ultimately exclusion. Take for instance the paying for labour in alcohol rather than money; clearly an arrangement in which the financially poor are exploited in a way that gives rise to outcomes that fit a narrative historically used to justify exclusion from better opportunity.

The authors refer to exclusion as a social process which reinforces the position of the privileged group over that of the dispossessed. Understanding such dispossession as subtle and persistent harm is a significant modern challenge. The way groups and individuals are dehumanised and dementalised embodies the myths used as charters for action. This writing goes some way in advancing the joined-up thinking that will allow us to get beyond the looking glass that privileges the siloed understandings that reinforce wicked problems. I would have liked to have seen more explicit mention of how family, friends and society can be the cause of mental ailment and withdrawal from other people.

Individuals adapt to the circumstances they find themselves in, and those adaptations allow them to survive the situation in which they are obliged to live. As people encounter disadvantage hardwired in the culture, the behaviours they must engage in to survive often alienate them from a place of opportunity in enfranchised culture. A consequence of this is that they become the focus of a professionalized, depersonalized gaze which places their humanity within a dehumanised rubric. They increasingly become spoken to and acted towards as a categorised pathology related to a sense of utilitarianism. Under-resourced, highly formalized services are left with the task of cleaning up after the excesses of private interest.

These complexes are picked up on here, acknowledging a tacit acceptance and complicity of certain socialised positions that lean on ersatz aphorisms of participation, agency and resilience. It is refreshing to see a discussion of structural violence that dogs so many people, hampering well-being and creating iatrogenic problems. Much more is to come in this expanding area as we see social justice movements like the Psychiatric Survivors Movement and Black Lives Matter philosophers detail modern forms of poverty, ailment and oppression, which lack articulating language.

In this writing, we find an account of Occupational Therapy being grounded in meaningful activity and opened out as a multi/interdisciplinary approach to processes of human development that strikes a balance between the practical and humane. A challenge will be to deliver such humanised support in the face of 'quality assurance' bureaucracies that permeate how services are resourced. Alongside this will be the challenges of professionals to live the values espoused by their profession whilst sufficiently resisting the depersonalization that formality encourages.

Alex Dunedin

REFERENCES

American Occupational Therapy Association. (2016). *Occupational therapy's distinct value: Mental health promotion, prevention, and intervention across the lifespan.* American Association of Occupational Therapists. www.aota.org.

Cloete, L. G., & Ramugondo, E. (2015). 'I drink'": Mothers' Alcohol Consumption as Both Individualized and Imposed Occupation. *South African Journal of Occupational Therapy, 45*(1), 34–40.

Cole, M. B., & Creek, J. (Eds.). (2016). *Global Perspectives in Professional Reasoning.* Thorofare, NJ: SLACK Inc.

Collins, P., Patel, V., Joestl, S. S., March, D., Insel, T., & Daar, A. S. (2011). Grand Challenges in Global Mental Health. *Nature, 475,* 27–30.

Corbett, S. (2017). *How to be a Craftivist.* London: Unbound.

Creek, J., & Cook, S. (2017). Learning from the Margins: Enabling Effective Occupational Therapy. *British Journal of Occupational Therapy, 80*(7), 423–431.

deBruyn, M., & Wright, J. (2017). Joining the Dots: Theoretically Connecting the Vona du Toit Model of Creative Ability (VdTMoCA) with Supported Employment. *South African Journal of Occupational Therapy, 47*(2), 49–52.

Duncan, M. (2016). Development Reasoning in Community Practice. In M. B. Cole, & J. Creek (Eds.), *International Perspectives on Professional Reasoning* (203–238). Thorofare, NJ: SLACK Inc.

Duncan, M., Swartz, L., & Kathard, H. (2011b). The Burden of Psychiatric Disability on Chronically Poor Households: Part 2 (Coping). *South African Journal of Occupational Therapy, 41*(3), 64–70.

Eberharter, V. V. (2012). *The Intergenerational Trauma of Occupational Preferences, Segregation and Wage Inequality - Empirical Evidence from Europe and the United States."* SOEPpaper506. http://www.diw.de/soeppapers.

Fossey, M. (2012). Unsung Heroes: Developing a Better Understanding of the Emotional Support Needs of Service Families. In *Report for Centre for Mental Health, the Royal British Legion and Combat Stress.* www.centreforementalhealth.org.uk/pdfs/unsung_heroes.pdf.

Galvaan, R. (2012). Occupational Choice. In G. Whiteford, & C. Hocking (Eds.), *Occupational Science: Society, Inclusion Participation* (Vols. 152–62). Chichester: Blackwell Publishing Ltd.

Gujendragad, J. M. (2015). Struggles of Women with Mental Illness. *Journal of Human and Social Sciences (IOSR-JHSS)*, 20(4), 37–41.

HM Government. (2019). *2018 UK Annual Report on Modern Slavery.* https://assets.publishing.service.gov.uk/government/uploads/system/uploads/attachment_data/file/749346/2018_UK_Annual_Report_on_Modern_Slavery.pdf. [Accessed 8 July 2019].

Johnston, D. W., Shurer, S., & Shields, M. A. (2012). Exploring Intergenerational Persistence of Mental Health: Evidence from Three Generations. *Journal of Health Economics*, 32(6), 1077–1089.

Kohrt, B. A., Asher, L., Bhardwaj, A., Fazel, M., Jordans, M. J. D., Mutamba, B. B., et al. (2018). The Role of Communities in Mental Health Care in Low- and Middle-Income Countries: A Meta-Review of Components and Competencies. *International Journal of Environmental Research and Public Health*, 15(6) (June): 1279.

Krishnan, L. (2015). Social Exclusion, Mental Health, Disadvantage and Injustice. *Psychology & Developing Societies*, 27(2), 155–173.

Krug, E. G., Dahlberg, L. L., Mercy, J. A., Zwi, A. B., & Lozano, R. (Eds.). (2002). *World Report on Violence and Health.* Geneva: World Health Organization.

Link, H. (2014). *The Unhealthy State of Homelessness: Health Audit results 2014.* http://www.homeless.org.uk/sites/default/files/site-attachments/The unhealthy state of homelessness FINAL.pdf. [Accessed 8 July 2019].

Lorenzo, T. (2016). Collaborative Reasoning: Teaching and Learning to Facilitate Disability Inclusion in Policy and Practice. In M. Cole, & J. Creek (Eds.), *Global Perspectives in Professional Reasoning* (pp. 99–116). Thorofare, NJ: SLACK Inc.

Mental Health Foundation. (2019). *Stigma and Discrimination.* www.mentalhealth.org.uk/a-to-z/s/stigma-and-discrimination. [Accessed 8 July 2019].

Miller, G. (2014). Is the Agenda for Global Mental Health a Form of Cultural Imperialism? *Medical Humanities*, 40, 131–134.

Mills, C. W. (1967). *Power, Politics and People: The Collected Essays of C. Wright Mills.* Oxford: Oxford University Press. Orig. 1957.

Mirza, M., Magasi, S., & Hammel, J. (2016). Soul Searching Occupations: Critical Reflections on Occupational Therapy's Commitment to Social Justice, Disability Rights, and Participation. In P. Block, D. Kasnitz, A. Nishida, & N. Pollard (Eds.), *Occupying Disability: Critical Approaches to Community,* Justice, and Decolonizing Disability, pp. 159–174. New York: Springer.

Mooney, M. A. (2016). Human Agency and Mental Illness. *Journal of Critical Realism*, 15(4), 376–390.

Morris, I. (2010). *Why the West Rules - for Now: The Patterns of history, and what They Reveal about the Future.* London: Profile Books Limited.

Murthy, R. S. (2011). Mental Health Services in Low and Middle-Income Countries. In G. Thornicroft, et al. (Ed.), *Oxford Textbook of Community Mental Health* (pp. 325–336). Oxford: Oxford University Press.

Narayan, D., Patel, R., Schafft, K., Rademacher, A., & Koch-Scultz, S. (2000). *Voices of the Poor: Can Anyone Hear Us?* New York: Oxford University Press for the World Bank.

Nell, M., & Shapiro, J. (2012). *No Place by the Fire: The Story of South African Ex-Combatants and the National Peace Accord Trust.* Atlantic Philanthropies. www.atlanticphilanthropies.org.

Nussbaum, M. C. (2000). *Women and Human Development: The Capabilities Approach.* Cambridge: Cambridge University Press.

Parker, I. (2004). Psychoanalysis and Critical Psychology. In D. Hook (Ed.), *Critical Psychology.* 139–61: Lansdowne: UCT Press.

Pooremamali, P., Morville, A., & Eklund, M. (2017). Barriers to Continuity in the Pathway towards Occupational Engagement Among Ethnic Minorities with Mental Illness. *Scandinavian Journal of Occupational Therapy*, 24(4), 259–268.

Ramugondo, E., & Kronenberg, F. (2015). Explaining Collective Occupations from a Human Relations Perspective: Bridging the Individual-Collective Dichotomy. *Journal of Occupational Science*, 22(1), 3–16.

Rathod, S., Pinninti, N., Irfan, M., Gorczynski, P., Rathod, P., Gega, L., et al. (2016). Mental Health Service Provision in Low- and Middle-Income Countries. *Health Services Insights*, 10, 1–7. https://doi.org/10.1177/1178632917694350. [Accessed 8 July 2019].

Richardson, P., & Duncan, M. (2013). A Context for Mental Health Research in Occupational Therapy. In E. Cara, & A. MacRae (Eds.), *Psychosocial Occupational Therapy: An Evolving Practice* (3rd ed.) (pp. 61–92). Delmar: Engage Learning.

Rose, D. (2018). A Hidden Activism and its Changing Contemporary Forms: Mental Health Service Users/Survivors Mobilising. *Journal of Social and Political Psychology*, 6(2), 728–744.

Rutten, B. P. F., Hammels, C., Geschwind, N., Menne-Lothmann, C., Pishva, E., et al. (2013). Resilience in Mental Health: Linking Psychological and Neurobiological Perspectives. *Acta Psychiatrica Scandinavica*, 128(1 (July)), 3–20.

Sakellariou, D., & Pollard, N. (2017). *Occupational Therapies without Borders: Integrating Justice with Practice* (2nd ed.). Elsevier.

Schulz, V., & Buys, A. (2011). In *From Dependency to Dignity: The A2B for Community Development* (2nd ed.). A2B Entrepreneurial Transformation Movement. http://www.a2btransformation.com. [Accessed 8 July 2019].

Sen, A. (1999). *Development as Freedom.* New York: Knopf.

Sodeke-Gregson, E. A., Holttum, S., & Billings, J. (2013). Compassion Satisfaction, Burnout, and Secondary Traumatic Stress in UK Therapists who Work with Adult Trauma Clients. *European Journal of Psychotraumatology*, *4*(10). www.ncbi.nlm.nih.gov/pmc/articles/PMC3877781/. [Accessed 8 July 2019].

Swarbrick, M., & Noyes, S. (2018). Effectiveness of Occupational Therapy Services in Mental Health. *American Journal of Occupational Therapy*, *72*(5), 1–4.

Tamm, J. W., & Luyet, R. J. (2004). *Radical Collaboration: Five Essential Skills to Overcome Defensiveness and Build Successful Relationships*. New York: Harper Business.

Trevedi, P. (2014). Nothing about Us, without Us - a User/Survivor Perspective of Global Mental Health. *International Review of Psychiatry*, *26*(5), 544–550.

United Nations. (2015). *Transforming our World: The 2030 Agenda for Sustainable Development*. A/RES/70/1. http://sustainabledevelopment.un.org. [Accessed 29 October 2018].

United Nations. (2018). *Sustainable Development Goal 6: Synthesis Report on Water and Sanitation*. New York: United Nations Publications.

Van Bruggen, H. (2016). Strategic thinking and reasoning in occupational therapy. In M. Cole, & J. Creek (Eds.), *Global Perspectives in Professional Reasoning* (pp. 99–116). Thorofare, NJ: SLACK Inc.

Van Den Tillaart, S., Kurtz, D., & Cash, P. (2009). Powerlessness, Marginalized Identity, and Silencing of Health Concerns: Voiced Realities of Women Living with a Mental Health Diagnosis. *International Journal of Mental Health Nursing, 18*, 153–163.

Varshney, M., Mahapatra, A., Krishnan, V., et al. (2016). Violence and Mental Illness: What is the True Story? *Journal of Epidemiology and Community Health, 70*, 223–225.

Veldman, K. (2016). *Mental health from a Life-Course Perspective: The Transition from School to Work*. Groningen: University of Groningen.

Watson, R. (2013). A Population Approach to Occupational Therapy. *South African Journal of Occupational Therapy, 43*(1), 34–39.

World Federation of Occupational Therapists. (2016). *Ethics, Sustainability and Global Experiences*. http://www.wfot.org. *Global Perspectives in Pofessional Reasoning*. [Accessed 8 July 2019].

World Federation of Occupational Therapists. (2019). *Position Statement on Human Rights*. http://www.wfot.org. [Accessed 8 July 2019].

World Federation of Occupational Therapists. (2019a). *Resource Manual: Occupational therapy and Community-Centred Practice*. http://www.wfot.org. [Accessed 8 July 2019].

World Federation of Occupational Therapists. (2019b). *Resource Manual: Occupational therapy for Displaced Persons*. http://www.wfot.org. [Accessed 8 July 2019].

World Federation of Occupational Therapists. (2019c). *Guide for Occupational therapy First Responders to Disasters and Trauma*. http://www.wfot.org. [Accessed 8 July 2019].

World Health Organisation. (2018). Accelerating Country Action on Mental Health. In *Report of the 10th meeting of the mhGAPForum*. Geneva: WHO.

World Health Organization. (2008). *Mental health Gap Action Programme: Scaling up Care for mental, Neurological, and Substance Use Disorders*. Geneva: WHO.

World Health Organization. (2013). *Mental health Action Plan 2013–2020*. Geneva: WHO.

Young, I. M. (2000). Five Faces of Oppression. In M. Adams, W. J. Blumenfeld, R. Castañeda, H. W. Hackman, M. L. Peters, & X. Zuñiga (Eds.), *Readings for Diversity and Social Justice* (pp. 35–49). New York: Routledge.

GLOSSARY

Activity adaptation The occupational therapist changes an activity so it is better suited for people engaging in occupational therapy by considering what each person values about the activity and how it can be adjusted (Creek 2003).

Activity analysis The occupational therapist evaluates the potential of an activity to meet therapeutic aims by systematically considering the usefulness and relevance of each component for the setting and for the service user (Creek 2003).

Activity grading To maintain progress, the occupational therapist adapts an activity to be more challenging as a person's occupational performance improves or easier when their capacity is reduced for any reason (Pentland et al. 2018).

Adherence Taking medications for periods of time, complying with instructions, and following a recommended regimen for administering them (National Institute for Health and Care Excellence (NICE) 2009).

Arts therapies Interventions to improve mental health that use creative and expressive processes associated with the arts including drama, music and dance. The titles of art therapist, drama therapist and music therapist are protected in law in some countries (e.g., in the United Kingdom under the category of Arts Therapies) (Health and Care Professions Council (HCPC) 2018).

Care coordinator A practitioner responsible for ensuring that an individual's mental healthcare plan is based on a holistic assessment of need, coordinated across all service provider agencies, and regularly reviewed and updated.

Care programme approach (CPA) A formal approach to care planning in UK mental health services in which an assigned care coordinator addresses and reviews the service users assessed needs in collaboration with them and others involved (Department of Health (DH) 2007).

Carer Anyone who supports a service user in a voluntary capacity, typically a family member, a close friend, work colleague or neighbour.

Consent Consent to any stage of the occupational therapy process means a person gives their permission for it to happen, when all relevant information has been shared with the person in a way that they understand (Royal College of Occupational Therapists (RCOT) 2021).

Continuing professional development A therapist's responsibility for their own learning and development, requiring a cyclical process of reflection and action which ensures they maintain their capacity to practice safely and legally (RCOT 2017).

Dual diagnosis The co-occurrence in the same individual of two psychiatric diagnoses, such as bipolar disorder and substance use disorder or intellectual disability and dementia (World Health Organization (WHO) 2020).

Dysfunction A person's temporary or enduring difficulties with occupational performance, affecting their capacity to adapt and competently engage in their daily life occupations (Creek 2003).

Forensic practice A multidisciplinary approach related to criminal and legal systems to support those who pose risk to others, aiming to improve their quality of life, prevent relapse and reduce re-offending (Connell 2016).

Goal setting A stage in the occupational therapy process in which service users identify their goals and plan with their occupational therapist how to achieve them, negotiating aims and objectives (Kessler et al. 2019).

Habit A performance pattern in daily life, acquired by frequent repetition, that does not require attention and allows efficient function (Creek 2010, p. 25).

Mental capacity A person's ability to make and communicate decisions autonomously (The National Archives 2005).

Motivation An energy source for action that 'directs a person's actions towards meeting needs' (Creek 2010, p. 25).

Occupation A group of activities that has personal and sociocultural meaning, is named within a culture and supports participation in society (Creek 2010, p. 25).

Occupational adaptation The service user's process of transforming what they do and how they perform occupations to master and/or respond to their environment (Grajo et al. 2018).

Occupational alienation The experience of having to do something in a way that does not satisfy needs, affecting occupational engagement (Bryant 2016).

Occupational apartheid Situations in which occupations are classified, paid and valued and enhance life for some, while in the same places and times occupations are taken for granted, exploited and trivialized for others (Townsend 2003).

Occupational balance The individual's perception of having the right amount of occupations and the right variation between occupations to maintain their health and well-being (Wagman et al. 2012).

Occupational deprivation Reduction of, or exclusion from, meaningful activities and limitation of roles and routines due to circumstances beyond the individual's control (Whiteford 2000).

Occupational performance The act of doing an occupation, which includes making choices, getting organized, being competent, and interacting with the environment (Creek 2010).

Occupational science The study of humans as occupational beings and the relationship between occupation and health (Molineux 2017).

Occupational therapy process The sequence of steps or actions taken by the therapist to enable service users to progress towards their goals (referral, information gathering, assessment, formulation, goal setting, plan, implementation and evaluation) (Pentland et al. 2018; American Occupational Therapy Association 2020).

Occupational therapy A profession which promotes health and well-being by 'enabling people and communities to engage in the occupations they want to, need to, or are expected to or by modifying the occupation or the environment to better support their occupational engagement' (World Federation of Occupational Therapists, (WFOT) 2012).

Outcome An observed or measured consequence of an intervention (Laver Fawcett 2007) or a service user's participation in a therapeutic process.

Peer support worker A person with direct experience of recovering from mental health problems who is employed to support service users (Penney 2018).

Person-centred care An approach used in older people's mental health services that gives ownership of a care plan to a service user, valuing their individuality and personal perspective (Kitwood 1997).

Person-centred practice An interdisciplinary approach to practice which aims to give priority to partnerships with service users to ensure services are safe, effective and relevant to their needs (Health Foundation 2016).

Positive risk-taking Enabling positive therapeutic outcomes by assessing risks and benefits, agreeing a management strategy, and facilitating a suitable activity (Morgan 2020).

Recovery A way of living a satisfying, hopeful and contributing life even with limitations caused by an illness (Anthony 2007).

Recovery-oriented practice An interdisciplinary approach to practice in which staff works in partnership with service users for recovery, holding onto hope for their future and focusing on how to improve the quality of diverse aspects of their lives (O'Hagan 2004).

Reflective practice Creating space to think about your practice systematically, routinely and critically to maximize learning from experience (WFOT 2016, p. 71).

Relapse prevention An approach that explores a person's history of mental health problems, particularly the triggers for their onset, and offers support to help develop strategies for preventing further episodes.

Resilience A protective factor against psychological distress in adverse situations which enables individuals to adapt successfully and handle challenges (Rutten et al. 2013).

Risk management Ensuring risks are identified and reduced whenever possible to maintain duty of care to the service users and the general public.

Safeguarding Protecting the health, well-being and human rights of individuals, which allows people to live free from harm, abuse and neglect.

Sensory processing The way the body receives, analyses and responds to information from the environment (Dunn 2009; Beyer et al. 2019).

Social exclusion Non-participation in the key activities of the society in which a person lives (Burchardt et al. 2002).

Social model of disability A model for social and political change, which sees disability as a consequence of attitudinal and physical barriers in society (Oliver 2013; Molineux 2017).

Supervision A meeting facilitated by an internal supervisor or independent mental health professional to focus on the professional practice of an individual or team with the aims of processing reflections, managing workload and fostering professional development.

Therapeutic use of self Ensuring the therapeutic nature of contact with service users is sustained by intentionally using personal qualities such as self-awareness and empathy to choose how to think and act, explore what is happening and communicate effectively, verbally and non-verbally.

Trauma-informed care An approach to service delivery focusing on a person's *story* and recognizing how trauma adversely affects people's lives, their needs and service usage. To care effectively, the staff creates a safe, accepting place and asks what *has happened* rather than what *is wrong* (Machtinger et al. 2018).

Triage An intensive process aiming to assess, stabilize and determine the best course of action for a person in an emergency or crisis situation.

Triggers Experiences that can be identified as sources of distress: occupational therapy can involve learning to recognize triggers and manage their impact to prevent relapse.

REFERENCES

Anthony, W. (2007). Toward a vision of recovery for mental health and psychiatric rehabilitation services. 2nd edition. https://cpr.bu.edu/wp-content/uploads/2011/11/Preview-Toward-a-Vision-of-Recovery-2nd-edition.pdf.

Beyer, O., Butler, S., Murphy, B., Olig, M., Skinner, S., & Moser, C. S. (2019). Sensory integration and sensory processing… what's in a name? *Journal of Occupational Therapy, Schools, & Early Intervention*, 12(1), 1–37. https://doi.org/10.1080/19411243.2019.1589702.

American Occupational Therapy Association. (2020). *Occupational Therapy Practice Framework: Domain and Process, 4th Edition.* [Bethesda, MD]: AOTA Press.

Bryant, W. (2016). The Dr Elizabeth Casson memorial lecture 2016: Occupational alienation – a concept for modelling participation in practice and research. *British Journal of Occupational Therapy*, 79(9), 521–529. https://doi.org/10.1177/0308022616662282.

Burchardt, T., Le Grand, J., & Piachaud, D. (2002). Degrees of exclusion: Developing a dynamic, multidimensional measure. In J. Hills, J. Le Grand, & D. Piachaud (Eds.), *Understanding social exclusion* (pp. 30–43). New York: Oxford University Press.

Connell, C. (2016). Forensic occupational therapy to reduce the risk of reoffending: A survey of practice in the United Kingdom. *The Journal of Forensic Psychiatry & Psychology*, 27(6), 907–928.

Creek, J. (2003). *Occupational therapy defined as a complex intervention*. London: College of Occupational Therapists.

Creek, J. (2010). *The core concepts of occupational therapy. A dynamic framework for practice.* London: Jessica Kingsley.

Deegan, P. (2001). Recovery as a self-directed process of healing and transformation. *Occupational Therapy in Mental Health*, 17(3/4), 5–21.

Department of Health (DH). (2007). *Making the CPA work for you. DH, Gov UK.* Available at: http://www.cpaa.org.uk/uploads/1/2/1/3/12136843/new_cpauserguide.pdf.

Dunn, W. (2009). Sensation and sensory processing. In E. B. Crepeau, E. S. Cohn, & B. A. Boyt Schell (Eds.), *Willard and Spackman's occupational therapy* (11th ed.) (pp. 777–791). Philadelphia: Lippincott Williams & Wilkins.

Grajo, L., Boisselle, A., & DaLomba, E. (2018). Occupational adaptation as a construct: A scoping review of literature. *Open Journal of Occupational Therapy*, 6, 1. https://scholarworks.wmich.edu/cgi/viewcontent.cgi?article=1400&context=ojot.

Health and Care Professions Council (HCPC). (2018). *Arts Therapies*. Available at: https://www.hcpc-uk.org/about-us/who-we-regulate/the-professions/.

Health Foundation. (2016). *Person-centred care made simple*. What Everyone Should Know.

About person-centred care. The Health Foundation, London.

Kessler, D., Walker, I., Sauvé-Schenk, K., & Egan, M. (2019). Goal setting dynamics that facilitate or impede a client-centered approach. *Scandinavian Journal of Occupational Therapy*, 26(5), 315–324. https://doi.org/10.1080/11038128.2018.1465119.

Kitwood, T. (1997). *Dementia reconsidered: The person comes first.* Buckingham: Open University Press.

Laver Fawcett, A. (2007). *Principles of assessment and outcome measurement for occupational therapists and physiotherapists: Theory, skills and application.* Chichester: Wiley.

Machtinger, E. L., Davis, K. B., Kimberg, L. S., et al. (2019). From treatment to healing: Inquiry and response to recent and past trauma in adult health care. *Women's Health Issues*, 29(2), 97–102. Available at: www.whijournal.com/article/S1049-3867(18)30550-4/fulltext.

Molineux, M. (2017). *Oxford dictionary of occupational science and occupational therapy.* Oxford: Oxford University Press.

Morgan, S. (2020). *Why positive risk-taking is so misunderstood.* Available at: https://strengthsrevolution.net/category/positive-risk-taking/.

National Institute for Care and Health Excellence (NICE). (2009). *Medicines adherence: Involving patients in decisions about prescribed medicines and supporting adherence.* https://www.nice.org.uk/guidance/cg76/chapter/introduction.

The National Archives. (2005). *The mental capacity act.* Available at: https://www.legislation.gov.uk/ukpga/2005/9/contents.

O'Hagan, M. (2004). *Guest Editorial, Australian e-Journal for the Advancement of Mental Health, 3*(1), 5–7. DOI: 10.5172/jamh.3.1.5.

Oliver, M. (2013). The social model of disability: Thirty years on. *Disability & Society, 28*(7), 1024–1026. https://doi.org/10.1080/09687599.2013.818773.

Penney, D. (2018). Who gets to define "peer support?" *Mad in America: Science, psychiatry, and social justice.* Available at: https://www.madinamerica.com/2018/02/who-gets-to-define-peer-support/.

Pentland, D., Kantartzis, S., Clausen, M. G., & Witemyre, K. (2018). *Occupational therapy and complexity: Defining and describing practice.* London: Royal College of Occupational Therapists.

Royal College of Occupational Therapists (RCOT). (2017). *Professional standards for occupational therapy practice.* London: RCOT.

Royal College of Occupational Therapists (RCOT). (2021). *Professional standards for occupational therapy practice, conduct and ethics.* Royal College of Occupational Therapists. Available at: https://www.rcot.co.uk/publications/professional-standards-occupational-therapy-practice-conduct-and-ethics.

Rutten, B. P. F., Hammels, C., Geschwind, N., et al. (2013). Resilience in mental health: Linking psychological and neurobiological perspectives. *Acta Psychiatrica Scandinavica, 128*(1), 3–20.

Townsend, E. (2003). Power and justice in enabling occupation. *Canadian Journal of Occupational Therapy, 70*(2), 74–87.

Wagman, P., Hakansson, C., & Bjorklund, A. (2012). Occupational balance as used in occupational therapy: A concept analysis. *Scandinavian Journal of Occupational Therapy, 19*, 322–327.

Wilcock, A. (1998). Occupation for health. *British Journal of Occupational Therapy, 61*(8), 340–345.

World Federation of Occupational Therapists (WFOT). (2012). *About occupational therapy.* Available at: https://wfot.org/about/about-occupational-therapy.

World Federation of Occupational Therapists (WFOT). (2016). *Minimum standards for the education of occupational therapists revised 2016.* Available at: https://wfot.org/resources/new-minimum-standards-for-the-education-of-occupational-therapists-2016-e-copy.

INDEX

Note: Page numbers followed by "f" indicate figures, "t" indicate tables and "b" indicate boxes.